T0195391

USMLE STEP 3

TED X. O'CONNELL, MD, FAAFP
Chief of Family and Community Medicine, Kaiser Permanente Vallejo, Founding
Program Director, Family Medicine Residency Program, Kaiser Permanente Napa-
Solano, Napa, California; Associate Clinical Professor, Department of Community
and Family Medicine, University of California–San Francisco, School of Medicine,
San Francisco, California

THOMAS E. BLAIR, MD
Acting Chief of Emergency Medicine, VA Greater Los Angeles Healthcare System,
Assistant Clinical Professor of Emergency Medicine, David Geffen School of Medicine
at UCLA, Los Angeles, California

RYAN A. PEDIGO, MD, MHPE
Associate Residency Program Director, Department of Emergency Medicine, Harbor-UCLA
Medical Center, Torrance, California; Assistant Professor of Emergency Medicine, David
Geffen School of Medicine at UCLA, Los Angeles, California

ELSEVIER

Elsevier
1600 John F. Kennedy Blvd.
Ste 1800
Philadelphia, PA 19103-2899

USMLE STEP 3 SECRETS, 2nd EDITION   ISBN: 978-0-323-87855-5

Notices

Knowledge and best practice in this field are constantly changing. As new research and experience broaden our understanding, changes in research methods, professional practices, or medical treatment may become necessary.

Practitioners and researchers must always rely on their own experience and knowledge in evaluating and using any information, methods, compounds or experiments described herein. Because of rapid advances in the medical sciences, in particular, independent verification of diagnoses and drug dosages should be made. To the fullest extent of the law, no responsibility is assumed by Elsevier, authors, editors or contributors for any injury and/or damage to persons or property as a matter of products liability, negligence or otherwise, or from any use or operation of any methods, products, instructions, or ideas contained in the material herein.

Content Strategist: James Meritt
Senior Content Development Manager: Somodutta Roy Choudhary
Senior Content Development Specialist: Malvika Shah
Publishing Services Manager: Shereen Jameel
Project Manager: Janish Ashwin Paul
Design Direction: Bridget Hoette

Printed in India

Last digit is the print number: 9 8 7 6 5 4 3 2

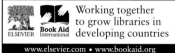

Working together
to grow libraries in
developing countries

www.elsevier.com • www.bookaid.org

To Nichole, Ryan, Sean, and Claire. I love you.
TED X. O'CONNELL

To my son, Rye. Your curiosity and love of exploration inspire me to ask more questions and seek more answers.
THOMAS E. BLAIR

To my wonderful wife Tiffany for always being supportive and being an amazing mother to Lucy.
RYAN A. PEDIGO

CONTENTS

REGARDING ERRATA

A list of errata for this book can be found at www.tedxoconnell.com and at BookRevision.com. We welcome you to visit these websites to submit errors, updates, or suggestions for this book. Thank you for helping to ensure the accuracy and high quality of *USMLE Step 3 Secrets*.

TED X. O'Connell, MD, FAAFP
Thomas E. Blair, MD
Ryan A. Pedigo, MD, MHPE

EDITORIAL REVIEW BOARD

PREFACE

A Note From the Authors

On the USMLE examinations, and throughout medical education, associations are often made between disease processes and certain racial and ethnic groups or even socioeconomic status. These associations become linked with individual groups and can perpetuate stereotypes, misinformation, and racism. In essence, physicians in training are taught to link key words, phrases, and ideas for the purposes of making associations on examinations and in clinical contexts.

Associations made with certain terms or disease processes, without qualifications or explanation, can cause those of us in health care to believe that being a part of a particular group causes one to have a predilection for health problems and disease processes. The reasons a disease process is more prevalent in certain racial, ethnic, and socioeconomic groups may be due in large part to long-standing social inequities, health disparities, structural racism, oppression, adverse childhood experiences, politics, environment, and likely many other factors. It is vitally important to remember that an increased prevalence should not be assumed to be intrinsically linked to being part of any particular group.

Because *USMLE Step 3 Secrets* is designed to help prepare you for success on the USMLE Step 3 exam, some of these keywords and linkages remain in this book out of necessity because the linkages are so prevalent on standardized exams. Despite this, we encourage you to consider the broader social issues outlined here and work within the health care system to call out and try to eliminate inappropriate associations between disease processes and individual groups of people. We owe it to our patients and to society to do this and to be better going forward.

TED X. O'Connell, MD, FAAFP
Thomas E. Blair, MD
Ryan A. Pedigo, MD, MHPE

CHAPTER 1

GENERAL PRINCIPLES

NORMAL DEVELOPMENT

INFANCY/CHILDHOOD

1. Name the commonly tested gross motor, fine motor, social, and verbal/cognitive childhood milestones for each age of development listed in the following table.

Age	Gross Motor	Fine Motor	Social	Verbal/Cognitive
3 mo	Roll	Grab	Smile	Laugh
6 *(Six)* mo	Sit up	Scraping/raking grasp Switch hands—move objects from one hand to the other	Stranger anxiety	Schmooze/coo incoherently
9 *(P)* mo *Because the letter P is just a 9 backwards*	Pull self up to standing position	Pincer grasp Able to play Pat-a-cake	Parent/separation anxiety	"Papa"—can say single words Personal—recognizes own name Object Permanence
12 *(Twelve)* mo	Stand Tall—stands under own power Walk *by* One *(it might not follow the "T" mnemonic, but it's a nice memory hook)*	Track/point at objects	Nothing special	Nothing special
18 mo	Climb stairs	Uses cups and cutlery	Complains—starts throwing tantrums	Calls objects by name (e.g., "book," "dog") Can't use toilet yet—potty training begins
2 yr	Uses 2 legs to run	Nothing special	2 people—will leave and return to parent but may not engage with peers yet ("two people" = *child* and *parent*)	200-word vocabulary 2-word sentences Follows 2-step commands

Continued on following page

Age	Gross Motor	Fine Motor	Social	Verbal/ Cognitive
3 *(Three)* yr	Able to ride Tricycle	Draw circle—*can draw a circle when they Tricycle*	3 people—start playing with peers ("three people" = *child, parent, child's friend*)	Toilet trained—successful potty training complete Thousand (1000) word vocabulary Constantly asks W-H-Y *(three letters)*
4 *(Four)* yr	Four-limb dexterity—able to hop and balance on one leg	Draw square and cross (Four sides in a square, four lines make a cross)	Figments—may have imaginary friends	Full sentences and storytelling Names at least two colors
5 *(Five fingers)* yr	Uses five fingers to play with a jump rope	Uses five fingers to dress and groom self (e.g., tie shoes, button a shirt)	Nothing special	Uses five fingers to start counting (up to 10)

Miscellaneous milestone pearls:

The "appropriate" number of stacked blocks is 3× their age starting at age 1 year (i.e., a toddler should be able to stack 3 blocks by age 1, 6 blocks by age 2, etc.).

For premature infants in their first 2 years of life, adjust their expected milestones by the number of weeks early they were delivered. For example, an infant born at a gestational age of 28 weeks (i.e., 12 weeks early) should be expected to reach the 6-month milestones around age 9 months (i.e., 12 weeks later), 12-month milestones around age 15 months, and so on until 2-year milestones around age 2 years and 3 months.

2. True or false: The overall trend or pattern of development is more important than the particular age at which any individual milestones is reached.

True. The exact age is not as important as the overall pattern when monitoring for dysfunctional development. When in doubt, use a formal developmental test such as the **M**odified **Ch**ecklist for **A**utism in **T**oddlers (M-CHAT).

3. What screening and preventive care measures should be done at every pediatric visit?

Height, weight, blood pressure, and developmental/behavioral assessment should be performed during every pediatric clinic visit. Also be prepared to provide anticipatory guidance (e.g., counseling/discussion about age-appropriate concerns) to the child's parents during each visit.

4. True or false: Screening and preventive care do not have to be addressed during a pediatric clinic visit if the chief complaint is unrelated to well-child development.

False. Screening and preventive care are important parts of every patient encounter—adult or child. Your exam questions may try to fool you on this point. For example, consider a mother who complains that her 4-year-old child sleeps 11 hours every night. The answer to the question, "What should you do next?" may not be about sleep patterns at all, but rather should be to perform any routine screening procedure that you would expect a 4-year-old child to receive (e.g., an objective hearing exam).

5. What are the frequently tested items under the umbrella of primary prevention using "anticipatory guidance"?

Tell parents the following:
- Keep the water heater under 120°F.
- Have functional smoke detectors in the home.
- Have the phone number for poison control handy.
- Advise smoking cessation if anyone in the home uses tobacco or vape products.
- Use proper car restraints (e.g., child safety seat until 2 years, booster seat until height is 4'9").
- Put the infant to sleep on the side or back ("Back to Sleep") to help prevent sudden infant death syndrome (SIDS).
- Advise against sharing a bed with the infant due to risk of SIDS or accidental smothering.
- Do not use infant walkers (they cause injuries).
- Watch out for small objects (they may be aspirated).
- Do not give honey before 1 year of age (risk of unintended botulinum poisoning).

- Do not give cow's milk before 1 year of age.
- Introduce solid foods gradually, starting at 4 to 6 months of age.
- Supervise children in bathtubs and swimming pools.
- Minimize screen time (televisions, computers, portable devices).
- Get plenty of physical activity (at least 60 minutes daily).

6. **How often should height, weight, and head circumference be measured? What do they signify? Which measurements will be the first and last to become abnormal if the child is not developing appropriately?**
Height and weight should be measured routinely during every clinic visit, well into adulthood. Head circumference should be measured at every visit until the patient is 2 years old. All three parameters are markers of general well-being; abnormal values may suggest disease. The first measurement to become abnormal is weight (a child can lose weight but cannot shrink); the last measurement to become abnormal is head circumference because you are essentially waiting for the child's body to outgrow the head.

7. **What if a child has low height, weight, or head circumference compared to peers?**
The trend or pattern over time along a plotted growth curve will tell you more than any single measurement. You may be asked to interpret these growth curves on the USMLE. If a child has always tended low or high compared to peers, the pattern is generally benign. A patient who crosses two or more growth curves is more worrisome. Parents commonly bring in a child who they believe is experiencing delayed physical growth or delayed puberty. You need to know when to reassure and when to do further testing and questioning.

8. **Define failure to thrive. What causes it?**
There is no consensus definition for failure to thrive, but commonly used definitions include a head circumference, height, or weight less than the 5th percentile for age, a weight less than 80% of ideal weight for age, or a weight that drops two or more major lines on the growth curve. Failure to thrive is most commonly due to psychosocial or functional problems. Watch for signs of neglect and child abuse. Organic causes usually have specific clues to trigger your suspicion.

9. **What conditions are suggested by obesity in children?**
Obesity is usually due to overeating and too little activity (>95% of cases). Less than 5% of cases are due to organic causes (e.g., Cushing syndrome, Prader-Willi syndrome).

10. **What conditions should you consider in a child with an abnormal head circumference?**
Increased head circumference may indicate hydrocephalus or tumor, whereas decreased head circumference may indicate microcephaly (e.g., TORCH infections: congenital *to*xoplasmosis, *o*ther [e.g., syphilis, HIV], *r*ubella, *c*ytomegalovirus, *h*erpes simplex infection or Zika virus or aneuploidy). Again the pattern of head circumference over time (plotted on a growth curve) is most helpful in defining pathology.

11. **When are hearing and vision screened?**
Hearing and vision should be measured objectively at least once by 4 years of age. After that initial screen, measure every few years until adulthood or more often if the history so dictates.

12. **In what clinical situations should you worry about hearing loss in pediatric patients?**
- Bacterial meningitis, especially by *Hemophilus influenzae*, which may cause sensorineural hearing loss of the vestibulocochlear nerve (cranial nerve [CN] 8)
- Congenital TORCH infections
- Measles or mumps
- Chronic middle ear effusions or chronic or recurrent otitis media
- Use of ototoxic drugs (e.g., aminoglycosides, furosemide)

13. **What is the red reflex? What does an abnormal red reflex suggest?**
When a penlight is shined at the pupil, you usually see red because of the underlying fundus. Check for the red reflex at birth and routinely thereafter to detect congenital cataracts, strabismus, or ocular tumors. If a cataract, strabismus, or ocular tumor is present, the red reflex disappears. For cataracts and tumors, you may see white instead of red—this finding is known as leukocoria and is classically due to retinoblastoma (Fig. 1.1).

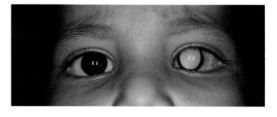

Fig. 1.1 Leukocoria (white pupillary reflex) is the most common presenting feature of retinoblastoma and may be first noticed in family photographs. (Courtesy of U. Raina.)

14. True or false: Before a certain age intermittent strabismus is normal.
True. It is normal for infants to have occasional ocular misalignment (strabismus) until 4 months of age. After 4 months (or with constant eye deviation), strabismus should be evaluated and managed by an ophthalmologist to prevent possible blindness in the affected eye.

15. How is strabismus managed if it persists beyond age 3 months?
Patch the **good eye** to force the abnormal eye to develop. Severe strabismus may require surgical intervention.

16. How and when should pediatric patients be screened for iron-deficiency anemia?
According to American Academy of Pediatrics (AAP) guidelines a risk assessment for iron-deficiency anemia should begin at 4 months of age, with hemoglobin and hematocrit measured at 1 year of age. Risk factors to assess for include prematurity, low birthweight, excessive ingestion of cow's milk before 1 year of age, low dietary iron intake, and low socioeconomic status.

17. Which infants should receive iron supplementation? At what age?
Iron supplements are recommended for exclusively breastfed infants beginning at 4 months of age. Infants receive enough iron during the third trimester of pregnancy to last for the first 4 months of life, but because breast milk contains so little iron, supplements are needed after 4 months. Formula-fed infants receive adequate iron for the first 12 months of life with standard infant formula.

18. True or false: Breastfed infants are more likely to require vitamin D supplements than formula-fed infants.
True. The AAP recommends that exclusively and partially breastfed infants receive **oral** vitamin **D** supplementation ("neonates **d**rink vitamin **D** but receive an inje'k'tion of vitamin **K**") shortly after birth and continue until they are weaned and begin consuming formula or whole milk. Formula-fed infants do not require vitamin D supplements in the United States because all formulas are already supplemented with vitamin D.

19. How and when do you screen for lead exposure?
Screening for lead toxicity is controversial. Routine screening is no longer recommended. However, all Medicaid-eligible children must be screened. Consider screening high-risk children (those who live in old buildings, have a sibling or playmate with lead toxicity, eat paint chips, live near a battery recycling plant, or have a parent who works at a battery recycling plant). Screen for lead exposure by ordering a serum lead level. If the initial lead level is abnormally high, closer follow-up and intervention are needed. The best first step is to stop the exposure.

20. True or false: Most children need fluoride supplementation.
False. Because most water is fluoridated, supplementation is not needed. However, if a child lives in an area where the water is inadequately fluoridated (rare) or the child is fed exclusively from premixed, ready-to-eat formulas (which use nonfluoridated water), fluoride supplements should be given.

21. When should children be screened for tuberculosis?
Universal screening for tuberculosis is not recommended. There is no need to screen children who have no risk factors. Risk assessment should occur regularly until 2 years of age, then annually. Test those at high risk (family member with tuberculosis or a positive tuberculosis test, a child born in a high-risk country, a child who has traveled to a high-risk country, or a child who has consumed unpasteurized milk or cheese).

22. True or false: Screening children for renal disease with a urinalysis is not recommended.
True. However, you should screen for congenital/anatomic abnormalities (e.g., vesicoureteral reflux) after a febrile urinary tract infection in children between the ages of 2 months and 2 years by getting an ultrasound plus either voiding cystourethrogram (VCUG) or radionuclide cystogram (RNC). Screening after 2 years of age is more controversial and likely will not be asked on the USMLE.

23. What high-yield information do you need to know about immunizations for the USMLE Step 3 exam?
High-yield information includes the recommendations for special patient populations (e.g., give pneumococcal vaccine to patients with sickle cell disease or splenectomy) and notable vaccine contraindications (no live vaccines such as measles-mumps-rubella or varicella for immunocompromised patients or pregnant patients).

24. Which vaccine is contraindicated in pediatric patients with a history of intussusception?
The **rotavirus** vaccine is contraindicated for pediatrics with a history of intussusception.

25. True or false: Pediatric immunizations for preterm infants should be given based on chronologic age.
True. The only exception is for the hepatitis B vaccine. If the birthweight is less than 2 kg, the infant should be immunized by hospital discharge or 1 month of age (whichever event is earlier).

26. When should you recommend that a child see a dentist for the first time?
The AAP and American Academy of Pediatric Dentistry (AAPD) both recommend that a child see a dentist within 6 months of first tooth eruption or at 12 months of age, whichever comes first.

27. When does the anterior fontanelle usually close? What disorder should you suspect if it fails to close?

The anterior fontanelle is usually closed by **18 months** of age. Delayed closure or an unusually large anterior fontanelle may indicate hypothyroidism, hydrocephalus, rickets, or intrauterine growth restriction (IUGR).

28. True or false: Milky-white and possibly blood-tinged vaginal discharge is usually abnormal in the first week of life for a female newborn.

False. This discharge is usually physiologic and due to maternal hormone withdrawal.

29. True or false: Children have the same range of normal vital signs as adults.

False. Children have *lower* baseline blood pressure and *higher* baseline heart and respiratory rates than do adults. In addition, children often have different acceptable ranges of lab values. For example, a healthy child's hemoglobin/hematocrit value is normally higher at birth and lower throughout childhood compared with that of an adult. In addition, the renal, pulmonary, hepatic, and central nervous systems are not fully mature or functional at birth.

30. When should the Moro and palmar grasp reflex disappear?

These primitive reflexes should disappear by 6 months of age.

31. True or false: A diagnosis of encopresis or enuresis cannot be made before a certain age.

True. Encopresis is considered normal until age 4 years, and enuresis is normal until age 5 years. This diagnostic point is obviously important when the parent complains because both are normal findings in a 3-year-old child. If the problem persists, rule out physical problems (e.g., Hirschsprung disease, urinary tract infection) and treat with behavioral modification (e.g., "gold star for being good" charts, alarms, biofeedback) as the first-line treatment. Desmopressin and imipramine may be used for refractory cases of enuresis.

32. What are some complications of constipation in young children?

Common complications include encopresis, enuresis, anal fissures, and hemorrhoids. Constipation can be associated with toilet training, entry to daycare/school, transition to solid diet, and introduction or excessive consumption of cow's milk.

ADOLESCENCE

1. What are the Tanner stages? When do they occur?

The Tanner stages measure the stages of puberty. Stage 1 is preadolescent; stage 5 is adult. Advancing stages are assigned for testicular and penile growth in boys and breast growth in girls. Both male and female stages also use pubic hair development. The average age of puberty (when a patient first has changes from the preadolescent stage 1) is earlier for girls than boys (10.5 years in girls compared to 11.5 years in boys). The classic first events of puberty are testicular enlargement in boys and breast development in girls.

2. True or false: A 1-month history of a painful nipple mass in a 13-year-old boy with Tanner stage 3 genitalia and who is otherwise healthy warrants further workup.

False. This situation is a common description of pubertal gynecomastia, which occurs in more than 50% of male adolescents. It usually presents with a palpable mass or lump behind one or both nipples and can be painful. It can be safely observed as the condition typically regresses substantially or self-resolves by 1 year.

3. What causes precocious puberty?

Precocious puberty is usually idiopathic but may be due to the **McCune-Albright syndrome** (triad includes precocious puberty, fibrous dysplasia of the bone, and the "coast of Maine" café-au-lait spots), ovarian tumors (e.g., granulosa, theca cell, or gonadoblastoma), testicular tumors (e.g., Leydig cell tumors), central nervous system disease or trauma, adrenal neoplasm, or congenital adrenal hyperplasia (CAH). CAH causes precocious puberty only in boys (due to elevated androgen levels) and is usually due to 21-hydroxylase deficiency. Obesity may also lead to precocious puberty in girls due to elevated adipose-related estrone levels.

4. True or false: If the underlying cause for precocious puberty is uncorrectable or idiopathic after diagnostic workup, patients should still receive treatment.

True. Most patients are given long-acting gonadotropin-releasing hormone (GnRH) agonists (e.g., leuprolide) to modulate the hypothalamic-pituitary-gonadal axis and ultimately suppress the progression of puberty. Among other benefits, this approach helps to prevent the short stature that may result from premature epiphyseal closure.

5. Define delayed puberty. What is the most common cause?

In boys, delayed puberty is defined as no enlargement of the testicles by age 14 or a time lapse of more than 5 years from the start to the completion of growth of the genitals. In girls, delayed puberty is defined as no breast development (thelarche) by age 13, a time lapse of more than 5 years from the beginning of breast growth to the first menstrual period, or no menstruation by age 16. The most common cause is **constitutional delay**, a normal variant. Watch for parents with a similar history of being "late bloomers." The child's growth curve consistently lags behind that of peers, but the line representing the child's growth curve is parallel to the normal growth curve. Treatment is reassurance only.

6. **What are other potential causes for delayed puberty?**
   Rarely, delayed puberty is due to primary testicular failure (Klinefelter syndrome, cryptorchidism, history of che-motherapy, gonadal dysgenesis) or ovarian failure (Turner syndrome, gonadal dysgenesis). Even more rarely, delayed puberty is due to a hypothalamic/pituitary defect such as Kallmann syndrome or tumor.

7. **What are the three leading causes of death in adolescents?**
   Accidents, homicide, and suicide together cause about 75% of teenage deaths.

8. **True or false: Sexually active teenaged girls need screening for chlamydial infection and gonorrhea.**
   True. There are high numbers of reported cases of chlamydia and gonorrhea in younger women. The Centers for Disease Control and Prevention (CDC) recommends annual screening for chlamydia for all sexually active females ages 25 years and under. The CDC recommends screening high-risk sexually active females for gonorrhea.

ADULTHOOD

1. Cover the right-hand column and give the indications for each of the following vaccines.

Vaccine	*Who Should Receive (and Other Information)*
Hepatitis B	Recommended for adults at increased risk of hepatitis B virus infection (e.g., health care workers, diabetics, patients with HIV, end-stage renal disease, chronic liver disease, or MSM). Infants should be vaccinated in a three-step series, starting the day they are born.
Influenza (inactivated)	Everyone age $\geq$6 mo, including pregnant women, adults age >50 yr, people with chronic medical conditions or immunocompromised status (and their caregivers), and health care workers should be vaccinated annually. *Note: The live attenuated influenza vaccine is contraindicated during preg-nancy and in patients with HIV, asplenia, complement deficiencies, or immu-nocompromised status. The inactivated vaccine has no contraindications.*
Pneumococcus	13-valent pneumococcal conjugate vaccine (PCV13) and 23-valent pneumo-coccal polysaccharide vaccine (PPSV23) is recommended for all adults age $\geq$65 yr. A four-step series of PCV13 is recommended for infants, starting at age 2 mo. Minimum age to receive PPSV23 is 2 yr. PPSV23 is recommended for adults ages 19–64 yr with chronic heart disease, chronic lung disease, chronic liver disease, diabetes mellitus, alcoholism, or cigarette use. Both PCV13 and PPSV23 should be given to immunocompromised adults ages 19–64 yr. Immunocompromised status includes HIV, chronic renal failure, asplenia, leukemia, lymphoma, Hodgkin disease, generalized ma-lignancy, multiple myeloma, and solid organ transplantation. *Note: When both are indicated, give PCV13 first. PCV13 and PPSV23 should not be given during the same visit.*
Rubella	All nonpregnant women of childbearing age and health care workers. Women of childbearing age who lack immunity or history of immunization. Do not give to pregnant women or immunocompromised patients, including those with HIV and CD4 <200 cells/mm^3. Women should avoid pregnancy for 4 wk after receiving the vaccine.
Tetanus	A five-step series of DTaP is recommended for children starting at age 2 mo, with the fifth dose received between age 4 and 6 yr. At age 11 yr, one dose of Tdap followed by a Td booster every 10 yr is recommended. Tdap should be given to women with every pregnancy regardless of their prior immunization history (preferably in the late second or the third trimester). When deciding whether a wound requires tetanus prophylaxis, first ask pa-tients about their immunization history then consider the severity of the wound. Patients with unknown or incomplete immunization status (i.e., <3 doses in their lifetime) should **always** be given a tetanus booster (preferably Tdap) no matter how clean or minor the wound. Patients with complete immunization history (i.e., $\geq$3 doses in their lifetime) should only receive a tetanus booster with clean, minor wounds if their last dose was >10 yr ago, or with unclean or major wounds (including burns) if their last dose was >5 yr ago. Coadministration of tetanus immune globu-lin is only recommended for patients with unknown or incomplete vacci-nation **and** unclean or major wounds.

DTaP, Diphtheria tetanus acellular pertussis; *HIV*, human immunodeficiency virus; *MSM*, men who have sex with men; *Tdap*, tetanus diphtheria acellular pertussis.

2. Cover all but the left-hand column, and give the appropriate screening recommendations for healthy, asymptomatic patients with average risk for the related cancers. Although other guidelines for cancer screening are in clinical use, the recommendations from the American Cancer Society (see table) are a good guideline to use for the USMLE. Controversial topics are typically not tested on the USMLE.

Cancer	Procedure	Age to Begin Screening	Age to Stop Screening	Frequency
Breast	Mammography **Note:** *Clinical breast exam is no longer recommended.*	45 yr **Note:** *Interested patients may begin annual screening at age 40 yr.*	Life expectancy <10 yr. No age specified.	Annually (age 45–54 yr) Every 2 yr (age ≥55 yr)
Cervical	Pap smear only (age 21–29) **or** Pap and HPV cotest (age 30–65 yr) **Note:** *HPV cotest only performed in age 21–29 yr if Pap is abnormal.* **Note:** *A woman with prior total hysterectomy should not be screened unless she has other risk factors.*	21 yr regardless of sexual activity	65 yr **Note:** *Women with cervical precancer should continue screening for at least 20 more years, even if they pass age 65.*	Every 3 yr (if screened by Pap only) Every 5 yr (if Pap and HPV cotest is used)
Colorectal	Colonoscopy **or** Flexible sigmoidoscopy (FS) **or** CT colonography **or** Multitarget stool DNA test (mt-sDNA) **or** Guaiac-based fecal occult blood test (gFOBT) **or** Fecal immunochemical test (FIT)	45 yr (qualified recommendation) **or** 50 yr (strong recommendation)	75 yr **or** Life expectancy <10 yr	Every 10 yr (colonoscopy) **or** Every 5 yr (FS or CT colonography) **or** Every 3 yr (mt-sDNA) **or** Annually (gFOBT or FIT)
Endometrial	Endometrial biopsy			Routine screening is not recommended unless the patient is symptomatic (e.g., unexplained vaginal bleeding)
Lung	Low-dose CT scan	55 yr **and** 30-pack-year smoking history **and** Currently smokes or quit within the last 15 yr	80 yr	Annually

Continued on following page

Cancer	Procedure	Age to Begin Screening	Age to Stop Screening	Frequency
Prostate	Prostate-specific antigen test (with or without DRE) *Note:* Have a risk/benefit discussion with patients before screening. Shared decision making. Consider DRE for PSA between 2.5 and 4 ng/mL	50 yr *Note:* Start screening at age 45 yr for all Black men or men with a first-degree relative diagnosed before age 65 yr.	75 yr **or** Life expectancy <10 yr	PSA 2.5 ng/mL or greater screened annually PSA <2.5 ng/mL screened every 2 yr

CT, Computed tomography; *DRE,* digital rectal exam; *HPV,* human papillomavirus; *Pap,* Papanicolaou.
*Start at age 45 in Blacks and at age 40 for patients with a first-degree relative diagnosed at an early age.

3. True or false: Tumor markers are generally not used for cancer screening.
True. Prostate-specific antigen is the exception to this rule. Alpha-fetoprotein (liver and testicular cancer), carcinoembryonic antigen (CEA), CA-125, and other serum markers are not used for screening the general population, although they may be used to monitor for cancer recurrence. While they may not be used for screening in clinical practice, look for abnormal lab values to show up in questions as a clue to diagnosis.

4. True or false: Urinalysis should not be used to screen the general population for bladder cancer.
True. Screening with urinalysis for urinary tract cancer (which causes hematuria) is not recommended. However, look for persistent, painless hematuria as a clue that urinary tract cancer may be present. On the USMLE, a mention of painless hematuria after extended use of the alkylating agent cyclophosphamide or exposure to the parasite *Schistosoma haematobium* should also make you suspect bladder cancer.

5. What specific problems are caused by obesity?
Obesity causes an increase in overall mortality (at any age) and increases the risk of insulin resistance and diabetes, hypertension, hypertriglyceridemia, coronary artery disease, gallstones, sleep apnea and hypoventilation, osteoarthritis, thromboembolism, varicose veins, and cancer (especially endometrial cancer).

SENESCENCE

1. What age group constitutes the most rapidly growing segment of the population?
Persons over the age of 85 years.

2. True or false: An 80-year-old person needs more calories than a 30-year-old person.
False. An 80-year-old person has half the lean body mass of a 30-year-old person and thus needs fewer calories. The basal metabolic rate is based on lean body mass. Elderly patients, however, need more vitamin B_{12}, vitamin D (and/or calcium), folate, and nonheme iron than do younger patients.

3. True or false: Hearing and vision changes are a normal part of aging.
True. **Presbyopia** (hardening of the lens that decreases the ability to accommodate) becomes almost universal after age 50, thus the common need for reading glasses after age 50. **Presbycusis**, the loss of ability to discriminate between sounds, most markedly at higher frequency, is also part of the normal process of aging. Hearing aids may help.

4. True or false: Brain atrophy is a normal part of aging.
True. Decreased brain weight, enlarged ventricles and sulci, and a slightly decreased ability to learn new material are normal parts of aging.

5. Describe the normal changes in male sexual function that occur with aging.
- Increased refractory period (after ejaculation, it takes longer before he can have another erection)
- Increased amount of time to achieve an erection
- Delayed ejaculation (an elderly man may ejaculate only one of every three times that he has sex)

6. Describe the normal changes in female sexual function that occur with aging.
- Decreased vaginal lubrication (estrogen cream or water-soluble lubricants can be helpful in treating symptoms)
- Dyspareunia (pain with intercourse) due to atrophy of clitoral, labial, and vaginal tissues (treated with estrogen cream)
- Delayed orgasm

7. True or false: Impotence and lack of sexual desire are normal in elderly people.
   False. Impotence in men and lack of sexual desire in either sex are not normal and should be investigated and treated. Look for psychiatric disorders (e.g., depression) as well as physical causes, such as medications (selective serotonin reuptake inhibitors [SSRIs] and antihypertensives are notorious culprits), vascular disease (watch for atherosclerosis risk factors), and neurologic disease (especially in diabetics).

8. Describe the normal changes in sleep habits in elderly people.
   Elderly persons require less sleep, sleep less deeply, sleep earlier in the evening, wake up more frequently during the night, and awaken earlier in the morning. It also takes longer for elderly persons to fall asleep (longer sleep latency), and they have less stage 3 and 4 and rapid eye movement sleep.

9. Define pseudodementia. How do you recognize it on the Step 3 exam?
   Depression in the elderly can resemble dementia. Look for a history that would trigger depression (e.g., loss of a spouse, change in living situation or level of independence, terminal or debilitating disease) and other symptoms of depression (e.g., frequent crying, suicidal thoughts).

10. True or false: Almost 50% of patients over the age of 65 suffer from some type of dementia.
    False. Roughly 15% of people over the age of 65 suffer from dementia, but the prevalence increases with age. Roughly 50% of people over age 80 have dementia or mild cognitive impairment. The most common types of dementias are Alzheimer dementia, dementia with Lewy bodies, vascular dementia, Parkinson dementia, and frontotemporal dementia. Other disorders that can cause dementia include HIV and Pick disease. Test for reversible causes of dementia and memory impairment such as electrolyte disturbances (classically hyponatremia), hypothyroidism, depression, neurosyphilis, and vitamin B_{12} deficiency.

11. What else do you need to know about dementia?
    The various types of dementia are discussed in detail in Chapter 2.

12. What is the best prophylaxis for pressure ulcers in an immobilized patient?
    Frequent turning and the use of special air mattresses.

MEDICAL ETHICS AND JURISPRUDENCE

CONSENT AND INFORMED CONSENT TO TREATMENT

1. What are the components of informed consent?
   Informed consent involves giving the patient information about the following:
   • Diagnosis (patient's condition and what it means)
   • Prognosis (the natural course of the condition without treatment)
   • Proposed treatment (description of the procedure and what the patient will experience)
   • Risks and benefits of the treatment
   • Alternative treatments
      Patient then must be allowed to make their own choice. The documents seen on the wards that patients are made to sign are not technically required or sufficient for informed consent. They are used for medicolegal purposes (i.e., lawsuit paranoia).

2. What should you do if a patient is in critical condition or in a coma and has made no advance directive or living will?
   Begin resuscitation of the patient. Contact the family, next of kin, or health care power of attorney, and follow their wishes. In cases of disagreement among family members, suspicion of ulterior motives, or uncertainty, involve the hospital's ethics committee. As a last resort, go to the courts for help.

3. True or false: A living will should not be respected if the next of kin asks you not to follow it.
   False. Such situations are tricky, but technically (and for the USMLE) living wills or patient-mandated "do-not-resuscitate" orders should be respected and followed if properly documented. The classic board question involves a patient who says in a living will that if he or she is unable to breathe independently, a ventilator should not be used. Do not put the patient on a ventilator, even if the husband, wife, son, or daughter tells you to do so.

4. What should you do if a patient lacks capacity to make decisions?
   A physician can determine capacity for decision making, but courts determine competency. If a patient lacks capacity for decision making, obtain consent from family (spouse, adult children, parents, and then adult siblings) and/or have the courts appoint a guardian (surrogate decision maker or health care power of attorney).

5. What should you do if a child has a medical emergency, and the parents are unavailable for decision making?
   Treat the child as you see fit; that is, act in the child's best interest.

6. What should you do if a patient requires emergency care, but the patient cannot communicate and no family members are available?
Treat the patient as you see fit unless you know that the patient wishes otherwise.

7. True or false: Adult patients of sound mind are allowed to refuse lifesaving treatments.
True. You should not force blood products, antibiotics, or any other treatments on a patient who does not want them.

8. What about depression in the context of end-of-life decisions?
Depression should always be evaluated as a reason for lack of capacity. Patients who are actively suicidal may not have capacity to consent to or refuse life-prolonging treatment.

9. True or false: In some circumstances, patients can be hospitalized against their will.
True. Psychiatric patients may be hospitalized against their will if they are deemed to be a danger to themselves or others or are "gravely disabled," meaning unable to care for themselves by meeting their basic needs of food, clothing, and shelter. Patients can be held only for a limited time (1–3 days) before they must have a hearing before a court official to determine whether they must remain in custody. These decisions are based on the principle of **beneficence** (the principle of doing good for the patient and avoiding harm).

10. True or false: Restraints can be used on patients against their will.
True. Chemical and/or physical restraints can be used on an agitated (e.g., delirious, psychotic) patient if needed, but their use should be brief and reevaluated often (at least once every 24 hours). Be aware that the use of restraints in delirious or demented patients rarely helps prevent falls and may cause injury.

11. When do patients under the age of 18 years not require parental consent for a medical decision?
In general, people under the age of 18 years do not require parental consent if they are emancipated (married, living on their own and financially independent, raising children, or serving in the armed forces); have a sexually transmitted disease, want contraception, or are pregnant; want treatment or counseling for substance use disorders; or have psychiatric illness. Some states have exceptions to these rules, but for Step 3 purposes, minors may make their own decisions in such situations.

PHYSICIAN–PATIENT RELATIONSHIP

1. With whom can you discuss your patient's condition?
Only with people who need to know because they are directly involved in the patient's care and with people authorized by the patient (e.g., authorized family members). In the case of a patient with a designated health care proxy, information may only be shared if a patient is deemed to lack capacity to make their own health care decisions, which is when the proxy comes into effect. Do not tell a medical colleague who is uninvolved with the patient's care how that patient is doing, even if the colleague is a friend of yours or of the patient.

2. In what situations are you allowed to breach patient confidentiality?
Break confidentiality only in the following situations:
- The patient asks you to do so.
- Child abuse is suspected (mandated reporting).
- The courts mandate you to do so.
- You must fulfill the duty to warn or protect (if a patient threatens to kill someone or oneself, you have to tell someone, the authorities, or both).
- The patient has a reportable disease.
- The patient is a danger to others (e.g., if a patient is blind or has seizures, let the proper authorities know so that they can revoke the patient's license to drive; if the patient is an airplane pilot with paranoid schizophrenia, then authorities need to know).

3. True or false: It is acceptable to hide a diagnosis from a patient if the family asks you to do so.
False. Do not hide a diagnosis from a patient (including a child) if the patient wants to know (even if the family asks you to do so). Do not lie to any patient because the family asks you to do so. Conversely, you should not force patients to receive information against their will; if they do not want to know the diagnosis, do not tell them.

4. What findings should make you suspect child abuse?
- Failure to thrive
- Multiple fractures, bruises, or injuries in different stages of healing
- Concentric cigarette-shaped burns
- Signs of intentional burns (e.g., scald injuries from intentional immersion that are symmetric with sharp lines of demarcation)
- Metaphyseal "bucket handle" or "corner" fractures (Fig. 1.2)
- Shaken baby syndrome (retinal hemorrhages or subdural hematomas with no external signs of trauma)

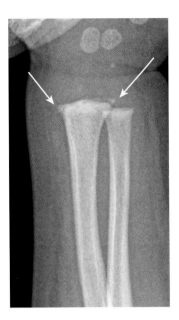

Fig. 1.2 There are metaphyseal corner fractures *(solid white arrows)*, small avulsion-type fractures of the distal radius, a finding characteristic of child abuse. (From Herring W. *Learning Radiology: Recognizing the Basics.* Philadelphia: Elsevier; 2020:324-338.)

- Behavioral, emotional, or interactional problems
- Sexually transmitted diseases
- Dissociative identity disorder (previously known as multiple personality disorder; classically due to sexual abuse)
- Whenever a parent's story does not fit the child's injury

5. True or false: You must have proof before you can report child abuse.
   False. In fact, reporting any suspicion of child abuse is mandatory. You do not need proof and cannot be sued for reporting your suspicion.

DEATH AND DYING

1. True or false: Adult patients of sound mind are allowed to refuse lifesaving treatments.
   True. You should not force blood products, antibiotics, or any other treatments on a patient who does not want them.

2. What is the difference between active and passive euthanasia?
   Active euthanasia is the intentional hastening of death, whereas passive euthanasia is withdrawing or opting not to initiate aggressive, "heroic" life-prolonging treatments (e.g., intubation or artificial nutrition) and "letting nature take its course."

3. True or false: Withdrawing care and withholding care are the same in the eyes of the law.
   True. It is important to communicate this principle to family members. The simple fact that a patient is on a respirator does not mean that you cannot turn the respirator off.

4. True or false: In a terminally ill patient with an incurable illness, one of the primary goals is to relieve pain.
   True. Opioids are commonly used, even though they may cause respiratory depression. If in keeping with a patient's wishes, it is more important to make the patient comfortable and pain free, even with the risk of respiratory depression in this setting.

APPLIED BIOSTATISTICS AND CLINICAL EPIDEMIOLOGY

UNDERSTANDING STATISTICAL CONCEPTS

1. How is the sensitivity of a test defined? What are highly sensitive tests used for clinically?
   Sensitivity is defined as the ability of a test to detect disease and mathematically as the number of true positives divided by the number of people with the disease. Tests with high sensitivity are used for disease screening. False positives occur, but the test does not miss many people with the disease (low false-negative rate). One way to remember this is the word *snout*, written "Sn-N-out," meaning with high **sen**sitivity (Sn) a **n**egative (N) test rules **out** (out) the disease.

2. **How is the specificity of a test defined? What are highly specific tests used for clinically?**
Specificity is defined as the ability of a test to detect health (or nondisease) and mathematically as the number of true negatives divided by the number of people without the disease. Tests with high specificity are used for disease confirmation. False negatives occur, but the test does not identify anyone who is actually healthy as sick (low false-positive rate). The ideal confirmatory test must have high sensitivity and high specificity; otherwise, people with the disease may be called healthy. One way to remember this is the word *spin*, written "Sp-P-in," meaning that with high **sp**ecificity (Sp) a positive (P) test rules **in** (in) the disease.

3. **Explain the concept of a trade-off between sensitivity and specificity.**
The trade-off between sensitivity and specificity is a classic statistics question. For example, you should understand how changing the cutoff glucose value in screening for diabetes (or changing the value of any of several screening tests) will change the number of true- and false-negative as well as true- and false-positive results. If the cutoff glucose value is raised, fewer people will be identified as diabetic (more false negatives, fewer false positives), whereas if the cutoff glucose value is lowered, more people will be identified as diabetic (fewer false negatives, more false positives). As an example, if the diagnostic threshold for a fasting blood sugar for diabetes were raised from greater than or equal to 125 mg/dL to greater than or equal to 300 mg/dL, most people with diabetes would be missed (low sensitivity because a patient with a blood sugar of 285 mg/dL would be negative for diabetes according to this criterion). In addition, the test would be very specific for patients with blood sugar greater than or equal to 300 md/dL (patients would certainly have diabetes if they had a positive test).

4. **Define positive predictive value (PPV). On what does it depend?**
When a test is positive for disease, the PPV measures how likely it is that the patient has the disease (probability of having a condition, given a positive test). PPV is calculated mathematically by dividing the number of true positives by the total number of people with a positive test. PPV depends on the prevalence of a disease (the higher the prevalence, the higher the PPV) and the sensitivity and specificity of the test (e.g., an overly sensitive test that gives more false positives has a lower PPV).

5. **Define negative predictive value (NPV). On what does it depend?**
When a test comes back negative for disease, the NPV measures how likely it is that the patient is healthy and does not have the disease (probability of not having a condition given a negative test). It is calculated mathematically by dividing the number of true negatives by the total number of people with a negative test. NPV also depends on the prevalence of the disease and the sensitivity and specificity of the test (the higher the prevalence, the lower the NPV). In addition, an overly sensitive test with many false positives leads to a higher NPV.

6. **Define attributable risk. How is it measured?**
Attributable risk is the number of cases of a disease attributable to one risk factor (in other words, the amount by which the incidence of a condition is expected to decrease if the risk factor in question is removed). For example, if the incidence rate of lung cancer is 1/100 in the general population and 10/100 in smokers, the attributable risk of smoking in causing lung cancer is 9/100 (assuming a properly matched control group).

7. **Develop the habit of drawing a 2 × 2 table for Step 3 statistics questions. Given the following 2 × 2 table, define the formulas for calculating the following test values:**

Disease	Test Name	Formula
Test	Sensitivity	A/(A + C)
or	Specificity	D/(B + D)
Exposure	PPV	A/(A + B)
	NPV	D/(C + D)
	Odds ratio	(A × D)/(B × C)
	Relative risk	[A/(A + B)]/[C/(C + D)]
	Attributable risk	[A/(A + B)] − [C/(C + D)]

NPV, Negative predictive value; *PPV*, positive predictive value.

8. **Define relative risk. From what types of studies can it be calculated?**
Relative risk compares the disease risk in people exposed to a certain factor with the disease risk in people who have not been exposed to the factor in question. Relative risk can be calculated only after prospective or experimental studies; it cannot be calculated from retrospective data. If a Step 3 question asks you to calculate the relative risk from retrospective data, the answer is "cannot be calculated" or "none of the above."

9. **What is a clinically significant value for relative risk?**
Any value for relative risk other than 1 is clinically significant. For example, if the relative risk is 1.5, a person is 1.5 times more likely to develop the condition if exposed to the factor in question. If the relative risk is 0.5, the person is only half as likely to develop the condition when exposed to the factor; in other words, the factor is protective.

10. **Define odds ratio. From what types of studies is it calculated?**
    Odds ratio attempts to estimate relative risk with retrospective studies (e.g., case control). An odds ratio compares two factors—(1) the incidence of disease in persons exposed to the factor and the incidence of nondisease in persons not exposed to the factor, and (2) the incidence of disease in persons unexposed to the factor and the incidence of nondisease in persons exposed to the factor—to see whether there is a difference between the two. As with relative risk, values other than 1 are significant. The odds ratio is a less than perfect way to estimate relative risk (which can be calculated only from prospective or experimental studies). You can remember that an **o**dds **r**atio is commonly used in **c**ase **c**ontrol studies through the mnemonic: **CC** (or **c**ritical **c**are) patients often go to the **OR** (**o**perating **r**oom).

11. **What do you need to know about standard deviation (SD) for the USMLE?**
    You need to know that for a normal or bell-shaped distribution, the mean ±1 SD contains 68% of the values, the mean ±2 SD contains 95% of the values, and the mean ±3 SD contains 99.7% of the values. A classic question gives the mean and SD and asks what percentage of values will be above a given value. For example, if the mean score on a test is 80 and the standard deviation is 5, 68% of the scores will be within 5 points of 80 (scores of 75–85), and 95% of the scores will be within 10 points of 80 (scores of 70–90). The question may ask what percentage of scores are over 90. The answer is 2.5% because 2.5% of the scores fall below 70 and 2.5% of the scores are over 90. Variations of this question are common.

12. **Define mean, median, and mode.**
    The mean is the average value, the median is the middle value, and the mode is the most common value. A question may give several numbers and ask for their mean, median, and mode. For example, if the question gives the numbers 2, 2, 4, and 8:
    The mean is the average of the four numbers: $(2 + 2 + 4 + 8)/4 = 16/4 = 4$.
    The median is the middle value. Because there are four numbers, there is no true middle value. Therefore take the average between the two middle numbers (2 and 4), so the median = 3.
    The mode is 2, because the number 2 appears twice (more times than any other value).
    Remember that in a normal distribution, mean = median = mode.

13. **What is a skewed distribution? How does it affect the mean, median, and mode?**
    A skewed distribution implies that the distribution is not normal; in other words, the data do not conform to a perfect bell-shaped curve. **Positive skew** is an asymmetric distribution with an excess of high values; in other words, the tail of the curve is on the right (mean > median > mode) (Fig. 1.3). **Negative skew** is an asymmetric distribution with an excess of low values; in other words, the tail of the curve is on the left (mean < median < mode). Because such distributions are not normal, the SD and mean are less meaningful values.

14. **Define test reliability. How is it related to precision? What reduces reliability?**
    Practically speaking, the reliability of a test is synonymous with its precision. Reliability measures the reproducibility and consistency of a test. For example, if the test has good interrater reliability, the person taking the test will get the same score even if two different people administer the same test. Random error reduces reliability and precision (e.g., limitation in significant figures).

15. **Define test validity. How is it related to accuracy? What reduces validity?**
    Practically speaking, the validity of a test is synonymous with its accuracy. Validity measures the trueness of measurement (i.e., whether the test measures what it claims to measure). For example, if a valid IQ test is administered to a genius, the test should not indicate that the person has an intellectual disability. Systematic error reduces validity and accuracy (e.g., when the equipment is miscalibrated).

16. **Define correlation coefficient. What is the range of its values?**
    A correlation coefficient measures to what degree two variables are related. The value of the correlation coefficient ranges from −1 to +1.

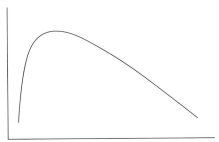

Fig. 1.3 Positive skew. An excess of higher values makes this a nonnormal distribution. (From O'Connell T. *USMLE Step 2 Secrets.* 4th ed. Philadelphia: Elsevier; 2014 [fig 3-2].)

17. **True or false: A correlation coefficient of –0.6 is a stronger correlation coefficient than +0.4.**
    True. The important factor in determining the strength of the relationship between two variables is the distance of the value from zero. A correlation coefficient of 0 equates to no association whatsoever; the two variables are totally unrelated. A correlation coefficient of +1 equates to a perfect positive correlation (when one variable increases, so does the other), whereas –1 corresponds to a perfect negative correlation (when one variable increases, the other decreases). Therefore the absolute value indicates the strength of the correlation (e.g., the strength of –0.3 is the same as that of +0.3).

18. **Define confidence interval. Why is it used?**
    When you take a set of data from a subset of the population and calculate the mean, you may want to say that it is equivalent to the mean for the whole population. In fact, however, the two means are usually not exactly equal. A confidence interval of 95% (the value used in most medical literature before data are accepted by the medical community) indicates that there is 95% certainty that the mean for the entire population is within a certain range (usually 2 SD of the experimental or derived mean, calculated from the subset of the population examined). For example, if the heart rate of 100 people is sampled and the mean is calculated as 80 beats per minute with an SD of 2, the confidence interval (also known as *confidence limits*) is written as $76 < X < 84 = 0.95$. In other words, there is 95% certainty that the mean heart rate of the whole population (X) is between 76 and 84 (within 2 SD of the mean).

19. **When are a chi-square test, *t*-test, and analysis of variance test used?**
    All of these tests are used to compare different sets of data.
    Chi-square test: used to compare percentages or proportions (nonnumeric or nominal data)
    t-test: used to compare two means
    Analysis of variance (ANOVA): used to compare three or more means

20. **What is the difference between nominal, ordinal, and continuous types of data?**
    Nominal data have no numeric value (e.g., the day of the week). Ordinal data give a ranking but no quantification (e.g., class rank, which does not specify how far number 1 is ahead of number 2). Most numeric measurements are continuous data (e.g., weight, blood pressure, and age). This distinction is important because of question 19: Chi-square tests must be used to compare nominal or ordinal data, whereas a *t*-test or ANOVA test is used to compare continuous data.

21. **Define the following rates commonly seen on the USMLE.**

Rate	Definition
Birth rate	Live births/1000 population
Fertility rate	Live births/1000 population
Death rate	Deaths/1000 population
Neonatal mortality rate	Neonatal deaths (first 28 days of life)/1000 live births
Perinatal mortality rate	Neonatal deaths + stillbirths/1000 total births
Infant mortality rate	Deaths (from 0–1 yr old)/1000 live births
Maternal mortality rate	Maternal pregnancy-related deaths (deaths while pregnant or in the first 42 days after delivery)/100,000 live births

22. **What five types of studies should you know for the Step 3 exam?**
    From highest to lowest quality and desirability: (1) experimental studies, (2) prospective studies, (3) retrospective studies, (4) case series, and (5) prevalence surveys.

23. **What are experimental studies?**
    Experimental studies are the gold standard. They compare two equal groups in which one variable is manipulated and its effect is measured. Experimental studies use double blinding (or at least single blinding) and well-matched controls to ensure accurate data. It is not always possible to do experimental studies because of ethical concerns.

24. **What are prospective studies? Why are they important?**
    Prospective studies (also known as *observational, longitudinal, cohort, incidence,* or *follow-up studies*) involve choosing a sample and dividing it into two groups based on the presence or absence of a risk factor and following the groups over time to see what diseases they develop. For example, individuals with and without asymptomatic hypercholesterolemia may be followed to determine if those with hypercholesterolemia have a higher incidence of myocardial infarction later in life. The relative risk and incidence can be calculated from this type of study. Prospective studies are time consuming and expensive but practical for common diseases.

25. **What are retrospective studies? Discuss their advantages and disadvantages.**
    Retrospective (case control) studies choose population samples after the fact according to the presence (cases) or absence (controls) of disease. Information can be collected about risk factors. For example, you can compare

individuals with lung cancer and individuals without lung cancer to determine if those with lung cancer smoked more before they developed lung cancer. In a retrospective study, an odds ratio can be calculated, but true relative risk cannot be calculated, and incidence cannot be measured. Compared with prospective studies, retrospective studies are less expensive, less time consuming, and more practical for rare diseases.

26. **What is a case series study? How is it used?**
A case series study simply describes the clinical presentation of people with a certain disease. This type of study is good for extremely rare diseases (as are retrospective studies) and may suggest a need for a retrospective or prospective study.

27. **What is a prevalence survey? How is it used?**
A prevalence (cross-sectional) survey looks at the prevalence of a disease and the prevalence of risk factors. When used to compare two different cultures or populations, a prevalence survey may suggest a possible cause of a disease. The hypothesis then can be tested with a prospective study. For example, researchers have found a higher prevalence of colon cancer and a diet higher in fat in the United States versus a lower prevalence of colon cancer and a diet lower in fat in Japan.

28. **What is the difference between incidence and prevalence?**
Incidence is the number of new cases of a disease in a unit of time (generally 1 year, but any time frame can be used). The incidence of a disease is equal to the absolute (or total) risk of developing a condition (as distinguished from relative or attributable risk).
Prevalence is the total number of cases of a disease (new or old) at a certain point in time.

29. **If a disease can be treated only to the point that people can be kept alive longer without being cured, what happens to the incidence and prevalence of the disease?**
This is the classic question about incidence and prevalence on the Step 3 exam. Nothing happens to the incidence (the same number of people contract the disease every year), but the prevalence will increase because people with the disease live longer. For short-term diseases (e.g., influenza), the incidence may be higher than the prevalence, whereas for chronic diseases (e.g., diabetes or hypertension), the prevalence is greater than the incidence.

30. **Define *P*-value.**
The significance of the *P*-value is high yield on the Step 3 exam. If *P* is less than 0.05 for a set of data, there is less than a 5% chance ($0.05 = 5\%$) that the data were obtained by random error or chance. If *P* is less than 0.01, the chance is less than 1%. For example, if the blood pressure in a control group is 180/100 mm Hg but falls to 120/70 mm Hg after drug X is given, a *P*-value less than 0.10 means that the chance that this difference was due to random error or chance is less than 10%. It also means, however, that the chance that the result is random and unrelated to the drug may be as high as 9.99%. A *P*-value less than 0.05 is generally used as the cutoff for statistical significance in the medical literature.

31. **What three points about *P*-value should be remembered for the Step 3 exam?**
   - A study with a *P* value less than 0.05 may still have serious flaws.
   - A low *P*-value does not imply causation.
   - A study that has statistical significance does not necessarily have clinical significance. For example, if drug X can lower blood pressure from 130/80 to 129/80 mm Hg with *P* less than 0.0001, drug X is unlikely to be used because the result is not clinically important given the minimal blood pressure reduction, the costs, and probable side effects.

32. **Explain the relationship of the *P*-value to the null hypothesis.**
The *P*-value is also related to the null hypothesis (the hypothesis of no difference). For example, in a study of hypertension, the null hypothesis says that the drug under investigation does not work, therefore any difference in blood pressure is due to random error or chance. If the drug works well and lowers blood pressure by 60 points, the null hypothesis must be rejected because clearly the drug works. When *P* is less than 0.05, the null hypothesis can be rejected with confidence because the *P*-value indicates that there is less than a 5% chance that the null hypothesis is correct. If the null hypothesis is wrong, the difference in blood pressure is not due to chance, therefore it must be due to the drug.
   In other words, the *P*-value represents the chance of making a type I error (i.e., claiming an effect or difference when none exists or rejecting the null hypothesis when it is true). If $P < 0.07$, there is a less than 7% chance of a type I error if a true difference (not due to random error) in blood pressure between the control and experimental groups is claimed.

33. **What is a type II error?**
In a type II error, the null hypothesis is accepted when in fact it is false. In the previous example, this would mean that the antihypertensive drug works but the experimenter says that it does not.

34. **What is the power of a study? How do you increase the power of a study?**
Power measures the probability of rejecting the null hypothesis when it is false (a good thing). The best way to increase power is to **increase the sample size.**

35. **What are confounding variables?**
Confounding variables are unmeasured variables that affect both the independent (manipulated, experimental) variable and dependent (outcome) variables. For example, an experimenter measures the number of ashtrays owned and the incidence of lung cancer and finds that people with lung cancer have more ashtrays. The experimenter concludes that ashtrays cause lung cancer. Smoking tobacco is the confounding variable because it causes the increase in ashtrays and lung cancer.

36. **Discuss nonrandom or nonstratified sampling.**
City A and City B can be compared, but they may not be equivalent. For example, if City A is a retirement community and City B is a college town, of course City A will have higher rates of mortality and heart disease if the groups are not stratified into appropriate age-specific comparisons.

37. **What is nonresponse bias?**
Nonresponse bias is a type of selection bias that occurs when people do not return printed surveys or answer the phone in a phone survey. If nonresponse accounts for a significant percentage of the results, the experiment will suffer. The first strategy in this situation is to visit or call the nonresponders repeatedly. If this strategy is unsuccessful, list the nonresponders as unknown in the data analysis and determine if any results can be salvaged. *Never* make up or assume responses.

38. **Explain lead-time bias.**
Lead-time bias is due to time differentials. The classic example is a cancer screening test that claims to prolong survival compared with older survival data, when in fact the difference is due only to earlier detection and *not* to improved treatment or prolonged survival.

39. **Explain admission rate bias.**
The classic admission rate bias occurs when an experimenter compares the mortality rates for myocardial infarction (or some other disease) in hospitals A and B and concludes that hospital A has a higher mortality rate. But the higher rate may be due to tougher admission criteria at hospital A, which admits only the sickest patients with myocardial infarction. Hence hospital A has higher mortality rates, although its care may be superior. The same bias can apply to morbidity and mortality rates for a surgeon if the surgeon takes on only difficult cases.

40. **Explain recall bias.**
Recall bias is a risk in all retrospective studies. When people cannot remember exactly, they may inadvertently overestimate or underestimate risk factors. For example, John died of lung cancer, and his angry widow remembers him as smoking "like a chimney," whereas Mike died of causes not related to smoking, and his loving wife denies that he smoked "much." In fact, both men smoked one pack per day.

41. **Explain interviewer bias.**
Interviewer bias occurs in the absence of blinding. The scientist receives a large amount of money to perform a study and wants to find a difference between cases and controls. Thus the scientist may inadvertently call the same patient comment or outcome "not significant" in the control group and "significant" in the treatment group.

42. **What is unacceptability bias?**
Unacceptability bias occurs when people do not admit to embarrassing behavior. For example, they may claim to exercise more than they do to please the interviewer, or they may claim to have taken experimental medications when they actually spat them out.

43. **What is attrition bias and intention to treat analysis?**
Attrition bias occurs in prospective studies when a substantial number of subjects are lost to follow-up. This type of bias may be minimized by conducting a study that will likely be important to participants, fostering good communication between participants and study staff, and by using intention-to-treat analysis. Intention-to-treat analysis dictates that all participants who are randomized are included in statistical analysis and are analyzed in the groups to which they were allocated regardless of which treatment (if any) they received. Generally, an attrition rate of less than 5% leads to little bias, whereas more than 20% likely threatens the validity of a study.

GENERAL EMERGENCY MEDICINE PRINCIPLES

1. **Explain the ABCDEs of trauma. How are they used?**
The ABCDEs of trauma are **a**irway, **b**reathing, **c**irculation, **d**isability, and **e**xposure. They are the keys to the initial management of trauma patients. Follow them in order if simultaneous management is not possible. For example, if a patient is bleeding to death and also has a blocked airway, address airway management first.

2. **What is the difference between airway and breathing in trauma protocol?**
Airway means provision, protection, and maintenance of an adequate airway at all times. If the patient can answer questions, the airway is fine for now. You can use an oropharyngeal airway in uncomplicated cases and give supplemental oxygen. When you are in doubt or the patient's airway is blocked, intubate. If intubation fails, do a cricothyroidotomy.

Breathing is similar to airway, but even patients with an open airway may not be breathing spontaneously. The end result is the same. When you are in doubt or the patient is not breathing, intubate. If intubation fails, do a cricothyroidotomy.

3. **Explain circulation, disability, and exposure.**
   Circulation refers to circulating blood volume. For practical purposes, it means that if the patient seems hypovolemic (tachycardic, bleeding, weak pulse, pale, diaphoretic, capillary refill >2 seconds), give intravenous fluids and/or blood products. Initially you should start two large-bore intravenous lines and give a bolus of 10 to 20 mL/kg ($\sim$1 L) of lactated Ringer solution or normal saline. Then reassess the patient after the bolus for improvement. Repeat the bolus, if needed.
   Disability refers to the need to check neurologic function. In practical terms, this translates into doing a Glasgow Coma Scale (GCS) assessment. Intubation is generally recommended for patients with GCS less than 8 as they are usually unable to reliably protect their airway.
   Exposure reminds you to expose and examine the entire body. In other words, remove all of the patient's clothes and "put a finger in every orifice" so that you do not miss any occult injuries.

4. **What imaging films are routinely ordered for most patients with at least moderately severe trauma?**
   Cervical spine, chest, and pelvic radiographs.

5. **What is a FAST exam? Explain what you are looking for when performing a FAST exam.**
   FAST is an acronym for **f**ocused **a**ssessment with **s**onography for **t**rauma. It is a bedside ultrasound exam used to search for free fluid where fluid should not be (i.e., pathologic pericardial, intrathoracic, and/or intraperitoneal free fluid). If detected, these fluids will appear darker than the surrounding tissue (hypoechoic or anechoic). The extended FAST exam (E-FAST) includes additional views to investigate for pneumothorax.

6. **What is the imaging study of choice for head trauma?**
   Noncontrast computed tomography (CT) (better than magnetic resonance imaging for acute trauma).

7. **What are the three zones of the neck? How is trauma in each of the different zones managed?**
   Zone I is the base of the neck from 2 cm above the clavicles to the level of the clavicles.
   Zone II is the midcervical region from 2 cm above the clavicle to the angle of the mandible.
   Zone III is the top of the neck from the angle of the mandible to the base of the skull.
   With zone I and III injuries, you generally should order an arteriogram before going to the operating room. Zone I injuries also warrant bronchoscopy, esophagoscopy, and contrast swallow study. With zone II injuries, proceed to the operating room for surgical exploration without an arteriogram. In patients with obvious bleeding or a rapidly expanding hematoma in the neck, proceed directly to the operating room no matter where the injury is located.

8. **What are toxidromes? Describe the toxidromes associated with cholinergic crisis, anticholinergic crisis, sympathomimetic toxicity, and opiate toxicity.**
   Toxidromes are clinical syndromes characterized by a particular constellation of classic presenting symptoms caused by exposure to toxic levels of well-documented causative substances.
   - Cholinergic crisis (e.g., organophosphates or insecticides) classically presents with SLUDGE: excessive **s**alivation, **l**acrimation, **u**rination, **d**iaphoresis, **g**astrointestinal upset, and **e**mesis. Also look for pinpoint pupils and decreased heart rate.
   - Anticholinergic crisis (e.g., tricyclic antidepressant overdose) presents as a patient who is blind as a bat (mydriasis), hot as a hare (temperature dysregulation), mad as a hatter (central nervous system disturbances), dry as a bone (dry mucous membranes), full as a flask (urinary retention), and red as a beet (flushing). Also look for decreased bowel sounds and increased heart rate. Note that in a question stem it may be easy to confuse the mydriasis, temperature dysregulation, and mental status change for sympathomimetic toxicity, so look for *dry skin* to distinguish anticholinergic crisis from the diaphoretic patient with sympathomimetic toxicity.
   - Sympathomimetic toxicity (e.g., cocaine or amphetamine use) can cause hypertension, tachycardia, increased activity, anxiety, dilated pupils, diaphoresis, and possibly altered mental status.
   - Opiate toxicity (e.g., heroin overdose) can cause pinpoint pupils and respiratory depression. Also look for decreased bowel sounds, bradycardia, and hypotension.

9. **On the USMLE, bizarre, unique, and fatal side effects are tested as well as common side effects of common drugs. Cover the right-hand column and name the side effects of the listed drugs.**

Drug or Drug Class	Side Effect(s)
Acetaminophen	Liver toxicity (in high doses)
Acetazolamide	Normal anion gap metabolic acidosis
Aminoglycosides	Hearing loss, renal toxicity

Continued on following page

Drug or Drug Class	Side Effect(s)
Amiodarone	Thyroid dysfunction, pulmonary toxicity, liver toxicity (mnemonic: TFTs, PFTs, LFTs), bradyarrhythmias, corneal microdeposits, blue-gray skin discoloration
Angiotensin-converting enzyme inhibitors	Cough, angioedema
Angiotensin receptor blockers	Angioedema
Aspirin	Gastrointestinal bleeding, hypersensitivity, early respiratory alkalosis with late high anion gap metabolic acidosis
Bleomycin	Pulmonary fibrosis
Bupropion	Seizures
Busulfan	Pulmonary fibrosis
Chloramphenicol	Aplastic anemia, gray-baby syndrome
Chlorpropamide	Syndrome of inappropriate antidiuretic hormone (SIADH)
Cisplatin	Nephrotoxicity
Clindamycin	Pseudomembranous colitis (can be caused by any broad-spectrum antibiotic)
Clofibrate	Increased gastrointestinal neoplasms
Clozapine	Agranulocytosis
Cyclophosphamide	Hemorrhagic cystitis
Cyclosporine	Renal toxicity
Demeclocycline	Diabetes insipidus
Didanosine (ddl)	Pancreatitis, peripheral neuropathy
Digitalis	Gastrointestinal disorders, hyperkalemia, vision changes, arrhythmias
Doxorubicin	Cardiomyopathy
Ethambutol	Optic neuritis
Halogen anesthesia	Malignant hyperthermia
Halothane	Liver necrosis
Heparin	Thrombocytopenia, thrombosis
HMG-CoA reductase inhibitors (e.g., simvastatin)	Liver and muscle toxicity
Hydralazine	Lupuslike syndrome
Hydroxychloroquine	Retinopathy
Isoniazid	Vitamin B_6 deficiency (leading to intractable seizures, neuropathy), lupuslike syndrome, liver toxicity
Isotretinoin	Terrible teratogen
Lithium	Diabetes insipidus, thyroid dysfunction
Local anesthetic	Seizures, cardiac arrhythmia
Methotrexate	Hepatotoxicity, pulmonary toxicity, and myelosuppression
Methyldopa	Hemolytic anemia (Coombs test positive)
Metronidazole	Disulfiram-like reaction with alcohol
Minoxidil	Hirsutism
Monoamine oxidase inhibitors (MAOIs)	Tyramine crisis (after eating cheese or wine)
Morphine	Sphincter of Oddi spasm
Niacin	Skin flushing, pruritus
Opiates	SIADH
Oxytocin	SIADH
Penicillins	Anaphylaxis; rash with Epstein-Barr virus
Phenytoin	Folate deficiency, teratogen, hirsutism
Procainamide	Lupuslike syndrome
Quinine	Cinchonism (tinnitus, vertigo), thrombocytopenia, QT prolongation
Quinolones	Teratogens (cartilage damage), QT prolongation, delirium
Rifampin	Orange-red body secretions
Selective serotonin reuptake inhibitors (e.g., fluoxetine)	Anxiety, agitation, insomnia, sexual dysfunction, serotonin syndrome
Succinylcholine	Malignant hyperthermia; do not use in the presence of hyperkalemia

Drug or Drug Class	Side Effect(s)
Sulfa drugs	Rash, acute interstitial nephritis, kernicterus in neonates
Tetracyclines	Photosensitivity, teeth staining in children
Thioridazine	Retinal deposits, cardiac toxicity
Trazodone	Priapism
Valproic acid	Neural tube defects in offspring
Vancomycin	Red man's syndrome (related to infusion rate)
Vincristine	Peripheral neuropathy
Warfarin	Skin necrosis, teratogen, increased risk for clots early (that is why heparin bridging is needed)
Zidovudine (AZT)	Bone marrow suppression

10. Cover the right-hand column of the table and name the antidote for each of the poisonings or overdoses listed.

Poisoning or Overdose	Antidote
Acetaminophen	N-acetylcysteine
Benzodiazepines	Flumazenil (can precipitate seizures or delirium tremens if the patient has chronic benzodiazepine dependence)
Beta-blockers	Glucagon
Carbon monoxide	Oxygen (hyperbaric if severe)
Cholinesterase inhibitors	Atropine (always first), pralidoxime
Copper or gold	D-penicillamine or trientine (zinc is an alternative)
Dabigatran	Idarucizumab
Digoxin	Replete potassium and other electrolytes; digoxin-specific antibodies
Direct Factor Xa inhibitors (apixaban, rivaroxaban)	Andexanet
Heparin	Protamine sulfate
Iron	Deferoxamine
Lead	Dimercaptosuccinic acid (DMSA, succimer), dimercaprol, calcium sodium edetate (EDTA)
Methanol or ethylene glycol	Fomepizole, ethanol
Muscarinic receptor blockers	Physostigmine
Opioids	Naloxone
Quinidine or tricyclic antidepressants	Sodium bicarbonate (cardioprotective)
Salicylic acid (aspirin)	Urine alkalinization, dialycic
Warfarin	Vitamin K, fresh frozen plasma, prothrombin complex concentrate (if life-threatening bleeding)

11. How do you manage suspected acetaminophen overdose or toxicity?

The first step is to secure the ABCs (airway, breathing, circulation). If it has been 4 hours or less since time of ingestion, administer activated charcoal for gastric decontamination. However, usually the timing of ingestion is unknown. In that case, the first step is to obtain a serum acetaminophen (APAP) level and liver function tests. Administer N-acetylcysteine if there is any evidence of liver injury, serum APAP levels are above the "treatment line" on the Rumack-Matthew nomogram, or APAP levels are greater than 10 μg/mL with unknown ingestion time.

12. What are the clinical signs of aspirin toxicity? How do you treat it?

Signs of aspirin toxicity include tinnitus, hyperventilation (stimulation of medullary respiratory center), nausea/vomiting, altered mental status, and sometimes pulmonary edema. Overdose initially causes a primary respiratory alkalosis that develops into a mixed respiratory alkalosis-anion gap metabolic acidosis. Treatment is via alkalinization of the urine with sodium bicarbonate. Dialysis is indicated in emergent scenarios (e.g., pulmonary edema, renal failure, severely elevated salicylate levels).

13. What complications should you monitor for in caustic ingestion (e.g., acid or alkali)? How should these patients be managed?

Complications of caustic ingestion include perforation, ulcers, strictures, and carcinoma. Stricture formation is the most common complication and typically develops over several weeks. In terms of management, the first step, as always, is to secure the ABCs. All sources of chemical contamination (e.g., clothing) should be removed. Obtain a chest x-ray if the patient has or develops any respiratory symptoms to rule out perforation. All patients should receive an esophagogastroduodenoscopy within 24 hours to evaluate damage and guide management.

14. **What substances can cause methemoglobinemia? How is methemoglobinemia treated?**
Methemoglobinemia is acquired via exposure to oxidizing substances, most commonly topical anesthetic agents (e.g., lidocaine, benzocaine), dapsone, nitrites (including nitroglycerin), and aniline dyes. Treatment includes oxygen supplementation and administration of methylene blue and vitamin C.

15. **What are the clinical signs of arsenic toxicity? What are the most common sources of exposure? How do you treat it?**
Acute arsenic toxicity can present with abdominal pain, nausea, vomiting, diarrhea, garlic odor breath, and QTc prolongation. The most common sources include pesticides, contaminated well water, and pressure-treated wood. Treat with dimercaprol or dimercaptosuccinic acid (DMSA, succimer).

16. **What are the clinical signs associated with cyanide toxicity? When should you be suspicious for such exposure?**
Cyanide toxicity is associated with headache, abdominal pain, flushed "cherry red" skin, altered mental status, seizures, and coma. Watch for signs if a patient recently had significant smoke exposure (e.g., fire) or is on a nitroprusside drip for blood pressure control.

17. **If the following medications are given at the same time, what may happen?**

Medications	*Possible Effect of Simultaneous Administration*
MAOI plus meperidine	Serotonin syndrome
Aminoglycoside plus loop diuretic	Enhanced ototoxicity
Thiazide plus lithium	Lithium toxicity
MAOI plus SSRI	Serotonin syndrome (hyperthermia, rigidity, myoclonus, and autonomic instability)

MAOI, monoamine oxidase inhibitor; *SSRI*, selective serotonin reuptake inhibitor.

CHAPTER 2

DISORDERS OF THE NERVOUS SYSTEM AND SPECIAL SENSES

1. Cover all but the left-hand column, then describe the classic findings of cerebrospinal fluid (CSF) analysis in the following conditions.

Condition	Appearance	Cells (mm)[a]	Glucose (mg/dL)	Protein (mg/dL)	Pressure (mm Hg)
Normal CSF	Clear	0–3 (L)	50–100	20–45	100–200
Bacterial meningitis	Clear, cloudy, or purulent	>1000 (PMN)	<50	Around 100	>200
Viral/aseptic meningitis	Clear	>100 (L)	Normal	Normal/slightly increased	Normal/slightly increased
Pseudotumor cerebri	Clear	Normal	Normal	Normal	>200
Guillain-Barré syndrome[b]	Clear	0–100 (L)	Normal	>100	Normal
Cerebral hemorrhage[c]	Xanthochromia, bloody, or clear	Bloody (RBC)	Normal	>45	>200
Multiple sclerosis[d]	Clear	Normal/slightly increased (L)	Normal	Normal/slightly increased	Normal

Note: Tuberculous and fungal meningitis have low glucose (<50) with increased cells (>100), which are predominantly lymphocytes. In patients with fungal meningitis, a positive India ink preparation equals *Cryptococcus neoformans*.
[a]Main cell type is in parentheses after number (*L*, lymphocytes; *PMN*, neutrophils; *RBC*, red blood cells).
[b]Guillain-Barré syndrome is also known as albuminocytologic dissociation.
[c]Think of subarachnoid hemorrhage, but this pattern also may occur after an intracerebral bleed.
[d]On electrophoresis of CSF look for oligoclonal bands due to increased IgG production and an increased level of myelin basic protein in the CSF during active demyelination.

2. Cover the right-hand column, then localize the neurologic lesion for each of the following signs and symptoms.

Symptom/Sign	Area
Decreased or no reflexes, fasciculations, atrophy	Lower motor neuron disease (or possibly muscle problem)
Hyperreflexia, clonus, increased muscle tone	Upper motor neuron lesion (cord or brain)
Apathy, inattention, disinhibition, labile affect	Frontal lobes
Broca (motor) aphasia	Dominant frontal lobe[a]
Wernicke (sensory) aphasia	Dominant temporal lobe[a]
Memory impairment, hyperaggression, hypersexuality	Temporal lobes
Inability to read, write, name, or do math	Dominant parietal lobe[a]
Ignoring one side of body, trouble with dressing	Nondominant parietal lobe[a]
Visual hallucinations/illusions	Occipital lobes
Cranial nerves 3 and 4	Midbrain
Cranial nerves 5, 6, 7, and 8	Pons
Cranial nerves 9, 10, 11, and 12	Medulla
Ataxia, dysarthria, nystagmus, intention, tremor, dysmetria, scanning speech, dysdiadochokinesia	Cerebellum

[a]The left side is dominant in >95% of population (99% of right-handed people and 60%–70% of left-handed people).

3. When evaluating a delirious or unconscious patient with no history of trauma, for what three common conditions should you think about giving empiric treatment?
   1. Hypoglycemia (give glucose)
   2. Opioid overdose (give naloxone)
   3. Thiamine deficiency (give thiamine before giving glucose in a suspected alcoholic)
   Other common causes are alcohol, illicit drugs, prescription drugs, diabetic ketoacidosis, stroke, and epilepsy or postictal state.
   Other common causes are alcohol, illicit drugs, prescription drugs, diabetic ketoacidosis, stroke, and epilepsy or postictal state. Remember the mnemonic **DON'T** for altered mental status: **d**extrose, **o**xygen, **n**aloxone, **t**hiamine.

4. Define spina bifida. How can it be prevented?
   Spina bifida is a congenital abnormality in which lack of fusion of the spinal column, specifically the posterior vertebral arches, allows protrusion of spinal membranes, with or without spinal cord. Spina bifida occulta, the mildest form of the disease (bone deficiency without dural membrane or cord protrusion), is often asymptomatic and should be suspected in patients with a triangular patch of hair over the lumbar spine. More serious defects are usually obvious and occur most often in the lumbosacral region. A **meningocele** is protrusion of the meninges outside the spinal canal, whereas a **myelomeningocele** is protrusion of meninges plus central nervous system (CNS) tissue outside the spinal canal. Patients with a myelomeningocele almost always have an associated Arnold-Chiari malformation. Giving folate supplementation to potential mothers reduces the incidence of spina bifida and other neural tube defects.

5. Define hydrocephalus. How is it recognized in children?
   Hydrocephalus is excessive accumulation of CSF in the cerebral ventricles. In children, look for increasing head circumference, increased intracranial pressure, bulging fontanelle, scalp vein engorgement, and paralysis of upward gaze. The most common causes include congenital malformations, tumors, and inflammation (e.g., hemorrhage, meningitis). Treat the underlying cause, if possible; otherwise, a surgical shunt is created to decompress the ventricles.

6. Define subclavian steal syndrome. What symptoms does it cause? How is it treated?
   Subclavian steal syndrome is usually due to left subclavian artery obstruction proximal to the vertebral artery origin. To perfuse an exercising arm, blood is "stolen" from the vertebrobasilar system; that is, it flows backward into the distal subclavian artery instead of forward into the brainstem. The typical presentation includes CNS symptoms (e.g., syncope, vertigo, confusion, ataxia, dysarthria) and upper extremity claudication during exercise. Treat with surgical bypass.

DEGENERATIVE/DEVELOPMENTAL DISORDERS

1. What treatable causes of dementia must always be ruled out?
   B_{12} deficiency and hypothyroidism, for which the American Academy of Neurology recommends screening. Other treatable causes of dementia for which you might consider screening in some patients with specific risk factors include hyperhomocysteinemia, endocrine disorders (thyroid and parathyroid), uremia, liver disease, hypercalcemia, syphilis, Lyme disease, brain tumors, and normal-pressure hydrocephalus. Treatment of Parkinson disease may reverse dementia if it is present.

2. Define pseudodementia.
   Depression can cause some clinical signs and symptoms of dementia, classically in the elderly. This type of dementia is reversible with treatment. Step 3 questions will give you other signs and symptoms of depression (e.g., sadness, loss of loved one, weight or appetite loss, suicidal ideation, poor sleep, feelings of worthlessness).

3. What are the classic differences between delirium and dementia?

	Delirium	*Dementia*
Onset	Acute and dramatic	Chronic and insidious
Common causes	Illness, toxin, withdrawal	Alzheimer disease, multiinfarct dementia, HIV/AIDS
Reversible	Usually	Usually not
Attention	Poor	Usually unaffected
Orientation	Impaired and fluctuating	Often normal but may be impaired
Arousal level	Fluctuates	Normal

HIV/AIDS, Human immunodeficiency virus/acquired immunodeficiency syndrome.

4. What signs and symptoms do delirium and dementia have in common?
   Both may have hallucinations, illusions, delusions, memory impairment (usually global in delirium, whereas remote memory is spared in early dementia), and sundowning (worse at night). However, a new pattern of sundowning should be presumed to be delirium.

5. **Describe the characteristics of Alzheimer dementia.**
   Alzheimer dementia is a neurodegenerative disorder primarily affecting older adults and characterized by memory impairment, particularly short-term memory for facts and events. Memory loss develops insidiously and progresses slowly over time. Language function, visuospatial skills, and executive function tend to be affected early in the disease process, and with progression patients may have difficulty with activities of daily living.

6. **Describe the characteristics of dementia with Lewy bodies.**
   Dementia with Lewy bodies is an increasingly recognized Parkinson plus syndrome characterized by dementia plus two of the three following distinctive clinical features: visual hallucinations (classically involving small animals or small human beings/children), later-onset parkinsonism (in contrast to Parkinson disease, which has later-onset dementia; bradykinesia, limb rigidity, and gait disorders), and cognitive fluctuations. In contrast to Alzheimer dementia, the memory loss in dementia with Lewy bodies presents later in the course of the disease. Early symptoms include driving difficulties (e.g., getting lost) and impaired job performance. Sleep disorders such as acting out dreams are common in patients with dementia with Lewy bodies.

7. **Describe a scenario that would make you suspect vascular dementia.**
   Look for a patient with vascular risk factors (e.g., hypertension, diabetes, dyslipidemia, coronary artery disease) who presents with dementia of abrupt onset and a stepwise deterioration.

8. **Describe the characteristics of frontotemporal dementia.**
   Frontotemporal dementia is characterized by focal deterioration of the frontal and/or temporal lobes, leading to changes in personality or social behavior, with an eventual progression to dementia. Age of onset is typically in the 50s or 60s.

9. **Define Parkinson disease. How do you recognize it on the Step 3 exam?**
   Parkinson disease has a classic tetrad of (1) slowness or poverty of movement, (2) muscular (lead pipe and cogwheel–like) rigidity, (3) pill-rolling tremor at rest (which disappears with movement and sleep), and (4) postural instability (manifested by the classic shuffling gait and festination). Patients may also have dementia and depression. The mean age of onset is around 60 years.

10. **Describe the pathophysiology of Parkinson disease. How is it treated pharmacologically?**
    The cause is thought to be a loss of dopaminergic neurons, especially in the **substantia nigra,** which project to the basal ganglia. The result is decreased dopamine in the basal ganglia. Drug therapy, which aims to increase dopamine, includes dopamine precursors (levodopa with carbidopa), dopamine agonists (bromocriptine, apomorphine, pergolide, pramipexole, and ropinirole), monoamine oxidase-B inhibitors (selegiline), COMT inhibitors (entacapone and tolcapone), anticholinergics (trihexyphenidyl and benztropine), and amantadine.

11. **What is the classic iatrogenic cause of parkinsonian signs and symptoms?**
    Antipsychotics may cause parkinsonian symptoms in schizophrenics. This is a favorite Step 3 question. Treat this side effect of antipsychotic medication with anticholinergics (benztropine, trihexyphenidyl) or antihistamines (diphenhydramine).

12. **True or false: Dementia is common in patients with Parkinson disease.**
    True. Dementia is a common feature of Parkinson disease. Factors that influence the incidence of dementia include older age, age 60 years or older at onset of Parkinson disease, longer duration of Parkinson disease, and severity of parkinsonism.

13. **Give a classic case description of multiple sclerosis.**
    Multiple sclerosis classically presents with an insidious onset of neurologic symptoms in white women aged 20 to 40 years with exacerbations and remissions. Common presentations include paresthesias and numbness, weakness and clumsiness, visual disturbances (decreased vision and pain due to optic neuritis, diplopia due to cranial nerve involvement), gait disturbances, incontinence and urgency, and vertigo. Also look for emotional lability, other mental status changes, scanning speech (spoken words are broken into syllables separated by a noticeable pause with stress occasionally on the wrong syllable), and worsening of symptoms with hot showers. The patient may have a positive Babinski sign. The patient's symptoms do not follow a single neurologic lesion. Classic initial symptoms to recognize include:
    1. **Internuclear ophthalmoplegia**—a disorder of conjugate gaze in which the affected eye shows impairment of adduction.
    2. **Transverse myelitis**—a disorder in which one or more continuous segments of the spinal cord (most commonly thoracic) becomes inflamed, leading to a motor and sensory loss below the level of the lesion, autonomic dysfunction (bowel and bladder dysfunction), and eventual spastic paralysis and hyperreflexia.
    3. **Optic neuritis**—a disorder characterized by unilateral vision loss, eye pain with movement, afferent pupillary defect, and red color desaturation.

14. **What is the most sensitive test for diagnosis of multiple sclerosis? How is it treated?**
    Magnetic resonance imaging (MRI) is the most sensitive diagnostic tool and shows demyelination plaques in the periventricular white matter. Also look for increased immunoglobulin G (IgG)/oligoclonal bands and possibly myelin

basic protein in the CSF. Treatment is not highly effective but includes interferon, glatiramer, mitoxantrone, natali-zumab, cyclophosphamide, and methotrexate. Acute exacerbations are treated with glucocorticoids.

15. **How do you recognize amyotrophic lateral sclerosis (ALS) on the Step 3 exam?**
ALS (Lou Gehrig disease) is the only condition that you are likely to be asked about that causes both upper and lower motor neuron lesion signs and symptoms. This idiopathic neurodegenerative disease is more common in men, and the mean age at onset is 55. The key is to notice a combination of upper motor neuron lesion signs (spasticity, hyperreflexia, positive Babinski sign) and lower motor neuron lesion signs (fasciculations, atrophy, flaccidity) present at the same time. Treatment is generally supportive, and riluzole may have survival benefit and increase time to tracheostomy. Fifty percent of patients die within 3 years of disease onset.

NEUROMUSCULAR/DEGENERATIVE DISORDERS

1. **Define Guillain-Barré syndrome (GBS).**
GBS is a postinfectious autoimmune polyneuropathy. Look for a history of mild infection, especially upper respi-ratory infection (*Campylobacter* infection is the most commonly identified precipitant of GBS), or immunization roughly 1 week before onset of symmetric, distal weakness or paralysis with mild paresthesia that starts in the feet and legs with loss of deep tendon reflexes in affected areas. The hallmark of the disease is that motor func-tion is often affected with intact or only minimally impaired sensation. As the ascending paralysis or weakness progresses, respiratory paralysis may occur. Watch carefully; usually spirometry is done to follow inspiratory ability. Intubation may be required. Diagnosis is by clinical presentation. CSF shows markedly increased protein with normal white blood cell count (albuminocytologic dissociation). Nerve conduction velocities are slowed. The disease usually resolves spontaneously. Plasmapheresis (for adults) and intravenous (IV) immunoglobulin (for children) reduce the severity and length of disease. Do *not* use steroids; they no longer have a role in the treat-ment of GBS.

2. **What causes nerve conduction velocity to be slowed?**
Demyelination. Watch for GBS and multiple sclerosis as causes.

3. **What causes an electromyography (EMG) study to show fasciculations or fibrillations at rest?**
A lower motor neuron lesion (i.e., a peripheral nerve problem).

4. **What causes an EMG study with no muscle activity at rest and decreased amplitude of muscle contraction on stimulation?**
Intrinsic muscle disease such as the muscular dystrophies or inflammatory myopathies (e.g., polymyositis). You now know enough about EMG for the USMLE.

5. **Describe the signs and symptoms of Huntington disease. How is it acquired? What is the classic computed tomography (CT) finding?**
Huntington disease is an autosomal dominant condition that usually presents between the ages of 35 and 50 years. Look for choreiform movements (irregular, spasmodic, involuntary movements of the limbs or facial mus-cles) and progressive intellectual deterioration, dementia, or psychiatric disturbances (suicidal ideation is com-mon). **Atrophy of the caudate nuclei** may be seen on CT or MRI scan. Treatment is supportive; tetrabenazine or atypical neuroleptics (olanzapine, risperidone, or aripiprazole) may help with the chorea and agitation/psychosis.

6. **Describe the pathophysiology of myasthenia gravis (MG). Who is affected? What are the classic physical findings?**
MG is an autoimmune disease that destroys acetylcholine receptors. Most patients have antibodies to acetylcho-line receptors in their serum. The disease usually presents in women between the ages of 20 and 40 years. Look for ptosis, diplopia, and general muscle fatigability, especially toward the end of the day or with repetitive use.

7. **How is MG diagnosed? What tumor is associated with it?**
Diagnosis is made with the Tensilon test. After injection of edrophonium (Tensilon), a short-acting anticholinester-ase inhibitor, muscle weakness improves. Nerve stimulation studies can also be used. Watch for associated **thymomas** (a tumor of the thymus). Thymectomy is generally recommended for patients under age 60 years without thymoma. Chronic medical treatment consists of long-acting anticholinesterase inhibitors (pyridostigmine) and immunotherapy (glucocorticoids, mycophenolate, azathioprine, and cyclosporine).

8. **What three conditions may cause an MG-like clinical picture?**
   1. **Eaton-Lambert syndrome** is a paraneoplastic syndrome (classically seen with small cell lung cancer) associ-ated with muscle weakness. The extraocular muscles are spared, whereas MG is almost always characterized by prominent involvement of extraocular muscles. Eaton-Lambert syndrome has a different mechanism of ac-tion (impaired release of acetylcholine from nerves) and a differential response to repetitive nerve stimulation. The weakness in MG worsens with repetitive use or stimulation, whereas the weakness in Eaton-Lambert syn-drome improves.

2. **Organophosphate poisoning** also causes MG-like muscle weakness. Poisoning is usually due to agricultural exposure. Look for symptoms of parasympathetic excess (e.g., miosis, excessive bronchial secretions, urinary urgency, and diarrhea). Edrophonium causes worsening of the muscular weakness. Treat with atropine and pralidoxime.
3. **Aminoglycosides in high doses** may cause MG-like muscular weakness and/or prolong the effects of muscular blockade after anesthesia.

CEREBROVASCULAR DISEASES

1. **In what common situation is a lumbar puncture contraindicated?**
   With acute head trauma, intracranial hypertension (signs include papilledema), coagulopathy, suspicion for intracranial hemorrhage, or suspicion for a spinal epidural abscess. You should do a lumbar tap only after you have a negative CT or MRI scan of the head in these settings. Otherwise you may cause uncal herniation and death.

2. **List the four major types of intracranial hemorrhages.**
   1. Subdural hematoma
   2. Epidural hematoma
   3. Subarachnoid hemorrhage
   4. Intracerebral hemorrhage

3. **What causes a subdural hematoma? How do you recognize and treat it?**
   Subdural hematomas are due to bleeding from veins that bridge the cortex and dural sinuses. On a CT scan, the hematoma is crescent shaped (Fig. 2.1). The blood does not cross the falx cerebri (midline) because the dura is attached to the skull. Subdural hematomas are common in alcoholics and victims of head trauma. They may present immediately after trauma or as long as 1 to 2 months later. The bleeding is relatively slow because it is venous blood. If the patient has a history of head trauma, always consider the diagnosis of subdural hematoma. If large, expanding, or accompanied by neurologic deficits, treat with surgical evacuation.

4. **What causes an epidural hematoma? How do you recognize and treat it?**
   Epidural hematomas are due to bleeding from meningeal arteries (classically, the middle meningeal artery). Bleeding tends to occur quickly because it is higher pressure arterial blood, and the hematoma pushes away the dura

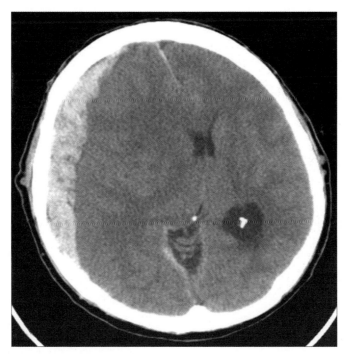

Fig. 2.1 Subdural hematoma. The crescent-shaped blood clot is causing a severe midline shift and brain herniation. (From Standring S. *Gray's Anatomy.* London: Elsevier; 2016:429-441.)

as it expands. On CT scan, the hematoma is lenticular in shape (Fig. 2.2). At least 85% of epidural hematomas are associated with a skull fracture (classically, a temporal bone fracture), and many patients have an ipsilateral "blown" pupil (dilated, fixed, nonreactive pupil on the side of the hematoma). The classic history includes head trauma with loss of consciousness, followed by a lucid interval of minutes to hours, and then neurologic deterioration. Treatment usually includes surgical evacuation.

5. **Define subarachnoid hemorrhage. What causes it? How is it treated?**
A subarachnoid hemorrhage describes bleeding between the arachnoid and pia mater. The most common cause is trauma, followed by ruptured berry aneurysms. Blood can be seen in the cerebral ventricles and surrounding the brain or brainstem on CT scan. The classic patient describes the "worst headache of my life," also known as a thunderclap headache, although many die or are unconscious before they reach the hospital. Patients who are awake have signs of meningitis (positive Kernig sign and Brudzinski sign). Remember the association between polycystic kidney disease and berry aneurysms. CT is the test of choice and should be performed before performing lumbar puncture (see question 1). A lumbar puncture shows grossly bloody CSF or xanthochromia (yellowish color of CSF due to breakdown of heme into bilirubin).

Treat with support of vital functions, anticonvulsants, and observation. Once the patient is stable, do a CT or magnetic resonance angiogram to look for aneurysms or arteriovenous malformations, which may be treatable with surgical clipping or catheter-directed angiographic procedures.

6. **What causes an intracerebral hemorrhage? How do you recognize and treat it?**
Intracerebral hemorrhage is bleeding into the brain parenchyma (Fig. 2.3). The most common cause is hypertension, but it also may be due to other forms of stroke, trauma, arteriovenous malformations, coagulopathies, or tumors. Two-thirds of intracerebral hemorrhages occur in the basal ganglia (especially with hypertension). The patient may present with coma or, if awake, contralateral hemiplegia and hemisensory deficits. Blood (which appears white on CT scan) can be seen in the brain parenchyma and may extend into the ventricles. Surgery is reserved for large, accessible hemorrhages, although usually it is not helpful.

7. **What causes strokes? How common are they?**
Cerebrovascular disease (stroke) is the most common cause of neurologic disability in the United States—and the third leading cause of death. Ischemia due to atherosclerosis (atherothrombotic ischemia) is by far the most common type of stroke (>85% of cases). Hypertension is another cause of stroke and typically causes hemorrhagic

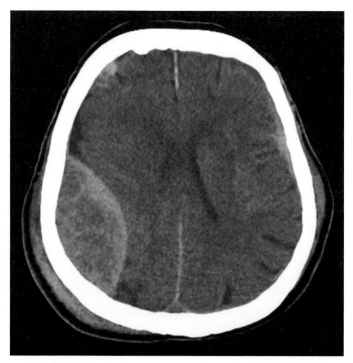

Fig. 2.2 A head computed tomography scan showing a right-sided epidural hematoma. The blood clot is biconvex. (From Standring S. *Gray's Anatomy.* London: Elsevier; 2016:429-441.)

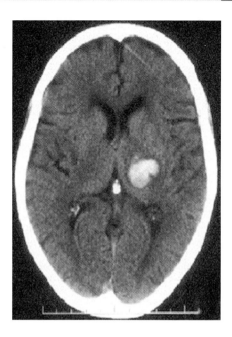

Fig. 2.3 Intracerebral hemorrhage. A computed tomography scan shows a parenchymal hemorrhage involving the left thalamus and posterior internal capsule. (From Goldman L. *Goldman's Cecil Medicine.* 24th ed. Philadelphia: Saunders; 2011 [fig. 415.4]. Courtesy Gregory W. Albers, Stanford University, Stanford, CA.)

stroke, most commonly in the basal ganglia, thalamus, or cerebellum. Having said this, be aware of more exotic causes of stroke, such as atrial fibrillation with resultant clot formation and emboli to the brain, septic emboli from endocarditis, paradoxic emboli through a patent foramen ovale, and sickle cell disease.

8. **How is an acute stroke treated?**
   Treatment for an acute ischemic stroke in evolution is supportive (e.g., airway, oxygen, IV fluids). The first step is to get a CT scan of the head without contrast to evaluate for bleeding or mass (Fig. 2.4). If no blood is seen on the CT scan, aspirin is usually the medication of choice. Heparin is not recommended for treatment of acute ischemic stroke and should be avoided on the USMLE. Thrombolysis with tissue plasminogen activator (t-PA) can be attempted if patients come to the hospital within 3 hours (up to 4.5 hours in certain circumstances) and meet strict criteria for its use.

9. **Define transient ischemic attack (TIA). How is it managed?**
   TIA is a brief episode of neurologic dysfunction resulting from temporary cerebral ischemia not associated with cerebral infarction. This newer definition is tissue based rather than time based. TIA is often a precursor to stroke

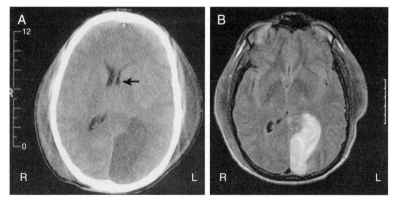

Fig. 2.4 Stroke on computed tomography (CT) and magnetic resonance imaging (MRI) scans. (A) The CT scan performed 3 days after a stroke shows a low-density area posteriorly on the left, with a mass effect and clear midline shift *(arrow)*. (B) The MRI scan performed on the same day shows the infarcted area much more clearly. (From Mettler Jr FA. *Essentials of Radiology.* 2nd ed. Philadelphia: Saunders; 2004 [fig. 2-17].)

and is due to ischemia. The classic presentation is ipsilateral blindness (amaurosis fugax) and/or unilateral hemiplegia, hemiparesis, weakness, or clumsiness that lasts less than 5 minutes.

Order a carotid duplex scan to look for carotid stenosis. The correct choice for long-term therapy is aspirin and antiplatelet medications. Choose carotid endarterectomy over aspirin if the degree of carotid stenosis is 70% to 99%.

10. **What clues suggest carotid stenosis? How is it diagnosed?**
The classic presentation of carotid stenosis is TIA—especially amaurosis fugax, which is the sudden onset of transient, unilateral blindness sometimes described as a "shade pulled over one eye." Physical exam may reveal a carotid bruit. Ultrasound of the carotid arteries (duplex scan of the carotids) is used to diagnose and quantify the degree of stenosis.

11. **How is carotid stenosis managed?**
In symptomatic patients, if the stenosis is **70% to 99%**, patients usually are advised to undergo carotid endarterectomy (CEA) for the best long-term prognosis—if their state of health allows them to tolerate the surgery. If stenosis is 50% to 69%, the data are less clear, and patient factors affect the decision. CEA is generally recommended for men, patients ages 75 or older, patients with recent stroke (not TIA), and patients with hemispheric symptoms other than transient monocular blindness (amaurosis fugax). Female patients, patients younger than 75 years, and those with mild symptoms generally do better with medical management if stenosis is 50% to 69%. If stenosis is less than 50%, medical management is indicated.

Patients should not undergo carotid endarterectomy after a stroke that leaves them severely disabled, but small, nondisabling strokes are not contraindications to surgery. Carotid endarterectomy should not be performed during a TIA or stroke in evolution. Surgery is always done electively, not on an emergent basis.

In asymptomatic patients, if the stenosis is 60% to 99%, CEA is indicated. If stenosis is less than 60%, medical management is indicated. Medical management includes antihypertensive agents, statins, and antiplatelet therapy.

The role of carotid angioplasty and carotid stenting in carotid stenosis is not yet clearly defined. Carotid endarterectomy remains the treatment of choice for suitable carotid stenosis.

Because medical therapy has improved since the initial studies comparing CEA with medical management were performed, medical management of lower-grade carotid stenosis and asymptomatic carotid stenosis is gaining favor. This is an area that is still being clarified in the medical literature and likely will not be tested on the USMLE.

12. **In what setting does dural venous sinus thrombosis occur? How is it diagnosed and treated?**
The risk factors are similar to those for deep venous thrombosis in other areas, including hypercoagulable state, trauma, dehydration, pregnancy, oral contraceptive use, infections (e.g., extension of sinusitis or mastoiditis intracranially), nephrotic syndrome, and local tumor invasion. The diagnostic test of choice is MRI. Though hemorrhagic infarcts are common with dural venous thrombosis, treatment with anticoagulation improves outcomes.

PERIPHERAL NERVE DISEASES

1. **What are the causes of lower motor neuron facial nerve paralysis?**
   - Bell palsy (discussed in more detail later in the chapter)
   - Herpes infection (Ramsay Hunt syndrome), which commonly involves the eighth nerve. Look for vesicles on the pinna and inside the ear; encephalitis or meningitis may be present.
   - Lyme disease (one of the most common causes of bilateral facial nerve palsy)
   - Stroke
   - Middle ear or mastoid infections
   - Meningitis
   - Temporal bone fracture (look for the Battle sign and/or bleeding from the ear)
   - Tumor, classically an acoustic schwannoma (i.e., neuroma) of the cerebellopontine angle

   Order a CT or MRI scan of the head if the cause is not apparent or if the history or physical exam raises suspicion, especially in the presence of additional neurologic signs.

2. **List the causative categories of peripheral neuropathy and give examples of each.**
   1. Metabolic/endocrine: diabetes mellitus (autonomic and sensory neuropathy), uremia, and hypothyroidism
   2. Nutritional: deficiencies of vitamin B_{12}, vitamin B_6 (look for history of isoniazid use), thiamine ("dry" beriberi), and vitamin E
   3. Toxins/medications: lead (the classic symptom is wrist or foot drop; look for coexisting CNS or abdominal symptoms) or other heavy metals, isoniazid, vincristine, ethambutol (optic neuritis), and aminoglycosides (especially CN VIII)
   4. Immunization and autoimmune disorders: GBS, lupus erythematosus, polyarteritis nodosa, scleroderma, sarcoidosis, and amyloidosis

5. Trauma: carpal tunnel syndrome (entrapment of the median nerve at the wrist; usually due to repetitive physical activity but may be a presentation of acromegaly or hypothyroidism; look for positive Tinel and Phalen signs), pressure paralysis (radial nerve palsy in alcoholics), and fractures (causing nerve compression)
6. Infectious: Lyme disease, diphtheria, human immunodeficiency virus, and leprosy

3. **What test can be used to prove the presence of a peripheral neuropathy, regardless of cause?**
Nerve conduction velocity is slowed with a peripheral neuropathy.

4. **Cover the right-hand columns, then specify the nerve root origin and the motor and sensory functions of the following peripheral nerves. In what common clinical scenarios are they often damaged?**

Nerve	Nerve Roots	Motor Function	Sensory Function	Clinical Scenario
Radial	C5-T1	Wrist, thumb, and finger extension (watch for wrist drop)	Back of forearm, back of hand (first 3 digits)	Supracondylar humeral fracture with anterolateral displacement
Ulnar	C8-T1	Finger abduction (watch for claw hand)	Front and back of last 2 digits	Elbow dislocation or fracture; supracondylar humeral fracture with posterior displacement
Median	C5-T1	Pronation of forearm, wrist flexion, thumb opposition	Palmar surface of hand (first 3.5 digits)	Carpal tunnel syndrome, humeral fracture, supracondylar humeral fracture with anteriomedial displacement (also consider brachial artery injury)
Axillary	C5-C6	Abduction and lateral rotation of arm	Lateral shoulder	Upper anterior humeral dislocation or fracture
Musculocutaneous	C5-C7	Flexion of the upper arm at the shoulder and elbow, supination of the forearm	Anterolateral forearm	Uncommon injury; penetrating trauma to the axilla
Peroneal	L4-S2	Dorsiflexion and eversion of foot (watch for foot drop)	Dorsal foot and lateral leg	Knee dislocation, fibula fracture

5. **What two diseases commonly cause isolated palsies of cranial nerves III, IV, and VI? How do you recognize them?**
Isolated palsies of cranial nerves III, IV, and VI are usually due to vascular complications of diabetes mellitus and hypertension. Symptoms generally resolve on their own within 2 months. In patients older than 40 years with a history of diabetes or hypertension and no other neurologic deficits or pain, observation is generally all that is required, because hypertension and/or diabetes is the most likely cause. If resolution does not occur within 8 weeks, if the patient is younger than 40 years, if neither hypertension nor diabetes is present, or if the patient starts to develop pain or other neurologic deficits, order an MRI scan of the head to rule out tumor or aneurysm (i.e., benign cause less likely).

HEADACHE AND MOVEMENT DISORDERS

1. **Differentiate among tension, cluster, and migraine headaches. How is each treated?**
Tension headaches are the most common; look for a long history of headaches and stress, plus a feeling of tightness or stiffness, usually frontal or occipital and bilateral. Treat with stress reduction and acetaminophen/nonsteroidal antiinflammatory drugs (NSAIDs).
Cluster headaches are unilateral, severe, and tender; they occur in clusters (e.g., three in 1 week, then none for 2 months) and are usually accompanied by autonomic symptoms such as ptosis, lacrimation, rhinorrhea, and nasal congestion. Supplemental oxygen and subcutaneous sumatriptan are first-line therapy for acute attacks.

Migraine headaches are classically associated with an aura (a peculiar sensation, such as a noise or a flash of light, that lets the patient know that an attack is about to start). Remember the mnemonic POUND: **p**ulsatile quality, **o**nset/duration of 4 to 72 hours, **u**nilateral, **n**ausea/vomiting, and **d**isabling. Often, signs and symptoms also include photophobia, phonophobia, and a positive family history. Occasionally neurologic symptoms are seen during attacks. Migraines usually begin between the ages of 10 and 30 years. Medications used for the acute treatment of migraines include NSAIDs, triptans, ergotamine, and antiemetics. Prophylaxis can be achieved with beta-blockers, tricyclic antidepressants, topiramate, valproic acid, and calcium channel blockers.

2. **How do you recognize a headache secondary to brain tumor or intracranial mass?**
By the presence of associated neurologic signs and symptoms of intracranial hypertension (papilledema; nausea/vomiting, which may be projectile; and mental status changes or ataxia). The classic headache occurs every day and is worse in the morning. Watch for a headache that wakes the patient from sleep. Headaches from an intracranial mass get worse with a Valsalva maneuver, exertion, or sex. Get a CT or MRI scan of the head.

3. **Define idiopathic intracranial hypertension (IIH; formerly pseudotumor cerebri). How is it diagnosed and treated?**
Idiopathic intracranial hypertension is a fairly benign condition that can mimic a tumor because both cause intracranial hypertension with papilledema and daily headaches that are classically worse in the morning and may be accompanied by nausea and vomiting. The difference, however, is that IIH is usually found in young, obese females who are unlikely to have a brain tumor. Negative CT and MRI scans rule out a tumor or mass. The main worrisome sequela is vision loss. Treatment is supportive; weight loss usually helps, and repeated lumbar punctures or a CSF shunt may be needed. Large doses of vitamin A, tetracyclines, and withdrawal from corticosteroids are possible causes of IIH.

4. **How do you recognize a headache due to meningitis?**
The adult patient has a fever, **Brudzinski sign** or **Kernig sign,** altered mental status, focal neurologic signs, seizures, vomiting, and positive CSF findings (the classic findings in bacterial meningitis are significantly elevated white blood cells, decreased glucose, protein around 100 mg/dL, and increased opening pressure) if a lumbar tap is done. Photophobia is also common.

5. **What causes the "worst headache" of a patient's life?**
This is a classic description for a subarachnoid hemorrhage. The most common causes are ruptured congenital berry aneurysm or trauma. Look for blood around the brain, within sulci, or within basal cisterns (star sign) on a CT/MRI scan or xanthochromic (pink-yellow coloration due to breakdown of hemoglobin >6 hours after onset) grossly bloody CSF on lumbar puncture. Treatment is supportive. Aneurysms require surgical treatment to prevent rebleeding and death.

6. **What are the common extracranial causes of headache?**
   - Eye pain (optic neuritis, eyestrain from refractive errors, iritis, glaucoma)
   - Middle ear pain (otitis media, mastoiditis)
   - Sinus pain (sinusitis)
   - Oral cavity pain (toothache)
   - Herpes zoster infection with cranial nerve involvement
   - Toxins (e.g., carbon monoxide poisoning)
   - Nonspecific headache (e.g., malaise from any illness)

7. **What are the two overarching types of seizures and their subtypes that you should be able to recognize?**
   1. Partial (focal) seizure
      a. Simple partial seizure
      b. Complex partial seizure
   2. Generalized seizure
      a. Absence (petit mal)
      b. Myoclonic
      c. Tonic-clonic
      d. Tonic
      e. Atonic

8. **Describe simple partial seizures. How are they treated?**
Simple partial (local or focal) seizures may be motor (e.g., Jacksonian march), sensory (e.g., hallucinations), or psychic (cognitive or affective symptoms). The key point is that consciousness is *not* impaired. The first-line agents for treatment are carbamazepine, lamotrigine, oxcarbazepine, and levetiracetam.

9. **Describe complex partial seizures. How are they treated?**
Complex partial (psychomotor) seizures are any simple partial seizure followed by impairment of consciousness. Patients perform purposeless movements and may become aggressive if restraint is attempted (however, people

who get in fights or kill other people are not having a seizure). The first-line agents for treatment are valproate, lamotrigine, and levetiracetam.

10. **Give the classic description of an absence seizure.**
Absence (petit mal) seizures are brief (10–30 seconds in duration) generalized seizures in which the main manifestation is loss of consciousness, often with eye or muscle fluttering. They do not begin after the age of 20 years. The classic description is a child in a classroom who stares into space in the middle of a sentence and then 20 seconds later resumes the sentence where they left off. The child is *not* daydreaming, but having a seizure. There is no postictal state (an important difference between absence and complex seizures). The first-line treatment agents are ethosuximide and valproate.

11. **How do you recognize a tonic-clonic seizure?**
Tonic-clonic (grand mal) seizures are the classic seizures that we knew about before we went to medical school. They may be associated with an aura. Tonic muscle contraction is followed by clonic contractions usually lasting 2 to 5 minutes. Associated symptoms may include incontinence and tongue lacerations. The postictal state is characterized by drowsiness, confusion, headache, and muscle soreness. The first-line agents for treatment are valproate, lamotrigine, or levetiracetam.

12. **Define febrile seizure and distinguish between a simple and complex febrile seizure.**
Children between the ages of 6 months and 5 years may have a seizure caused by fever. Always assume another cause outside this age range. Simple febrile seizures are of the tonic-clonic, generalized type, are less than 15 minutes in duration, and occur only once in a 24-hour period. A febrile seizure that is longer than 15 minutes, is associated with focal neurologic signs, or recurs within 24 hours is considered complex. For simple febrile seizures, no specific seizure treatment is required, but you should treat the underlying cause of the fever, if possible, and give acetaminophen to reduce fever. Such children do *not* have epilepsy, and the chances of their developing it are slightly higher than in the general population. For all febrile seizures, but especially for those classified as complex, make sure that the child does not have meningitis, tumor, or another serious cause of the seizure. The Step 3 question will give clues in the case description if you should pursue workup for a serious condition.

13. **What are the common causes of secondary seizures? How are they treated?**
- Mass effect (tumor, hemorrhage)
- Metabolic disorder (hypoglycemia, hypoxia, phenylketonuria, hyponatremia)
- Toxins (lead, cocaine, carbon monoxide poisoning)
- Drug withdrawal (alcohol, barbiturates, benzodiazepines, withdrawing anticonvulsants too rapidly)
- Cerebral edema (severe or malignant hypertension; also watch for pheochromocytoma and eclampsia)
- CNS infections (meningitis, encephalitis, toxoplasmosis, cysticercosis)
- Trauma
- Stroke

Treat the underlying disorder, and use a benzodiazepine (lorazepam or diazepam) and/or phenytoin or fosphenytoin acutely to control seizures. For all seizures (primary or secondary), secure the airway, and, if possible, roll the patient onto side to prevent aspiration.

14. **Define status epilepticus. How is it treated?**
Status epilepticus is defined as a seizure that lasts for a sufficient length of time (usually 30 minutes or longer, though considering the need for rapid evaluation and intervention to avoid cardiovascular morbidity and refractory status, an accepted operation definition is ≥5 minutes of continuous seizures) or is repeated frequently enough that the individual does not regain consciousness between seizures. Status epilepticus may occur spontaneously or result from withdrawing anticonvulsants too rapidly. Treat with IV lorazepam. Give fosphenytoin if the seizures persist. As with all seizures, remember your ABCs (**a**irway, **b**reathing, **c**irculation). Protect the airway. Intubate if necessary, and roll the patient onto side to prevent aspiration.

15. **True or false: Hypertension can cause seizures**
True. Always remember hypertension as a cause of seizures or convulsions, headache, confusion, stupor, and mental status changes.

16. **What do you need to remember when prescribing anticonvulsants to women?**
All anticonvulsants are teratogenic, and women of reproductive age need counseling about the risks of pregnancy. Do a pregnancy test before starting an anticonvulsant, and offer birth control. Polypharmacy increases the risk of teratogenicity. Valproic acid is well known for its association with an increased incidence of neural tube defects. There is limited human information on the risks to the fetus with the newer antiepileptic medications.

17. **What does CN V (trigeminal nerve) innervate? What classic peripheral nerve disorder affects its function?**
CN V innervates the muscles of mastication and facial sensation, including the afferent limb of the corneal reflex. Watch for **trigeminal neuralgia** (tic douloureux), which is classically described as unilateral shooting pains in the

face in older adults and often triggered by activity (e.g., brushing the teeth). This condition is best treated with antiepilepsy medications (e.g., carbamazepine). If the patient is younger and female or the symptoms are bilateral, consider multiple sclerosis, and rule out other causes, such as tumor or stroke.

18. **What is the most common cause of lower motor neuron facial nerve paralysis? How does it present?**
The most common cause is Bell palsy. Look for sudden-onset unilateral total facial paralysis (vs. upper motor paralysis, which spares the forehead due to bilateral innervation of the forehead), usually occurring after an upper respiratory infection. The cause is thought to be a reactivation of latent herpes simplex I infection in most cases. Patients may have *hyperacusis,* in which everything sounds loud because the stapedius muscle in the ear is paralyzed. In severe cases, patients may be unable to close the affected eye; if so, use drops to protect the eye. Most cases resolve spontaneously in about 1 month, although some have permanent sequelae. Oral prednisone and antiviral treatment for herpes (e.g., valacyclovir, acyclovir) may improve outcomes and lessen duration of symptoms.

19. **What structures does CN VII innervate? What is the difference between an upper and lower motor neuron lesion of the facial nerve?**
CN VII (facial nerve) innervates the muscles of facial expression, taste in the anterior two-thirds of the tongue, skin of the external ear, lacrimal and salivary glands (except the parotid gland), and stapedius muscle. With an upper motor neuron lesion of CN VII, the forehead is spared on the affected side, and the cause is usually a stroke or tumor. With a lower motor neuron lesion, the forehead is involved on the affected side, and the cause is usually Bell palsy or tumor.

20. **What brain lesions cause a resting tremor and an intention tremor? What about hemiballismus?**
A resting tremor, if due to a brain lesion, is generally a sign of basal ganglia disease, as is chorea. An intention tremor is usually due to cerebellar disease. Hemiballismus (random, violent, unilateral flailing of the limbs) is classically due to a lesion in the **subthalamic nucleus.**

21. **What other common conditions other than Parkinson disease cause a resting tremor?**
A resting tremor may be due to hyperthyroidism, anxiety, or drug withdrawal or intoxication. A common action tremor is called benign (essential) hereditary tremor. Benign hereditary tremor is usually autosomal dominant; look for a positive family history or improvement with consumption of alcohol, and use beta-blockers to reduce the tremor. Also watch for Wilson disease (hepatolenticular degeneration), which can cause chorea-like movements; asterixis (slow, involuntary flapping of outstretched hands) may be seen in patients with liver failure.

22. **Describe Tourette syndrome. How is it treated?**
Tourette syndrome is a motor tic disorder (eye-blinking, grunting, throat-clearing, grimacing, barking, or shoulder shrugging) that is exacerbated by stress and remits during activity or sleep. Although part of the classic description of Tourette syndrome, coprolalia (swearing) affects only 10% to 30% of patients. Males are affected more often than females. Of interest, Tourette syndrome can be caused or unmasked by the use of stimulants (e.g., for presumed attention deficit hyperactivity disorder). Antipsychotics (haloperidol) or dopamine receptor blockers (e.g., fluphenazine, pimozide) can be used if the symptoms are severe. Tourette syndrome tends to be a lifelong problem.

SLEEP DISORDERS

1. **Describe the hallmark findings of narcolepsy. How is it treated?**
Narcolepsy is a sleep disorder characterized by daytime sleepiness in spite of a normal daily sleep regimen. Patients have decreased latency for rapid-eye-movement (REM) sleep (patients go into REM as soon as they fall asleep); sleep paralysis (paralysis upon awakening); cataplexy (random loss of muscle tone that causes patients to fall down); and hallucinations as they awaken (hypnopompic) or fall asleep (hypnagogic). Patients may have a hypocretin deficiency. Treat with **modafinil** (a nonamphetamine stimulant), methylphenidate, or amphetamines.

NEOPLASMS

1. **Describe the common presentations of brain tumors.**
CNS tumors are the second most common tumors in children (second to leukemia); be suspicious in this age group. In adults, two-thirds of primary tumors are supratentorial (i.e., above the tentorium cerebelli, a portion of dura that separates the cerebellum from the cerebral hemispheres), whereas in children two-thirds are infratentorial (i.e., lower brainstem or cerebellum [posterior fossa]). In either group, look for new-onset seizures, neurologic deficits, or signs of intracranial hypertension (headache, blurred vision, papilledema, nausea, projectile vomiting). In children, also look for hydrocephalus (manifested as an inappropriately increasing head circumference), new clumsiness, ataxia, loss of developmental milestones, or a change in school performance or personality.

2. **What are the most common histologic types of primary CNS tumors in children and adults? How are primary brain tumors treated?**
The most common primary type in **adults** is **glioma**. Most gliomas are astrocytomas, which are intraparenchymal and have little or no calcification. The second most common type in adults is **meningioma**, which is often calcified and is external to the brain substance. In **children** the most common types are **cerebellar astrocytoma** (benign pilocytic astrocytoma) and **medulloblastoma**, followed by ependymoma. Treat with surgical removal (if possible), followed by radiation and/or chemotherapy, depending on the tumor.

3. **Which cancers tend to metastasize to the brain?**
Lung cancer, breast cancer, and melanoma are the most common; together they account for 75% of brain metastases.

4. **Metastatic cancer to the spine can cause spinal cord compression. How do you recognize and treat this medical emergency?**
Spinal cord compression causes local spinal pain and neurologic symptoms (reflex changes, weakness, sensory loss, paralysis, incontinence, urinary retention). In rare cases it may be the first indication of a malignancy. The first step is to start high-dose corticosteroids and order an MRI scan. Surgery, external beam radiation therapy, and stereotactic body radiotherapy are the treatment options for a tumor compressing the spinal cord. Prompt intervention is essential, and outcome is closely linked to pretreatment function.

5. **What causes spinal cord compression? How do patients present?**
Spinal cord compression is usually defined as acute or subacute. Most cases of acute cord compression result from trauma. Look for the appropriate history. Subacute compression is often due to metastatic cancer but may also result from a primary neoplasm, subdural or epidural abscess (classically seen in diabetics and due to *Staphylococcus aureus*), or hematoma (especially after a lumbar tap or epidural/spinal anesthesia in a patient with a bleeding disorder or a patient taking anticoagulation).
    Patients present with local spinal pain (especially with bone metastases) and neurologic deficits below the lesion (e.g., hyperreflexia, positive Babinski sign, weakness, sensory loss).

6. **How should patients with subacute spinal cord compression be diagnosed and treated?**
The first step in the emergency department is to give high-dose corticosteroids and order an MRI scan (preferred over CT). If the cause is cancer or tumor, give local radiation if the metastases are from a known primary tumor that is radiosensitive. Surgical decompression can be used if the tumor is not radiosensitive. For a hematoma or subdural/epidural abscess, surgery is indicated for decompression and drainage. Prognosis is related most closely to pretreatment function; the longer you wait to treat, the worse the prognosis.

7. **What diseases should come to mind in children with cerebellar findings?**
    • Brain tumor (cerebellar astrocytoma, medulloblastomas)
    • Hydrocephalus (enlarging head in an infant age <6 months, Arnold-Chiari or Dandy-Walker malformation)
    • Friedreich ataxia (starts between ages 5 and 15 years; autosomal recessive; look for areflexia, loss of vibration/position sense, and cardiomyopathy)
    • Ataxia-telangiectasia (progressive cerebellar ataxia, oculocutaneous telangiectasias, and immune deficiency)

8. **What diseases should come to mind for adults with cerebellar findings?**
Alcohol abuse, brain tumor, ischemia or hemorrhage, and multiple sclerosis.

9. **What tumor should you suspect in an adult with signs of CN VIII damage and increased intracranial pressure?**
An acoustic neuroma (especially in the setting of neurofibromatosis). Coinvolvement of the facial nerve is not uncommon.

10. **What tumor should you suspect in children with intracranial calcifications on skull radiographs?**
Craniopharyngioma (benign tumor that arises from remnants of the Rathke pouch and grows slowly from birth).

11. **What is the classic physical finding for a pituitary tumor? What is the most common type?**
The classic physical finding is **bitemporal hemianopsia** caused by compression of the tumor on the optic chiasm. Order an MRI scan of the brain in any patient with this finding. Patients may also have signs and symptoms of increased intracranial pressure. The most common type of pituitary tumor is a prolactinoma, which is associated with high prolactin levels, galactorrhea, and menstrual or sexual dysfunction. Other types of pituitary tumors may cause hyperthyroidism, Cushing disease, or acromegaly, or they may be nonfunctional (i.e., they do not secrete hormones).

INFECTIOUS DISEASES

1. **What is the classic age group for meningitis? Describe the physical findings.**
Neonates are the classic age group for meningitis; 75% of all cases occur in children younger than 2 years. Deciding when to do a lumbar tap is difficult because patients often do not have classic physical findings (Kernig

sign and Brudzinski sign). Look for lethargy, hyper- or hypothermia, poor muscle tone, bulging fontanelle, vomiting, photophobia, altered consciousness, and signs of sepsis (e.g., hypotension, jaundice, respiratory distress). Seizures may also be seen, but simple febrile seizures are common in the absence of meningitis if the patient is between 5 months and 6 years old. The maximum height of a fever, as opposed to the rate of rise, is felt to be the main determinant of risk in febrile seizures.

2. **What should you do if you suspect meningitis?**
In the absence of trauma, do a lumbar puncture immediately and begin broad-spectrum antibiotics and IV fluids. Do *not* wait for culture or other results to start antibiotics.

3. **What is the most common neurologic sequela of meningitis?**
Hearing loss. All pediatric and many adult patients need formal hearing evaluation after recovering from meningitis. Vision testing is also recommended. Other sequelae include intellectual disability, motor deficits/paresis, epilepsy, and learning/behavioral disorders. Dexamethasone may help reduce the incidence of hearing loss in patients with meningitis.

4. **What are the common viral (aseptic) causes of meningitis in children?**
Mumps and measles meningitis may be seen in children who are not immunized. The best treatment is prevention via immunization. Watch for neonatal herpes encephalitis (HSV-2) if the mother has genital lesions of herpes simplex virus at the time of delivery. Other children and adults can develop HSV-1 herpes encephalitis, which classically affects the **temporal lobes** on a head CT or MRI scan. Give IV acyclovir.

5. **Which types of bacterial meningitis require antibiotic prophylaxis in contacts?**
N. meningitidis and *H. influenzae.* If a case of meningitis is due to *Neisseria,* give all contacts rifampin, ciprofloxacin, ceftriaxone, or azithromycin as prophylaxis; rifampin is used for *H. influenzae* meningitis prophylaxis.

TRAUMA AND TOXIC EFFECTS

1. **What are the two classic causes of a "floppy" (flaccid) baby? How do you differentiate the two?**
Genetic disorders, the most common of which is Werdnig-Hoffmann disease (WHD), and infant botulism. History easily differentiates the two. WHD is an autosomal recessive degeneration of anterior horn cells in the spinal cord and brainstem (lower motor neuron disease). Most infants are hypotonic at birth, and all are affected by 6 months. Look for a positive family history and a long, slowly progressive disease course. Treatment is supportive only.

   Infant botulism is caused by a *Clostridium botulinum* toxin. Look for sudden onset and a history of ingesting honey or other home-canned foods. Diagnosis is made by finding *C. botulinum* toxin or organisms in the feces. Treatment involves inpatient monitoring and support with a close watch of respiratory status. The child may need intubation for respiratory muscle paralysis. Spontaneous recovery usually occurs within 1 week, and supportive care is all that is needed.

2. **What does a unilateral, dilated, nonreactive pupil after head trauma suggest?**
A unilateral, dilated, nonreactive pupil in the setting of head trauma most likely represents impingement of the ipsilateral third cranial nerve and impending uncal herniation due to increased intracranial pressure. Of the different intracranial hemorrhages, this scenario is seen most commonly with epidural hemorrhages. Do *not* do a lumbar puncture in any patient with a blown pupil because you may precipitate uncal herniation and death. Instead, order a CT or MRI scan of the head.

3. **List four classic signs of a basilar skull fracture.**
   1. Periorbital ecchymosis (raccoon eyes)
   2. Postauricular ecchymosis (Battle sign)
   3. Hemotympanum (blood behind the eardrum)
   4. CSF otorrhea or rhinorrhea (leakage of CSF, which is clear in appearance, from the ears or nose)

4. **What is the imaging test of choice for skull fractures of the calvarium? How are they managed?**
Skull fractures of the calvarium (roof of the skull) are best seen on CT scan (preferred over plain x-rays). Surgical indications include contamination (surgical cleaning and debridement), depression with impingement on brain parenchyma, or open fracture with CSF leak. Otherwise, such fractures can be observed and generally heal on their own.

5. **True or false: Severe, permanent neurologic deficits may occur after head trauma, even with a negative CT or MRI scan of the head.**
True. Head trauma can cause cerebral contusion or shear injury of the brain parenchyma (diffuse axonal injury), both of which may not show up on a CT or MRI scan but may cause temporary or permanent neurologic deficits.

6. **What finding suggests increased intracranial pressure?**
Increased intracranial pressure (intracranial hypertension) is highly suggested in the setting of bilaterally dilated and fixed pupils. Normal intracranial pressure is between 5 and 15 mm Hg. Less specific symptoms include headache, papilledema, nausea and vomiting, and mental status changes. Look also for the classic Cushing triad, which consists of increasing blood pressure, bradycardia, and respiratory irregularity.

7. **How should increased intracranial pressure be managed?**

The first step is to elevate the head of the bed and intubate the patient. Once intubated, the patient should be hyperventilated for rapid lowering of intracranial pressure through decreased intracranial blood volume (due to cerebral vasoconstriction). **Mannitol** diuresis or boluses of hypertonic saline (3% normal saline) can be tried to lessen cerebral edema. Furosemide is also used but is less effective. Ventriculostomy should be performed if hydrocephalus is identified. Therapeutic hypothermia can be used to protect the brain from secondary injury. Barbiturate coma and decompressive craniotomy (burr holes) are last-ditch measures. Anticonvulsant therapy should be started if seizures are suspected; prophylactic anticonvulsants are controversial but may be warranted in some cases.

Remember that cerebral perfusion pressure equals blood pressure minus intracranial pressure. In other words, do *not* treat hypertension initially in a patient with increased intracranial pressure, because hypertension is the body's way of trying to increase cerebral perfusion. Lowering blood pressure in this setting may worsen symptoms or even cause a stroke.

8. **True or false: Lumbar puncture is the first test that should be performed in a patient with increased intracranial pressure.**

False. *Never* do a lumbar puncture in any patient with signs of increased intracranial pressure until a CT scan is done first. If the CT is totally negative, you can proceed to a lumbar puncture, if needed. If you do a lumbar puncture first, you may precipitate uncal herniation and death.

9. **How do patients with spinal cord trauma present? How are they managed?**

Patients with spinal cord trauma often present with "spinal shock" (loss of reflexes and motor function, hypotension). Order standard trauma radiographs (cervical spine, chest, pelvis) as well as additional spine radiographs or CT scans based on physical exam. Also give corticosteroids (proven to improve outcome). Moderate hypothermia is increasingly being utilized in the management of patients with spinal cord trauma. Surgery is done for incomplete neurologic injury (some residual function maintained) with external compression (e.g., subluxation, bone chip). MRI can visualize cord injury noninvasively.

10. **What causes spinal cord compression? How do patients present?**

Spinal cord compression is usually defined as acute or subacute. Most cases of acute cord compression result from trauma. Look for the appropriate history. Subacute compression is often due to metastatic cancer but may also result from a primary neoplasm, subdural or epidural abscess (classically seen in diabetics and due to *S. aureus*), or hematoma (especially after a lumbar tap or epidural/spinal anesthesia in a patient with a bleeding disorder or a patient taking anticoagulation).

Patients present with local spinal pain (especially with bone metastases) and neurologic deficits below the lesion (e.g., hyperreflexia, positive Babinski sign, weakness, sensory loss).

11. **How should patients with subacute spinal cord compression be diagnosed and treated?**

The first step in the emergency department is to give high-dose corticosteroids and order an MRI scan (preferred over CT). If the cause is cancer or tumor, give local radiation if the metastases are from a known primary tumor that is radiosensitive. Surgical decompression can be used if the tumor is not radiosensitive. For a hematoma or subdural/epidural abscess, surgery is indicated for decompression and drainage. Prognosis is related most closely to pretreatment function; the longer you wait to treat, the worse the prognosis.

DISORDERS OF THE EYE

1. **What causes bitemporal hemianopsia until proven otherwise?**

A pituitary tumor (or other neoplasm) pressing on the optic chiasm.

2. **Use the visual field defect to localize the site of the brain lesion (Fig. 2.5).**

Visual Field Defect	*Lesion Location*
Right anopsia (monocular blindness)	Right optic nerve
Bitemporal hemianopsia	Optic chiasm
Left homonymous hemianopsia	Right optic tract
Left upper quadrant anopsia	Right optic radiations in the right temporal lobe
Left lower quadrant anopsia	Right optic radiations in the right parietal lobe
Left homonymous hemianopsia with macular sparing	Right occipital lobe (from posterior cerebral artery occlusion)

3. **How do you distinguish between a benign and serious cause of CN III deficit?**

With benign causes (i.e., hypertension and diabetes) of a CN III palsy, the pupil is normal in size and reactive; no treatment is needed. With serious causes (i.e., aneurysm, tumor, or uncal herniation), the pupil is dilated and nonreactive (blown). Urgent diagnosis and treatment are required. Additional neurologic symptoms also indicate a serious cause.

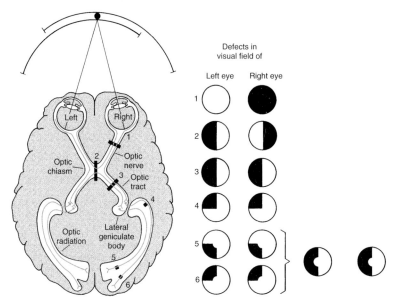

Fig. 2.5 Visual field defects produced by lesions at various levels of the visual pathway. *1*, Right optic nerve; *2*, optic chiasm; *3*, optic tract; *4*, Meyer loop; *5*, cuneus; *6*, lingual gyrus; *bracket*, occipital lobe (with macular sparing). (From Berne R, et al. *Physiology*. 5th ed. Philadelphia: Mosby; 2003 [fig. 8-10].)

The first step in serious cases is to get a CT/MRI scan of the head. Careful observation is preferred in benign cases, but if the patient does not improve within a few months or does not have hypertension or diabetes, you should order a CT/MRI scan of the head just in case.

4. Describe the classic presentation of a retinoblastoma.
   Retinoblastoma classically presents in a child younger than 3 years old with leukocoria (the pupillary red reflex changes to white) and/or unilateral exophthalmos. It may be bilateral in the inherited form.

5. What is the hallmark of conjunctivitis?
   Hyperemia of the conjunctival vessels.

6. Distinguish allergic, viral, and bacterial conjunctivitis.

Etiology	Signs and Symptoms	Treatment
Allergic	Itching, bilateral, seasonal, long duration	Vasoconstrictors or topical antihistamines/mast cell stabilizers
Viral*	Preauricular adenopathy, highly contagious (look for affected contacts); clear, watery discharge	Supportive, hand washing to prevent spread
Bacterial**	Purulent discharge; classic in neonates	Topical antibiotics ± systemic antibiotics

*The number-one viral cause is adenovirus.
**The number-one bacterial cause in adults is *Staphylococcus aureus*.

7. True or false: Conjunctivitis frequently causes loss of vision.
   False. Other than transient blurriness (due to tear film debris) that resolves with blinking, conjunctivitis should not affect vision. If vision is affected, think of other, more serious conditions.

8. Define glaucoma. What are the risk factors for developing it? What are the two general types?
   Glaucoma is best thought of as ocular hypertension (or elevated intraocular pressure, measured with a tonometer). Effects of glaucoma include visual field defects and blindness. The risk factors are age over 40, black race, and positive family history. The two main types are open-angle and closed-angle glaucoma.

9. Describe physical findings of open-angle glaucoma. How common is it? How is it treated?

Open-angle glaucoma causes 90% of the cases of glaucoma; it is painless and does not have acute attacks. The only signs are elevated intraocular pressure (usually 20–30 mm Hg), a gradually progressive visual field loss, and optic nerve changes (increased cup-to-disc ratio "cupping" on funduscopic exam). Treatment may involve several different classes of medications, including beta-blockers, prostaglandins, alpha-adrenergic agonists, carbonic anhydrase inhibitors, and cholinergic agonists, as well as laser therapy and surgery.

10. How does closed-angle glaucoma present? What should you do if you recognize it?

Closed-angle glaucoma presents with sudden ocular pain, seeing halos around lights, red eye, high intraocular pressure (>30 mm Hg), nausea and vomiting, sudden decreased vision, and a fixed, middilated pupil. Patients aged 55 to 70 years are most commonly affected. Dark environments, such as movie theaters, that trigger pupillary dilation are commonly the trigger in USMLE Step 3 question stems. It is an ophthalmologic emergency. Treat the patient immediately with **pilocarpine,** timolol, brimonidine, and/or acetazolamide to abort the attack. If these therapies fail, you can consider IV mannitol or oral glycerin. Definitive surgery (peripheral iridectomy) is used to prevent further attacks. In rare cases, anticholinergic medications can trigger an attack of closed-angle glaucoma in a susceptible, previously untreated patient. Medications do not cause acute attacks in patients with open-angle glaucoma or in patients with surgically treated closed-angle glaucoma.

11. How do steroids affect the eye?

Steroids, whether topical or systemic, can cause glaucoma and cataracts. Topical ocular steroids can worsen ocular herpes and fungal infections. For the Step 3 exam, do *not* give topical ocular steroids, especially if the patient has a dendritic corneal ulcer that is stained green by fluorescein. Such an ulcer represents herpes.

12. Define ultraviolet keratitis. How is it treated?

Excessive exposure to ultraviolet light can cause keratitis (corneal inflammation) with pain, foreign body sensation, red eye, tearing, and temporarily decreased vision. Patients have a history of welding, using a tanning bed or sunlamp, or snow-skiing (snow-blindness). Treat with an eye patch (for 24 hours) and topical antibiotic. You can reduce pain with an anticholinergic eye drop that causes paralysis of the ciliary muscle (cycloplegia).

13. What pediatric rheumatologic condition is commonly associated with uveitis?

Juvenile idiopathic arthritis (especially the pauciarticular form). Patients with juvenile idiopathic arthritis need periodic ophthalmologic examination to check for uveitis.

14. What is the most common cause of painless, slowly progressive loss of vision?

Cataracts, especially in the elderly. Treatment is surgical removal of the affected lens(es) and replacement with an artificial lens.

15. What should cataracts in a neonate suggest?

Cataracts in a neonate may indicate a TORCH (**t**oxoplasmosis, **o**ther, **r**ubella, **c**ytomegalovirus, and **h**erpes simplex virus) infection or an inherited metabolic disorder (the classic example is galactosemia).

16. What changes in the retina and fundus are seen in diabetes and hypertension?

Diabetes is associated with dot-blot hemorrhages, microaneurysms, and neovascularization of the retina. **Hypertension** is associated with arteriolar narrowing, copper/silver wiring, and cotton-wool spots. Papilledema may be seen with severe hypertension and should alert you to the presence of a hypertensive emergency.

17. What is the most common cause of blindness in patients under and over the age of 55 years? In black patients?

Diabetes is the number-one cause of blindness in younger adults in the United States, and senile macular degeneration (look for macular drusen) is the most common cause of blindness in adults over age 55. Glaucoma is the number-one cause of blindness in blacks of any age and the third overall cause of blindness in the United States.

18. Define proliferative diabetic retinopathy. How is it treated? How is nonproliferative diabetic retinopathy treated?

Proliferative diabetic retinopathy occurs after many years of established diabetes and is defined by the development of neovascularization (new, abnormal growth of vessels in the retina). Treatment involves application of a laser beam to the periphery of the entire retina (**panretinal photocoagulation**). Surgical or medical vitrectomy is used in some cases. Medical therapy for proliferative diabetic retinopathy is investigational but is used in some circumstances. The most promising are the vascular endothelial growth factor (VEGF) inhibitors (bevacizumab, ranibizumab, pegaptanib).

Focal laser treatment and anti-VEGF is common for nonproliferative (background) retinopathy when macular edema is present; the laser is applied only to the affected area. In severe cases, panretinal photocoagulation may be used. Otherwise, nonproliferative retinopathy is treated supportively—primarily with tight control of blood glucose and follow-up eye exams to watch for development of macular edema or neovascularization.

19. **What is the key to managing chemical burns to the eye? Which is worse—acid or alkaline burns?**
With chemical burns to the eye (acid or alkaline), the key to management is copious irrigation with the closest source of water. The longer you wait, the worse the prognosis. Do not wait to get additional history. Alkali burns have a worse prognosis because they go through liquefactive necrosis and tend to penetrate more deeply into the eye.

20. **Distinguish between a hordeolum (stye) and a chalazion. How are they treated?**
A hordeolum is a painful red lump near the eyelid margin. A chalazion is a painless lump away from the eyelid margin. Treat both with warm compresses. For chalazions, use intralesional steroid injection or incision and drainage if warm compresses do not work.

21. **How do you recognize and treat herpes simplex keratitis?**
Herpes simplex keratitis usually begins with conjunctivitis and vesicular lid eruption and then progresses to the classic dendritic keratitis (seen with fluorescein stain) (Fig. 2.6). Treat with topical antivirals (e.g., idoxuridine, trifluridine). Corticosteroids are generally contraindicated in dendritic keratitis because they may make the condition worse.

22. **What findings suggest an ophthalmic herpes zoster infection?**
Ophthalmic herpes zoster infection should be suspected in patients with involvement of the tip of the nose (Hutchinson sign) and/or medial eyelid, a typical zoster dermatomal skin rash, and eye complaints. Treat with oral acyclovir. Complications include loss of vision, uveitis, keratitis, and glaucoma.

23. **How do you recognize a central retinal artery occlusion? What causes it?**
Central retinal artery occlusion presents with sudden (within a few minutes), painless, unilateral loss of vision. The classic funduscopic appearance includes a pale, opaque fundus with a cherry red spot in the fovea (center) of the macula. The most common cause is emboli (from carotid plaque or heart), but watch for temporal arteritis as a cause on the Step 3 exam. No satisfactory treatment is available. However, treatment options include ocular massage, timolol, hyperventilation, and surgical therapies.

24. **Describe the symptoms of temporal arteritis (giant cell arteritis). What should you do if you suspect it?**
Temporal arteritis is a vasculitis seen in individuals over 50 years of age. Symptoms include jaw claudication, unilateral headache, loss of vision (due to central retinal artery occlusion), tortuous temporal artery (as seen or palpated on exam), markedly elevated erythrocyte sedimentation rate, and coexisting **polymyalgia rheumatica** (in 50%; causes proximal muscle pain and stiffness). If temporal arteritis is suspected in the setting of vision complaints, administer high-dose corticosteroids immediately before confirming the diagnosis with a temporal artery biopsy. Withholding treatment until a formal diagnosis can be made may cause the patient to lose vision in the other eye.

25. **How do you recognize central retinal vein occlusion? Describe the cause and treatment.**
Central retinal vein occlusion also presents with sudden (within a few hours), painless, unilateral loss of vision. The classic funduscopic appearance includes distended, tortuous retinal veins, retinal hemorrhages, cotton wool exudates, and a congested, edematous fundus. No satisfactory treatment is available. The most common causes are hypertension, diabetes, glaucoma, and increased blood viscosity (e.g., leukemia). Complications are related to neovascularization, which commonly develops and leads to vision loss and glaucoma.

26. **Describe the classic history of a patient with retinal detachment.**
The classic history of a patient with retinal detachment includes a sudden (instant), painless, unilateral loss of vision with floaters (little black spots that are seen no matter where the patient looks) and flashes of light. It is sometimes described as a "curtain or veil coming down in front of my eye." This history should prompt

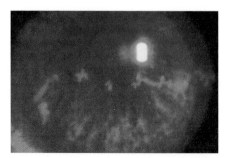

Fig. 2.6 Varicella dendritic keratitis. Numerous dendrites are seen in this slit-lamp photograph with fluorescein staining of the dendritic lesions from active viral growth in the corneal epithelium. (From Krachmer JH, et al. *Cornea.* 3rd ed. Philadelphia: Mosby; 2010 [Fig. 80.2, plate 2].)

immediate referral to an ophthalmologist. On exam, you may see a gray, elevated retina. Risk factors include trauma, diabetes, and cataract surgery. Surgery may save the patient's vision by reattaching the retina.

27. **True or false: Cataracts and macular degeneration are common causes of bilateral, painless loss of vision in the elderly.**
True. Although one side may be worse than the other, bilateral complaints are not uncommon. The red reflex typically becomes black with a significant cataract. Those with macular degeneration typically have focal yellow-white deposits called **drusen** in and around the macula on funduscopic exam. Treat cataracts with surgery; most cases (90%) of macular degeneration are the dry or nonexudative subtype, which is treated supportively (e.g., magnification aids). Wet or exudative macular degeneration is treated with IV VEGF inhibitors, thermal laser photocoagulation in selected patients, and photodynamic therapy.

28. **How do optic neuritis and papillitis present? What are the common causes?**
Optic neuritis and papillitis typically present with a fairly quick (over hours to days), painful, unilateral or bilateral loss of vision. The pain is exacerbated with eye movements. Patients with optic neuritis will fail a red desaturation test and see red objects as pink or lighter red. The optic disc margins may appear blurred on funduscopic exam with papillitis, just as in papilledema.

    Multiple sclerosis (which can also cause internuclear ophthalmoplegia) is a very common cause of optic neuritis, especially in 20- to 40-year-old women. Lyme disease, malignancy, and syphilis are other causes.

29. **What is strabismus? Beyond what age is it abnormal in children?**
Strabismus is the medical term for a lazy eye. The affected eye deviates, most commonly inward. Strabismus is normal only if intermittent and during the first 3 months of life. When strabismus is constant or persistent beyond 3 months, it requires ophthalmologic referral to prevent blindness (known as amblyopia) in the affected eye.

30. **Why does blindness develop in patients with strabismus?**
The visual system is still developing until the age of 7 or 8 years. For this reason, visual screening of both eyes is important in children. If one eye does not see well or is turned outward, the brain cannot fuse the two different images that it sees. Thus it suppresses the so-called bad eye, which does not develop the proper neural connections. This eye will never see well and cannot be corrected with glasses because the problem is neural rather than refractive. This condition is called amblyopia and is treatable with special glasses, eye patching of the unaffected eye, or surgery if it is caught in time; the goal of treatment is to allow normal neural connections (and thus vision) to develop.

31. **What is presbyopia? When does it occur?**
Presbyopia is the loss of lens ability to accommodate; it is why aging adults need reading glasses for near vision. Presbyopia occurs between the ages of 40 and 50 years and is a normal part of aging.

DISORDERS OF THE EAR

1. **Describe how otitis externa typically presents. What causes it?**
Patients have erythematous, swollen skin in the auditory canal and pain on manipulation of the auricle. A foul-smelling discharge and conductive hearing loss may also be present. Swimming is a known risk factor for otitis externa (inflammation of the outer ear). It is most often due to infection with *Pseudomonas aeruginosa.* Treat with topical antibiotics (e.g., ofloxacin, neomycin, polymyxin B) and possibly topical steroids to reduce swelling.

2. **What causes otitis media? How do you recognize it?**
Otitis media (inflammation of the middle ear) is an extremely common pediatric infection, most often due to infection with *Streptococcus pneumoniae, Haemophilus influenzae,* or *Moraxella catarrhalis.* Patients have no pain with manipulation of the auricle; positive symptoms include earache, fever, erythematous and bulging tympanic membranes (the light reflex and landmarks are difficult to see with otoscopy), and nausea and vomiting.

3. **What are the complications of otitis media? How are they avoided?**
Complications include tympanic membrane perforation (bloody or purulent discharge), mastoiditis (fluctuance and inflammation over the mastoid process, often with anterior displacement of the affected ear, roughly 2 weeks after the onset of otitis media), labyrinthitis, hearing loss (conductive hearing loss is more common than sensorineural hearing loss but both may occur), palsies of cranial nerves VII and VIII, meningitis, cerebral abscess, dural sinus thrombosis, and chronic otitis media (due to permanent perforation of the tympanic membrane). Patients with chronic otitis media may develop cholesteatomas with marginal perforations that require surgical excision.

    Otitis media is generally treated with antibiotics to avoid these complications (e.g., amoxicillin, second-generation cephalosporin such as cefuroxime, or a macrolide).

4. **What is the problem with recurrent otitis media? How is it treated?**
Recurrent otitis media is a common pediatric problem (along with prolonged secretory otitis, a result of incompletely resolved otitis media) and can cause hearing loss with resultant developmental problems (speech, cognitive functions). Treat with prophylactic antibiotics or tympanostomy tubes. Adenoidectomy is controversial but may help in some cases; it is thought to help prevent blockage of the eustachian tubes.

5. **What causes infectious myringitis? How do you recognize and treat it?**
Infectious myringitis, also known as bullous myringitis, is an inflammation of the tympanic membranes that can be diagnosed when otoscopy reveals vesicles on the tympanic membrane. Infectious myringitis is classically caused by *Mycoplasma* species, but *S. pneumoniae* or viruses may also be the culprit. Treat with erythromycin or clarithromycin to cover *Mycoplasma* species and *S. pneumoniae*.

6. **What are the common causes of hearing loss?**
The most common cause is **aging** (presbycusis); prescribe a hearing aid if needed. The history may suggest other causes:
   - Prolonged or intense exposure to loud noise (e.g., work related)
   - Congenital TORCH infection
   - Ménière disease (accompanied by severe vertigo, tinnitus, nausea and vomiting; treat acute episodes with benzodiazepines, anticholinergics [scopolamine], and antihistamines [meclizine or dimenhydrate]; diuretics are often used for ongoing treatment; surgery may be used for refractory cases)
   - Drugs (e.g., aminoglycosides, aspirin, quinine, loop diuretics, cisplatin)
   - Tumor (classically, acoustic neuroma)
   - Labyrinthitis (may be viral or follow or extend from meningitis or otitis media)
   - Miscellaneous causes (diabetes, hypothyroidism, multiple sclerosis, sarcoidosis, pseudotumor cerebri)

7. **In what situations should you worry about hearing loss?**
   - A bout of meningitis (hearing loss is the most common neurologic complication)
   - Congenital TORCH infections
   - Measles or mumps
   - Chronic middle ear effusions or chronic or recurrent otitis media
   - Use of ototoxic drugs (e.g., aminoglycosides)

8. **Define otosclerosis. How is it treated?**
In otosclerosis, the otic bones become fixed together and impede hearing. The cause is unclear. Otosclerosis is the most common cause of progressive conductive hearing loss in adults, whereas presbycusis is the most common cause of sensorineural hearing loss in adults. Treat with a hearing aid or surgery.

9. **What is the Weber test used to evaluate? How is it performed and interpreted?**
The Weber test compares bone conduction in the two ears. A vibrating tuning fork is placed on the center of the forehead, and the patient is asked where the vibrating sound is heard best. The normal response is to hear the vibration in the middle (or equally in both ears). In patients with conductive hearing loss, the sound is heard best in the affected ear, whereas in patients with sensorineural hearing loss, the sound is heard best in the unaffected ear.

10. **What is the Rinne test used to evaluate? How is it performed and interpreted?**
The Rinne test compares air conduction with bone conduction. A vibrating tuning fork is placed on the tip of the mastoid process. When the patient can no longer hear the sound, the tuning fork is removed from the mastoid and placed next to the auditory meatus of the external ear, and the patient is asked if the sound can be heard.
Because air conduction is normally greater than bone conduction, patients can hear the tuning fork when it is placed next to the auditory meatus (air conduction) even after they can no longer hear it vibrating on the mastoid (bone conduction). In patients with conductive hearing loss, bone conduction is greater than air conduction, thus they cannot hear the tuning fork when it is placed next to the external auditory meatus. In patients with sensorineural hearing loss, both air and bone conduction are impaired, but the normal ratio (air conduction > bone conduction) is maintained. Thus they still hear the tuning fork next to the ear after they can no longer hear it on the mastoid.

11. **What is the usual cause of sudden deafness?**
Sudden sensorineural hearing loss (SSNHL) involves acute unexplained hearing loss that is usually unilateral and occurs over hours (usually <72 hours). More than 90% of patients with SSNHL report tinnitus. Most cases are idiopathic but have been postulated to be due to viral causes, microvascular events, or autoimmune causes. Physical examination is unremarkable. MRI is indicated to rule out etiologies such as acoustic neuroma, multiple sclerosis, or vascular insufficiency. Glucocorticoids (administered orally or by intratympanic injection) are considered first-line therapy; antiviral agents are sometimes used, though there is not much evidence to support their use. Two-thirds of patients will experience recovery, though the resolution is often not complete. Among those who recover, hearing usually returns within 2 weeks.

12. **What is the most common cause of acquired hearing loss in children? What is the most common cause of congenital hearing loss in children?**
Bacterial meningitis. All children should receive a formal hearing test after a bout of meningitis. Congenital cytomegalovirus (CMV) infection is the most common cause of congenital hearing loss in children.

13. What are the common causes of vertigo?

    Vertigo can result from the same eighth cranial nerve lesions that cause hearing loss (Ménière disease, tumor, infection, multiple sclerosis). Another common cause is benign positional (paroxysmal) vertigo, which is induced by certain head positions, may be accompanied by horizontal nystagmus (never vertical nor rotatory), and is not associated with hearing loss. This condition often resolves spontaneously; no treatment is required. Epley maneuver, or modified Epley maneuvers, may help with resolution of symptoms.

14. Describe the function of CN VIII. What symptoms do lesions cause?

    CN VIII (the vestibulocochlear nerve) is needed for hearing and balance. Lesions can cause deafness, tinnitus, and/or vertigo. In children, think of meningitis as a cause. In adults, symptoms may be due to a toxin or medication (e.g., aspirin, aminoglycosides, loop diuretics, cisplatin), infection (labyrinthitis), tumor, or stroke.

CHAPTER 3

DISORDERS OF THE RESPIRATORY SYSTEM

1. **What should you know about pulmonary function in the setting of surgery?**
   A baseline chest radiograph is not part of the standard preoperative evaluation but is often used for patients over age 60 years or patients with known pulmonary or cardiovascular disease. Preoperative pulmonary function testing (PFT) is somewhat controversial, and the question probably will not appear on Step 3. Overall, the best indicator of possible postoperative pulmonary complications is preoperative pulmonary function. The best way to reduce pulmonary complications postoperatively is to **stop smoking** preoperatively, especially if it is stopped at least 8 weeks prior to surgery. Aggressive pulmonary toilet, incentive spirometry, adequate but not overly aggressive pain control, and early ambulation help to prevent or minimize postoperative pulmonary complications. Lastly, remember that the most common cause of a postoperative fever in the first 24 hours is atelectasis.

2. **Describe the effect of smoking on the lung.**
   Lung cancer and chronic obstructive pulmonary disease (emphysema, chronic bronchitis, and bronchiectasis) are due to smoking. Emphysema almost always results from smoking; if the patient is very young or has no smoking history, you should consider **alpha$_1$-antitrypsin deficiency.** Although the changes of emphysema are irreversible, the risk of death still decreases if the patient stops smoking.

3. **What about secondhand smoke?**
   Secondhand smoke has been proven to be a risk factor for lung cancer and other lung disease. The risk increases linearly with increasing exposure. When parents smoke, their exposed children are at an increased risk for asthma and upper respiratory infections, including otitis media.

4. **What other bad things does smoking do?**
   Smoking retards the healing of peptic ulcer disease, and cessation stops the development of **Buerger disease** (Raynaud symptoms in a young male smoker). Smoking by a pregnant woman increases the risk of low birthweight, prematurity, spontaneous abortion, stillbirth, and infant mortality. Cessation of smoking preoperatively is the best way to decrease the risk of postoperative pulmonary complications, especially if it is stopped at least 8 weeks before surgery.

OBSTRUCTIVE AIRWAYS DISEASE

1. **What is the most common lethal genetic disease in whites? How do you recognize it?**
   Cystic fibrosis, which is an autosomal recessive disease. Always suspect cystic fibrosis in pediatric patients with rectal prolapse, meconium ileus, esophageal varices, recurrent pulmonary infections, or failure to thrive. The classic complaint from the mother is a "salty-tasting" baby. Patients also commonly have pancreatic insufficiency and infertility (98% of affected males and 50% of females); they also may develop cor pulmonale (right-heart failure). Most states now screen for cystic fibrosis in the standard newborn screening.

2. **How is cystic fibrosis diagnosed and treated?**
   Diagnosis is made by an abnormal increase in the electrolytes of the patient's sweat (sodium and chloride) and/or deoxyribonucleic acid (DNA) testing. Treat with chest physical therapy, annual influenza vaccine, fat-soluble vitamin supplements, pancreatic enzyme replacement, bronchodilators, dornase alfa, and aggressive treatment of infections with antibiotics that cover *Staphylococcus, Haemophilus influenzae*, and *Pseudomonas* spp. *Staphylococcus* is the predominant organism in children and *Pseudomonas* spp. in adults. Eventually these patients will need lung transplantation.

3. **What is chronic obstructive pulmonary disease (COPD)?**
   COPD is a progressive, inflammatory lung disease that causes air flow obstruction. The disease encompasses both chronic bronchitis, which refers to inflammation of the bronchi and bronchioles, and emphysema, which is characterized by destruction of alveoli and poor gas exchange. Patients usually present with chronic productive cough and shortness of breath. Tobacco smoking is the main cause, though air pollution (especially indoor air pollution such as from wood-burning stoves), genetics, and aging contribute to COPD. Typical exam findings include diminished breath sounds, rhonchi, and wheezing. On x-ray, look for hyperinflated, hyperlucent lungs, an elongated and narrow mediastinum, and flattened diaphragms.

4. **How is COPD diagnosed and treated?**
COPD is diagnosed by PFT or spirometry, and severity is graded by the GOLD criteria. The diagnosis is made by an FEV_1/FVC ratio less than 70% predicted, and severity is determined based on degree of limitation in FEV_1.
    Initial treatments include use of an inhaled long-acting beta-agonist (LABA; e.g., salmeterol) or long-acting anticholinergic (e.g., tiotropium). Inhaled corticosteroids are sometimes used in more severe cases or with peripheral eosinophilia. Chronically hypoxic patients with ambulatory oxygen saturations less than 88% or arterial PaO_2 measurements less than 55 may be prescribed home oxygen therapy. Smoking cessation, of course, should be recommended and can significantly slow the progression of the disease. Routine influenza and pneumonia vaccines should be administered.

5. **What do you need to think of if you have a young patient with COPD?**
If you have a patient younger than 45 years with minimal smoke exposure, think of alpha$_1$-antitrypsin deficiency.

6. **What are the treatment goals for chronic stable COPD? What are the treatment options?**
The main treatment goals for stable COPD are symptom relief, improved exercise tolerance, prevention of disease progression, prevention of exacerbations, and reduced mortality. The general medication classes used to treat COPD are short-acting beta$_2$-agonists (e.g., albuterol), long-acting beta$_2$-agonists (e.g., salmeterol, formoterol), short-acting anticholinergics (e.g., ipratropium), long-acting anticholinergics (e.g., tiotropium), and inhaled corticosteroids (e.g., beclomethasone, fluticasone, budesonide). The selective phosphodiesterase-4 inhibitor roflumilast can be used in selected patients. Oxygen can be given to patients who are chronically hypoxemic. Do not forget to provide influenza and pneumococcal vaccinations for all patients with COPD.

7. **What is a COPD exacerbation? How is it treated?**
A COPD exacerbation is an acute event characterized by worsening of respiratory symptoms beyond the normal day-to-day variations in a patient with COPD. It is most commonly caused by a viral infection of the upper respiratory tract. A chest x-ray is usually ordered to assess other contributing factors (e.g., pneumonia). The decision to hospitalize is based on the patient's overall status. Treatment includes a short-acting inhaled beta$_2$-agonist (albuterol) with a short-acting inhaled anticholinergic drug (ipratropium). Patients should also be given systemic steroids, typically prednisone 40 mg daily for 5 days. Antibiotics are indicated for patients with increased dyspnea, sputum volume, and sputum purulence, as well as those who have a need for mechanical ventilation. Oxygen is provided as needed.

8. **Describe the difference between obstructive and restrictive pulmonary disease on PFT.**
In COPD, the functional expiratory volume in 1 second divided by the total forced vital capacity (FEV_1/FVC) is less than normal (<0.7). In restrictive lung disease (classically fibrotic lung disease, chest wall deformities, neuromuscular disease, obesity), FEV_1/FVC is often normal or increased. FEV_1 may be equal in both conditions, but the ratio of FEV_1/FVC is always different.

9. **How do you recognize and treat asthma?**
Watch for chronic wheezing in allergic (atopic) children with a family history of asthma, allergies, or eczema. In the acute setting, treat with beta$_2$ agonists. Use steroids if the attack is severe or does not respond to beta$_2$-agonists. Inhaled glucocorticoids (preferred agent), leukotriene modifiers (zafirlukast, montelukast, zileuton), long-acting beta-agonists, omalizumab, and cromolyn sodium are prophylactic agents and are not used for acute attacks. Phosphodiesterase inhibitors (theophylline, aminophylline) are older agents that are now used infrequently. Do *not* prescribe beta-blockers for asthmatics or patients with COPD; they block the beta$_2$-receptors that are needed to open the airways.

10. **What is the concern with the use of LABAs in the treatment of asthma?**
The US Food and Drug Administration has recommended that LABAs not be used as solo agents in the treatment of asthma in children or adults due to an increased risk of death. The advisory recommends that LABAs not be used alone as initial therapy for asthma of any severity, that they not be added when asthma control is actively deteriorating, that they only be used long term in patients whose asthma cannot be adequately controlled with other asthma controller medications, and that the LABA be discontinued, if possible, once asthma control is achieved.

11. **What should you think if a patient with acute asthma stops hyperventilating or has a normal carbon dioxide (CO_2) level?**
Beware the asthmatic who is no longer hyperventilating or whose CO_2 is normal or rising. The patient should be hyperventilating, which causes low CO_2. If the patient seems calm or sleepy, do *not* assume that the patient is okay. Such patients are probably crashing; they need an immediate arterial blood gas (ABG) analysis and possible intubation. Fatigue alone is sufficient reason to intubate. Remember also that any patient with COPD may normally live with a higher CO_2 and lower oxygen (O_2) level. Treat the patient, not the lab value. If the patient is asymptomatic and talking to you, the lab value should not cause panic.

12. **When should you intubate?**
As a rough rule of thumb, think about intubation in any patient whose CO_2 is greater than 50 mm Hg or whose O_2 is less than 50 mm Hg, especially if the pH in either situation is less than 7.30 while the patient is breathing

room air. Usually, unless the patient is crashing rapidly, a trial of oxygen by nasal cannula, face mask, or BiPAP (biphasic positive airway pressure) is given first. If it does not work or if the patient becomes too tired (use of accessory muscles is a good clue to the work of breathing), intubate. Clinical correlation is always required; patients with chronic lung disease may be asymptomatic at lab value levels that seem to defy reason. Alternatively, lab values may look great, but if the patient is becoming tired from increased work of breathing or is significantly altered (e.g., Glasgow Coma Scale <8), intubation may be needed.

PNEUMOCONIOSIS/FIBROSING OR RESTRICTIVE PULMONARY DISORDERS

1. **What is interstitial lung disease (ILD)?**
   ILD refers to a broad group of restrictive lung diseases with decreased diffusing capacity (DLCO) and elevated alveolar-arterial gradient in addition to reduced lung volumes (FVC and TLC). Many patterns exist on computed tomography (CT) of the chest, including honeycombing, ground glass, and mosaicism. Etiologies include pneumoconiosis/inhalational exposures, connective tissue diseases (CTD), sarcoidosis, hypersensitivity pneumonitis, and drug toxicities. Immunosuppression may be considered for patients with CTD-ILD. Similar to patients with COPD, chronic home oxygen therapy should be considered if patients have ambulatory oxygen saturations less than 88% or ABG PaO_2 measurements less than 55. Depending on age, comorbidities, and timeline of disease progression, patients with ILD should be considered for lung transplantation. Step 3 questions will center around clinical scenarios:
   - Asbestosis: prior occupational history will include some level of construction, usually with shipyards or plumbing. Patients may have pleural plaques and are at increased risk of bronchogenic carcinoma (more so than mesothelioma).
   - Berylliosis: classically in aerospace industry exposures.
   - Coal miner lung: from coal dust exposure. May have concomitant rheumatoid arthritis in Caplan syndrome.
   - Silicosis: from sandblasting exposures. Silica has an association with increased susceptibility to *Mycobacterium tuberculosis* from disruption of macrophages.
   - CTD-ILD: CTDs include rheumatoid arthritis, systemic lupus erythematosus, Sjögren syndrome, systemic sclerosis, mixed CTD, and myositides. Look out for physical exam hints (digital fissures/ulcerations/ashes, arthropathies, Raynaud phenomenon) and autoimmune serologies.
   - Sarcoidosis: classically black female with enlarged lymph nodes with noncaseating granulomas and bilateral hilar adenopathy on chest radiograph.
   - Hypersensitivity pneumonitis: look broadly for exposures to molds (farmer's lung) and birds (Bird fancier's lung).
   - Drug toxicities: look for use of amiodarone, methotrexate, bleomycin, and nitrofurantoin

2. **What symptoms do patients with ILD exhibit?**
   Look for progressive dyspnea with exertion, a persistent nonproductive cough, a history of appropriate occupational exposure (e.g., dust, chemicals), a history of CTD, an abnormal chest x-ray, and/or lung function abnormalities on spirometry. On examination, look for pulmonary crackles and clubbing of the digits.

3. **How do you evaluate suspected ILD?**
   The workup is quite involved because of all the possible causes of pulmonary fibrosis. Most patients should have a complete blood count (CBC), a chemistry panel, liver function tests, creatine kinase, urinalysis, chest x-ray and high-resolution CT of the chest, PFTs, and bronchoalveolar lavage. Other typical laboratory tests include rheumatoid factor, antibodies against cyclic citrullinated peptide, antinuclear antibody, antisynthetase antibody, aldolase, scleroderma antibodies, and Sjögren antibodies.

4. **What is sarcoidosis? What symptoms do patients exhibit?**
   Sarcoidosis is a multisystem granulomatous disorder of unknown cause. Affected individuals exhibit bilateral hilar lymphadenopathy, pulmonary reticular opacities, and skin, joint, and/or eye lesions. Sarcoidosis is three to four times more common in black populations and typically affects young adults. In approximately half of cases it is detected in asymptomatic patients because of incidental radiographic abnormalities. In symptomatic patients, look for fever, cough, malaise, dyspnea, chest pain, weight loss, and arthritis. The features of sarcoidosis can be remembered by the mnemonic GRUELING: **g**ranulomas, **r**heumatoid arthritis, **u**veitis, **e**rythema nodosum, **l**ymphadenitis, **i**nterstitial fibrosis, **n**egative purified protein derivative (PPD), **g**ammaglobulinemia. Look for bilateral hilar lymphadenopathy and/or infiltrates on chest x-ray. Hypercalcemia is common. PFTs reveal a restrictive or mixed restrictive-obstructive pattern.

5. **How is the diagnosis of sarcoidosis made?**
   Sarcoidosis is a diagnosis of exclusion. Evaluate for other causes such as lymphoma, tuberculosis, human immunodeficiency virus (HIV), fungal infection, and idiopathic pulmonary fibrosis. Do a complete physical examination and order a chest x-ray, PFTs, CBC, serum chemistries, including calcium, serum angiotensin-converting enzyme (ACE) level (classically elevated), urinalysis, electrocardiogram (ECG), PPD, and ophthalmologic evaluation. PFTs typically show a restrictive pattern. Diagnosis is made on the basis of a tissue biopsy revealing noncaseating granulomas without organisms.

6. **How is sarcoidosis treated?**
Most cases of sarcoidosis do not require treatment because patients are often asymptomatic and nonprogressive and some experience spontaneous remission. Treat symptomatic patients with prednisone.

7. **What is pneumoconiosis?**
Pneumoconiosis is an interstitial lung disease that results from dust inhalation and is almost always occupational. The main types of pneumoconiosis are coal worker's pneumoconiosis, asbestosis, and silicosis. Look for a patient with chronic shortness of breath, the right occupational exposure, a restrictive pattern on PFTs, and a chest x-ray revealing patchy, subpleural, bibasilar interstitial infiltrates or honeycombing.

8. **What is asbestosis? What are the symptoms? With what malignancy is asbestos exposure associated?**
Asbestosis is pneumoconiosis caused by inhalation of asbestos fibers that results in a slowly progressive pulmonary fibrosis. There is usually a latency period of 20 to 30 years between exposure and the development of symptoms, most commonly dyspnea with exertion. There is usually no cough, wheezing, or sputum production. Asbestos exposure is associated with an increased risk of mesothelioma, which is discussed in more detail later in this chapter.

9. **How is asbestosis diagnosed? What is the treatment?**
Asbestosis is a clinical diagnosis based on a history of exposure, certain findings on high-resolution chest CT, the presence of interstitial fibrosis, and the absence of other causes of parenchymal lung disease. There is no specific treatment, but supportive measures should be instituted. These include avoidance of further exposure to asbestos, smoking cessation, pneumococcal and influenza vaccines, and oxygen supplementation if needed.

RESPIRATORY FAILURE AND PULMONARY VASCULAR DISEASE

1. **What is pulmonary hypertension (PHTN)? How is it classified and treated?**
PHTN is defined as an elevated mean pulmonary arterial pressure ($\geq$20 mm Hg) as assessed on right heart catheterization. PHTN represents increased stress on the right ventricle, leading to dysfunction and potential right ventricular failure. The World Health Organization (WHO) classifies PHTN into five groups, which assists with understanding diagnostic workup and treatment.

Who Classification	Workup	Treatment
Group I: Pulmonary arterial hypertension	History of intravenous drug use (methamphetamine), connective tissue disease evaluation, human immunodeficiency virus	Prostacyclins (epoprostenol); endothelin receptor antagonists (macitentan, bosentan); phosphodiesterase-5 inhibitors (sildenafil, tadalafil)
Group 2: PHTN from left-sided heart disease	Elevated pulmonary capillary wedge pressure on right heart catheterization, transthoracic echo	Optimize heart failure medications; diuresis
Group 3: PHTN from chronic hypoxemic lung disease	Pulmonary function tests; high-resolution computed tomography	Oxygen supplementation; smoking cessation
Group 4: Chronic thromboembolic pulmonary hypertension	Ventilation-perfusion lung scanning	Anticoagulation; pulmonary thromboendarterectomy
Group 5: Unclear/miscellaneous	Evaluate for hematologic diseases as well as systemic and metabolic disorders	Treat the underlying disorder

2. **How do you recognize and treat acute respiratory distress syndrome (ARDS)?**
ARDS results from acute lung injury and causes noncardiogenic pulmonary edema, respiratory distress, and hypoxemia. Common risk factors are sepsis, pneumonia, aspiration of gastric contents, major trauma, pancreatitis, shock, near-drowning, drug overdose, major burns, and blood transfusions. Look for ARDS to develop within 24 to 48 hours of the initial insult. The classic patient has mottled/cyanotic skin, intercostal retractions, rales or rhonchi, and no improvement of hypoxia with oxygen administration. Radiographs show pulmonary edema with a normal cardiac silhouette (no cardiomegaly). Treat with intubation, mechanical ventilation with low tidal volumes (6–8 cc/kg of ideal body weight), and positive end-expiratory pressure, while addressing the underlying cause (if possible). Patients with worsening hypoxemia despite this may be paralyzed with cisatracurium and placed prone, with conservative fluid management to avoid volume overload as an additional contributor to hypoxemia.

3. **What is the most common cause of fever in the first 24 hours after surgery?**
   Atelectasis. Prevent and treat atelectasis with early ambulation, chest physiotherapy/percussion, incentive spirometry, and proper pain control. Too much pain or excessive narcotic administration (both can decrease respiratory effort) increases the risk of atelectasis.

4. **In what clinical settings might pulmonary embolus (PE) occur?**
   PE commonly follows deep vein thrombosis, obstetric delivery (amniotic fluid embolus), or long-bone fractures (fat emboli). The classic patient in an exam vignette recently went on a long car ride, took a long airplane flight, or has been immobilized. Symptoms include sudden-onset tachypnea, dyspnea, chest pain, hemoptysis (if a lung infarct has occurred), hypotension, syncope, or death in severe cases. In rare instances, the chest radiograph or CT scan shows a wedge-shaped defect due to pulmonary infarct, and the ECG shows evidence of right-heart strain such as the classic S1Q3T3 of a prominent S wave in lead 1 and both a Q wave and inverted T wave in lead 3.

5. **How is PE diagnosed?**
   Use a CT pulmonary angiogram or ventilation/perfusion (V/Q) scan to evaluate for PE. If either test is positive, PE is diagnosed, and treatment is started. If the test is indeterminate, a conventional pulmonary angiogram is used to clinch the diagnosis. Conventional pulmonary angiography is the gold standard, but it is invasive and carries substantial risks. If a CT angiogram or V/Q scan is negative, it is highly unlikely that the patient has a significant PE, thus no treatment is needed. In the setting of a low-probability V/Q scan and high clinical suspicion, a CT angiogram or conventional pulmonary angiogram is needed.

6. **How is PE managed?**
   Oxygenation is essential to PE management. Anticoagulants (e.g., low-molecular-weight heparin or intravenous unfractionated heparin) are also critical in PE management to prevent further clots and emboli. The patient should be gradually switched to oral warfarin, which must be continued for at least 3 to 6 months. In patients with recurrent clots while on anticoagulation or patient with contraindications to anticoagulation, an inferior vena cava filter (e.g., Greenfield filter) should be placed. In patients with massive PE, embolectomy (surgical or catheter embolectomy) or pharmacologic thrombolysis (e.g., giving t-PA) may be attempted.

UPPER RESPIRATORY TRACT CONDITIONS

1. **What are the three common causes of rhinitis?**
   Viral, allergic, and bacterial.

2. **How do you recognize and treat viral rhinitis?**
   Viral rhinitis (the common cold) may be due to rhinovirus (the most common cause), influenza, parainfluenza, coxsackievirus, adenovirus, respiratory syncytial virus (RSV), coronavirus, or echovirus. Treatment is symptomatic. Vasoconstrictors such as phenylephrine can be used for short-term symptomatic relief, but they may cause rebound congestion when discontinued.

3. **How do you recognize and treat allergic rhinitis?**
   Allergic rhinitis (hay fever) is associated with seasonal flare-ups, boggy and bluish turbinates, onset before 20 years of age, nasal polyps, sneezing, pruritus, conjunctivitis, wheezing or asthma, eczema, positive family history, eosinophils in nasal mucus, and elevated serum immunoglobulin E. Skin tests may identify an allergen. Treat with avoidance of known antigens (e.g., pollen). Antihistamines, nasal steroids, and/or cromolyn may be used for more severe symptoms. Desensitization is also an option.

4. **What causes bacterial rhinitis? How is it treated?**
   Group A streptococci, pneumococci, or staphylococci are the most common culprits. Bacterial rhinitis is not usually due to infection of the nasal mucosa alone but is more commonly due to infection of an adjacent compartment complicated by inflammation of the nasal mucosa, hence the term *bacterial rhinosinusitis*. Look for coexisting sore throat, lymphadenopathy, fever, and tonsillar exudate. Do streptococcal throat cultures, and treat with antibiotics, if appropriate.

5. **By what age are the frontal sinuses well developed in children?**
   The frontal sinuses may not be well developed until the age of 10 years.

6. **How is a deviated nasal septum treated in patients with recurrent bacterial sinusitis?**
   Surgical correction.

7. **What causes nosebleeds?**
   The most common cause of nosebleed is trauma; for example, nose-picking is a common cause in children. Environmental changes also commonly cause nosebleeds. Watch out for the following causes:
   - Local tumor (nasopharyngeal angiofibroma; seen in adolescent boys with no history of trauma or blood dyscrasia; signs include recurrent nosebleeds and/or obstruction)

- Leukemia (from pancytopenia; typically in children with associated fever and anemia)
- Other causes of thrombocytopenia (e.g., idiopathic thrombocytopenic purpura, hemolytic uremic syndrome)

8. **How do you recognize a nasal fracture? What complication may result?**
A nasal fracture can be seen on radiographs or CT scan. Watch for a septal hematoma, which must be surgically removed to prevent pressure-induced septal necrosis.

9. **How does streptococcal pharyngitis present? How do you diagnosis and treat it?**
Look for sore throat with fever, tonsillar exudate, enlarged tender cervical nodes, and leukocytosis. A positive streptococcal throat culture confirms the diagnosis. Elevated titers of antistreptolysin O (ASO) and anti-DNase antibody can be used for a retrospective diagnosis in patients with rheumatic fever or postinfectious glomerulonephritis. Treat streptococcal pharyngitis with penicillin, amoxicillin, cephalosporin, macrolide, or clindamycin to avoid rheumatic fever and scarlet fever.

10. **What are the symptoms of peritonsillar abscess (PTA)?**
PTA typically has symptoms of severe sore throat, fever, and a muffled voice. Drooling may be present, and patients often have trismus. On examination, look for a swollen and fluctuant tonsil with deviation of the uvula to the opposite side.

11. **How is PTA evaluated and treated?**
PTA is a clinical diagnosis by history and physical examination. No specific testing may be required. Bedside ultrasound can confirm the presence of a PTA, and definitive treatment is needle aspiration or incision and drainage. PTAs are usually polymicrobial, so ampicillin-sulbactam or clindamycin are usually the preferred agents. In otherwise healthy patients, once a PTA is drained, the patient can be discharged on oral antibiotics.
    In cases that are not as straightforward, CT of the neck with IV contrast may be required to confirm the diagnosis and/or establish the presence of other diagnoses (e.g., retropharyngeal abscess). Throat swabs for rapid group A streptococcal (GAS) antigen or a throat culture can confirm the presence of GAS but will not rule in or out PTA.

NEOPLASMS

1. **What should you do if a patient has a solitary pulmonary nodule on chest radiograph?**
The first step is to compare the current film with old films (if available). If the lesion has not changed in more than 2 to 3 years, it is very likely to be benign. A nodule that has increased in size on serial imaging should be biopsied or excised. CT scans are used to evaluate and follow a solitary pulmonary nodule. A nodule that has a low probability of being malignant can be followed with serial CT scans. A positron emission tomography scan is used to evaluate intermediate probability nodules. A nodule that has a high probability of being malignant should be excised.

2. **What classic clues on the Step 3 exam point to the cause of a solitary pulmonary nodule?**
    - Immigrant: think of tuberculosis; do a PPD skin test or interferon gamma release assay (IGRA; QuantiFERON) if suspicion is low to moderate. If there is concern that the patient has active pulmonary tuberculosis, the patient should be placed on isolation with acid-fast bacilli smears and *M. tuberculosis* polymerase chain reaction tests, as a negative IGRA *does not* rule out active tuberculosis.
    - Southwest US exposure: think of *Coccidioides immitis*.
    - Cave explorer, exposure to bird droppings or Ohio/Mississippi river valleys (Midwest): think of histoplasmosis.
    - Smoker over the age of 50: think of lung cancer; order bronchoscopy if central, or biopsy if peripheral.
    - Person under 40 with none of the previous: think of hamartoma.

3. **What clinical vignette should make you suspect lung cancer?**
The classic clue is a change in the chronic cough of a smoker. The greater the pack-years of tobacco use, the more suspicious you should be. Patients may also present with hemoptysis, pneumonia, or weight loss. The chest radiograph may show a mass or pleural effusion. Perform thoracentesis to examine for malignant cells. A less common presentation is recurrent or unresolving pneumonia in the same lung lobe, which would be suspicious for a postobstructive bronchogenic carcinoma.

4. **How do you diagnose and treat lung cancer?**
As with all cancers, you need a tissue biopsy (e.g., via bronchoscopy, CT-guided biopsy, open lung biopsy) to confirm malignancy and to define the histologic type. Non–small cell lung cancer may be treated with surgery if the cancer remains within the lung parenchyma (i.e., without involvement of the opposite lung, pleura, chest wall, spine, or mediastinal structures). Small cell lung cancer is inoperable and is treated with chemotherapy. Non–small cell lung cancer and extensive non–small cell lung cancer are treated with chemotherapy with or without radiation. Usually a platinum-containing chemotherapy regimen (e.g., cisplatin) is used, and bevacizumab can be added for non–small cell lung cancer.

5. **What consequences can result from an apical (Pancoast) lung cancer?**
Horner syndrome: from invasion of the cervical sympathetic chain. Look for unilateral ptosis, miosis, and anhidrosis (no sweating).

Superior vena cava syndrome: due to compression of superior vena cava with impaired venous drainage. Look for edema and plethora (redness) of the neck and face and central nervous system symptoms (headache, visual symptoms, and altered mental status).

Unilateral diaphragm paralysis: from phrenic nerve involvement (apical tumor not required), which will result in an elevated hemidiaphragm on chest x-ray.

Hoarseness: from recurrent laryngeal nerve involvement (apical tumor not required).

6. **What is a paraneoplastic syndrome? What are the commonly tested paraneoplastic syndromes of lung cancer?**

A paraneoplastic syndrome is a condition caused by a malignancy but not due directly to destruction or invasion by the tumor. Classic examples in lung cancer include:

Cushing syndrome: from production of adrenocorticotropic hormone (histologic type: small cell carcinoma).

Syndrome of inappropriate antidiuretic hormone secretion (SIADH): from production of antidiuretic hormone (histologic type: small cell carcinoma).

Hypercalcemia: from production of parathyroid-like hormone (histologic type: squamous cell carcinoma).

Lambert-Eaton syndrome: myasthenia gravis–like disease from lung cancer that spares the ocular muscles. The muscles become stronger with repetitive stimulation, which is the opposite of myasthenia gravis (histologic type: small cell carcinoma).

7. **What are the symptoms of mesothelioma? What is the typical x-ray finding? How is mesothelioma diagnosed?**

Look for gradual-onset chest pain, dyspnea, cough, fatigue, and weight loss, particularly in a patient with a history of asbestos exposure. A chest x-ray typically reveals a unilateral pleural abnormality with a large unilateral pleural effusion. Perform thoracentesis and send the fluid for cytology. Pleural biopsy is usually indicated to establish a tissue diagnosis.

8. **What two points do you need to know about nasopharyngeal cancer?**

It usually is seen in Asians (particularly those who are from Asia), and it is associated with **Epstein-Barr virus.**

9. **What cancers are more likely in smokers?**

Smoking increases the risk of cancers of the lung (smoking causes 85%–90% of cases); oral cavity (90% of cases); esophagus (70%–80% of cases); larynx, pharynx, bladder (30%–50% of cases); kidney (20%–30%); pancreas (20%–25%); cervix, stomach, colon, and rectum.

LUNG INFECTIONS

1. **Cover the right-hand column, then describe the preferred treatment for tuberculosis based on the clinical scenario.**

Clinical Setting/Findings	*Treatment*
Exposed adult with negative PPD skin test	None
Exposed child <5 yr old with negative PPD Treatment for PPD conversion (negative to positive), no active disease	Isoniazid (INH) for 3 mo, then repeat PPD INH for 9 mo
Active pulmonary disease/positive culture	INH/rifampin/pyrazinamide/ethambutol for 2 mo, then INH/rifampin for 4 mo in most patients

PPD, Purified protein derivative.

2. **Name some other important tuberculosis treatment issues.**

- Multidrug-resistant strains are an increasing problem and require four-drug therapy (pyrazinamide, isoniazid, ethambutol, and rifampin) in most circumstances.
- If the patient is nonadherent, directly observed therapy (someone watches the patient take medications every day) is recommended.
- Consider supplementation with vitamin B_6 (pyridoxine) for patients on isoniazid (INH), or watch for signs of deficiency, such as neuropathy, confusion, angular cheilitis, or a seborrheic dermatitis-like rash.
- Watch for liver dysfunction in patients on therapy. Patients should be advised to abstain from alcohol while on treatment and should have their transaminase levels monitored.

3. **How is pneumonia diagnosed?**

The diagnosis of pneumonia is usually based on clinical findings (fever, rales, or rhonchi) plus elevated white blood cell count and an abnormal chest radiograph consistent with pneumonia. Sputum and blood cultures may be obtained, preferably before empiric antibiotic therapy is begun.

4. What is the difference between typical and atypical pneumonia?

Typical pneumonia is usually caused by bacteria such as *Streptococcus pneumoniae* or *Staphylococcus aureus*, the most common causes of pneumonia. Atypical pneumonia may be caused by viral infection (e.g., influenza or adenovirus), *Mycoplasma*, *Chlamydia* spp., *Legionella*, *Moraxella*, or *Haemophilus*.

	Typical Pneumonia	*Atypical Pneumonia*
Prodrome	Short (<2 days)	Long (>3 days) (headache, malaise, body aches)
Fever	High (>102°F)	Low (<102°F)
Age	>40 yr	<40 yr
Chest radiograph	One distinct lobe involved	Diffuse or multilobe involvement
Bug	*Streptococcus pneumoniae*	Many (*Haemophilus, Mycoplasma, Chlamydia* spp.)
Antibiotic*	Ceftriaxone, broad spectrum	Macrolides (e.g., azithromycin), doxycycline, or certain fluoroquinolones (e.g., levofloxacin, moxifloxacin)

*Avoid the temptation to pull out the "bigger-gun" antibiotics (very wide spectrum, potent) unless the patient is crashing or unstable.

5. What are the classic clinical clues for the different causative bugs in pneumonia?

College student: *Mycoplasma* sp. (look for cold agglutinins) or *Chlamydia* sp.

Alcoholic: *Klebsiella* sp. ("currant jelly" sputum), *S. aureus,* other enteric bugs (aspiration)

Cystic fibrosis: *Pseudomonas* sp. or *S. aureus*

Immigrant: tuberculosis

COPD: *H. influenzae, Moraxella* sp.

Known tuberculosis with pulmonary cavitation: *Aspergillus* sp.

Silicosis (metal, granite, pottery workers): tuberculosis

Exposure to air conditioner or aerosolized water: *Legionella* sp.

HIV/acquired immunodeficiency syndrome (AIDS): *Pneumocystis jirovecii* or cytomegalovirus (CMV) (if you are shown koilocytosis and the patient is very immunosuppressed), although *S. pneumoniae* is still the most common cause of pneumonia in HIV-positive patients.

Exposure to bird droppings: *Chlamydia psittaci* or histoplasmosis

Child less than 1 year old: RSV

Child 2 to 5 years old: parainfluenza (croup)

6. What should you suspect if a child has recurrent pneumonias?

If the pneumonia always occurs in the same spot (especially the right middle and/or right lower lobe), it most likely is due to foreign body aspiration. Remember that a foreign body is most likely to go down the right mainstem bronchus. This diagnosis should be considered especially if the child has no other signs of immunodeficiency (e.g., other types of infections, symptoms of cystic fibrosis) before or during the episodes. If immunodeficiency is the cause of recurrent pneumonias, the child should have a history of chronic bilateral lung problems and other types of infection.

7. What is "round" pneumonia?

Pneumonia may appear round, typically in children, which causes it to simulate a mass. In such cases involving children, assume pneumonia and treat appropriately. A follow-up x-ray can be obtained to confirm resolution, which is not usually required in children, who almost never develop lung malignancies. In an adult, a round pneumonia should be viewed with suspicion (more likely to be a malignancy), and further workup with a CT scan is typically employed.

8. Why should you get a follow-up chest x-ray in all smokers over age 50 who develop pneumonia?

A follow-up chest x-ray is indicated in smokers over age 50 who develop pneumonia to make sure it clears after appropriate antibiotic treatment. If pneumonia does not clear by 4 to 6 weeks, suspect something other than bacterial pneumonia. The classic culprit is malignancy, specifically **bronchoalveolar carcinoma,** which is a subtype of adenocarcinoma. In addition, recurrent pneumonias in the same location in an adult may be due to an endobronchial mass, whether benign or malignant.

9. What is the most common cause of pneumonia? How does it classically present?

S. pneumoniae. Look for rapid onset of shaking chills after 1 to 2 days of upper respiratory infection symptoms (sore throat, runny nose, dry cough), followed by fever, pleurisy, and productive cough (yellowish-green or rust-colored from blood), especially in older adults. Chest radiograph shows lobar consolidation (Fig. 3.1), and the white blood cell count is high with a large percentage of neutrophils. Treat with a macrolide (e.g., azithromycin, clarithromycin), doxycycline, third-generation cephalosporin plus a macrolide or doxycycline, or a fluoroquinolone that provides atypical pathogen coverage (e.g., levofloxacin, moxifloxacin).

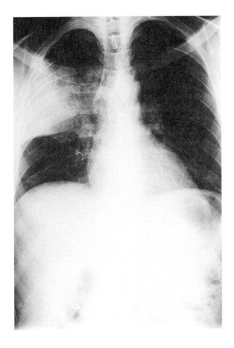

Fig. 3.1 Pneumococcal pneumonia with lobar consolidation. (From Mason RJ, Broaddus VC, Martin TR, et al. *Murray and Nadel's Textbook of Respiratory Medicine.* 5th ed. Philadelphia: Saunders; 2010 [fig. 32-1].)

10. **What is the best prevention against *S. pneumoniae*?**
    Vaccination. Give pneumococcal vaccine to all children as well as adult patients over 65 years old, asplenia (splenectomized patients, patients with sickle cell disease who have autosplenectomy, or splenic dysfunction), immunocompromised patients (HIV, malignancy, organ transplant), and all patients with chronic disease (e.g., diabetes, cardiac disease, asthma and other pulmonary disease, renal disease, liver disease, or tobacco use).

11. **How do you recognize and treat *H. influenzae* pneumonia?**
    H. influenzae is now uncommon in children due to vaccination, but it is still an important cause of pneumonia in the elderly and in those with underlying lung disease such as COPD. It often resembles pneumococcal pneumonia clinically, but look for gram-negative coccobacilli on sputum Gram stain. Treat with amoxicillin or a second- or third-generation cephalosporin.

12. **Describe the hallmarks of *S. aureus* pneumonia**
    S. aureus tends to cause hospital-acquired (nosocomial) pneumonia and pneumonia in patients with cystic fibrosis (along with *Pseudomonas* sp.), IV drug abusers, and patients with chronic granulomatous disease (look for recurrent lung abscesses). Empyema and lung abscesses are relatively common with *S. aureus* pneumonia. *S. aureus* pneumonia can be a complication of influenza.

13. **In what clinical situations do you tend to see gram-negative pneumonias?**
    Pseudomonas infection is classically associated with cystic fibrosis. *Klebsiella* infection is associated with people with alcohol use disorder and people who are homeless (watch for classic description of currant jelly sputum). Enteric gram-negative organisms (e.g., *Escherichia coli*) are associated with aspiration, neutropenia, and hospital-acquired pneumonia. These types of pneumonias often have a high mortality rate because of the types of patients affected and the severity of the pneumonia (abscesses are common). Treat empirically with an antipseudomonal penicillin (e.g., ticarcillin, piperacillin) with or without a beta-lactamase inhibitor (e.g., clavulanate, tazobactam). Alternatives include ceftazidime or ciprofloxacin.

14. **How do you recognize *Mycoplasma* pneumonia?**
    Mycoplasma infection is most common in adolescents and young adults (the classic patient is a college student or soldier who lives in a dormitory/barracks and has sick contacts). It is one of the atypical pneumonias because it presents differently from a typical pneumonia due to *S. pneumoniae*. For example, it has a long prodrome with gradual worsening of malaise, headaches, dry nonproductive cough, and sore throat; the fever tends to be low grade. Chest radiograph shows a patchy, diffuse bronchopneumonia and classically looks terrible, although the patient often does not feel that bad (which is why it is sometimes called "walking pneumonia"). Look for positive **cold-agglutinin antibody titers,** which may cause hemolysis or anemia. Atypical pneumonia is treated empirically with a macrolide antibiotic (azithromycin), doxycycline, or broad-spectrum fluoroquinolone (e.g., levofloxacin or moxifloxacin).

15. **What about chlamydial pneumonia?**

Chlamydia sp. is second only to *Mycoplasma* sp. as the cause of atypical pneumonia in adolescents and young adults. It presents similarly but has negative cold-agglutinin antibody titers. Treat with erythromycin in children under 8 years of age and either azithromycin or doxycycline in children over 8 years of age, adolescents, and adults.

16. **What kind of pneumonia should you suspect in a patient with alcohol use disorder?**

Aspiration pneumonia. Look for enteric organisms (anaerobes, *E. coli*, streptococci, staphylococci) as the cause. Think of *Klebsiella* spp. if the sputum resembles currant jelly or thick mucoid capsules are mentioned in culture reports.

17. **How do you recognize *P. jirovecii* pneumonia (PCP)?**

For the Step 3 exam, think of PCP first in any patient with HIV and pneumonia, even though community-acquired pneumonia is more common, even in patients with AIDS. Look for severe hypoxia with normal radiographs or diffuse, bilateral interstitial infiltrates (Fig. 3.2). Patients usually have a dry, nonproductive cough. PCP may be detected with silver stains (Wright-Giemsa, Giemsa, or methenamine silver) applied to induced sputum; if not, you can use bronchoscopy with bronchoalveolar lavage and brush biopsy to make the diagnosis. High levels of lactate dehydrogenase (LDH) are suspicious in the appropriate setting. PCP is now usually treated presumptively (typically with trimethoprim-sulfamethoxazole), with diagnostic testing reserved for those in whom the diagnosis is unclear or initial treatment fails. Corticosteroids are added in the treatment of suspected PCP in patients with (1) hypoxemia on pulse oximetry, (2) PaO_2 less than or equal to 70 mm Hg on room air, or (3) an alveolar-arterial gradient greater than or equal to 35 mm Hg for ABG.

18. **In what setting do you see PCP and CMV pneumonia?**

HIV-positive patients with CD4 counts less than 200/mm³ (AIDS) and other severely immunosuppressed patients (e.g., organ transplant recipients taking powerful immunosuppressants or patients on cancer chemotherapy) are susceptible to PCP. In patients with AIDS, PCP is the most common opportunistic pneumonia and may require bronchoalveolar lavage for diagnosis. PCP can be seen with silver stains and typically causes bilateral interstitial lung infiltrates. Chest x-ray may show a bat-wing appearance, which represents bilateral interstitial infiltrates. LDH may be elevated, and ABG may show an increased A-a gradient. Treat with trimethoprim-sulfamethoxazole plus corticosteroids. CMV pneumonia is characterized by intracellular inclusion bodies. Treat with ganciclovir or valganciclovir.

19. **What is the best time to treat PCP?**

Before it happens. PCP is acquired when the CD4 count is below 200/mm³. At that point you should institute PCP prophylaxis with trimethoprim-sulfamethoxazole. Alternatives include dapsone or atovaquone.

20. **What is a common cause of wheezing in children under age 2 years?**

Reactive airway disease due to viral infection, commonly RSV infection, which classically occurs in the winter and causes a fever. Asthma may also be the cause but is usually associated with a chronic history.

21. **What are the "big three" respiratory infections in patients younger than 5 years?**

Croup, epiglottitis, and RSV infection (bronchiolitis). These three diseases are high yield on the USMLE.

22. **How do you recognize croup (acute laryngotracheitis)? Describe the cause and treatment.**

The disease begins with symptoms of viral upper respiratory infection (e.g., rhinorrhea, cough, fever). Roughly 1 to 2 days later, patients develop a barking cough, hoarseness, and inspiratory stridor. The **steeple sign** (reflects subglottic narrowing of the trachea) (Fig. 3.3) is classic on a frontal radiograph of the chest or neck. Look for a child 1 to 2 years of

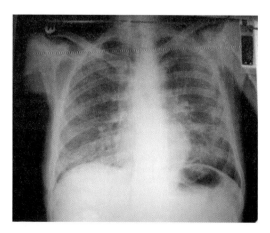

Fig. 3.2 Chest radiograph in a patient with *Pneumocystis* pneumonia. (From Kumar P. *Kumar & Clark's Cases in Clinical Medicine*. Philadelphia: Saunders Elsevier; 2013:325-381.)

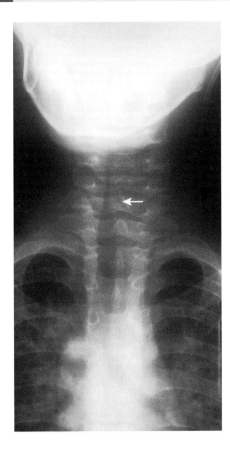

Fig. 3.3 Anteroposterior radiograph of the neck region of child with croup. Note the steeple sign *(white arrow)*. (From Wetmore RF. *Pediatric Otolaryngology: The Requisites in Pediatrics.* 1st ed. Philadelphia: Mosby; 2007 [fig. 11-1].)

age. Croup usually occurs in the fall or winter. Fifty to 75% of cases are due to infection with parainfluenza virus; the other common causative agent is influenza virus. Treat with dexamethasone, racemic epinephrine, and humidified oxygen.

23. **How do you recognize epiglottitis? Describe the cause and treatment.**
    Epiglottitis usually occurs in children 2 to 5 years old. The main cause is *H. influenzae* type b, thus widespread vaccination has significantly reduced the incidence of this condition. *S. aureus, S. pyogenes*, and *S. pneumoniae* are other potential causes. Look for little or no prodrome, with rapid progression to high fever, toxic appearance, drooling, and respiratory distress with no coughing (the "three Ds"—drooling, dysphagia, and distress) in unvaccinated children less than 2 to 5 years old. The **thumb sign** (describes a swollen, enlarged epiglottis) (Fig. 3.4) is classic on lateral radiographs of the neck. Do not examine the throat or irritate the child in any way. You may precipitate airway obstruction. When a case of epiglottitis is diagnosed, the first step is to be prepared to establish an airway (intubation and, if needed, tracheostomy). Treat with a combination of oxacillin or cefazolin or clindamycin or vancomycin plus cefotaxime or ceftriaxone.

24. **Describe the classic clinical vignette for bronchiolitis. What is the cause? How is it treated?**
    Bronchiolitis generally affects children aged 0 to 18 months and usually occurs in the fall or winter. More than 75% of cases are caused by RSV; other causes are parainfluenza and influenza viruses. Patients first develop symptoms of viral upper respiratory infection, followed 1 to 2 days later by rapid respirations, intercostal retractions, and expiratory wheezing. The child may have crackles on auscultation of the chest. Diffuse hyperinflation of the lungs is classic on chest radiograph; look for flattened diaphragms. Treat supportively (e.g., oxygen, mist tent, bronchodilators, IV fluids).

25. **What "old-school" pediatric infection causes pseudomembranes and myocarditis? What about whooping cough?**
    Diphtheria (*Corynebacterium diphtheriae*) and pertussis (*Bordetella pertussis*), respectively. Diphtheria is quite uncommon in the United States because of mandatory vaccination. Pertussis was uncommon, but the incidence has

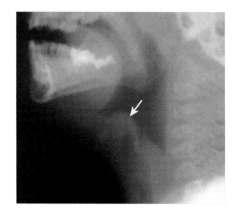

Fig. 3.4 Lateral neck radiograph demonstrating epiglottis with the thumb sign. (From Zaoutis LB, Chiang VW. *Comprehensive Pediatric Hospital Medicine.* 1st ed. Philadelphia: Mosby; 2007 [fig. 66-3].)

been increasing significantly over the past 20 years. If a child is unimmunized, don't forget these two entities. Diphtheria causes grayish pseudomembranes (necrotic epithelium and inflammatory exudate) on the pharynx, tonsils, and uvula as well as myocarditis. Pertussis is associated with severe paroxysmal coughing and a high-pitched whooping inspiratory noise (traditionally called "whooping cough"), particularly in children and especially those under 1 year of age. Treat diphtheria with antitoxin and either penicillin or erythromycin. Treat pertussis with azithromycin or erythromycin.

TRAUMA AND TOXIC EFFECTS

1. **How are patients managed after a near-drowning episode?**
   Some, but not all, physicians believe that drowning in fresh water is worse than saltwater because aspiring fresh water may cause hypervolemia, electrolyte disturbances, and hemolysis. After a near-drowning episode, unconscious patients should be intubated, whereas conscious patients should have their ABG monitored due to its hypotonicity. Death due to a near-drowning episode is typically due to hypoxia and/or cardiac arrest. Remember to look for head or neck trauma and consider potential reasons why the near-drowning episode occurred (e.g., intoxication, seizure, syncope, suicide attempt).

2. **Which six thoracic injuries can be rapidly fatal?**
   1. Airway obstruction
   2. Open pneumothorax
   3. Tension pneumothorax
   4. Cardiac tamponade
   5. Massive hemothorax
   6. Flail chest
   You may be asked to recognize and/or treat any of these six conditions on the USMLE.

3. **How do you recognize and treat airway obstruction?**
   Patients with airway obstruction have no audible breath sounds, cannot answer questions even if awake, and may be gurgling. Treat with intubation. If intubation fails, do a cricothyroidotomy (or a tracheostomy in the operating room if time allows).

4. **How do you recognize and treat an open pneumothorax?**
   An open pneumothorax presents with an open defect in the chest wall and decreased or absent breath sounds on the affected side. This condition causes poor ventilation and oxygenation. Treat with intubation, positive pressure ventilation, and closure of the defect in the chest wall. To close the defect, use gauze and tape it on three sides only. This approach allows excessive pressure to escape so that you do not convert an open pneumothorax into a tension pneumothorax.

5. **How do you recognize and treat a tension pneumothorax?**
   A tension pneumothorax may occur after blunt or penetrating trauma to the chest. Air forced into the pleural space cannot escape and collapses the affected lung, and then shifts the mediastinum and trachea to the opposite side of the chest (Fig. 3.5). Findings include absent breath sounds on the affected side and a hypertympanic percussion sound. Hypotension and/or distended neck veins may result from impaired cardiac filling. Treat with needle thoracostomy followed by insertion of a chest tube.

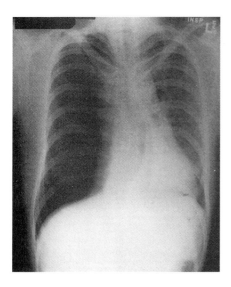

Fig. 3.5 Radiograph of tension pneumothorax. The right hemithorax is dark (lucent) because the mediastinum has shifted to the left. (From Marx JA. *Rosen's Emergency Medicine.* 7th ed. Philadelphia: Mosby; 2009 [fig. 75-3].)

6. **Define massive hemothorax. How is it diagnosed and treated?**

   Massive hemothorax is defined as a loss of more than 1 L of blood into the thoracic cavity. Patients have decreased (not absent) breath sounds in the affected area, dull note on percussion, hypotension, collapsed neck veins (from blood leaving the vascular tree), and tachycardia. Placement of a chest tube allows the blood to come out. Give intravenous fluids and/or blood before you place the chest tube if the diagnosis is known in advance. If the bleeding stops after the initial outflow, order a chest radiograph or CT scan to check for remaining blood or pathology. If blood is left behind, the patient is at risk for forming empyema. Treat supportively. If the bleeding does not stop, emergent thoracotomy is required.

7. **How do you recognize and treat flail chest?**

   Flail chest occurs when several adjacent ribs are broken in multiple places, causing the affected part of the chest wall to move paradoxically during respiration (inward during inspiration, outward during expiration). Almost all patients have an associated pulmonary contusion, which, combined with pain, may make respiration inadequate. When you are in doubt or the patient is not doing well, intubate and give positive pressure ventilation. The patient should also be evaluated for aortic damage.

8. **What clues suggest a diagnosis of diaphragmatic rupture? How is it treated?**

   Diaphragm rupture usually occurs after blunt trauma and on the left side (because the liver protects the right side of the diaphragm). You may hear bowel sounds when listening to the chest or see bowel that has herniated into the chest on the chest radiograph. Treatment is surgical repair of the diaphragm.

9. **How should a choking victim be managed?**

   Always leave choking patients alone if they are speaking, coughing, or breathing. If they stop doing all of these, perform the Heimlich maneuver.

10. **What should you do if a patient has a pleural effusion?**

    If you do not know the cause of the effusion (Fig. 3.6), consider thoracocentesis to examine the fluid in an attempt to determine its etiology. Common tests ordered on pleural fluid include Gram stain, culture and sensitivity testing (including tuberculosis culture), cell count with differential, glucose (low with infection), protein (high with infection), cytology (to look for malignancy), amylase (if pancreatitis is a suspected cause of effusion), triglycerides (if a chylous effusion is suspected), albumin, and LDH (the last two tests help to determine whether the fluid is an exudate or transudate by using Light criteria).

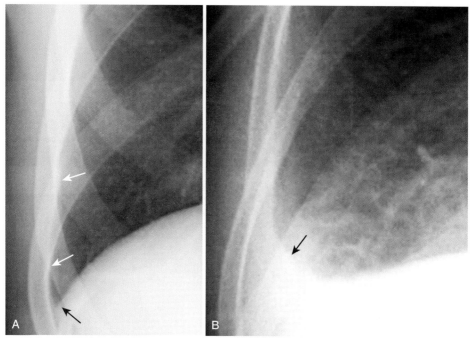

Fig. 3.6 Normal and blunted right lateral costophrenic sulcus. (A) The hemidiaphragm usually makes a sharp and acute angle as it meets the lateral chest wall on the frontal projection to produce the lateral costophrenic sulcus *(black arrow)*. Notice how aerated lung normally extends to the inner margin of each of the ribs *(white arrows)*. (B) When an effusion reaches about 300 mL in volume, the lateral costophrenic sulcus loses its acute angulation and becomes blunted *(black arrow)*. (From Herring W. *Learning Radiology: Recognizing the Basics*. Philadelphia: Elsevier; 2020:60-69 [fig. 8.5].)

CHAPTER 4

CARDIOVASCULAR DISORDERS

1. **What is the most common cause of syncope? What other conditions should you consider?**
   Vasovagal syncope is the most common cause and is classically seen after stress or fear. Arrhythmias and ortho-static hypotension are also common. Always remember to consider hypoglycemia as a cause. The other main categories to worry about include:
   1. **Cardiac problems** (arrhythmias, hypertrophic cardiomyopathy [HCM], valvular disease, tamponade). Always check an electrocardiogram (ECG). Further testing with echocardiography or treadmill stress testing can be performed based on the ECG findings and degree of suspicion for cardiac etiology for syncope.
   2. **Neurologic disorders** (e.g., seizures, migraine headache, brain tumor, stroke). Consider an electroencephalo-gram or computed tomography (CT)/magnetic resonance imaging (MRI) scan if history suggests seizures or intracranial lesion.
   3. **Vascular disease** (consider transient ischemic attacks [TIAs] or carotid stenosis, which can be ruled out with carotid artery ultrasound/duplex scanning, though this is not a common cause of syncope).
   4. **Medication effects** (e.g., anticholinergic agents, beta-blockers, narcotics, vasodilators, alpha-agonists, antipsychotics).
   5. **Sleep disturbances** (e.g., narcolepsy and cataplexy).
      As many as half of patients have syncope of unknown cause after a standard diagnostic evaluation.

HYPOTENSION

1. **What class of antihypertensive agents is best known for severe, first-dose orthostatic hypotension?**
   $Alpha_1$-antagonists such as terazosin.

2. **Define shock.**
   Shock is a state of life-threatening circulatory insufficiency in which blood flow to and perfusion of peripheral tis-sues are inadequate to sustain proper organ or cellular function. Initial effects of shock are reversible, but as it progresses both in duration and severity, rapid organ failure and death may result. Although they are not explicitly mentioned in a rigid definition of shock, for USMLE purposes you may consider hypotension with either oliguria or anuria to be associated findings. Reflex tachycardia is also often present.

3. **List the four primary classifications of shock.**
   The four primary classifications of shock are:
   1. Distributive
   2. Hypovolemic
   3. Cardiogenic
   4. Obstructive

4. **Which four hemodynamic factors are used to distinguish the four types of shock from one another?**
   Cardiac output (CO), preload, afterload, and tissue perfusion are used to distinguish the four types of shock from one another.

5. **Describe how cardiac output, preload, afterload, and tissue perfusion are measured or estimated in a clinical setting.**
   In a clinical setting CO is measured by cardiac index, preload is measured by pulmonary capillary wedge pressure (PCWP), afterload is measured by systemic vascular resistance (SVR), and tissue perfusion is estimated by sys-temic venous oxygen saturation (SVO_2).

6. **What are the normal physiologic ranges for CO, PCWP, SVR, and SVO_2 in a healthy recumbent adult?**
   - **CO**: 2.8 to 4.2 $L/min/m^2$
   - **PCWP**: 9 to 23 mm Hg
   - **SVR**: 900 to 1400 dyn $\times$ s/cm^5 or 11.3 to 17.5 Wood units
   - **SVO_2**: approximately 65%

7. List the characteristic hemodynamic changes that occur in each type of shock.

Type of Shock	CO	PCWP	SVR	SVO$_2$
Distributive	Increased	Early: WNL Late: Low	Low	Increased
Hypovolemic	Early: WNL Late: Low	Early: WNL Late: Low	Increased	Early: Increased Late: Low
Cardiogenic	Low	Increased	Increased	Low
Obstructive	Early: WNL Late: Low*	Early: WNL Late: Low	Increased	Increased*

CO, Cardiac output; PCWP, pulmonary capillary wedge pressure; SVR, systemic vascular resistance; SVO$_2$, systemic venous oxygen saturation; WNL, within normal limits.

*In obstructive shock due to **cardiac tamponade**, cardiac output is *increased* and SVO$_2$ is *low*. This can be used to distinguish cardiac tamponade from other potential etiologies of obstructive shock.

8. List three examples of distributive shock.
Neurogenic, septic, and anaphylactic shock are all examples of distributive shock.

9. How do you recognize neurogenic shock?
Patients experiencing neurogenic shock typically have a history of severe central nervous system trauma or hemorrhage and often present with flushed skin because the loss of sympathetic tone causes extensive vasodilation. The lack of sympathetic tone may also cause the heart rate to remain normal in a hypotensive patient (because of the impaired sympathetic tone, reflex tachycardia cannot occur).

10. How do you recognize septic shock?
Look for fever, tachycardia, tachypnea, skin that is flushed and warm to the touch, extremes of age, and leukocytosis. (*Note:* leukocytosis may be absent if the patient is immunosuppressed.) Start broad-spectrum antibiotics after "pan-culturing" the patient's blood, sputum, and urine.

11. What clues suggest anaphylactic shock?
Look for a history of recent exposure to the common culprits: bee stings, peanuts, shellfish, penicillins, sulfa drugs, or any new medication. Anaphylactic shock is mediated by immunoglobulin E (IgE). Treat with **epinephrine** (typically administered intramuscularly) and fluids. Administer oxygen and intubate if necessary. A tracheostomy or cricothyroidotomy should be performed if laryngeal edema or another contraindication prevents intubation. Bronchodilators, corticosteroids, and antihistamines are all second-line agents in anaphylaxis. Monitor all patients for at least 6 hours after the initial reaction.

12. List six potential etiologies of hypovolemic shock.
Hemorrhage, burns, heat-related dehydration, profuse vomiting or diarrhea, salt-wasting renal dysfunction, and third spacing are all potential etiologies of hypovolemic shock.

13. How do you recognize hypovolemic shock?
Look for a history of fluid loss as described previously. Patients usually have orthostatic hypotension, tachycardia, sunken eyes, and tenting of the skin, with infants additionally having a sunken fontanelle. Patients in hypovolemic shock may also present with cold, clammy, pale skin.

14. List three potential etiologies of cardiogenic shock. Give three examples of each etiology.
Arrhythmias, cardiomyopathies, and mechanical dysfunction are three potential etiologies of cardiogenic shock. Arrythmias that may lead to cardiogenic shock include atrial fibrillation or flutter, ventricular fibrillation, and heart block. Cardiomyopathies include myocardial infarction (MI), myocarditis, and heart failure. Examples of mechanical dysfunction include valvular stenosis or rupture, ventricular septal defect, and atrial myxoma.

15. What clues on physical exam suggest cardiogenic shock?
Most patients in cardiogenic shock have cold, clammy skin and look pale due to the lack of tissue perfusion. Distended neck veins and pulmonary congestion (e.g., crackles heard when auscultating lung bases) are usually present on physical exam.

16. List five potential etiologies of obstructive shock.
Pulmonary embolism, pulmonary hypertension, tension pneumothorax, hemothorax, and cardiac tamponade are all potential etiologies of obstructive shock.

17. What clues suggest pulmonary embolus as a cause of obstructive shock?
Look for deep venous thrombosis (DVT; positive **Homan sign** with painful, swollen leg) or risk factors for DVT. Remember the **Virchow triad:** endothelial damage, stasis, and hypercoagulable state. Watch for common risk factors, including postoperative status (especially after orthopedic or pelvic surgery), recent delivery (amniotic fluid embolus), traumatic long bone fractures (fat emboli), or malignancy. Patients classically have acute onset of chest

pain, tachypnea, shortness of breath, right-axis shift on ECG (as a sign of right-heart strain), and positive CT pulmonary angiography or ventilation/perfusion scan.

18. **How do you recognize pericardial tamponade as a cause of shock?**
Look for a history of a stab wound or significant blunt trauma to the left chest, often presenting with distended neck veins. Bedside cardiac ultrasound is a quick way to assess for tamponade. Perform pericardiocentesis emergently before obstructive shock begins to set in.

19. **Explain toxic shock syndrome.**
Toxic shock syndrome usually presents in a woman of reproductive age who leaves her tampon in place too long or in a patient with wound packing that has been in for too long. Look for skin desquamation. Toxic shock syndrome may be caused by the *Staphylococcus aureus* toxin TSST-1 or by an invasive group A *Streptococcus pyogenes* infection.

20. **What clues suggest Addison disease as a cause of shock?**
Patients with Addison disease usually have a history of therapeutic corticosteroid use and/or autoimmune disease and typically have lab results indicating hyperkalemia and hyponatremia. These patients may present with advanced neurologic symptoms, including confusion, delirium, or coma. Treat with glucocorticoids such as hydrocortisone plus aggressive normal saline fluid resuscitation.

21. **What is the most important point to remember when managing a patient who is in shock? In addition to vital signs, which additional physiologic parameters should you monitor?**
The most important point to remember is to monitor the ABCs (**a**irway, **b**reathing, **c**irculation). Patients in shock often need immediate lifesaving intervention. Do not hesitate to intubate, do not feed the patient, and, if possible, do not give narcotics. Treat the underlying condition. Mental status changes are often an important clue indicating clinical deterioration. Also monitor by ECG, urine output, arterial blood gas, hemoglobin/hematocrit, and Swan-Ganz parameters. (Swan-Ganz is not commonly used in clinical practice but may still be tested on the USMLE.)

22. **After the ABCs are secured, what should you do for a patient in shock?**
After establishing the ABCs, quickly give oxygen and begin fluid resuscitation unless the patient is in congestive heart failure (CHF). If CHF is present, avoid fluids or you will worsen the volume overload that your patient is already experiencing. Once you have administered oxygen and started fluid resuscitation, you may proceed to treating the underlying condition.

23. **How should fluids be given if a patient is in shock?**
"Two large-bore IVs" is the phrase you will commonly hear on the wards and see on your exams. "Large bore" typically means either 14 or 16 gauge. Infuse 1 to 2 L as fast as it will go (the standard bolus is 10–20 mL of normal saline or lactated Ringer solution per kg body weight). After the bolus, reassess the patient to determine if the bolus helped; this is called a fluid challenge. Positive signs include increases in blood pressure and urine output after the bolus. Do not be afraid to give a second (or third) bolus if your patient does not improve after the first one. Remember to watch for fluid overload so you do not cause or exacerbate CHF. Consider placing a Foley catheter to ensure accurate monitoring of urine output.

24. **What should you do if multiple fluid challenges fail to resolve your patient's hypotension?**
Use invasive hemodynamic monitoring (i.e., central line placement or Swan-Ganz catheter) to help determine the cause of the shock and to guide therapeutic decisions. The patient may require vasopressor medications to elevate the blood pressure.

25. **Discuss the use of dobutamine, dopamine, norepinephrine, and isoproterenol to support blood pressure in the setting of shock.**
Dobutamine is a beta$_1$-agonist used to increase CO by increasing cardiac contractility; it also has mild beta$_2$ activity that may result in peripheral vasodilation.
Dopamine activates dopamine receptors at low doses, which results in selective vasodilation (the traditional use for renal perfusion is questionable). At moderate doses, its beta$_1$-agonist effects dominate, which increases contractility. At the highest doses, dopamine has alpha$_1$-agonist effects and therefore may cause vasoconstriction. Note that these dose-dependent effects are hotly debated in clinical practice but may still be tested on the USMLE.
Norepinephrine is used for its vasoconstrictive alpha$_1$-agonist effects, but it also has inotropic beta$_1$ effects. It is primarily given to patients with hypotension to increase peripheral resistance and improve perfusion of vital organs.
Isoproterenol is primarily an inotropic and chronotropic agent rather than a vasopressive agent. It is used for hypotension caused by bradycardia and is effective due to its beta$_1$ and beta$_2$ adrenergic effects.

26. **What about the use of phenylephrine, epinephrine, and phosphodiesterase inhibitors in the setting of shock?**
Phenylephrine is used for its vasoconstrictive alpha$_1$-agonist effects. It is similar to norepinephrine in this way, except phenylephrine has no beta-adrenergic effects.
Epinephrine is a strong beta$_1$-agonist with moderate beta$_2$- and alpha$_1$-agonist activity. It is typically used in patients experiencing cardiac arrest or anaphylactic shock.

Milrinone and **inamrinone** are phosphodiesterase inhibitors. They are used in patients with refractory heart failure (they are not first-line agents) because they have a positive inotropic effect by reducing the metabolism of cyclic adenosine monophosphate (cAMP) and therefore increasing cAMP concentration. They cannot be used in hypotensive patients, however, as they may exacerbate fluid overload and precipitate cardiogenic shock.

ISCHEMIC HEART DISEASE AND ATHEROSCLEROSIS

1. Define hypertension.
   Hypertension was redefined in the updated American College of Cardiology/American Heart Association (ACC/AHA) guidelines, published in 2017. There are now four blood pressure categories for adults, based on systolic blood pressure (SBP) and diastolic blood pressure (DBP):
   - **Normal**: SBP *less than* 120 mm Hg **and** DBP *less than* 80 mm Hg
   - **Elevated**: SBP between 120 and 129 mm Hg **and** DBP *less than* 80 mm Hg
   - **Hypertension stage 1**: SBP between 130 and 139 mm Hg **or** DBP between 80 and 89 mm Hg
   - **Hypertension stage 2**: SBP 140 mm Hg and higher **or** DBP 90 mm Hg and higher
        Note that patients with SBP and DBP in two separate categories are considered to be in the higher of the two categories.

2. What is the "two-measurement" rule in the diagnosis of hypertension?
   Blood pressure should be measured on two separate office visits before the diagnosis of hypertension can be made. However, if asked, recommend nonpharmacologic measures after the first abnormal measurement.

3. How often should you screen for hypertension?
   According to the 2017 ACC/AHA guidelines, adults with no prior history of hypertension should be screened on an annual basis. It is recommended that patients with risk factors such as obesity (e.g., body mass index [BMI] $\geq$30) be screened every 6 months.

4. What is the target blood pressure for patients with hypertension?
   A blood pressure *below* 130/80 mm Hg is the target blood pressure for all hypertensive adults, according to the 2017 ACC/AHA guidelines. This includes patients with comorbidities such as atherosclerotic or cardiovascular disease, diabetes mellitus, chronic kidney disease, heart failure, and peripheral artery disease (PAD).

5. What are the conservative (i.e., nonpharmacologic) treatments for hypertension? When should you recommend these interventions?
   A healthy diet with regular exercise is the mainstay of nonpharmacologic therapy. Dietary recommendations include reduced sodium intake (e.g., <1500 mg/day), enhanced potassium intake (3500–5000 mg/day), moderate alcohol intake (men $\leq$2 drinks/day; women $\leq$1 drink per day), and adoption of the DASH diet (little-known fact: DASH is an acronym for Dietary Approaches to Stop Hypertension). Regular exercise should include 90 to 150 minutes/week of aerobic or dynamic resistance activity, aiming to lose weight until the patient achieves a BMI of 27 or less. This is the first-line-treatment for patients in the "elevated" category but should also be recommended to patients with hypertension stages 1 and 2 even if planning to begin pharmacotherapy.

6. What are the primary pharmacologic treatments for hypertension?
   The 2017 ACC/AHA guidelines split pharmacotherapies into two categories: **primary** and **secondary** agents. Primary agents include thiazide diuretics, angiotensin-converting enzyme (ACE) inhibitors, angiotensin receptor blockers (ARBs), or calcium channel blockers (CCBs; both dihydropyridine and nondihydropyridine).

7. What are the secondary pharmacologic treatments for hypertension?
   Secondary agents include loop diuretics, potassium-sparing diuretics, aldosterone antagonist diuretics, direct renin inhibitors, beta-blockers, alpha-blockers, and direct vasodilators.

8. In patients with hypertension stage 1, how do you decide when to treat with pharmacotherapy versus nonpharmacologic intervention alone?
   Pharmacotherapy should be initiated in patients with hypertension stage 1 who also have one of the following comorbidities: diabetes mellitus, chronic kidney disease, or history of atherosclerotic cardiovascular disease (ASCVD) such as a prior MI, acute coronary syndrome (ACS), PAD, TIA, stroke, prior revascularization procedure, stable angina, or serum low-density lipoprotein (LDL) greater than 190 mg/dL. These patients should be reevaluated in 1 month to assess response to pharmacotherapy. Patients with hypertension stage 1 without these comorbidities should begin with nonpharmacologic therapy alone and be reevaluated in 3 to 6 months.

9. How do thiazide diuretics affect serum levels of sodium, potassium, calcium, and uric acid?
   Thiazide diuretics will lower the serum levels of sodium and potassium and will raise the serum levels of calcium and uric acid. Monitor your patients for clinical signs of hyponatremia, hypokalemia, and hyperuricemia when starting a thiazide. Thiazide-related hypokalemia may be managed by adding a potassium-sparing diuretic (e.g., amiloride, triamterene).

10. **In which two clinical scenarios should you be cautious about administering a thiazide diuretic?**
Be cautious when administering a thiazide in patients with a history of gout or who are currently taking lithium for a mood disorder. Thiazides may induce a hyperuricemic gouty attack or lithium toxicity due to reduced renal excretion.

11. **Which diuretic medications are preferred over thiazides to treat hypertension in patients with heart failure or chronic kidney disease?**
Loop diuretics (e.g., furosemide, bumetanide, torsemide). Besides these two clinical scenarios, loop diuretics are considered secondary antihypertensive agents.

12. **Which primary agents may precipitate acute renal failure in hypertensive patients with bilateral renal artery stenosis (RAS)? Why?**
ACE inhibitors, due to their vasodilatory effect on the efferent glomerular arterioles that causes further reduction in the glomerular filtration rate (GFR).

13. **Which hypertensive medications should not be combined with ACE inhibitors? Why?**
ARBs (sartans) and direct renin inhibitors (aliskiren), due to similar mechanisms of action.

14. **What is the most significant electrolyte change to watch for in patients starting an ACE inhibitor?**
Hyperkalemia, which may also be caused by ARBs or aliskiren.

15. **Which life-threatening condition must you watch for when starting an ACE inhibitor? If this occurs, how is it managed?**
Watch for life-threatening angioedema when starting a patient on an ACE inhibitor. Patients experiencing angioedema should immediately discontinue the ACE inhibitor, allow 6 weeks to pass, then begin an ARB.

16. **In which clinical situations are ACE inhibitors the preferred antihypertensive medication?**
ACE inhibitors are preferred to control hypertension in patients with stable heart failure, history of MI, proteinuric chronic kidney disease, or albuminuric diabetes mellitus. ACE inhibitors are the only antihypertensive medication proven to reduce mortality associated with CHF as well as reduce the progression to nephropathy and neuropathy in diabetic patients.

17. **Name two dihydropyridine and two nondihydropyridine calcium channel blockers used to treat hypertension.**
Two major dihydropyridine CCBs used to treat hypertension are amlodipine and nifedipine. Two major nondihydropyridine CCBs are verapamil and diltiazem.

18. **In which patient population could you consider calcium channel blockers as first-line hypertensive monotherapy?**
In the general black population, including those with diabetes, initial antihypertensive monotherapy should include either a thiazide diuretic or CCB.

19. **In which clinical situation should antihypertensive calcium channel blockers be avoided? Why?**
Heart failure with reduced ejection fraction (HFrEF), as CCBs may reduce CO by decreasing cardiac contractility and heart rate, thereby exacerbating the existing heart failure. Watch out for clinical signs of heart failure such as pedal edema in patients taking CCBs, especially dihydropyridines (e.g., amlodipine, nifedipine).

20. **Coadministration of which antihypertensive agent should be avoided in patients taking nondihydropyridine calcium channel blockers? Why?**
Beta-blockers, due to the increased risk of bradycardia or heart block.

21. **Which antihypertensive medications should be considered in patients with comorbid atrial fibrillation or atrial flutter?**
Nondihydropyridine CCBs **or** beta-blockers, although remember not to give these medications together.

22. **True or False: Beta-blockers may be used as monotherapy in hypertensive patients with no additional medical conditions.**
False. Beta-blockers have proven to be either ineffective or inferior to primary antihypertensive agents when used as monotherapy in patients with no additional medical conditions.

23. **In which clinical situations might you consider a beta-blocker as first-line antihypertensive pharmacotherapy?**
Beta-blockers may be considered first-line antihypertensive pharmacotherapy in patients with atrial fibrillation or flutter, hyperthyroidism, migraines, and essential tremor. Beta-blockers may also be used as first-line agents in patients with heart failure or with history of ischemic heart disease, although ACE inhibitors are also considered

first-line agents in these conditions. On your exam, you are unlikely to be asked to choose between an ACE inhibitor and a beta-blocker.

24. **Which antihypertensive medications may exacerbate preexisting asthma or chronic obstructive pulmonary disease (COPD)? Why?**
Noncardioselective beta-blockers (e.g., propranolol), due to the bronchoconstrictive effects of blocking beta$_2$-receptors in smooth muscle along the airway.

25. **Which antihypertensive medications are contraindicated during pregnancy?**
ACE inhibitors, ARBs, and aliskiren are contraindicated during pregnancy.

26. **Which medications are recommended for women of reproductive age and pregnant women with hypertension?**
Labetalol, hydralazine, and alpha-methyldopa are safe during pregnancy. If preeclampsia is present (e.g., new-onset hypertension with frequent headaches, vision problems, or end-organ damage), remember that magnesium sulfate can be used to lower the mother's blood pressure.

27. **Define hypertensive urgency. How is it distinguished from hypertensive emergency?**
Hypertensive urgency and hypertensive emergency both present with blood pressure greater than 180/120 mm Hg. The key difference is that hypertensive **emergency** also includes evidence of end-organ damage, while hypertensive **urgency** does not. Examples of the end-organ damage that may be seen in hypertensive emergencies include acute renal failure, acute ischemic stroke, intracerebral hemorrhage, dissecting aortic aneurysm, acute left ventricular failure (presenting with pulmonary edema), unstable angina, acute MI, or encephalopathy. When considering encephalopathy, watch for headaches, confusion, retinal hemorrhages, papilledema, mental status changes, vomiting, blurry vision, dizziness, and/or seizures.

28. **What are the most common causes of secondary hypertension?**
In younger adults, a common cause of secondary hypertension is excessive alcohol intake. In younger women specifically, birth control pills may be the cause of their apparent hypertension. Renovascular disease (classically seen in young women with fibromuscular dysplasia) may cause secondary hypertension and can be identified by auscultating an abdominal bruit. Obstructive sleep apnea and primary aldosteronism are also common causes of secondary hypertension.

29. **List the less common (but commonly tested) causes of secondary hypertension.**
Pheochromocytoma. Look for paroxysmal spikes in blood pressure associated with acute diaphoresis, headache, flushing, and confusion. As a screening test, order a 24-hour urine collection to assess catecholamine products (metanephrines, vanillylmandelic acid, homovanillic acid). The definitive treatment for pheochromocytoma requires surgical intervention.
Renal artery stenosis. Unlike young patients with fibromuscular dysplasia, elderly patients typically have RAS due to atherosclerosis. A renal artery bruit is classically present (although not sensitive); magnetic resonance or conventional angiography makes the definitive diagnosis. Remember that giving ACE inhibitors to patients with bilateral RAS may precipitate acute renal failure. RAS is definitively treated with angioplasty or stenting.
Polycystic kidney disease (PCKD). Look for a palpable flank mass, positive family history (autosomal dominant pattern of inheritance), and elevations in serum creatinine and blood urea nitrogen when suspecting PCKD.
Cushing syndrome. Look for classic stigmata of Cushing syndrome on physical exam (e.g., central obesity, moon facies, striae, proximal muscle weakness, buffalo hump). Order a 24-urine collection to assess free cortisol or a dexamethasone suppression test. Treat with surgical resection of the tumor.
Conn syndrome. The cause is an aldosterone-secreting adrenal neoplasm. Look for high aldosterone levels despite low renin levels, hypernatremia, hypokalemia, metabolic alkalosis, and/or an adrenal mass seen on abdominal CT. The screening test of choice is the plasma aldosterone to plasma renin activity ratio; a ratio greater than 30 is indicative of primary hyperaldosteronism. Definitive treatment is surgical resection of the tumor.
Coarctation of the aorta. Look for hypertension *in the upper extremities only*, with unequal pulses, radiofemoral delay, and rib notching on chest radiograph. In a female patient, it may be associated with Turner syndrome. MRI or angiography makes a definitive diagnosis. Treat with surgical repair of the coarctation.
Renal failure from any cause. In children, think poststreptococcal glomerulonephritis or hemolytic uremic syndrome.

30. **Which tests should be ordered for every patient with a diagnosis of hypertension? Why?**
    1. **ECG:** to assess for cardiac arrhythmias or structural changes (e.g., left ventricular hypertrophy).
    2. **Chemistry 7 panel** (i.e., basic metabolic panel): investigate for possible signs of secondary hypertension (e.g., electrolyte disturbances in Conn syndrome) and evaluate for diabetes.
    3. **Urinalysis:** investigate for possible signs of secondary hypertension (e.g., red blood cell casts in poststreptococcal glomerulonephritis) and assess for kidney damage (proteinuria).
    4. **Hemoglobin and hematocrit:** to evaluate for anemia or polycythemia.
    5. **Lipid panel:** to evaluate for dyslipidemia, which may suggest an underlying atherosclerotic disease.

31. **When is cholesterol screening done in adults? In children?**
Although no protocol is universally accepted, measurement of total cholesterol and high-density lipoprotein (HDL) cholesterol every 5 years once a person turns 35 years old for men and 45 for women is considered reasonable by most authorities. Start sooner and screen more frequently for obese patients and patients with a family history of hypercholesterolemia.
   Children without risk factors for cardiovascular disease should be screened once between the ages of 9 and 11 and a second time between the ages of 17 to 21. Children with risk factors should be screened when the risk factor is first identified.

32. **Why is cholesterol so important?**
Cholesterol is one of the main known modifiable risk factors for atherosclerosis. Atherosclerosis is involved in about one-half of all deaths in the United States and one-third of deaths between the ages of 35 and 65 years. Atherosclerosis is the most important cause of permanent disability and accounts for more hospital days than any other illness. (*Translation: Atherosclerosis and high cholesterol are high-yield USMLE topics.*)

33. **What physical findings will the Step 3 test use as clues to hypercholesterolemia?**
Xanthelasma, tendon xanthomas (cholesterol deposits in the skin, classically over tendons in the lower extremities), corneal arcus in younger patients, milky-appearing serum, and obesity are possible markers for familial hypercholesterolemia. Family members should be tested if a case of familial hypercholesterolemia is found. Pancreatitis in the absence of obvious risk factors may be a marker for familial hypertriglyceridemia.

34. **What are the current recommendations for management of cholesterol levels?**
The following information is from the 2019 ACC/AHA Guidelines on the Treatment of Blood Cholesterol to Reduce Atherosclerotic Cardiovascular Risk in Adults. This new guideline differs from the previous recommendations in that it moves away from specific LDL targets. Instead, overall LDL reductions are recommended.

Group	LDL Reduction Goal	Recommended Statin Therapy
Anyone with an LDL level ≥190 mg/dL	Reduce by >50%	High-intensity statin
Patients with diabetes aged 40–75 yr and LDL ≥70 mg/dL	Reduce by 30%–50%	Moderate-intensity statin
Anyone with 7.5%–20% chance of developing atherosclerotic CVD in the next 10 yr, using a specific calculator*	Reduce by 30%–50%	Moderate-intensity statin
Anyone with ≥20% ASCVD	Reduce LDL by ≥50%	High-intensity statin

ASCVD, Atherosclerotic cardiovascular disease; *CVD*, cardiovascular disease; *LDL*, low-density lipoprotein; *MI*, myocardial infarction; *PAD*, peripheral arterial disease.
*The Pooled Cohort Equations. Available at http://my.americanheart.org/professional/StatementsGuidelines/Preventin-Guidelines_UCM_457698_SubHomePage.jsp.

35. **What is meant by high-intensity and moderate-intensity statins?**
High-dose statin means a statin at a sufficient dose to reduce LDL by at least 50%. This includes atorvastatin 40 to 80 mg and rosuvastatin 20 to 40 mg. Moderate-dose statin means a statin at a sufficient dose to reduce LDL by 30% to 50%. This includes atorvastatin 10 to 20 mg, simvastatin 20 to 40 mg, rosuvastatin 5 to 10 mg, pravastatin 40 to 80 mg, and lovastatin 40 mg.

36. **List the major risk factors for coronary heart disease (CHD).**
Although elevated levels of LDL and total cholesterol are risk factors for CHD, do not count them as risk factors when deciding to treat or not to treat high cholesterol. The following factors should be counted:
   1. **Age** (men aged ≥45 years; women aged ≥55 years or with premature menopause and no estrogen replacement therapy)
   2. **Family history of premature heart attacks** (defined as definite MI or sudden death in father or first-degree male relative <55 years old or mother or first-degree female relative <65 years old)
   3. **Cigarette smoking**
   4. **Hypertension** (≥140/90 mm Hg or prescription for antihypertensive medications)
   5. **Diabetes mellitus**
   6. **Low HDL** (<40 mg/dL)
      Note: An HDL level ≥60 mg/dL is considered protective and negates one risk factor.

37. **Discuss other possible risk factors for heart disease.**
The 2019 ACC/AHA cholesterol guidelines address other factors that may indicate an elevated risk for ASCVD. In selected individuals who are in one of the four statin benefit groups and for whom a decision to initiate statin

therapy is otherwise unclear, additional factors may be considered to inform treatment decision making. These factors include:
1. Primary LDL ≥160 mg/dL
2. Family history of premature ASCVD with onset younger than 55 years in a first-degree male relative or younger than 65 years in a first-degree female relative
3. Comorbid conditions such as chronic kidney disease, metabolic syndrome, inflammatory diseases (e.g., rheumatoid arthritis, psoriasis, human immunodeficiency virus)
4. Ethnicity (e.g., South Asian ancestry)
5. Triglycerides ≥175 mg/dL
6. Lipoprotein(a) >50 mg/dL or 125 nmol/L
7. Apolipoprotein B (apoB) ≥130 mg/dL
8. High-sensitivity C-reactive protein ≥2 mg/L
9. Coronary artery calcium (CAC) score ≥100 Agatston units or ≥75th percentile for age, sex, and ethnicity
10. Ankle-brachial index >0.9
11. Elevated lifetime risk of ASCVD (yes, this is vague)

38. **How is high-density lipoprotein affected by alcohol? Estrogens? Exercise? Smoking? Progesterone?**
High HDL is protective against atherosclerosis and is increased by moderate alcohol consumption (1–2 drinks/day) but not by high alcohol intake, exercise, and estrogens. HDL is decreased by smoking, androgens, progesterone, and hypertriglyceridemia.

39. **What causes hypercholesterolemia?**
Genetics certainly plays a role, but most cases are thought to be multifactorial. The most common secondary causes of increased cholesterol are uncontrolled diabetes and excessive alcohol intake. Other secondary causes include hypothyroidism, uremia, nephrotic syndrome, obstructive liver disease, excessive alcohol intake (which increases triglycerides), and medications (e.g., birth control pills, glucocorticoids, thiazides, beta-blockers).

40. **What are some other medications that affect cholesterol metabolism?**

Medication Class	Examples	Mechanism of Action	Lipid Effect	Side Effects
Fibrates	Gemfibrozil, fenofibrate	Lipoprotein lipase activator	↓ TGs, ↑HDL	Myositis (↑ risk with concomitant statin use), hepatitis, GI upset, cholelithiasis
Cholesterol absorption inhibitors	Ezetimibe	Inhibits absorption of cholesterol in small intestine	↓ LDL	Diarrhea, abdominal pain
Bile acid resins	Cholestyramine, colestipol, colesevelam	Binds bile in the gastrointestinal tract to prevent reabsorption	↓ LDL	GI side effects
Niacin	Niacin, Niaspan (extended release)		↓ TGs, ↓ LDL, ↑ HDL	Facial flushing (can be prevented with aspirin)
PCSK9 inhibitors	Evolocumab, alirocumab	Inhibit PCSK9, which is a protein responsible for degrading LDL-Rs	↓↓ LDL	Injection site swelling, rash, myalgias

TG, triglycerides; *HDL*, high-density lipoprotein; *LDL*, low-density lipoprotein; *LDL-Rs*, low-density lipoprotein receptor; *GI*, gastrointestinal; *PCSK9*, proprotein convertase subtilisin/kexin type 9

41. **What elements of the history and physical exam steer you away from a diagnosis of myocardial infarction?**
Wrong age: A patient under the age of 40 is very unlikely to have an MI without known heart disease, strong family history, or multiple risk factors for coronary artery disease.
Lack of risk factors: A 60-year-old marathon runner who eats well and has a high level of HDL and no cardiac risk factors (other than age) is unlikely to have an MI.

Physical characteristics of pain: If the pain is reproducible by palpation, it is from the chest wall, not the heart. If the pain worsens with inspiration, that is pleuritic chest pain, not the heart. If the pain is associated with meals or certain foods, it is likely a gastrointestinal cause such as gastroesophageal reflux disease (GERD), not the heart. The pain associated with an MI is usually not sharp or well localized.

Many physicians still want to make sure that a heart attack has not occurred by obtaining an ECG and possibly one or more sets of cardiac enzyme levels. For your licensing exams, however, the above-mentioned clues should steer you toward an alternative diagnosis.

42. **What clues suggest the common causes of chest pain other than myocardial infarction?**
   Gastroesophageal reflux/peptic ulcer disease: Look for a relation to certain foods (e.g., spicy foods, chocolate), smoking, caffeine, or lying down. Pain is relieved by antacids or acid-reducing medications. Patients with peptic ulcer disease often test positive for *Helicobacter pylori*.
   Chest wall pain (costochondritis, bruised or broken ribs): Pain is well localized and reproducible with chest wall palpation or with inspiration.
   Esophageal problems (achalasia, nutcracker esophagus, or esophageal spasm): This is often a difficult differential. The question will probably give a negative workup for MI or mention the lack of atherosclerosis risk factors. Look for abnormalities with barium swallow (achalasia) or esophageal manometry. Achalasia is treated with pneumatic dilatation or botulism toxin administration. Treat nutcracker esophagus or esophageal spasm with CCBs (e.g., diltiazem). If medical treatments are ineffective, endoscopic or surgical myotomy may be needed.
   Pericarditis: Look for a history suggesting viral upper respiratory infection prodrome within the last month. The ECG shows diffuse ST-segment elevation in all leads, the erythrocyte sedimentation rate is elevated, and a low-grade fever will likely be present. Classically, the pain is positional and is relieved by sitting forward. A triphasic pericardial rub is heard on auscultation. The most common cause is infection with Coxsackie B virus. Other causes include tuberculosis, uremia, malignancy, and lupus erythematosus or other autoimmune diseases (Fig. 4.1).
   Pneumonia: Pneumonia-related chest pain is due to pleuritis. Patients may also present with cough, fever, and/or sputum production. Ask about possible sick contacts and obtain a chest radiograph.
   Aortic dissection: This is associated with severe tearing or ripping pain that may radiate to the back. Look for hypertension or evidence of Marfan syndrome (tall, thin patient with hyperextensible joints). Blunt chest trauma can cause aortic laceration and pseudoaneurysm, which are different conditions that are often managed similarly. Look for a widened mediastinum on chest radiograph.

43. **What historical points should steer you toward a diagnosis of myocardial infarction?**
   Patients often have a history of angina or previous chest pain, murmurs, arrhythmias, risk factors for coronary artery disease, hypertension, or diabetes. They may also be taking digoxin, furosemide, cholesterol medications (e.g., statins), antihypertensives, or other cardiac medications.

44. **Describe the classic pattern of myocardial infarction chest pain.**
   The pain is classically described as a crushing or pressure sensation; it is a poorly localized substernal pain that may radiate to the shoulder, arm, or jaw. The pain is usually not reproducible on palpation and in patients with a

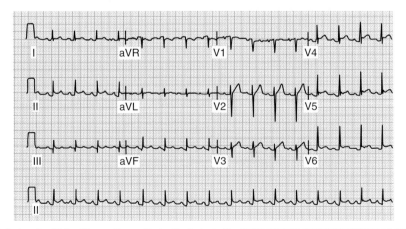

Fig. 4.1 Acute pericarditis in a 30-year-old man with pleuritic chest pain. The electrocardiogram demonstrates ST-segment elevation most clearly seen in leads I, II, aVF, and V3 to V6, diffuse PR-segment depression, and PR-segment elevation in lead aVR. (From Demangone D. ECG manifestations: noncoronary heart disease. *Emerg Med Clin North Am.* 24:113-131.)

heart attack often does not resolve with nitroglycerin (as it often does in angina). The pain usually lasts at least 30 minutes.

45. **Describe the classic physical exam findings in patients with myocardial infarction.**
Patients are often diaphoretic, anxious, tachycardic, tachypneic, pale, and appear anxious; they may also have nausea and vomiting. A large MI can cause heart failure; look for bilateral pulmonary rales in the absence of other pneumonia-like symptoms, distended neck veins, a new S3 or S4 heart sound, new murmurs, and/or cardiogenic shock.

46. **What findings on ECG should make you suspect a myocardial infarction?**
Inverted or flattened T waves, ST-segment elevation (depression means ischemia; elevation means injury), and/or Q waves in a segmental distribution (e.g., leads II, III, and aVF for an inferior infarct) suggest MI has or is occurring (Fig. 4.2). A new left bundle branch block is also considered an MI equivalent.

47. **What tests are used to diagnose a myocardial infarction?**
Other than an ECG, serum levels of the troponin enzyme levels are typically drawn three times in 8-hour intervals for the first 24 hours after presentation before MI is ruled out. Troponin levels stay elevated for more than 24 hours but take about 2 hours to reach their peak. Do not be fooled by an initial troponin measurement in the normal range if the patient's chest pain began only a few minutes ago. Chest radiographs may show cardiomegaly and/or pulmonary congestion; echocardiography may show ventricular wall motion abnormalities.

48. **Describe the management of a myocardial infarction.**
These patients should be admitted to the intensive or cardiac care unit. Several basic principles should be kept in mind:
1. Early reperfusion is indicated if the time from onset of symptoms is less than 12 hours, and choice of reperfusion therapy is determined by patient and medical center criteria. Early reperfusion (<4–6 hours) is preferred to try to salvage myocardium ("time is myocardium"). Reperfusion may be accomplished by fibrinolysis or percutaneous coronary intervention (i.e., balloon angioplasty or stent). Coronary artery bypass grafting (CABG) may be required.
2. ECG monitoring is essential. If ventricular tachycardia occurs, use amiodarone.
3. Use the mnemonic **MONA BASH** to remember the eight medications that may be used to manage MI:
   1. Control pain with **morphine,** which may improve pulmonary edema, if present.
   2. Give **oxygen** by nasal cannula, and maintain an oxygen saturation greater than 90%.
   3. Administer **nitroglycerin** unless there is evidence of right-sided heart failure; nitroglycerin in these patients will cause their blood pressure to bottom out.
   4. Administer **aspirin** (or clopidogrel).
   5. **Beta-blockers,** which patients without contraindications should take for life, reduce the mortality rate of MI as well as the incidence of a second MI.
   6. An **ACE inhibitor** or **ARB** should be started within 24 hours.
   7. Administer an HMG-CoA reductase inhibitor (**statin**).
   8. Administer unfractionated or low-molecular-weight **heparin.**

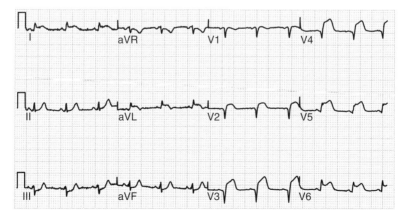

Fig. 4.2 An anterolateral acute myocardial infarction caused by a lesion in the proximal left anterior descending artery. ST-segment elevation is seen in leads I, aVL, and V2 through V6. (From Marx J, Hockberger R, Walls R. *Rosen's Emergency Medicine: Concepts and Clinical Practice.* 6th ed. Philadelphia: Mosby; 2006 [fig. 77-6].)

49. **When is heparin indicated in the setting of chest pain and myocardial infarction?**
For unstable angina, a cardiac thrombus or (if severe) CHF is seen on echocardiogram. The USMLE Step 3 will not ask about other indications, which are not as clear-cut. Do not give heparin to patients with contraindications to its use (e.g., active bleeding).

50. **How can you recognize stable angina?**
The chest pain of stable angina begins with exertion or stress, is reproduced predictably at the same level of exertion, and does *not* occur at rest or after calming down. The pain is described as a pressure or squeezing pain in the substernal area and may radiate to the shoulders, neck, and/or jaw. It is often accompanied by shortness of breath, diaphoresis, and/or nausea. The pain is usually relieved by nitroglycerin. An ECG done during an acute attack often shows ST-segment depression, but in the absence of pain, the ECG is often normal. In angina, the pain should last less than 20 minutes or be relieved after a sublingual nitroglycerin; otherwise, suspect progression to unstable angina or MI.

51. **Define unstable angina. How is it diagnosed and treated?**
Unstable angina is similar to the presentation of stable angina, but chest pain is present at rest. Unstable angina typically presents with normal or only minimally elevated cardiac enzymes, minor ECG changes (e.g., ST depression without evidence of ST elevation), and prolonged chest pain that may not respond to nitroglycerin. Management for unstable angina is similar to that for MI. The patient is admitted to the coronary or intensive care unit and typically receives the MONA BASH medications (see question 48). Consider emergent percutaneous transluminal coronary angioplasty (PTCA) if the pain does not resolve. Almost all patients have a history of stable angina with risk factors for coronary artery disease.

52. **Describe vasospastic angina (previously called Prinzmetal or variant angina).**
This rare type of angina is characterized by pain at rest (unrelated to exertion), often occurs in the middle of the night or early morning, and presents with ST-segment elevation; cardiac enzymes are normal. Patients are usually younger, and the cause is coronary artery spasm. Vasospastic angina usually responds to nitroglycerin and is managed chronically with CCBs, which reduce arterial spasm.

53. **Define silent myocardial infarction. How common is it?**
Patients with a silent MI do not develop chest pain. They present with CHF, shock, or confusion and delirium (especially elderly patients). MIs are silent in up to 25% of cases (especially in diabetics with neuropathy). Diabetic, elderly, and female patients are more likely to experience silent or atypical MI symptoms, so have a lower threshold for checking an ECG and troponins if these patients present with vague symptoms such as abdominal discomfort, nausea, or diaphoresis.

54. **True or False: Patients should be given aspirin as soon as possible in the emergency department for a suspected myocardial infarction or unstable angina.**
True, but beware the patient with chest pain who ends up having an aortic dissection (aspirin should be avoided in such patients).

55. **How is smoking related to heart disease?**
Smoking is the best risk factor to eliminate for prevention of deaths related to heart disease; it is responsible for 30% to 45% of such deaths in the United States. This risk is decreased by 50% within 1 year of quitting; by 15 years after quitting, the risk is the same as someone who has never smoked.

56. **What is the most common cause of death during vascular surgery?**
MI, regardless of the procedure performed. Peripheral vascular and aortic disease are generalized markers for atherosclerosis, and almost all patients have significant coronary artery disease. Always evaluate patients for modifiable and treatable atherosclerosis risk factors (i.e., cholesterol, hypertension, smoking, diabetes).

57. **Describe the classic presentation of chronic mesenteric ischemia.**
The classic patient has a long history of postprandial abdominal pain (also known as intestinal angina; eating is "exercise" for the intestines), which causes "fear" of food and extensive weight loss. This diagnosis is difficult because, like all atherosclerotic disease, it presents in patients over age 40 who have other conditions that may cause the same problem (e.g., peptic ulcer disease, pancreatic cancer, stomach cancer). Look for a history of extensive atherosclerosis (known coronary artery disease, peripheral vascular disease, stroke, or multiple risk factors), abdominal bruit, hemoccult-positive stool, and lack of jaundice (jaundice suggests pancreatic cancer). Most patients get a CT scan of the abdomen; negative results raise the suspicion of ischemia. Diagnosis can be made with selective angiography of the superior mesenteric artery. Magnetic resonance angiography and CT angiography are emerging tools, but angiography is still the preferred modality. Patients are treated with surgical revascularization because of the risks of bowel infarction and malnutrition.

58. **How does an acute bowel infarction present?**
Classically, a patient with a history of extensive atherosclerosis, multiple atherosclerosis risk factors, or atrial fibrillation presents with abdominal pain or tenderness (the classic presentation is "pain out of proportion to the

exam"), bloody diarrhea, and possibly peritoneal signs (e.g., rebound tenderness, guarding). Watch for thumb-printing (thickened bowel walls that resemble thumbprints) on abdominal radiographs. Patients may also have tachycardia, hypotension, and/or shock.

CONGESTIVE HEART FAILURE

1. What are the typical signs and symptoms of congestive heart failure?
   Typical signs and symptoms of CHF include:
   - Fatigue
   - Ventricular hypertrophy on ECG
   - Dyspnea
   - S3 or S4 heart sounds
   - Cardiomegaly on chest radiograph
   - Specific left- and right-sided findings (discussed in the next question)

2. What signs and symptoms help to determine whether congestive heart failure is due to left or right ventricular failure?
   Left ventricular failure (HFrEF; heart failure with reduced ejection fraction): orthopnea (shortness of breath when lying down; the patient sleeps on more than one pillow or even sitting up); paroxysmal nocturnal dyspnea (patients may sleep with either multiple pillows or in a reclining chair to keep themselves propped up); pulmonary congestion (bilateral basilar rales on auscultation); Kerley B lines on chest radiograph; pulmonary vascular congestion and edema; bilateral pleural effusions.
   Right ventricular failure (HFpEF; heart failure with preserved ejection fraction): peripheral edema, jugular venous distention, hepatomegaly, ascites, underlying lung disease (cor pulmonale).
   Note: Both ventricles are commonly affected in CHF, so a mixed pattern is commonly seen. Remember that the most common cause of right-sided heart failure is left-sided heart failure.

3. How is chronic congestive heart failure treated?
   Chronic CHF is treated on an outpatient basis, with dietary modifications (e.g., sodium restriction) and medical management the mainstays of therapy. ACE inhibitors (first-line agents proven to reduce mortality rate by preventing cardiac myocyte remodeling), beta-blockers (somewhat counterintuitive but proven to effectively manage left-sided CHF), diuretics (e.g., furosemide, spironolactone, metolazone), digoxin (not used in diastolic dysfunction; usually reserved for moderate to severe CHF with low ejection fraction or systolic dysfunction), and vasodilators (arterial and venous) may all be used.

4. How is acute congestive heart failure treated?
   Acute CHF is treated on an inpatient basis with oxygen, diuretics, and positive inotropes as the mainstays of therapy. Digoxin may be used if the patient is stable. Intravenous sympathomimetics (dobutamine, dopamine, amrinone) may be considered for severe CHF.

5. What factors precipitate congestive heart failure exacerbations in previously stable patients?
   The most common precipitator of CHF exacerbation is dietary or mediation nonadherence, but watch for **myocardial infarction,** severe hypertension, arrhythmias, infections and fever, pulmonary embolus, anemia, thyrotoxicosis, and myocarditis.

6. Define cor pulmonale. With what clinical scenarios is it associated?
   Cor pulmonale is right ventricular enlargement, hypertrophy, and right-sided heart failure due to primary lung disease. Chronic lung disease leads to right heart strain, which eventually becomes right-sided heart failure. Common causes are COPD and pulmonary embolism, which lead to pulmonary hypertension and then cor pulmonale. Sleep apnea and obesity hyperventilation syndrome may also lead to cor pulmonale; look for an obese snorer who reports feeling sleepy during the day. Patients with cor pulmonale may have tachypnea, cyanosis, digital clubbing, parasternal heave, loud P2, and a right-sided S4 in addition to the signs and symptoms of pulmonary disease. Cor pulmonale can be managed with prostacyclins (e.g., parenteral epoprostenol), antiendothelins (e.g., bosentan), phosphodiesterase-5 inhibitors (e.g., sildenafil), and CCBs (e.g., diltiazem) while awaiting heart-lung transplantation.

DYSRHYTHMIAS

1. What ECG abnormalities do you need to know about for the Step 3 exam? How are they treated?
   Figs. 4.3 through 4.15 demonstrate ECG strips of the arrhythmias described here. Always check for electrolyte disturbances (e.g., potassium, calcium) as a cause for any arrhythmia.

Arrhythmia	*Treatment and Warnings*
Atrial fibrillation	In symptomatic patients, first control the ventricular rate with a beta-blocker, nondihydropyridine calcium channel blocker, or digoxin: • If **acute** (onset <24 hr), cardiovert with amiodarone, procainamide, or DC cardioversion. • If **chronic**, first anticoagulate, then cardiovert; if this approach fails or atrial fibrillation recurs, leave the patient on rate control medications (beta-blocker, calcium channel blocker, or digoxin) and anticoagulation.
Atrial flutter	Treat like atrial fibrillation. You may try to stop the arrhythmia with vagal maneuvers (e.g., carotid massage, Valsalva maneuver).
First-degree heart block	No treatment; avoid beta-blockers and calcium channel blockers, both of which slow conduction and may worsen a first-degree block.
Second-degree heart block	For Mobitz type I (Wenckebach), use pacemaker or atropine only in symptomatic patients; remember the characteristic PR interval changes with "*longer, longer, longer, drop; now you've got a Wenckebach.*" Use pacemaker in all patients with Mobitz type II.
Third-degree heart block	Use pacemaker.
WPW syndrome	Use **procainamide** or quinidine; avoid digoxin and verapamil.
Ventricular tachycardia	If pulseless, treat with immediate defibrillation followed by epinephrine, vasopressin, amiodarone, or lidocaine as you initiate CPR. If a pulse is present, treat with amiodarone and synchronized cardioversion.
Ventricular fibrillation	Immediate defibrillation followed by epinephrine, vasopressin, amiodarone, or lidocaine as you initiate CPR.
PVCs	Usually not treated; if severe and symptomatic, consider beta-blockers or amiodarone.
Sinus bradycardia	Usually not treated; use atropine or pacing if severe and symptomatic (e.g., after myocardial infarction). Avoid beta-blockers, calcium channel blockers, and other conduction-slowing medications.
Sinus tachycardia	Usually none; correct the underlying cause. Use beta-blocker or calcium channel blocker if symptomatic.

CPR, Cardiopulmonary resuscitation; *DC,* direct current; *PVCs,* premature ventricular complexes; *WPW,* Wolff-Parkinson-White.

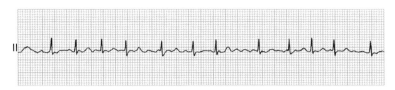

Fig. 4.3 Atrial fibrillation. There are no true P waves, and the ventricular rate is irregular. (From Goldberger AL. *Clinical Electrocardiography: A Simplified Approach.* 7th ed. Philadelphia: Mosby; 2006 [fig. 15-4].)

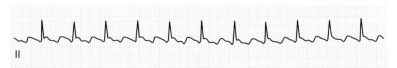

Fig. 4.4 An example of atrial flutter. In contrast to atrial fibrillation, atrial flutter is regular. The baseline has a sawtooth shape. (From Walsh D. *Palliative Medicine.* 1st ed. Philadelphia: Saunders; 2008 [fig. 80-2].)

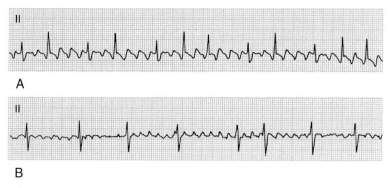

Fig. 4.5 Atrial flutter with variable block (A) and coarse atrial fibrillation (B) may be easily confused. Notice that for atrial fibrillation the ventricular rate is erratic, and the atrial waves are not identical from segment to segment, whereas these atrial waves are identical for atrial flutter. (From Goldberger A. *Clinical Electrocardiography: A Simplified Approach.* 7th ed. Philadelphia: Mosby; 2006 [fig. 23-3].)

First-degree AV block

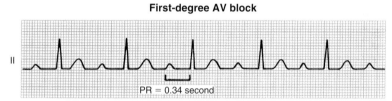

Fig. 4.6 First-degree atrioventricular block with a PR interval that is prolonged to more than 0.20 second with each electrical cycle (0.12–0.20 second is normal). (From Goldberger A, Goldberger ZD, Shvilkin A. *Goldberger's Clinical Electrocardiography: A Simplified Approach.* 8th ed. Philadelphia: Saunders; 2012 [fig. 17-2].)

Mobitz type I (Wenckebach) second-degree AV block

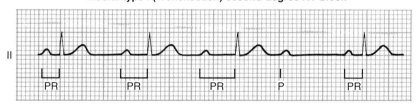

Fig. 4.7 Mobitz type I second-degree atrioventricular (AV) block (Wenckebach; a second-degree AV block in which the PR interval progressively lengthens from cycle to cycle until the AV node no longer conducts a stimulus from above). Notice the progression of the PR interval before the impulse is completely blocked. (From Goldberger A, Goldberger ZD, Shvilkin A. *Goldberger's Clinical Electrocardiography: A Simplified Approach.* 8th ed. Philadelphia: Saunders; 2012 [fig. 17-3].)

Mobitz II AV block with sinus rhythm

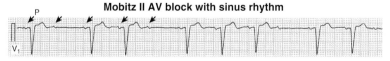

Fig. 4.8 Mobitz type II second-degree atrioventricular block (an intermittent dropped QRS). Note the abrupt appearance of sinus P waves that are not followed by QRS complexes (nonconducted or dropped beats). (From Goldberger A, Goldberger ZD, Shvilkin A. *Goldberger's Clinical Electrocardiography: A Simplified Approach.* 8th ed. Philadelphia: Saunders; 2012 [fig. 17-5].)

Third-degree (complete) AV block

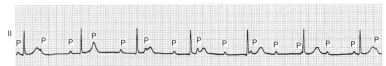

Fig. 4.9 A third-degree atrioventricular block (none of the atrial depolarizations conduct to the ventricles) is characterized by independent atrial *(P)* and ventricular (QRS complex) activity. The atrial rate is always faster than the ventricular rate. (From Goldberger A, Goldberger ZD, Shvilkin A. *Goldberger's Clinical Electrocardiography: A Simplified Approach.* 8th ed. Philadelphia: Saunders; 2012 [fig. 17-7].)

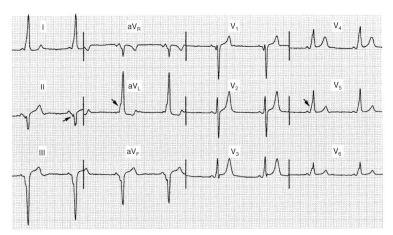

Fig. 4.10 Wolff-Parkinson-White syndrome. Triad of a wide QRS complex, a short PR interval, and delta waves *(arrows)*. (From Goldberger AL. *Clinical Electrocardiography: A Simplified Approach.* 7th ed. Philadelphia: Mosby; 2006 [fig. 12-3].)

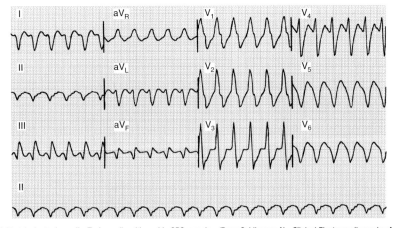

Fig. 4.11 Ventricular tachycardia. Tachycardia with a wide QRS complex. (From Goldberger AL. *Clinical Electrocardiography: A Simplified Approach.* 7th ed. Philadelphia: Mosby; 2006 [part 4, case 3].)

Ventricular fibrillation

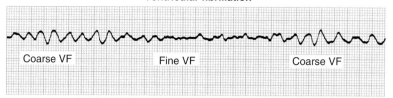

Coarse VF   Fine VF   Coarse VF

Fig. 4.12 Ventricular fibrillation *(VF)*. Fibrillatory waves in an irregular pattern. (From Goldberger AL. *Clinical Electrocardiography: A Simplified Approach.* 7th ed. Philadelphia: Mosby; 2006 [fig. 16-13].)

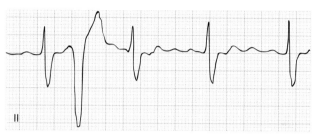

Fig. 4.13 A single premature ventricular complex. (From Marx J, Hockberger R, Walls R. *Rosen's Emergency Medicine.* 7th ed. Philadelphia: Mosby; 2009 [fig. 77-22].)

Sinus bradycardia

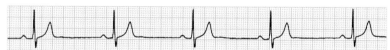

Fig. 4.14 Sinus bradycardia at a rate of about 40 beats/minute. (From Goldberger A, Goldberger ZD, Shvilkin A. *Goldberger's Clinical Electrocardiography: A Simplified Approach.* 8th ed. Philadelphia: Saunders; 2013 [fig. 20-1].)

Sinus tachycardia

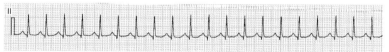

Fig. 4.15 Sinus tachycardia at a rate of about 150 beats/minute. (From Goldberger A, Goldberger ZD, Shvilkin A. *Goldberger's Clinical Electrocardiography: A Simplified Approach.* 8th ed. Philadelphia: Saunders; 2013 [fig. 13-2].)

2. What endocrine disease is suggested when a patient presents with sinus tachycardia or atrial fibrillation?
   Hyperthyroidism. Check the level of thyroid-stimulating hormone (TSH) as a screening test.

3. Which patients with atrial fibrillation should receive anticoagulation? What medications are recommended for this purpose?
   The **CHADS$_2$-VASc** score is used to estimate the risk of stroke in patients with nonrheumatic atrial fibrillation. The score is used to determine whether the patient should be managed with anticoagulation.
   The points in the following table are added to determine the CHADS$_2$-VASc score.
   - A **score of 0** is low risk for stroke; no anticoagulant therapy is recommended in most cases.
   - A **score of 1** is moderate risk; oral anticoagulation therapy or aspirin should be considered.
   - A **score of 2** or greater is high risk; oral anticoagulant therapy is recommended unless contraindicated (e.g., significant fall risk; bleeding risk; use HASBLED score).
   When indicated for a CHADS$_2$-VASc score of 2 or higher, anticoagulation by medical management has transitioned toward preferring **n**onvitamin K antagonist **o**ral **antic**oagulants (NOACs; e.g., apixaban, rivaroxaban, dabigatran) over warfarin.

	Condition	Points
C	**C**ongestive heart failure	1
H	Current **h**ypertension or taking antihypertensive medication	1
A	**A**ge >75 yr	2
D	**D**iabetes mellitus	1
S$_2$	Prior **s**troke or transient ischemic attack	2
V	**V**ascular disease	1
A	**A**ge 65–74 yr	1
Sc	Female **s**ex confers higher risk	1

4. **How does Wolff-Parkinson-White (WPW) syndrome classically present?**
A child becomes dizzy, dyspneic, or passes out after playing and then recovers and has no other symptoms. The cause is a transient reentrant tachyarrhythmia via an accessory pathway (bundle of Kent). ECG shows the pathognomonic sloping delta wave with shorted PR interval. The treatment of choice for these patients is radiofrequency catheter ablation of the pathway, but look for mentions of **procainamide** for medical management on your licensing exams.

DISORDERS OF THE GREAT VESSELS

1. **What is the most common cause of immediate death after an automobile accident or a fall from a great height?**
Aortic rupture. Look for a widened mediastinum on a chest radiograph and an appropriate history of trauma. Order a CT scan or angiogram if a contained aortic rupture is suspected (of those who survive to be admitted to the hospital, 50% will die in the first 24 hours). Aortic laceration, traumatic aortic injury, and traumatic pseudoaneurysm all describe the phenomenon seen in initial survivors: an aortic rupture contained by a hematoma or an inadequate amount of surrounding tissue (e.g., adventitia only). Treat with immediate surgical repair.

2. **What are the classic findings in a patient with an abdominal aortic aneurysm? How is it evaluated?**
Abdominal aortic aneurysm (AAA) classically presents as a pulsatile abdominal mass that may cause abdominal pain or back pain. If pain is present, rupture/leak of the aneurysm should be suspected, although an unruptured aneurysm may cause some degree of pain. Presumed ruptured AAA is a surgical emergency. Ultrasound or CT scan is used for initial evaluation and diagnostic confirmation in stable patients, as well as for serial monitoring.

3. **How is an abdominal aortic aneurysm managed? What clues indicate that the aneurysm has ruptured?**
If the aneurysm is smaller than 5 cm, you can follow it with serial ultrasound examinations to ensure that it is not enlarging. These smaller aneurysms should be managed with risk factor reduction (smoking cessation and treatment of hypertension and dyslipidemia). If the aneurysm is larger than 5 cm (or if you are told that it is enlarging rapidly), surgical correction should be advised if the patient can tolerate the surgery.

A **pulsatile abdominal mass plus hypotension** requires emergent laparotomy for a presumed ruptured aneurysm, which carries a mortality rate of roughly 80%. The management of an abdominal aortic aneurysm dissection depends on the location of the dissection. Patients who survive the initial tear typically present with a severe sharp or tearing sensation in the back or chest. Acute dissections involving the ascending aorta are considered surgical emergencies. Dissections confined to the descending aorta are treated medically unless the dissection progresses or continues to bleed.

VALVULAR HEART DISEASE

1. **Describe the etiology and classic history of the various heart valve abnormalities.**

Valve Problem	Etiology	History
Mitral stenosis	Rheumatic fever is most common etiology	Dyspnea, orthopnea, and PND
Mitral regurgitation	Typically results from rheumatic fever or chordate tendineae rupture after myocardial infarction	Fatigue, dyspnea, orthopnea

Valve Problem	Etiology	History
Aortic stenosis	Typically seen in the elderly due to valvular calcification Bicuspid or unicuspid valves may present with symptoms in childhood	Usually asymptomatic for years and begins with dyspnea on exertion Progresses to angina, syncope, and heart failure, with the mortality rate increasing through this progression
Aortic regurgitation	**CREAM** mnemonic: **c**ongenital **r**heumatic damage, **e**ndocarditis, **a**ortic dissection/**a**ortic root dilatation, **M**arfan syndrome	Can present acutely with severe dyspnea, acute pulmonary congestion, and cardiogenic shock. Can also present chronically with DOE, orthopnea, and PND

DOE, Dyspnea on exertion; *PND,* paroxysmal nocturnal dyspnea.

2. What physical exam findings are associated with various heart valve abnormalities?

Valve Problem	Physical Characteristics	Other Findings
Mitral stenosis	Late diastolic blowing murmur (best heard at apex)	Opening snap, loud S1, AF, LAE, PH
Mitral regurgitation	Holosystolic murmur (radiates to axilla)	Soft S1, LAE, PH, LVH
Aortic stenosis	Harsh systolic ejection murmurs (best heard in aortic area; radiates to carotids)	Slow pulse upstroke, S3/S4, ejection click, LVH, cardiomegaly; syncope, angina, heart failure. Murmur will *increase with increased preload* (e.g., hand grip; sitting position) to distinguish AS from hypertrophic cardiomyopathy (HCM)
Aortic regurgitation	Early diastolic decrescendo murmur (best heard at apex); patient may be described in a vignette as "bobbing" the head	Widened pulse pressure, LVH, LV dilatation, S3, Waterhammer pulse
Mitral prolapse	Midsystolic click, late systolic murmur	Panic disorder

AF, Atrial fibrillation; *LAE,* left atrial enlargement; *LV,* left ventricle; *LVH,* left ventricular hypertrophy; *PH,* pulmonary hypertension.

3. Describe the treatment of each of the aforementioned valvular disorders.
Mitral stenosis is a mechanical problem that requires balloon valvotomy or surgery if it becomes severe. Medical management (diuretics, digoxin, beta-blockers) is only adjunctive to either percutaneous or surgical intervention. **Mitral regurgitation** is treated with corrective surgery if certain indications such as flail leaflet or severe regurgitation are present. Vasodilators (e.g., nitroprusside, hydralazine) may be used in symptomatic patients. Atrial fibrillation is common due to the resulting left atrial enlargement, which should be managed medically, if present. Patients with **aortic stenosis** should almost universally receive surgical aortic valve replacement. Aortic valve replacement or repair is also indicated in symptomatic patients with chronic **aortic regurgitation.** Aortic valve replacement or repair may be indicated for asymptomatic patients under certain circumstances, such as progressive left ventricular enlargement (along with specific echocardiographic findings that are beyond the scope of the USMLE). Vasodilators may be used to reduce the hemodynamic burden and possibly delay the need for surgery in asymptomatic patients.

4. True or False: An understanding of the pathophysiology behind the various changes associated with long-standing valvular heart disease is high yield for the Step 3 exam.
True. This is not memorization but rather the ability to fundamentally understand which physiologic or anatomic changes are associated with each type of valvular dysfunction. For example, it is advisable to understand why right-heart failure may occur with long-standing mitral stenosis.

5. Who should receive endocarditis prophylaxis?
The 2017 AHA/ACC recommendations conclude that a minimal number of cases of infective endocarditis might be prevented by antibiotic prophylaxis for dental procedures. Antibiotic prophylaxis should only be considered if one of the following cardiac conditions is present prior to the dental procedure:
- Prosthetic cardiac valve or prosthetic material used in valve repair
- History of previous endocarditis

- Cardiac transplantation recipients with cardiac valvular disease
- Congenital heart disease only in the following categories:
  - Unrepaired cyanotic congenital heart disease, including those with palliative shunts and conduits
  - Completely repaired congenital heart disease with prosthetic material or device, whether placed by surgery or catheter intervention, during the first 6 months after the procedure
  - Repaired congenital heart disease with residual defects at the site or adjacent to the site of a prosthetic patch or prosthetic device (which inhibit endothelialization)
- Based on these AHA/ACC recommendations there is no evidence to support antibiotic prophylaxis prior to genitourinary or gastrointestinal procedures.

6. Describe the protocols for endocarditis prophylaxis, if indicated.

An antibiotic for prophylaxis should be administered in a single dose before the procedure. Amoxicillin is the preferred choice for oral therapy; cephalexin, clindamycin, azithromycin, or clarithromycin may be used in patients with penicillin allergy. Ampicillin, cefazolin, ceftriaxone, or clindamycin may be used for patients who cannot tolerate oral medication.

7. Describe the two clinical types of endocarditis. What are the causative organisms?

- **Acute** (fulminant) endocarditis, which typically affects normal heart valves and most commonly is caused by *S. aureus.*
- **Subacute,** which has an insidious onset and typically affects previously damaged or prosthetic valves. The most common cause is viridans streptococci, but other streptococcal and staphylococcal species also may cause endocarditis (e.g., *Staphylococcus epidermis, Streptococcus bovis,* and enterococci). Suspect colon cancer if *S. bovis* turns up on blood culture.

8. What elements of the history point to endocarditis?

Look for patients who are more likely to be affected by endocarditis:

- Intravenous drug abusers, who usually have right-sided lesions (Left-sided lesions are much more common in the general population.)
- Patients with abnormal heart valves (e.g., prosthetic valves, rheumatic valvular disease, congenital heart defects such as ventricular septal defects or tetralogy of Fallot)
- Postoperative patients (especially after dental surgery)
- Immunocompromised patients

9. What are the classic signs and symptoms of endocarditis?

Look for general signs of infection (e.g., fever, tachycardia, malaise) plus new-onset heart murmur, embolic phenomena (stroke and other infarcts), **Osler nodes** (painful nodules on tips of fingers), **Janeway lesions** (nontender, erythematous lesions on palms and soles), **Roth spots** (round retinal hemorrhages with white centers), and septic shock (more likely with acute than subacute disease).

10. How is endocarditis diagnosed and treated?

The diagnosis is generally made by blood cultures. Empiric treatment is begun until the culture and sensitivity results are known. An antistaphylococcal penicillin (such as oxacillin or nafcillin) plus an aminoglycoside is a good choice for native valve endocarditis. A third-generation penicillin or cephalosporin plus an aminoglycoside is a reasonable choice. Empiric treatment for prosthetic valve endocarditis is vancomycin plus gentamicin plus either cefepime or a carbapenem.

11. What are the major and minor Jones criteria for rheumatic fever? Why is rheumatic fever less common today?

The five major Jones criteria include migratory polyarthritis, carditis, central nervous system involvement (chorea), erythema marginatum, and subcutaneous nodules. The minor Jones criteria include fever, arthralgia, elevation in erythrocyte sedimentation rate or C-reactive protein (CRP), and prolonged PR interval on ECG. The diagnosis of rheumatic fever requires a history of streptococcal infection and the presence of two of the major criteria or one major criterion plus two minor criteria. Treatment of streptococcal pharyngitis with antibiotics markedly reduces the incidence of rheumatic fever, thus it is less common today. Give all patients affected by rheumatic fever endocarditis prophylaxis before surgical procedures.

PERIPHERAL ARTERIAL VASCULAR DISEASES

1. What are the symptoms of thoracic outlet obstruction? How is it treated?

Thoracic outlet obstruction refers to symptoms caused by obstruction of the nerves or blood vessels that serve the arm as the neurovascular bundle passes from the thoracocervical region to the axilla. Affected patients have upper extremity paresthesias (nerve impingement), weakness, cold temperature (arterial compromise), edema, and/or venous distention (venous compromise). The absence of central nervous system symptoms helps to differentiate this condition from subclavian steal syndrome. Causes include trauma, pregnancy, cervical ribs (ribs arising from a cervical vertebra that are usually asymptomatic but may compromise subclavian blood flow) or muscular hypertrophy (classic in young male weightlifters). Treat with surgical intervention (e.g., cervical rib resection).

2. **Define Leriche syndrome. What pathology does it indicate?**
   Leriche syndrome is the combination of claudication in the buttocks, buttock atrophy, and impotence in men due to aortoiliac occlusive disease. Most patients need an aortoiliac bypass graft.

3. **Define claudication. What are the associated physical findings?**
   Claudication is pain, usually in the lower extremity, brought on by exercise and relieved by rest. It occurs with severe atherosclerotic disease and is the equivalent of angina for the extremities. Associated physical findings include cyanosis (with dependent rubor), atrophic changes (thickened nails, loss of hair, shiny skin), decreased temperature, and decreased (or absent) distal pulses.

4. **How are patients with claudication managed?**
   The best treatment is conservative: cessation of smoking, exercise, and good control of cholesterol, diabetes, and hypertension. Antiplatelet agents are warranted in patients with claudication. Aspirin is preferred, but clopidogrel may be used for patients who cannot tolerate aspirin. Cilostazol may be used for the treatment of intermittent claudication. Beta-blockers may worsen claudication (as a result of $beta_2$-receptor blockade), but benefits may outweigh the risks in some patients (e.g., prior MI). If claudication progresses to rest pain (forefoot pain, generally at night, which is classically relieved by hanging the foot over the edge of the bed) or interferes with lifestyle or work obligations, perform an arterial duplex for diagnosis and use angioplasty or surgical revascularization procedure for treatment. Because claudication and peripheral vascular disease are generalized markers for atherosclerosis, check for other atherosclerosis risk factors.

5. **What is the probable cause of severe, sudden onset of foot pain in patients with no previous history of foot pain, trauma, or associated chronic physical findings?**
   This scenario may indicate an embolus (look for atrial fibrillation; the pulse may be absent in the affected area) or compartment syndrome (common after revascularization procedures).

DISEASES OF VEINS

1. **True or False: The lupus anticoagulant causes a clotting tendency.**
   True. Although the lupus anticoagulant may cause a prolonged partial thromboplastin time (PTT), the patient has a tendency toward thrombosis. Look for associated lupus symptoms, positive results on the Venereal Disease Research Laboratory (VDRL) or rapid plasma reagin (RPR) tests for syphilis, or a history of recurrent miscarriages to help you recognize this condition.

2. **What genetic and acquired causes of an increased tendency toward clot forming may appear on the Step 3 exam?**
   The list keeps growing. Watch for factor V Leiden mutation (or activated protein C resistance), prothrombin G20210A mutation, hyperhomocysteinemia, elevated factor VIII level, deficiencies in protein C, protein S, or antithrombin III as genetic causes of an increased tendency toward thrombosis. Acquired causes include antiphospholipid syndrome (lupus anticoagulant and anticardiolipin antibody), hyperhomocysteinemia, pregnancy, cancer, and estrogen-containing medications. Note that hyperhomocysteinemia can be genetic or acquired. All are treated with anticoagulant therapy to prevent DVT and pulmonary embolus. Suspect these conditions if a patient develops recurrent clots or develops a clot in the absence of risk factors for clot development. Women desiring contraception should not use oral estrogen-containing contraceptives, which increase thrombotic risk; favor nonhormonal methods such as an intrauterine device.

3. **What is the Virchow triad?**
   The Virchow triad describes three key predisposing factors that may lead to DVT: endothelial damage, venous stasis, and hypercoagulability. These three broad categories should help you remember when to think about the possibility of DVT.

4. **List the common clinical scenarios leading to the development of deep venous thrombosis.**
   - Surgery (especially orthopedic, pelvic, abdominal, or neurosurgery)
   - Malignancy
   - Trauma
   - Immobilization (e.g., hospitalization)
   - Pregnancy
   - Use of birth control pills
   - Disseminated intravascular coagulation
   - Hypercoagulable states such as factor V (Leiden), antithrombin III deficiency, protein C deficiency, protein S deficiency, prothrombin *G20210A* gene mutation, hyperhomocysteinemia, or antiphospholipid syndrome

5. **Describe the physical signs and symptoms of deep venous thrombosis. How is it definitively diagnosed?**
   Signs and symptoms of DVT include unilateral leg swelling, unilateral calf pain or tenderness, and/or **Homan sign** (calf tenderness with passive ankle dorsiflexion; present in 30% of cases). Superficial palpable cords imply

superficial thrombophlebitis as a more likely diagnosis. DVT is best diagnosed by Doppler compression ultrasonography or by impedance plethysmography of the veins of the affected extremity. The gold standard is venography, but this invasive test is reserved for situations in which the diagnosis is not clear.

6. **How is deep venous thrombosis managed? For how long?**
Systemic anticoagulation is necessary to manage DVT. Use intravenous heparin or subcutaneous low molecular weight heparin (LMWH) initially, followed by crossover to oral anticoagulation. Patients should be maintained on anticoagulation for at least 3 months and possibly for life if more than one episode of clotting occurs or other risk factors are present.

7. **What is the best way to prevent deep venous thrombosis in patients undergoing surgery?**
Prophylactic measures for patients undergoing surgery depend on the risk for developing DVT or pulmonary embolism. Early ambulation is recommended for low-risk patients. LMWH, low-dose unfractionated heparin, or fondaparinux is recommended for patients at moderate risk. High-risk patients should be given LMWH, fondaparinux, or an oral vitamin K antagonist. If the patient is at a high risk of bleeding, pneumatic compression stockings should be used instead.

8. **True or False: Deep venous thrombosis typically leads to a stroke.**
False, with one rare exception. Embolization of left-sided heart clots (due to atrial fibrillation, ventricular wall aneurysm, severe congestive heart failure, or endocarditis) may cause arterial infarcts (e.g., cerebral, renal, gastrointestinal, or extremity infarcts). DVT, on the other hand, may embolize to cause pulmonary emboli—**not** arterial emboli. The one rare exception occurs in patients with a right-to-left shunt (e.g., patent foramen ovale, atrial or ventricular septal defect, or pulmonary arteriovenous fistula). In such patients, a DVT may embolize, cross through the anatomic defect, and advance into the arterial circulation, causing an arterial infarct.

9. **Describe the usual history of a patient with superficial thrombophlebitis. How is the condition treated?**
Patients often have a history of varicose veins and exhibit localized leg pain with superficial cordlike induration, reddish discoloration, and mild fever. Superficial thrombophlebitis is not a significant risk factor for pulmonary embolus, and patients do not need anticoagulation. Treatment is usually conservative and includes nonsteroidal antiinflammatory drugs (NSAIDs) and warm compresses. The condition generally subsides on its own within a few days. A thrombectomy under local anesthesia can be performed for severe or nonresolving symptoms.

10. **True or False: Superficial thrombophlebitis is a risk factor for pulmonary embolus.**
False. Superficial thrombophlebitis (erythema, tenderness, edema, and a palpable clot in a superficial vein) affects superficial veins and does not cause pulmonary emboli. It is considered a benign condition, although recurrent superficial thrombophlebitis can be a marker for underlying malignancy (e.g., Trousseau syndrome, or migratory thrombophlebitis, is a classic marker for pancreatic cancer). Treat affected patients with NSAIDs and warm compresses.

11. **What are the signs and symptoms of venous insufficiency? How is it treated?**
Venous insufficiency generally occurs in the lower extremities. Patients may have a history of DVT, varicose veins, and/or swelling in the extremity with pain, fatigability, or heaviness. Symptoms are relieved by elevating the extremity. Patients may also have increased skin pigmentation around the ankles with possible skin breakdown and ulceration.
  Treatment is at first conservative, including elastic compression stockings, elevation with minimal standing, and treatment of ulcers with cleaning, wet-to-dry dressings, and antibiotics, if cellulitis occurs.

CONGENITAL DISEASE

1. **What do you need to know about the common congenital heart defects?**

Defect	*Symptoms, Treatment, and Other Information*
Patent ductus arteriosus (PDA)	Constant, **machine-like** murmur in upper left sternal border; dyspnea and possible CHF. Close with indomethacin or surgery (if indomethacin fails). Keep the ductus open with prostaglandin E_1. Associated with congenital rubella and high altitudes. *Preserve the PDA with **p**rostaglandins; **end** the PDA with **ind**omethacin.*
Ventricular septal defect (VSD)	*Most common congenital heart defect.* Characterized by a holosystolic murmur next to sternum. Most cases resolve on their own. Watch for fetal alcohol, TORCH, or Down syndrome.
Atrial septal defect (ASD)	Often asymptomatic until adulthood. Characterized by fixed, split S2 and palpitations. Most defects do not require correction (unless very large).

Defect	Symptoms, Treatment, and Other Information
Tetralogy of Fallot	*Most common cyanotic congenital heart defect.* Characterized by four anomalies: pulmonary stenosis, RVH, overriding aorta, and VSD (mnemonic: PROVe the tetralogy). Look for "tet" spells (children whose oxygenation improves with squatting).
Coarctation of aorta	Upper extremity hypertension only; radiofemoral delay; systolic murmur heard over mid-upper back; possibly cyanotic lower extremities; rib notching on radiograph; associated with Turner syndrome.

CHF, Congestive heart failure; *RVH*, right ventricular hypertrophy; *TORCH*, toxoplasma, other, rubella, cytomegalovirus, and herpes simplex.

2. Name the noncyanotic congenital heart defects.
Noncyanotic heart diseases result in left-to-right shunts in which oxygenated blood from the lungs is shunted back into the pulmonary circulation, resulting in a "pink baby." These noncyanotic heart conditions can be remembered by the three Ds: VS**D**, AS**D**, and P**D**A. These risk conversion to cyanotic right-to-left shunts (Eisenmenger syndrome) if the right ventricle hypertrophies to the point that it becomes stronger than the left ventricle.

3. Name the cyanotic congenital heart defects.
Cyanotic heart disease causes right-to-left shunts in which deoxygenated blood is shunted into the systemic circulation, resulting in a "blue baby." These cyanotic heart conditions can be remembered by the mnemonic **1-2-3-4-5**:
   1. Truncus arteriosus: there is just **one** common vessel leaving both ventricles
   2. Transposition of the great vessels: the **two** great vessels (aorta and pulmonary artery) are transposed
   3. Tricuspid atresia: **three** for **tri**cuspid
   4. Tetralogy of Fallot: **four** for **tetra**logy
   5. Total anomalous pulmonary venous return (TAPVR): there are **five** words in TAPVR

DISEASES OF THE MYOCARDIUM

1. What causes restrictive cardiomyopathy? How is it different from constrictive pericarditis?
Restrictive cardiomyopathy involves a problem with the ventricle musculature (e.g., myocardium) itself and is typically due to pathologic deposition/infiltrative disease such as amyloidosis, sarcoidosis, hemochromatosis, or myocardial fibroelastosis. A ventricular biopsy will be abnormal in all of these conditions. Cardiac MRI may also be useful. **Constrictive pericarditis** occurs in a setting of completely normal myocardium, but an irritated pericardium is preventing proper ventricular filling. Constrictive pericarditis can be fixed simply by removing an abnormal pericardium; look for a pericardial knock on exam, with calcification of the pericardium, and a normal ventricular biopsy. Watch for an S4 heart sound (which indicates stiff ventricles) and signs of right-sided heart failure (e.g., jugular venous distention and peripheral edema) in both conditions. These two disorders are mentioned together because both can cause a "restrictive"-type cardiac physiology, but the etiologies and management strategies are quite different.

2. What is the most common type of cardiomyopathy? What causes it?
Dilated cardiomyopathy is the most common type of cardiomyopathy. It is most commonly caused by chronic coronary artery disease or ischemia, though by strict definition this is not a true cardiomyopathy. On the USMLE Step 3, watch for Chagas disease, alcohol abuse, myocarditis, or chronic doxorubicin use as the cause of dilated cardiomyopathy.

3. Which type of cardiomyopathy most likely causes a young person to pass out or die while exercising or playing sports? How is this condition managed?
Hypertrophic cardiomyopathy, which may be autosomal dominant. This idiopathic condition causes an asymmetric ventricular hypertrophy that partially obstructs left ventricular outflow, reducing CO and causing diastolic dysfunction. Look for a systolic ejection murmur along the left sternal border (similar to aortic stenosis) that *decreases with increased preload* (e.g., squatting, hand grip) and *increases with decreased preload* (e.g., standing, Valsalva maneuver). Note that this is the opposite of how aortic stenosis murmurs change with the same maneuvers. Manage HCM with beta-blockers or disopyramide (to allow the ventricle more time to fill). Competitive sports should be avoided. Surgical correction may be considered. Positive inotropes (e.g., digoxin), diuretics, and vasodilators are contraindicated because they worsen the condition.

DISEASES OF THE PERICARDIUM

1. Describe the usual symptoms of cardiac tamponade. How is it diagnosed and treated?
Cardiac tamponade is classically associated with penetrating trauma to the left chest. Patients classically have the Beck triad: hypotension (caused by impaired cardiac filling), distended neck veins, and muffled heart sounds.

Patients will have normal breath sounds, which can distinguish tamponade from tension pneumothorax. **Pulsus paradoxus** is an exaggerated fall in blood pressure on inspiration that occurs in tamponade. If the patient is unstable, treat with pericardiocentesis; put a catheter through the skin and into the pericardial sac and aspirate blood and fluid. If the patient is stable, you can first perform echocardiography to confirm the diagnosis.

TRAUMA AND TOXIC EFFECTS

1. **What are the side effects of diuretics?**
   Thiazide diuretics cause calcium retention, hyperglycemia, hyperuricemia, hyperlipidemia, hyponatremia, hypokalemic metabolic alkalosis, and hypovolemia; because they are sulfa drugs, watch out for sulfa allergy. Think of the acronym **hyperGLUC** for high **g**lucose, **l**ipids, **u**ric acid, and **c**alcium.
   Loop diuretics cause hypokalemic metabolic alkalosis, hypovolemia (more potent than thiazides), ototoxicity, and calcium excretion; with the exception of ethacrynic acid, they also are sulfa drugs.
   Carbonic anhydrase inhibitors cause metabolic acidosis.
   Potassium-sparing diuretics (e.g., spironolactone) may cause hyperkalemia.

2. **What are the side effects of beta-blockers?**
   Like many antihypertensive agents, beta-blockers can cause sedation, depression, and sexual dysfunction. They also cause bradycardia and heart block in susceptible patients and should be avoided in patients with these conditions, as should central-acting CCBs (e.g., verapamil and diltiazem). Beta-blockers can also precipitate asthmatic attacks (via beta$_2$-receptor) and mask the symptoms of hypoglycemia and sepsis, thus they should be avoided or used with caution in asthmatics and those with COPD. A beta$_1$-selective beta-blocker (atenolol, metoprolol) or a combined beta- and alpha-blocker (carvedilol) is preferred if a beta-blocker is needed to treat another condition such as heart disease. Use in diabetic patients requires an analysis of the risks and benefits; if other equivalent medications are available, use them instead.

3. **What antihypertensive is best known for causing depression?**
   Methyldopa. Beta-blockers may also cause depression.

NUTRITIONAL AND DIGESTIVE SYSTEM DISORDERS

CHAPTER 5

MOUTH, SALIVARY GLANDS, AND ESOPHAGUS

1. **What causes parotid gland swelling?**
   The classic cause of multifocal parotid gland swelling is mumps. The best treatment for mumps and the complication of infertility is prevention through immunization. Multifocal parotid gland swelling may also be due to Sjögren syndrome, sarcoidosis, and bulimia. Alcoholism can cause parotid gland hypertrophy as well. Unifocal parotid gland swelling may be due to bacterial infection, sialolithiasis (a stone in the parotid duct), or neoplasm (of which pleomorphic adenoma is the most common type). Remember too that the parotid gland contains lymph nodes within its parenchyma (unique in this regard), which can become enlarged in a number of conditions, as with lymph nodes elsewhere.

2. **Define stomatitis. What does it suggest?**
   Stomatitis is an inflammation of the mucous membranes of the mouth. The classic finding is fissuring of the corners of the mouth (angular stomatitis). Watch for deficiencies of B-complex vitamins (riboflavin, niacin, pyridoxine) or vitamin C. Additional causes include drugs such as methotrexate and sulfasalazine.

3. **What factors increase the risk for oral cancers? Describe the typical appearance.**
   Smoking or chewing tobacco, alcohol consumption, and human papillomavirus (HPV) infection are the main risk factors for oral cancer, and their effects are synergistic. Also look for poor oral hygiene. Lesions often begin as leukoplakia (white patch) or malakoplakia (red patch). Oral hairy leukoplakia can resemble leukoplakia somewhat but is an unrelated condition affecting human immunodeficiency virus (HIV)–positive patients that is associated with the Epstein-Barr virus (which is the main risk factor for nasopharyngeal cancer).

4. **What are the common causes of a neck mass?**
   In **children**, watch for thyroglossal duct cysts, which have a *midline* location and elevate with tongue protrusion; branchial cleft cysts, which are *lateral* in location and often become infected; cystic hygroma, a benign tumor also known as lymphangioma that is associated with Turner syndrome and treated with surgical resection; and cervical lymphadenitis. Cervical lymphadenitis is usually due to streptococcal pharyngitis, Epstein-Barr virus (common in the second and third decades), cat-scratch disease, or mycobacterial infection (scrofula). In terms of malignancy in children, leukemia or lymphoma may present with cervical lymphadenopathy.

   In **adults,** suspect malignancy (particularly if the mass is firm, nonmobile, and >2 cm), either lymphadenopathy from a primary tumor (lymphoma) or metastatic neoplasm (usually squamous cell carcinoma). The mass may also represent the tumor itself (especially with thyroid cancer).

5. **Describe the workup for an unknown cancer in the neck.**
   The workup includes random biopsy of the nasopharynx, palatine tonsils, and base of the tongue as well as laryngoscopy, bronchoscopy, and esophagoscopy (with biopsies of any suspicious lesions). This approach is known as triple endoscopy with triple biopsy.

6. **How are bleeding esophageal varices treated?**
   First, think of the ABCs (**a**irways, **b**reathing, and **c**irculation). Stabilize the patient with intravenous fluids and blood if needed. If indicated, correct clotting factor deficiencies with fresh frozen plasma, fresh blood, and vitamin K. Patients with cirrhosis and upper gastrointestinal (GI) bleeding should be given prophylactic antibiotics to reduce all-cause mortality, bacterial infection, and rebleeding. Somatostatin analogues (octreotide) can be given intravenously to inhibit release of vasodilator hormones and indirectly decrease portal blood flow through splanchnic vasoconstriction. Next, upper endoscopy is performed to determine the cause of the upper GI bleed (there are many possibilities for the bleeding). Once varices are identified on endoscopy, sclerotherapy of the veins is attempted with cauterization, banding, or vasopressin. The mortality rate is high, and rebleeding is common. If you must choose, try a transjugular intrahepatic portosystemic shunt (TIPS) over an open surgical portacaval shunt for more definitive management, if needed. The most physiologic shunt type among surgical options is the splenorenal shunt. However, open surgical shunt procedures are now rarely performed.

7. **How are varices with no history of bleeding treated?**
   With nonselective beta-blockers (e.g., propranolol, nadolol, timolol) to relieve portal hypertension provided there is no contraindication to the use of beta-blockers.

8. **Define gastroesophageal reflux disease (GERD). What causes it?**
GERD is stomach acid refluxing into the esophagus. It is due to inappropriate, intermittent relaxation of the lower esophageal sphincter. Patients with a hiatal hernia have a much greater incidence of GERD (see later).

9. **Describe the classic symptoms of GERD. How is it treated? What are red flag symptoms?**
The main complaint is usually "heartburn," often related to lying supine after eating. GERD may also cause abdominal or chest pain. More rarely, it can cause cough from laryngeal irritation. Initial treatment is behavioral, including elevating the head of the bed and avoiding coffee, alcohol, tobacco, spicy and fatty foods, chocolate, and medications with anticholinergic properties. If this approach fails, antacids, histamine-2 (H2) blockers, and proton-pump inhibitors (PPIs) may be tried. Many patients have already tried over-the-counter remedies before presentation, and many physicians begin empiric treatment at the first visit since "lifestyle modifications" usually fail. Surgery (Nissen fundoplication) is reserved for severe or refractory cases. Red flag symptoms for GERD include dysphagia/odynophagia, anemia/melena/hematemesis, weight loss, pneumonia, high-risk patients (men age >50 or those with symptoms >5 years), or no response to PPI. Patients with these symptoms warrant an upper endoscopy for evaluation.

10. **What are the sequelae of GERD?**
Sequelae of GERD include esophagitis, esophageal stricture (which may mimic esophageal cancer), esophageal ulcer, hemorrhage, Barrett esophagus, and esophageal adenocarcinoma.

11. **What is a hiatal hernia? How is it different from a paraesophageal hernia?**
A hiatal hernia is a sliding hernia, which means that the entire gastroesophageal junction moves above the diaphragm, pulling the stomach with it. This common and benign finding may predispose to GERD. In a paraesophageal hernia, the gastroesophageal junction stays below the diaphragm, but the stomach herniates through the diaphragm into the thorax. This type of hernia is uncommon but serious; it may become strangulated and should be surgically repaired. Both can be seen on chest x-ray as a round retrocardiac density with air-fluid levels and are often incidental findings.

12. **What are the classic symptoms of esophageal disease?**
Dysphagia (difficulty in swallowing) and/or odynophagia (painful swallowing). Patients may also have atypical chest pain.

13. **Define achalasia. How is it diagnosed and treated?**
Achalasia is caused by incomplete relaxation of a hypertensive lower esophageal sphincter and loss or derangement of peristalsis. It is usually idiopathic but may be secondary to **Chagas disease** (South America; due to *Trypanosoma cruzi*). Patients have intermittent dysphagia for solids and liquids but no heartburn because the lower esophageal sphincter stays tightly closed and does not allow acid reflux. Barium swallow reveals a dilated esophagus with distal "bird-beak" narrowing. The diagnosis is often confirmed with esophageal manometry. Treat with calcium channel blockers, nitrates, pneumatic balloon dilatation, or botulinum toxin injection; in severe cases, treat with peroral endoscopic myotomy or surgical myotomy with fundoplication. Surgery (myotomy) is a last resort. Patients have an increased risk for esophageal carcinoma.

14. **What are the signs and symptoms of esophageal spasm? How is it treated?**
Both diffuse esophageal spasm and nutcracker esophagus (best thought of as a special variant of esophageal spasm) are characterized by irregular, forceful, and painful esophageal contractions that cause intermittent chest pain. Diagnose with esophageal manometry (decreased lower esophageal pressure) or barium swallow, which will show a "corkscrew" esophagus. Treat with calcium channel blockers, nitrates, and, if needed, surgery (myotomy).

15. **What clues suggest scleroderma as the cause of esophageal complaints?**
Scleroderma may cause aperistalsis due to esophageal fibrosis and atrophy of smooth muscle. The lower esophageal sphincter often becomes incompetent, and many patients have heartburn (opposite of achalasia). Look for positive antinuclear antibody and masklike facies as well as other autoimmune symptoms. Remember also the **CREST** syndrome, which consists of **c**alcinosis, **R**aynaud phenomenon, **e**sophageal dysmotility, **s**clerodactyly, and **t**elangiectasias.

16. **What do you need to know about the epidemiology of esophageal cancer?**
First, the epidemiology has recently changed, as adenocarcinoma is now more common than squamous cell carcinoma. Adenocarcinoma is due to the long-standing effects of gastric acid reflux and thus occurs in the distal esophagus. Barrett esophagus is the precursor lesion. Squamous cell carcinoma is usually caused by alcohol and tobacco (synergistic effect) and is classically seen in black men over the age of 40 years who smoke and drink alcohol. Patients complain of weight loss and food "sticking" in the chest (progresses solids to liquids). The tumor is usually in the proximal esophagus.

17. **What is the relationship between Barrett esophagus and esophageal cancer?**
Barrett esophagus, which is usually caused by long-standing GERD, predisposes to esophageal adenocarcinoma. Barrett esophagus describes a columnar metaplasia with goblet cells of the normally squamous cell esophageal

mucosa. Once Barrett esophagus is seen on endoscopy and confirmed with endoscopic biopsy, periodic biopsies must be done to monitor for the development of esophageal cancer.

18. **Describe the classic presentation of esophageal cancer. What is the most common cell type?**
The presentation depends on the histologic type. The classic patient with squamous cell carcinoma is a chronic smoker and alcohol drinker between the ages of 40 and 60 years (blacks more than whites) who presents with weight loss, anemia, and the complaint that "food is sticking in my throat," which progresses to dysphagia for liquids. The other cell type is adenocarcinoma, which is typically due to malignant degeneration of Barrett esophagus (columnar metaplasia of esophageal squamous epithelium due to acid reflux); thus patients typically have a long history of acid reflux and heartburn. Prognosis is usually quite poor in either type due to late presentation. Squamous cell carcinomas used to predominate, but squamous cell carcinoma and adenocarcinoma now occur with almost equal frequency.

19. **Distinguish between Mallory-Weiss and Boerhaave tears in the esophagus. How are they diagnosed?**
Mallory-Weiss tears are superficial erosions in the esophageal mucosa, whereas Boerhaave tears are full-thickness esophageal ruptures. Both may cause a GI bleed and are usually seen with vomiting and retching (alcoholics and bulimic patients) if they are not iatrogenic (due to endoscopy). Diagnosis of a Mallory-Weiss tear is usually made with endoscopy, during which bleeding vessels should be sclerosed, and/or from contrast radiographs. A Boerhaave tear may manifest as pneumothorax, pneumomediastinum, or pleural effusion on chest x-ray. Diagnosis can be made with a Gastrografin-contrast esophagram or computed tomography (CT) scan (barium is more inflammatory and should not be used). Findings of a Boerhaave tear include epigastric crepitus (Hamman crunch) on examination. Mallory-Weiss tears usually stop bleeding on their own or with endoscopic treatment, but Boerhaave tears require immediate surgical repair and drainage.

20. **What is the rule about bowel contrast when a gastrointestinal perforation is suspected?**
For all GI studies, barium is preferred because it provides higher-quality images. However, with suspected GI perforation, do not use barium because it can cause chemical peritonitis or mediastinitis when a perforation/leak is present. Instead, use water-soluble contrast (e.g., Gastrografin). Things get tricky in patients with a significant risk for aspiration because the lungs tolerate barium well but develop chemical pneumonitis from water-soluble contrast. When in doubt, give water-soluble contrast, followed by barium once perforation has been excluded.

STOMACH

1. **What are the risk factors for stomach cancer? What are the symptoms?**
Risk factors include Asian race, increasing age, smoking history, ingestion of smoked meat, and *Helicobacter pylori* infection. Signs and symptoms include anemia, weight loss, early satiety, abdominal pain, and a nonhealing gastric ulcer. All gastric ulcers must be biopsied to exclude malignancy. Consider follow-up endoscopy to document resolution of an ulcer, though this is somewhat controversial. Be especially suspicious if the question describes a nonhealing ulcer in a patient with weight loss.

2. **What is a Virchow node?**
A Virchow node is a left supraclavicular node enlargement due to the spread of visceral cancer (classically stomach cancer).

3. **How does peptic ulcer disease (PUD) present?**
PUD classically presents with chronic, intermittent, epigastric pain (burning, gnawing, or aching) that is localized and often relieved by antacids or milk. Look for epigastric tenderness. Other signs and symptoms include occult blood in the stool and nausea or vomiting. PUD is more common in men. The two types of PUD are gastric and duodenal ulcers.

4. **Explain the classic differences between duodenal and gastric ulcers.**

	Duodenal	**Gastric**
% of cases	75	25
Acid secretion	Normal to high	Normal to low
Main cause	*Helicobacter pylori*	Use of nonsteroidal antiinflammatory drugs, including aspirin
Peak age	40s	50s
Blood type	0	A
Eating food	Pain gets better, then worse 2–3 hr later	Pain not relieved or made worse

5. **What is the diagnostic study of choice for peptic ulcer disease?**
Endoscopy for visualization and biopsy of ulcers is the gold standard (most sensitive test), but an upper GI barium swallow study is cheaper and less invasive. Empiric treatment with medications may be trialed in the absence of

diagnostic studies if the symptoms are typical. If endoscopy is done, a biopsy of any gastric ulcer is mandatory to exclude malignancy. Duodenal ulcers do not have to be biopsied initially because malignancy is rare.

6. **What is the most feared complication of peptic ulcer disease? What should you suspect if an ulcer does not respond to treatment?**
Perforation is the most feared complication of PUD. Look for peritoneal signs (severe abdominal pain with rebound tenderness and involuntary guarding), history of PUD, and free air on an abdominal radiograph, which can be checked with an abdominal x-ray or CT. Treat with antibiotics that cover enteric organisms (such as ceftriaxone and metronidazole) and laparotomy with repair of the perforation. If ulcers are severe, atypical (e.g., located in the jejunum), or nonhealing, think about stomach cancer or Zollinger-Ellison syndrome (gastrinoma; check gastrin level). PUD is also the most common cause of upper GI bleeding in noncirrhotic patients, which can be severe in some cases.

7. **How is peptic ulcer disease treated initially?**
First, remember that diet changes are not thought to help heal ulcers, although reduced alcohol and tobacco use may speed healing. Stop all nonsteroidal antiinflammatory drug (NSAID) use. Start treatment with a PPI, test for *H. pylori* infection (biopsy, stool antigen testing, or urea breath test), and treat with antibiotics if positive. Many regimens exist, but the most commonly used is triple therapy with a PPI, clarithromycin, and amoxicillin. An alternative treatment in areas of high clarithromycin resistance is quadruple therapy: a PPI, bismuth subsalicylate, metronidazole, and tetracycline.

8. **Name the surgical options for ulcer treatment. What complications may occur?**
Surgical options are generally considered only if medical treatment has failed or if complications are present (perforation, bleeding). Surgical procedures for PUD include antrectomy, vagotomy, and Billroth I or II procedures. After surgery (especially with Billroth procedures), watch for dumping syndrome (weakness, dizziness, sweating, and nausea or vomiting after eating due to emptying of hypertonic gastric contents into the duodenum). Dumping syndrome can be managed with smaller, more frequent meals that are higher in complex carbohydrates, high-fiber foods, and protein-rich foods instead of simple sugars. Patients may also develop hypoglycemia 2 to 3 hours after a meal, which causes recurrence of the same symptoms, as well as afferent loop syndrome (bilious vomiting after a meal relieves abdominal pain), bacterial overgrowth (malabsorption, abdominal pain, and altered bowel habits), and vitamin deficiencies (vitamin B_{12} and/or iron, causing anemia).

9. **Define Zollinger-Ellison syndrome. What clues point to the diagnosis?**
Zollinger-Ellison syndrome is a gastrinoma that causes acid hypersecretion (gastrin stimulates acid secretion) and PUD. Peptic ulcers are often multiple and resistant to therapy and may be found in unusual locations (distal duodenum or jejunum). More than one-half of these pancreatic islet cell tumors are malignant. Diagnosis is made with an elevated fasting serum gastrin level or a secretin stimulation test.

10. **Define achlorhydria. What causes it?**
Achlorhydria is absence of hydrochloric acid (HCl) secretion. It is due most commonly to **pernicious anemia,** in which autoantibodies destroy acid-secreting parietal cells, causing achlorhydria and vitamin B_{12} deficiency. Achlorhydria is often associated with other endocrine autoimmune disorders (e.g., hypothyroidism, vitiligo, diabetes, hypoadrenalism). Achlorhydria may also be caused by surgical gastric resection and rarely a VIPoma.

11. **What are classic differences between upper and lower gastrointestinal bleeds?**

	Upper GI Bleed	*Lower GI Bleed*
Location	Proximal to ligament of Treitz	Distal to ligament of Treitz
Common causes	Gastritis, ulcers, varices, esophagitis	Vascular ectasia, diverticulosis, colon cancer, colitis, inflammatory bowel disease, hemorrhoids
Stool	Tarry, black stool (melena)	Bright red blood seen in stool (hematochezia)
NGT aspirate	Positive for blood	Negative for blood

GI, Gastrointestinal; *NGT,* nasogastric tube.
Additionally, an upper GI bleed more commonly presents with an increased blood urea nitrogen (BUN) level as the blood gets digested and absorbed.

12. **How is a gastrointestinal bleed treated?**
The first step is to *make sure that the patient is stable* by checking the ABCs (**a**irways, **b**reathing, **c**irculation) and giving intravenous fluids and blood, if needed, before searching for a cause. Start a PPI intravenously. Other supportive measures include oxygen and bowel rest. **Endoscopy** is usually the first test performed (upper or lower, depending on symptoms and nasogastric tube aspirate). Endoscopically treatable lesions include ulcers, polyps, vascular ectasias, and varices.

13. **What radiologic imaging studies can be done to localize a gastrointestinal bleed? Does surgery have a role?**
Radionuclide (i.e., nuclear medicine) scans can detect slow or intermittent bleeds if a source cannot be found with endoscopy. Angiography can detect more rapid bleeds, and embolization of bleeding vessels can be done

during the procedure. Surgery is reserved for severe or resistant bleeds and typically involves resection of the affected bowel (usually colon).

14. **Define the acute abdomen. What physical exam signs suggest its presence?**
Acute abdomen generally refers to sudden-onset, severe abdominal pain. The most common causes include pathologies of the GI tract such as cholecystitis, appendicitis, pancreatitis, and diverticulitis. Acute abdomen is commonly a sign of an inflamed peritoneum (peritonitis), which is often due to a surgically correctable problem. Patients with an acute abdomen often receive a laparotomy and/or laparoscopy because it signifies a potentially life-threatening condition. The best physical exam confirmations of peritonitis are **rebound tenderness** and **involuntary guarding.** Rebound tenderness is elicited by letting go quickly after deep palpation of the abdomen. Pain occurs in the area of palpation (with generalized peritonitis) or at the location of localized inflammation (e.g., Rovsing sign in appendicitis). Involuntary guarding describes abdominal wall muscle spasm that cannot be controlled. Voluntary guarding (person reflexively or willfully tenses the abdomen during attempted palpation) and tenderness to palpations are softer signs often present in benign diseases.

15. **What should you do if you are not sure whether a stable patient has an acute abdomen?**
When you are in doubt and the patient is stable, use as-needed pain medications (studies have shown that pain control does not delay diagnosis significantly but does improve the patient's experience), perform serial abdominal exams, and consider CT scan. If the patient becomes unstable, proceed to laparoscopy and/or laparotomy. You do not need to have a specific diagnosis before, just make sure that you rule out problems that act as mimics of acute abdomen (e.g., GERD, pulmonary embolism, myocardial ischemia, pneumonia) before proceeding.

16. **Name a few causes of peritonitis that do not require laparotomy or laparoscopy.**
Pancreatitis, many cases of diverticulitis, renal stones, and spontaneous bacterial peritonitis.

17. **Specify which conditions are associated with pain and peritonitis in the listed abdominal areas.**

Area	Organ (Conditions)
Right upper quadrant	Gallbladder/biliary (cholecystitis, cholangitis) or liver (abscess)
Left upper quadrant	Spleen (rupture with blunt trauma)
Right lower quadrant	Appendix (appendicitis), pelvic inflammatory disease (PID)
Left lower quadrant	Sigmoid colon (diverticulitis), PID
Epigastric area	Stomach (peptic ulcer) or pancreas (pancreatitis)

SMALL INTESTINE/COLON AND RECTUM

1. **Specify the classic differences between Crohn disease and ulcerative colitis.**

	Crohn Disease	Ulcerative Colitis
Place of origin	Distal ileum, proximal colon	Rectum
Thickness of pathology	Transmural	Mucosa/submucosa only
Progression	Irregular (skip-lesions)	Proximal, continuous from rectum; no skipped areas
Location	From mouth to anus	Involves only colon, rarely extends to ileum
Bowel habit changes	Obstruction, abdominal pain	Bloody diarrhea
Classic lesions	Fistulas/abscesses, cobblestoning, creeping fat, string sign on barium x-ray	Pseudopolyps, lead-pipe colon on barium x-ray, toxic megacolon
Histology	Noncaseating granulomas	Crypt abscesses
Colon cancer risk	Slightly increased	Markedly increased
Surgery	No (may make worse)	Yes (proctocolectomy with ileoanal anastomosis)

2. **Describe the extraintestinal manifestations of inflammatory bowel disease.**
Both forms of inflammatory bowel disease can cause uveitis, arthritis, ankylosing spondylitis, erythema nodosum, erythema multiforme, primary sclerosing cholangitis, failure to thrive or grow in children, toxic megacolon, anemia of chronic disease, and fever. Toxic megacolon is more common in ulcerative colitis; look for markedly distended colon on abdominal radiograph.

3. **How is inflammatory bowel disease treated?**
Patients with ulcerative colitis are treated with 5-aminosalicylic acid (5-ASA), with or without a sulfa drug (e.g., sulfasalazine), when stable. For both Crohn disease and ulcerative colitis, steroids and other immune modulators (e.g., azathioprine, cyclosporine, methotrexate) are used during severe disease flare-ups. Maintenance therapy depends on disease severity but often includes biologic agents such as tumor necrosis factor-alpha inhibitors.

4. **What causes toxic megacolon? How is it treated?**

   Toxic megacolon is classically seen with inflammatory bowel disease (especially ulcerative colitis) and infectious colitis (especially *Clostridium difficile*). In patients with HIV/acquired immunodeficiency syndrome (AIDS), tissue-invasive cytomegalovirus is the most common cause. It may be precipitated by the use of antidiarrheal medications, for which reason they are usually not given for infectious diarrhea. Most patients have a high fever, leukocytosis, abdominal pain, rebound tenderness, and a dilated segment of colon on abdominal radiograph. Toxic megacolon is an emergency! Start treatment by discontinuing all antidiarrheal medications. Do not allow the patient to eat, place a nasogastric tube, and start intravenous fluids. Give antibiotics to cover bowel flora (such as ceftriaxone and metronidazole). Give steroids if the cause is inflammatory bowel disease. Surgery is required if perforation occurs (free air is seen on abdominal radiograph).

5. **True or False: Children may develop inflammatory bowel disease and irritable bowel syndrome.**

   True. Abdominal pain may be the result of inflammatory bowel disease or irritable bowel syndrome. Diarrhea, fever, bloody stools, anemia, joint pains, and poor growth are more concerning for inflammatory bowel disease. GI complaints may be due to anxiety or psychiatric problems. Watch for separation anxiety, children who do not want to go to school, depression, and child abuse.

6. **Define diverticulosis. What are its complications?**

   Diverticulosis is characterized by saclike mucosal projections through the muscular layer of the colon and/or rectum. It is extremely common, and the incidence increases with age. It is thought to be caused in part by a low-fiber, high-fat diet, which in turn leads to constipation and increased luminal pressure. It is most common in the sigmoid colon. Complications include diverticular GI bleeding (common cause of painless lower GI bleeds and is most commonly found in the right colon) and diverticulitis (inflammation of a diverticulum). Diverticulitis can lead to abscess formation, fistula formation, sepsis, or large bowel obstruction.

7. **What is the cause of left lower quadrant pain and fever in a patient over 50 years old until proven otherwise? How is it treated?**

   Diverticulitis. Treat medically with broad-spectrum antibiotics (e.g., ciprofloxacin plus metronidazole), intravenous fluids, initial bowel rest with gradual advancement of diet, and a nasogastric tube if nausea and vomiting are present. For disease that recurs or is refractory to medical therapy, consider sigmoid colon resection.

8. **How do you diagnose and treat diverticulitis? What test should a patient have after a treated episode of diverticulitis?**

   Signs and symptoms of diverticulitis include left lower quadrant pain or tenderness, fever, diarrhea or constipation, and leukocytosis. The pathophysiology is similar to appendicitis: stool or other debris impacts within the out-pouched mucosa (the diverticulum) and causes obstruction, leading to bacterial overgrowth and inflammation. The diagnosis can be confirmed with a CT scan, if needed, which can also help to rule out complications such as perforation or abscess. A kidney, ureter, bladder (KUB) x-ray can be used to assess for ileus or perforation. In the absence of complications, the treatment is antibiotics that cover bowel flora (e.g., a fluoroquinolone plus metronidazole) and bowel rest (i.e., no oral intake). Antibiotics in complicated diverticulitis become more broad spectrum and include piperacillin/tazobactam or one of the -penems. Surgery in the form of a bowel resection may be needed when diverticulitis is complicated by perforation or abscess. Percutaneous CT drainage of an abscess is indicated if greater than 3 cm.

   After a treated episode of diverticulitis, all patients need colon cancer screening with colonoscopy (colon carcinoma with perforation can mimic diverticulitis clinically and on CT). These studies should be avoided during active diverticulitis, however, due to an increased risk for perforation. Patients should maintain a high-fiber diet.

9. **Define irritable bowel syndrome. How do you recognize it? How do you treat it?**

   Irritable bowel syndrome is a common cause of GI complaints. Patients may have psychiatric comorbidities and a history of diarrhea aggravated by stress, bloating, abdominal pain relieved by defecation, and/or mucus in the stool. There is a female-to-male predominance of 3:1, and patients are usually younger. Look for psychosocial stressors in the history and normal exam findings and test results. Irritable bowel syndrome is diagnosed via the Rome III criteria of abdominal pain plus two of the following: pain related to defecation, pain associated with a change in stool frequency, or pain associated with a change in stool form. You must do at least basic lab tests to rule out inflammatory bowel disease, celiac disease, and infectious causes; endoscopy should only be performed if alarm features are present.

   Treatment is a combination of nonpharmacologic management and medications. Depending on the type (predominantly diarrheal [IBS-D], predominantly constipation [IBS-C], or mixed), medications can be chosen. For IBS-C, choices include osmotic laxatives (PEG), lubiprostone (a chloride channel activator), or linaclotide (guanylate cyclase agonists). For IBS-D, loperamide is first-line therapy when nonpharmacologic treatment fails. For the abdominal pain, use antispasmodics (i.e., dicyclomine or hyoscyamine) and antidepressants (i.e., tricyclic antidepressants [TCAs]).

10. **How is diarrhea categorized?**
    According to etiology:
    - Systemic (Any illness can cause diarrhea as a systemic symptom, especially in children [e.g., infection].)
    - Osmotic
    - Secretory
    - Malabsorptive
    - Infectious
    - Exudative
    - Altered intestinal transit

11. **Define osmotic diarrhea. How can an easy diagnosis be made?**
    Osmotic diarrhea is caused by nonabsorbable solutes that remain in the bowel, where they retain water (e.g., lactose or other carbohydrate intolerance). It presents with a stool osmolar gap greater than 50 mOsm/kg, no blood or mucus in stool, and positive fecal fat. The stool osmolar gap is calculated with the following equation: $290 - [2 \times (stool\ Na^+ + stool\ K^+)]$. When the patient stops ingesting the offending substance (e.g., avoidance of milk or a trial of fasting), the diarrhea stops—an easy diagnosis.

12. **What causes secretory diarrhea?**
    Secretory diarrhea results when the bowel secretes too much fluid. It presents with a stool osmolar gap less than 50 mOsm/kg, no blood or mucus in stool, and no fecal fat. It is often due to bacterial toxins (cholera, some species of *Escherichia coli*), VIPoma (pancreatic islet cell tumor that secretes vasoactive intestinal peptide), or bile acids (after ileal resection). VIPomas can cause WDHA (watery diarrhea, hypokalemia, achlorhydria) syndrome. Secretory diarrhea persists even when the patient stops eating.

13. **What are the common causes of malabsorptive diarrhea?**
    Celiac disease (look for chronic diarrhea, weight loss, abdominal distention, and dermatitis herpetiformis; avoid gluten in the diet), Crohn disease, and postgastroenteritis (due to depletion of brush-border enzymes). Malabsorptive diarrhea improves with bowel rest (i.e., when the patient is not eating).

14. **What are the common clues to infectious diarrhea? What are the common causes?**
    Look for fever and white blood cells in the stool (only with invasive bacteria such as *Shigella, Salmonella, Yersinia,* and *Campylobacter* spp.; not found with toxigenic bacteria). Fecal inflammatory markers such as fecal calprotectin or fecal lactoferrin are typically elevated. Differentiating between potential causes of infectious diarrhea is difficult. History plays a role. Travel history (Montezuma's revenge caused by *E. coli*) is also a tip-off. *Shigella* infection tends to present with tenesmus. *Salmonella* is associated with consumption of raw chicken or eggs. *E. coli* O157:H7 infection is often spread via uncooked hamburger meat and often does not present with a fever. *C. perfringens* often presents with predominantly crampy abdominal pain. Hikers and stream-drinkers may have *Giardia* infection, which presents with steatorrhea (fatty, greasy, malodorous stools that float) due to small bowel involvement and unique protozoal cysts in the stool. Treat *Giardia* with metronidazole. Also watch for *C. difficile* diarrhea in patients with a history of antibiotic use. Test the stool for *C. difficile* toxin, and if the result is positive, treat with oral vancomycin (fidaxomicin is another option). Intravenous metronidazole may be added in more severe cases. Fecal microbiota transplantation is employed in recurrent cases.

15. **What causes exudative diarrhea?**
    Exudative diarrhea results from inflammation in the bowel mucosa that causes seepage of fluid. Mucosal inflammation is usually due to inflammatory bowel disease (Crohn disease or ulcerative colitis; see question 1) or cancer. Patients commonly have fever as well as white blood cells and other inflammatory markers (e.g., fecal calprotectin) in the stool, as in infectious diarrhea, but a *lack* of pathogenic organisms, chronicity, and extraintestinal symptoms are clues.

16. **What are the common causes of diarrhea due to altered intestinal transit?**
    This type of diarrhea is seen after bowel resections, in patients taking medications that interfere with bowel function, and in patients with thyroid disease (hypo- or hyperthyroidism) or neuropathy (e.g., diabetic diarrhea). Watch for factitious diarrhea, which is caused by secret laxative abuse (endoscopy may reveal pigmented colonic mucosa called melanosis coli). Impaired motility can also occur in autoimmune diseases such as systemic lupus erythematous or amyloidosis.

17. **What should you do if a patient has diarrhea?**
    In all patients with diarrhea, watch for and treat dehydration and electrolyte disturbances, especially metabolic acidosis and hypokalemia. Diarrhea is a common and preventable cause of death in underdeveloped countries. Do a rectal exam, look for occult blood in stool, and examine the stool for bacteria (Gram stain and culture), ova and parasites, fat content (steatorrhea), and white blood cells. If inflammatory bowel disease is suspected, fecal calprotectin is both specific and sensitive.

18. **What should you watch for in children after a bout of diarrhea?**
    After bacterial (especially *E. coli* or *Shigella* sp.) diarrhea in children, watch for **hemolytic uremic syndrome,** which is characterized by thrombocytopenia, microangiopathic hemolytic anemia (schistocytes, helmet cells, and

fragmented red blood cells on peripheral blood smear), and acute renal failure. Treatment is supportive. Patients may need dialysis and/or transfusions.

19. **What is the most common cause of diarrhea in children?**
As a primary cause, viral gastroenteritis is probable (e.g., Norwalk virus, rotavirus). Remember, however, that diarrhea is often a nonspecific sign of any systemic illness (e.g., otitis media, pneumonia, urinary tract infection).

20. **Describe the classic presentation of appendicitis. How is it treated?**
Appendicitis classically presents in 10- to 30-year-olds with a history of crampy, poorly localized periumbilical pain followed by nausea and vomiting. Then the pain localizes to the right lower quadrant, and peritoneal signs develop with worsening of nausea and vomiting. It is said that a patient who is hungry and asking for food does not have appendicitis (called the hamburger sign). A classic clue to the diagnosis is **Rovsing sign:** When you palpate the left lower quadrant and then quickly release your hand, the patient feels increased pain in the right lower quadrant. McBurney point, two-thirds of the way from the umbilicus to the anterior superior iliac spine, is the area of maximal tenderness in the right lower quadrant and the site where an open appendectomy incision is made. Ultrasound and CT are increasingly used to confirm the diagnosis before surgery in stable patients.

21. **What are the hallmarks of small bowel obstruction? How is it treated?**
Small bowel obstruction commonly causes bilious vomiting (early symptom), abdominal distention, constipation, hyperactive bowel sounds (high-pitched, rushing sounds), and usually poorly localized abdominal pain. Radiographs show multiple air-fluid levels. Patients often have a history of previous surgery.
Start treatment by withholding food, placing a nasogastric tube, and giving intravenous fluids. If the obstruction does not resolve or if peritoneal signs develop, laparotomy is usually needed. CT scanning can confirm an uncertain diagnosis in stable patients and may reveal the underlying cause of obstruction.

22. **What are the common causes of a small bowel obstruction?**
In adults, the most common cause is **adhesions,** which usually develop from prior surgery. Incarcerated hernias, Crohn disease, and malignancy are other common causes. Other causes include Meckel diverticulum and intussusception (both typically seen in children) and meconium ileus in newborns with cystic fibrosis.

23. **Describe the signs and symptoms of large bowel obstruction. What causes it? How is it treated?**
Large bowel obstruction usually presents with gradually increasing abdominal pain, abdominal distention, constipation, and feculent vomiting (late symptom). In older adults, the most common causes are diverticulitis, colon cancer, and volvulus (sigmoid most common, followed by cecal). In children, watch for Hirschsprung disease. Treat early by withholding food and placing a nasogastric tube for nausea and vomiting. Sigmoid volvulus can often be decompressed with an endoscope. Other causes or refractory cases require surgery to relieve the obstruction.

24. **What is the rule about occult blood in the stool of a patient over age 40 years?**
Occult blood in the stool of a person older than 40 years should be considered colon cancer until proven otherwise. To rule out colon cancer, do a colonoscopy.

25. **List the primary risk factors for colon cancer.**
Age: incidence begins to increase after age 40 years; peak incidence between 60 and 75 years
Family history: especially with familial polyposis or Gardner, Turcot, Peutz-Jeghers, or Lynch syndrome
Inflammatory bowel disease: ulcerative colitis more than Crohn disease, but both are associated with increased risk
Low-fiber, high-fat diet

26. **How do patients with colon cancer tend to present?**
Patients may present with asymptomatic blood in the stool (visible streaks of blood in stool or positive fecal occult blood test). Anemia is classic with right-sided colon cancer. Change in stool caliber ("pencil stool") or frequency (alternating constipation and frequency) is a classic presentation of left-sided colon cancer. Colon cancer is also a common cause of large bowel obstruction in adults. As with any cancer, look for unintentional weight loss.

27. **How is colon cancer treated?**
Treatment is primarily surgical, with resection of involved bowel. Adjuvant chemotherapy is usually recommended if there is lymph node involvement. Distant metastases frequently go to the liver first (as with all GI tumors). Surgical resection of a solitary liver metastasis is often attempted. With metastases elsewhere, chemotherapy is the only option, and prognosis is poor.

28. **What is the classic tumor marker for colon cancer? How is it used clinically?**
Carcinoembryonic antigen (CEA) may be elevated with colon cancer, and if a patient is found to have colon cancer, the CEA level is usually measured before surgery. If it is elevated preoperatively (not always), the CEA level should return to normal after surgical removal of the tumor. Periodic monitoring of CEA after surgery may help to

detect recurrence before it is clinically apparent. CEA is *not* used as a screening tool for colon cancer; it is used only to follow known cancer because it is neither sensitive nor specific (can be elevated with other visceral tumors).

29. **What are the symptoms of carcinoid tumors? Where are they most commonly found?**
Carcinoid tumors secrete serotonin-like products that can cause symptoms, but the liver breaks down serotonin and other vasoactive secretions to make the tumor initially asymptomatic. Once a carcinoid tumor metastasizes to the liver and vasoactive products reach the systemic circulation, symptoms begin (carcinoid syndrome): epi-sodic cutaneous flushing, abdominal cramps, diarrhea, and right-sided heart valve damage. The most common location is in the small bowel, but carcinoid tumors are also the most common appendiceal tumor (sometimes found at the time of appendectomy in patients with appendicitis).

30. **What lab test detects carcinoid tumors?**
Urinary levels of 5-hydroxyindoleacetic acid (5-HIAA; a serotonin breakdown product) are increased.

GALLBLADDER AND BILE DUCT

1. **What are the classic signs and symptoms of gallstone disease?**
Classic gallstone symptoms include postprandial, colicky pain in the right upper quadrant with bloating and/or nausea and vomiting. The pain usually begins 15 to 60 minutes after a meal (especially a fatty meal). Look for **Murphy sign** (palpation of the right upper quadrant under the rib cage causes arrest of inspiration due to pain) as the main physical exam finding for cholecystitis.

2. **What are the six Fs of cholecystitis? How are the demographics of patients with pigment stones different from those with cholesterol stones?**
The first five Fs summarize the demographics of people with cholesterol gallstones: **f**at, **f**orty, **f**ertile, **f**emale, and **f**latulent; the sixth F is **f**ebrile, which indicates that such patients have now developed acute cholecystitis. Patients with pigment (i.e., calcium bilirubinate) stones, which are brown in color, are classically young patients with hemolytic anemia (e.g., sickle cell disease, hereditary spherocytosis).

3. **How is a clinical suspicion of cholecystitis confirmed and treated?**
Ultrasound is the best first imaging study for suspected gallbladder disease. It may show gallstones, a thin layer of fluid around the gallbladder, and/or a thickened gallbladder wall. A more specific ultrasonographic Murphy sign using direct visualization of the gallbladder can be obtained (variant anatomy and significant obesity can create uncertainty). A nuclear hepatobiliary scintigraphic study (e.g., hepatobiliary iminodiacetic acid [HIDA] scan) clinches the diagnosis with nonvisualization of the gallbladder. The treatment is pain control and cholecystectomy (antibiotics may be indicated if infection is suspected); a laparoscopic approach is generally preferred over an open procedure.

4. **Define cholangitis. How does it differ from cholecystitis? How is it treated?**
Cholangitis is an inflammation of the bile ducts, whereas cholecystitis is an inflammation of the gallbladder. Cholangitis is classically due to biliary obstruction with subsequent bile stasis and infection, and it is much more deadly than cholecystitis. Choledocholithiasis (a gallstone in the common bile duct) and malignancy are common causes of obstruction. Autoimmune cholangitis (e.g., sclerosing cholangitis) and primary infection (e.g., *Clonorchis sinensis* and other parasite infections common in some parts of Asia) are other causes. Cholangitis classically presents with the **Charcot triad:** (1) right upper quadrant pain, (2) fever or shaking chills, and (3) jaundice. Pa-tients may have a history of gallstones. Start broad-spectrum antibiotics to cover bowel flora (e.g., piperacillin with tazobactam), and then manage more definitively depending on the circumstances (e.g., cholecystectomy with evacuation of any common duct stones for gallstone disease, biliary stent placement for unresectable malignant obstruction). If the patient becomes sicker, they may develop the **Reynold pentad**, which includes the Charcot triad plus (4) altered mental status and (5) hypotension.

5. **What usually precipitates acute cholangitis? What is the tip off to its presence? How is it treated?**
Cholangitis is usually precipitated by a gallstone that blocks the common bile duct with subsequent infection of the bile duct system. The tip-off is the presence of **Charcot triad:** fever, right upper quadrant pain, and jaundice. Treat with antibiotics (e.g., piperacillin-tazobactam), and remove gallstones surgically or endoscopically after the acute infection has resolved. The presence of **Reynold pentad** (Charcot triad plus hypotension and altered mental status) implies a more severe presentation requiring more urgent treatment.

6. **Who gets primary sclerosing cholangitis? What clues can help with diagnosis?**
Primary sclerosing cholangitis usually occurs in young adults (M>F) with inflammatory bowel disease (usually ulcerative colitis). It presents similarly to bacterial cholangitis. Fever, chills, pruritis, and right upper quadrant abdominal pain are common. Peripheral antineutrophil cytoplasmic antibodies (P-ANCA) can help with diagnosis. On biopsy, concentric bile duct fibrosis in an "onion-skin" pattern is seen. Sclerosing cholangitis is associated with ulcerative colitis and cholangiocarcinoma.

7. **What signs and symptoms suggest biliary tract obstruction as a cause of jaundice?**
   - Elevated conjugated bilirubin. Conjugated bilirubin is more elevated than unconjugated bilirubin because the liver still functions and can conjugate bilirubin, but conjugated bilirubin cannot be excreted because of biliary tract disease.
   - Markedly elevated alkaline phosphatase
   - Pruritus
   - Clay-colored stools
   - Dark urine that is strongly positive for conjugated bilirubin. Unconjugated bilirubin is not excreted in the urine because it is tightly bound to albumin.

8. **What are the commonly tested types of biliary tract obstructions?**
   Bile duct obstruction, cholestasis, cholangitis, primary biliary cholangitis, and primary sclerosing cholangitis.

9. **What are the two major causes of common bile duct obstruction? How are they distinguished?**
   The most common cause is obstruction with a gallstone (choledocholithiasis). Look for a history of gallstones or the four *F*s (female, forty, fertile, and fat). Ultrasound often identifies the stone; if not, use magnetic resonance cholangiopancreatography (MRCP) or endoscopic retrograde cholangiopancreatography (ERCP). ERCP can be therapeutic. Treatment is endoscopic removal of the stone. The second major cause of common bile duct obstruction is cancer. Look for weight loss. Pancreatic cancer is the most common type; look for **Courvoisier sign** (painless jaundice with a palpably enlarged gallbladder). Sometimes cholangiocarcinoma or bowel cancer blocks the common bile duct.

10. **What are the two common causes of cholestasis?**
    Medications (e.g., birth control pills, trimethoprim-sulfamethoxazole, phenothiazines, androgens) and pregnancy.

11. **What clues suggest a diagnosis of primary biliary cholangitis (formerly primary biliary cirrhosis)?**
    This condition is usually seen in middle-aged women with no risk factors for liver or biliary disease. It causes marked pruritus, jaundice, and positive **antimitochondrial antibodies.** It is also associated with cutaneous xanthomas and osteoporosis. The rest of the workup is negative. Cholestyramine can help with symptoms. Ursodeoxycholic acid can delay progression, but the only treatment is liver transplantation.

12. **Which diseases can cause elevated levels of alkaline phosphatase? What additional lab tests may be used to distinguish among these diseases?**
    Alkaline phosphatase may be elevated in biliary disease, bone disease, or pregnancy (the placenta produces alkaline phosphatase). If the elevation is due to biliary disease, gamma-glutamyltranspeptidase (GGT; also called gamma-glutamyl transferase) and/or 5'-nucleotidase (5'-NT) will also be elevated. In bone disease and pregnancy, however, GGT and 5'-NT will be within normal limits.

LIVER

1. **List the common findings of acute liver disease.**
   - Elevated liver function tests (aspartate aminotransferase [AST], alanine aminotransferase [ALT], bilirubin, alkaline phosphatase, and/or prothrombin time [PT] and international normalized ratio [INR])
   - Jaundice
   - Dark urine
   - Pale stools
   - Nausea and vomiting
   - Right upper quadrant pain or tenderness
   - Hepatomegaly

2. **List the common causes of acute liver disease.**
   - Alcohol
   - Medications
   - Infection (usually viral hepatitis such as HBV or HCV)
   - Reye syndrome
   - Biliary tract disease
   - Autoimmune disease
        A helpful mnemonic to remember potential causes of liver disease/cirrhosis is **ABCDEFGHI: a**utoimmune hepatitis, hepatitis **B**, hepatitis **C, d**rugs/toxins, **e**thanol, **f**atty liver (nonalcoholic steatohepatitis), **g**rowths, **h**emodynamic congestive heart failure, **i**ron/copper/A1AT deficiency.

3. **What are the classic causes of drug-induced hepatitis?**
   Acetaminophen, isoniazid, and other tuberculosis drugs (e.g., rifampin and pyrazinamide), halothane, HMG-CoA reductase inhibitors, and carbon tetrachloride. The first step in treatment is to stop the drug.

4. When should you suspect idiopathic autoimmune hepatitis? What is the serologic marker?

Idiopathic autoimmune hepatitis is classically seen in 20- to 40-year-old women with anti–smooth muscle or antinuclear antibodies and no risk factors or lab markers for other causes of hepatitis. Treat with steroids.

5. What are the usual causes of chronic liver disease?

Alcohol, hepatitis, and metabolic diseases. Watch for the stigmata of chronic liver disease: jaundice, gynecomastia, testicular atrophy, palmar erythema, spider angiomata on skin, asterixis, and ascites.

6. What is the most common cause of cirrhosis and esophageal varices?

Alcohol.

7. Define hemochromatosis. How do you recognize it?

Hemochromatosis, in its primary form, is usually autosomal recessive; look for a family history. Nearly 1 in 250 people in the United States are homozygous for this condition, although penetrance and clinical expression are variable. The pathophysiology is incompletely understood but includes excessive iron absorption by the intestine caused by *HFE* gene mutations, which prevents transferrin from binding to its receptor, ultimately exposing the blood to excessive iron levels. Excessive iron is deposited in the liver (potentially causing cirrhosis and/or hepato-cellular carcinoma), pancreas (potentially causing diabetes), heart (resulting in dilated or restrictive cardiomyopa-thy), skin (causing hyperpigmentation classically known as **bronze diabetes**), hypogonadism, and joints (arthritis). Men are symptomatic earlier and more often, because women lose iron with menstruation. Treat with phlebotomy and/or deferoxamine. Secondary iron overload can cause secondary hemochromatosis, which is classically due to an anemia that results in ineffective erythropoiesis (e.g., thalassemia) and excessive iron intake.

8. Define Wilson disease. How do you recognize it? How is it treated?

Wilson disease is an autosomal recessive disease caused by the effects of excessive serum copper. Serum **ceru-loplasmin** (a copper transport protein) is usually low or absent, and serum copper may be normal. Biopsy shows excessive copper in the liver. Patients classically have liver disease with central nervous system and psychiatric manifestations (due to copper deposits in the basal ganglia; another name for this disease is hepatolenticular degeneration) and **Kayser-Fleischer** rings in the eye. Treat with penicillamine (copper chelator).

9. What are the clues to a diagnosis of alpha$_1$-antitrypsin (AAT) deficiency?

The classic description is a young adult who develops cirrhosis and/or emphysema without risk factors for either. AAT deficiency has an autosomal recessive inheritance pattern; look for a positive family history. It is also associ-ated with panniculitis. Diagnosis requires a serum AAT less than 11 μmol/L as well as a severely deficient geno-type. Treatment involves intravenous pooled human AAT.

10. What metabolic derangements accompany liver failure?

Coagulopathy: prolonged PT. In severe cases, partial thromboplastin time (PTT) also may be prolonged. Vitamin K does not resolve the coagulopathy because it cannot be utilized by the damaged liver. Symptomatic patients must be treated with fresh frozen plasma.

Jaundice/hyperbilirubinemia: elevated conjugated and unconjugated bilirubin with hepatic damage (vs biliary tract disease; see later).

Hypoalbuminemia: the liver synthesizes albumin.

Ascites: due to portal hypertension and/or hypoalbuminemia. Ascites can be detected on physical exam by shifting dullness or a positive fluid wave. A possible complication is **spontaneous bacterial peritonitis** due to infected ascitic fluid that can lead to sepsis. Look for fever and/or change in mental status in a patient with known ascites. Perform a paracentesis, examine the ascitic fluid for elevated white blood cell count (a level >250 neutrophils is diagnostic), and do Gram stain, culture and sensitivity tests, glucose (low with infection), and protein (<1 g/dL). The usual causes are *E. coli, Streptococcus pneumoniae,* and other enteric bugs. Treat with broad-spectrum antibi-otics (cefotaxime is a common choice). A serum ascites albumin gradient (SAAG) of greater than 1.1 implicates portal hypertension as the etiology. Prophylaxis includes diuretics and, in certain cases, fluoroquinolones.

Portal hypertension: seen with cirrhosis (chronic liver disease); causes hemorrhoids, esophageal varices, and caput medusae (engorged veins on the abdominal wall).

Hyperammonemia: the liver clears ammonia. Treat with decreased protein intake (source of ammonia) and lactulose (a laxative that alters luminal pH to disfavor ammonia absorption). The last choice is rifaximin, which kills bowel flora that make ammonia.

Hepatic encephalopathy: mostly due to hyperammonemia; often precipitated by high protein intake, GI bleed, or infection. Look for asterixis (the flapping of outstretched hands) and/or mental status changes. Additionally, it can be precipitated by hypokalemia, metabolic alkalosis, and the placement of a TIPS. In addition to treating hyperammonemia, look for and treat the underlying cause.

Hepatorenal syndrome: liver failure may cause kidney failure. This portends a poor prognosis. The pathophysiol-ogy is complicated, but it is due to portal hypertension causing increased nitric oxide production in the splanchnic circulation. This leads to systemic vasodilation and renal hypoperfusion. The renin-aldosterone-angiotensin system is activated and causes local renal vasoconstriction. It is treated with albumin and splanchnic vasoconstrictors (i.e., octreotide or midodrine).

Hypoglycemia: the liver stores glycogen.

Disseminated intravascular coagulation: activated clotting factors are cleared by the liver.

11. **What are the classic physical stigmata of liver disease in those with alcohol use disorder?**
    - Abdominal wall varices (caput medusae)
    - Testicular atrophy
    - Esophageal varices
    - Encephalopathy
    - Hemorrhoids (internal)
    - Asterixis
    - Jaundice
    - Scleral icterus
    - Ascites
    - Edema
    - Palmar erythema
    - Spider angiomas
    - Gynecomastia
    - Terry nails (white nails with a ground-glass appearance and no lunula)
    - Fetor hepaticus ("breath of the dead," which is a sweet, fecal smell)
    - Dupuytren contractures

12. **What are the classic laboratory findings of liver disease in those with alcohol use disorder?**
    - Anemia (classically macrocytic)
    - Prolonged prothrombin time
    - Hyperbilirubinemia
    - Hypoalbuminemia
    - Thrombocytopenia
    - Leukocytosis (predominantly neutrophils)

13. **Describe the classic derangement of AST and ALT in alcoholic hepatitis.**
    The ratio of AST (also known as serum glutamate oxaloacetate transaminase [SGOT]) to ALT (also known as serum glutamate pyruvate transaminase [SGPT]) is at least 2:1, although levels of both may be elevated. Other causes of hepatitis are usually associated with the opposite ratio or equal elevation of both AST and ALT.

14. **What increases the risk for hepatocellular cancer? What is the classic tumor marker for liver cancer?**
    The same factors that increase the risk for cirrhosis. The big three are alcohol, chronic hepatitis (hepatitis C is now a more likely culprit than hepatitis B), and hemochromatosis. **Alpha-fetoprotein** is often elevated and can be measured postoperatively to detect recurrences. It can also be used for screening, along with ultrasound, in high-risk populations (e.g., those with cirrhosis).

15. **How do patients with liver cancer present? How is liver cancer treated?**
    Patients often have a history of alcoholism, hepatitis, and/or hemochromatosis or other causes of cirrhosis. They present with weight loss, right upper quadrant pain, and an enlarged liver. Surgery (e.g., resection, transplantation) is the only hope for cure. The prognosis is poor.

16. **What other tumors of the liver may appear on the USMLE? What clues suggest their presence?**
    Hemangioma: most common primary tumor of the liver; benign and generally left alone. Surgery is done only if symptomatic (pain, bleeding).
    Hepatic adenoma: benign tumor in women of reproductive age who take **birth control pills.** Stop the birth control pills, and the tumor may regress. If not, surgery is usually preferred to prevent hemorrhage and rare malignant transformation.
    Cholangiocarcinoma: malignant. Fifty percent of patients have inflammatory bowel disease (especially ulcerative colitis). Liver flukes (*Clonorchis* sp.) increase the risk in some immigrant populations (China, Japan, Taiwan, Vietnam, Korea, far eastern Russia).
    Angiosarcoma: malignant. Look for industrial exposure to vinyl chloride.
    Hepatoblastoma: malignant; the most common primary liver malignancy in children.

17. **Name three medications that cause hepatic enzyme induction and two that cause hepatic enzyme inhibition.**
    Barbiturates, antiepileptics (AEDs), and rifampin are the classic enzyme inducers; cimetidine, erythromycin, and ketoconazole are classic enzyme inhibitors. The end result may be ineffectiveness or toxicity of other administered drugs (e.g., warfarin, oral contraceptives, and antiepileptics).

18. **What happens with an overdose of acetaminophen?**
    High doses of acetaminophen cause liver toxicity due to the toxic metabolite NAPQI, which causes depletion of glutathione by overloading glutathione stores. Treat with **N-acetylcysteine** to decrease liver injury by regenerating glutathione.

PANCREAS

1. **Describe the classic presentation of pancreatic cancer. How is it treated? What is the cell of origin?**
   The classic patient is a 40- to 80-year-old smoker who has lost weight and has painless jaundice. Other signs and symptoms include depression, epigastric pain, migratory thrombophlebitis (**Trousseau syndrome,** which may also be seen with other visceral cancers), and a palpable, nontender gallbladder (**Courvoisier sign**). Pancreatic cancer is more common in men than in women, in diabetics than in nondiabetics, and in blacks than in whites. Surgery (Whipple procedure) is rarely curative, and the prognosis is generally dismal. Chemotherapy is minimally successful at prolonging survival. The cell of origin in pancreatic cancer is ductal epithelium.

2. **What is the most common islet cell tumor of the pancreas? How is it diagnosed?**
   Insulinomas (beta cell tumor) are the most common islet cell tumors. Look for two-thirds of the **Whipple triad:** hypoglycemia (glucose <50 mg/dL) and central nervous symptoms due to hypoglycemia (confusion, stupor, loss of consciousness). As a good doctor, you provide the third part of the Whipple triad: administration of glucose or glucagon to relieve symptoms. Ninety percent of insulinomas are benign and can be cured with resection, if possible. In your workup, take a history and check the C-peptide level first to make sure that the patient is not a diabetic who is taking too much insulin or a patient with factitious disorder. C-peptide levels are high with insulinoma and low with the other disorders.

3. **Name the other two islet cell tumors. What should islet cell tumors make you think about?**
   1. **Glucagonomas** (alpha cell tumor) cause hyperglycemia with high glucagon levels and necrolytic migratory erythema.
   2. **VIPomas** (tumors that secrete vasoactive intestinal peptide [VIP]) cause watery diarrhea, hypokalemia, and achlorhydria.
   Watch for multiple endocrine neoplasia (MEN) syndromes in patients with islet cell tumors.

4. **What are the signs and symptoms of acute pancreatitis?**
   Patients classically have epigastric abdominal pain that radiates to the back and decreases when leaning forward, nausea with vomiting that fails to relieve the pain, leukocytosis, and elevated amylase and lipase (more specific) levels. Watch for **Grey Turner sign** (blue-black flanks) and **Cullen sign** (blue-black umbilicus), both of which are due to a hemorrhagic pancreatic exudate and indicative of severe pancreatitis. Remember that perforated ulcers are also associated with elevated amylase and lipase levels and present similarly. However, patients usually have free air on abdominal radiographs and a history of PUD. Diagnosis of acute pancreatitis requires two of the following: characteristic abdominal pain, elevated amylase or lipase three times the upper limit of normal, and characteristic appearance on CT.

5. **Other than pancreatic disease, what else can cause elevated levels of amylase?**
   Damage to the salivary glands or bowel, renal failure, and ruptured tubal pregnancy may cause elevated amylase levels. Lipase is more specific for pancreatic pathology, and elevation of both amylase and lipase levels in the same patient is usually due to pancreatitis. The boards may try to trick you with isolated elevation of the amylase level.

6. **What causes acute pancreatitis?**
   More than 80% of cases are due to alcohol or gallstones. Remember the mnemonic **I GET SMASHED:**
   I = idiopathic
   G = gallstones
   E = ethanol
   T = trauma
   S = steroids
   M = mumps (and other infections) or malignancy
   A = autoimmune
   S = scorpion sting
   H = hypercalcemia or hypertriglyceridemia
   E = ERCP trauma
   D = drugs (e.g., isoniazid, furosemide, simvastatin, steroids, azathioprine)

7. **How is acute pancreatitis treated?**
   Patients are not allowed to eat, a nasogastric tube is often placed, and intravenous fluids and narcotics are given. For pain control, hydromorphone or fentanyl is often used. Other options include meperidine (which has a risk of seizures) or morphine (which causes sphincter of Oddi spasm, which increases pancreatitis risk, though clinical evidence of this is lacking).

8. **What are the complications of acute pancreatitis?**
   Early complications include acute respiratory distress syndrome, pleural effusion, and pancreatic ascites. Late complications include pseudocyst formation (drain surgically if symptomatic, persistent for several weeks, or >6 cm), abscess or infection (treat with antibiotics and drainage if needed), and chronic pancreatitis (calcifications of the pancreas may be seen on CT or plain abdominal films).

9. What causes chronic pancreatitis? How is it treated?

Chronic pancreatitis in the United States is almost always due to alcoholism and usually results from repeated bouts of acute pancreatitis. Gallstones do not cause chronic pancreatitis. Chronic pancreatitis may lead to diabetes, steatorrhea (excessive fat in the stool due to lack of pancreatic enzymes), calcification of the pancreas (which may be seen on a plain abdominal radiograph), and fat-soluble vitamin deficiencies (due to malabsorption). The incidence of pancreatic cancer is slightly increased in patients with pancreatitis, although smoking is a greater risk factor than alcohol for pancreatic cancer.

Treat chronic pancreatitis with alcohol abstinence, oral pancreatic enzyme replacement, and fat-soluble vitamin supplements.

NUTRITIONAL DISORDERS

1. What may happen if you give glucose to a person with alcohol use disorder without giving thiamine first?

You may precipitate Wernicke encephalopathy. Always give thiamine before glucose to avoid this complication.

2. What is the difference between Wernicke and Korsakoff syndromes? What causes each?

Wernicke syndrome is an acute encephalopathy characterized by ophthalmoplegia (paralysis of extraocular muscles), nystagmus, ataxia, and/or confusion. It can be fatal but is often reversible with thiamine.

Korsakoff syndrome is a chronic psychosis characterized by anterograde amnesia (inability to form new memories) and confabulation (making up stories) to cover up the amnesia. Korsakoff syndrome is generally irreversible and is thought to be due to damage to the mammillary bodies and thalamic nuclei. Both conditions result from thiamine deficiency.

3. Which vitamin deficiencies may lead to neurologic signs or symptoms?

Vitamin B_{12}: dementia, peripheral neuropathy, loss of vibration sense in the lower extremities, loss of position sense, ataxia, spasticity, hyperactive reflexes, and positive Babinski sign.

Thiamine: peripheral neuropathy, confusion, ophthalmoplegia, nystagmus, ataxia, confusion, delirium, and dementia.

Vitamin E: loss of proprioception/vibratory sensation, areflexia, ataxia, and gaze palsy.

Vitamin A: vision loss.

Vitamin B_6: peripheral sensory neuropathy (watch for isoniazid as a cause, and give prophylactic B_6 to patients taking isoniazid, if given the choice).

4. Specify the signs and symptoms of the various vitamin deficiencies and toxicities.

Vitamin	Deficiency	Toxicity
A	Nyctalopia (night blindness), xerosis cutis (dry skin) and scaly rash, xerophthalmia (dry eyes), Bitot spots (debris on conjunctiva); increased infections	Pseudotumor cerebri, bone thickening, teratogenic (craniofacial and heart defects)
C (ascorbic acid)	Scurvy (hemorrhages, skin petechiae, gingivitis, loose teeth), poor wound healing, hyperkeratotic hair follicles, bone pain (from periosteal hemorrhages)	Nephrolithiasis; can worsen hemochromatosis by promoting iron absorption
D	Rickets, osteomalacia, hypocalcemia	Hypercalcemia, nausea, renal toxicity
E	Anemia, peripheral neuropathy, ataxia	Necrotizing enterocolitis (infants)
K	Hemorrhage, prolonged prothrombin time	Hemolysis (can lead to kernicterus)
B_1 (thiamine)	Wet beriberi (high-output cardiac failure), dry beriberi (peripheral neuropathy), Wernicke and Korsakoff syndromes	
B_2 (riboflavin)	Angular stomatitis, dermatitis	
B_3 (niacin)	Pellagra (dementia, dermatitis, diarrhea), stomatitis	
B_6 (pyridoxine)	Peripheral neuropathy, stomatitis, convulsions in infants, microcytic anemia, seborrheic dermatitis	Peripheral neuropathy (only B vitamin with toxicity)
B_{12} (cobalamin)	Megaloblastic anemia *plus* neurologic symptoms (subacute combined degeneration, dementia, ataxia)	
Folic acid	Megaloblastic anemia *without* neurologic symptoms	

5. Specify the signs and symptoms of the various mineral deficiencies and toxicities.

Mineral	Deficiency	Toxicity
Iron	Microcytic anemia, koilonychia (spoon-shaped fingernails)	Hemochromatosis
Iodine	Goiter, cretinism, hypothyroidism	Myxedema
Fluoride	Dental caries (cavities)	Fluorosis with mottling of teeth and bone exostoses

Mineral	Deficiency	Toxicity
Zinc	Hypogeusia (decreased taste), rash, slow wound healing	
Copper	Menkes syndrome (X-linked; kinky hair, intellectual disability)	Wilson disease
Selenium	Cardiomyopathy and muscle pain	Loss of hair and nails
Manganese	Dermatitis	Manganese madness in miners of ore (behavioral changes/psychosis)
Chromium	Impaired glucose tolerance	

6. **What are the fat-soluble vitamins? In what general category of patients are they deficient?**
Vitamins A, D, E, and K are fat soluble. Deficiency of any of these vitamins may be due to malabsorption (e.g., cystic fibrosis, cirrhosis, celiac disease, duodenal bypass, bile-duct obstruction, pancreatic insufficiency, chronic giardiasis). In such patients, parenteral supplements are required if high-dose oral supplements fail.

7. **What vitamin, mineral, and electrolyte deficiencies are classically seen in patients with alcohol use disorder?**
Any can be seen, but watch especially for folate, thiamine, phosphorus, and magnesium deficiencies.

8. **What is the most common cause of vitamin B_{12} deficiency?**
Pernicious anemia, in which antiparietal cell antibodies destroy the ability to secrete intrinsic factor. Conditions associated with pernicious anemia include autoimmune disease such as hypothyroidism, type 1 diabetes, and vitiligo. Removal of the ileum and the tapeworm *Diphyllobothrium latum* are exotic causes of B_{12} deficiency. Diagnosis of pernicious anemia is clinched by a low serum B_{12} level. The presence of antiintrinsic factor antibodies is highly confirmatory for pernicious anemia. There is emerging evidence that medications, such as PPIs, H2 blockers, and metformin, increase the risk of B_{12} deficiency. Diagnosis of B_{12} deficiency can be confirmed by elevated levels of methylmalonic acid (MMA), especially in cases of borderline levels of B_{12}. Of note, increased levels of MMA also help to distinguish B_{12} deficiency from folate deficiency, both of which can present as megaloblastic anemia. The Schilling test is of historical interest but is no longer commonly employed in the diagnosis of B_{12} deficiency.

9. **How is vitamin B_{12} deficiency treated?**
Vitamin B_{12} supplements are given. The usual replacement is via parenteral (intramuscular) injection or high-dose oral replacement. Because of the potential for erratic absorption, oral replacement may be best utilized after levels have been normalized via the parenteral route. Supplementation may be required for life.

10. **What is the classic iatrogenic cause of vitamin B_6 deficiency?**
Prolonged therapy with isoniazid (especially in young people). Pyridoxine supplementation is recommended for patients on isoniazid therapy for tuberculosis.

11. **What causes folate deficiency? In what patient populations is it commonly seen?**
Folate deficiency is commonly seen in those with alcohol use disorder (poor folate intake) and pregnant women (increased need). All women of reproductive age should take folate supplements (ideally before pregnancy occurs) to prevent neural tube defects in their offspring. Rare causes of folate deficiency include poor diet (e.g., "tea and toast" diet), methotrexate, prolonged therapy with trimethoprim-sulfamethoxazole, anticonvulsant therapy (especially phenytoin), and malabsorption. Look for macrocytes and **hypersegmented neutrophils** with no neurologic signs or symptoms and low folate levels in serum or red blood cells. Treat with oral folate.

12. **Which medications may cause folate deficiency?**
Anticonvulsants (especially phenytoin), methotrexate, and trimethoprim.

13. **What are the physical findings of rickets (vitamin D deficiency) in children?**
   - Craniotabes (poorly mineralized skull; bones feel like a ping-pong ball)
   - Rachitic rosary (costochondral beading; small round masses on anterior rib cage)
   - Delayed fontanelle closure
   - Bossing of the skull
   - Kyphoscoliosis
   - Bow-legs and knock-knees
Bone changes appear first at the lower ends of the radius and ulna.

14. **Describe the relationship between vitamin K and broad-spectrum antibiotics.**
Prolonged therapy with broad-spectrum antibiotics is a potential cause of vitamin K deficiency. These medications can eliminate the normal gut bacteria that synthesize much of the vitamin K required daily.

15. **What is the classic Step 3 description of a vitamin C–deficient patient?**
An elderly person with a diet of "hot dogs and soda" or "tea and toast" who presents with bleeding gums and bone pain.

INFECTIONS

1. **What clues suggest hepatitis A? Describe the diagnostic serology.**
   Look for outbreaks from a foodborne source, commonly during or after travel. There are no long-term sequelae of infection, although acute liver failure is a remote possibility. Immunoglobulin M (IgM) antihepatitis A virus (HAV) is positive during jaundice or shortly thereafter. The incubation period for hepatitis A is about 4 weeks, though IgM may be detected by the time symptoms begin. Treatment is supportive. Infection can be prevented with vaccination.

2. **How is hepatitis B acquired? What is the best treatment?**
   Hepatitis B is acquired through needles, sex, or perinatal transmission. Transfused blood is now screened for hepatitis B, but this risk of transmission is still about 1/200,000 according to the American Red Cross. A history of transfusion years prior is still a risk factor (screening by blood banks began in 1972 in the United States). Prevention is the best treatment via vaccination. Interferon alfa-2b, peginterferon alfa-2a, adefovir, dipivoxil, entecavir, telbivudine, or tenofovir can be tried in patients with chronic hepatitis and elevated liver enzymes.

3. **Describe the serology of hepatitis B infection, including the surface, core, and "e" markers.**
   The hepatitis B surface antigen (HBsAg) is positive with any unresolved infection (acute or chronic). The hepatitis B "e" antigen (HBeAg) is a marker for infectivity; patients positive for the hepatitis B "e" antibody (HBeAb) have a low likelihood of spreading disease. The first antibody to appear is the IgM hepatitis B core antibody (HBcAb), which appears during the so-called window phase when both HBsAg and hepatitis B surface antibody (HBsAb) are negative. Positive HBsAb means that the patient is immune (as a result of either recovery from infection or vaccination); HBsAb never appears if the patient has chronic hepatitis.
   Make sure you know and understand the following table as it is high yield.
   Serologic Markers at Different Stages of Disease

	HBsAg	HBeAg	HBeAb	HBsAb	HBcAb
Incubation	+	+	−	−	−
Acute stage	+	+	−	−	+
Persistent carrier	+	+/−	−/+	−	+
Recovery (immune)	−	−	+	+	+
Immunization	−	−	−	+	−

The presence of HBeAg and HBeAb depends on the degree of infectivity.
Adapted from Cohen J, Powderly WG, Berkley SF, et al. *Infectious Diseases.* 2nd ed. Edinburgh: Mosby; 2004:2015, with permission.

4. **What are the possible sequelae of chronic HBV or hepatitis C virus (HCV) infection?**
   Cirrhosis and hepatocellular cancer (only with chronic, not acute, infection).

5. **What should be given to persons acutely exposed to hepatitis B?**
   Hepatitis B immunoglobulin and hepatitis B vaccination alone have been demonstrated to be effective in preventing transmission after exposure to HBV.

6. **Which type of viral hepatitis is the most common cause of chronic hepatitis?**
   Hepatitis C. HCV is the most likely cause of hepatitis after a blood transfusion. Although blood is now screened for hepatitis B and C, the hepatitis C test was developed later (screening in the United States began in 1972 for hepatitis B and 1992 for hepatitis C). Hepatitis C is also more likely than hepatitis B to progress to chronic hepatitis, cirrhosis, and cancer. The US Preventive Services Task Force now recommends that all adults ages 18 to 79 years be screened for hepatitis C.

7. **Describe the serology and treatment for hepatitis C.**
   A positive hepatitis C antibody means that the patient has had an infection in the past but does not mean the infection has been cleared. Most patients become chronic carriers of the virus. A test for HCV RNA is available to detect and quantify the viral load. Patients with hepatitis C should also be tested for HIV and hepatitis B. They should be tested for antibodies to hepatitis A and B to determine if vaccination is required.
   Treatment of hepatitis C is rapidly evolving since the development of direct-acting antiviral medications. These medications are highly effective and offer the potential to avoid treatment with interferon and sometimes ribavirin. All patients with a detectable HCV level over a 6-month period should be considered for treatment. Treatment regimens depend on the hepatitis C genotype. Genotype 1 is the most common in the United States. Specific treatment regimens are likely beyond the scope of USMLE Step 3 but are included here for thoroughness:
   - Ledipasvir-sofosbuvir
   - Elbasvir-grazoprevir with or without ribavirin
   - Ombitasvir-paritaprevir-ritonavir plus dasabuvir with or without ribavirin
   - Simeprevir plus sofosbuvir
   - Daclatasvir plus sofosbuvir
     A virologic response to treatment is assessed by measuring the viral load at 12 weeks following completion of therapy. A sustained virologic response is defined as an undetectable viral load at 24 weeks posttreatment.

8. When is hepatitis D seen? Describe the serology.

Hepatitis D is seen only in patients with hepatitis B. It may become chronic (with hepatitis B coinfection) and is acquired in the same ways as hepatitis B. It can either be acquired in a coinfection with hepatitis B or in a superinfection (hepatitis D infection after hepatitis B infection). The superinfection tends to lead to worse outcomes. IgM antibodies to the hepatitis D antigen demonstrate resolution of recent infection. Presence of the hepatitis D antigen, hepatitis D virus (HDV) RNA, and high levels of IgM antibodies to hepatitis D indicate chronicity.

9. How is hepatitis E transmitted? What is special about the infection in pregnant women?

Hepatitis E is transmitted like hepatitis A (via food and water; no chronic state). It is often fatal in pregnant women (for unknown reasons).

10. Which hepatitis viruses can lead to chronic liver disease?

HBV, HCV, and HDV. HDV can cause infection only in the setting of coexisting HBV.

TRAUMA AND TOXIC EFFECTS

1. What are the common gastrointestinal malformations in children? How are they distinguished?

Name*	Presenting Age	Vomit Description	Findings/Key Words
Pyloric stenosis	0–3 mo	Nonbilious, projectile	Males $>>$ females; palpable olive-shaped mass in the epigastrium; low Cl/low K metabolic alkalosis
Intestinal atresia	0–1 wk	Bilious	Double-bubble sign, Down syndrome
TE fistula†	0–2 wk	Food regurgitation	Respiratory compromise with feeding, aspiration pneumonia, inability to pass a nasogastric tube into the stomach, gastric distention (from air)
Hirschsprung disease	0–1 yr	Feculent	Abdominal distention, obstipation, no nerve ganglia seen on rectal biopsy; males $>>$ females
Anal atresia	0–1 wk	Late, feculent	Detected on initial exam in the nursery; males $>$ females
Choanal atresia	0–1 wk	—	Cyanosis with feeding, relieved by crying; inability to pass a nasogastric tube through nose

Cl, Chloride; *K*, potassium; *TE*, tracheoesophageal.
*Treat each of these conditions with **surgical repair**.
†The most common variant (85% of cases) has esophageal atresia with a fistula from the bronchus to the distal esophagus. The result is gastric distention, as each breath transmits air to the GI tract. Be able to recognize a sketch of this most common variant (Fig. 5.1).

2. What other pediatric gastrointestinal conditions are commonly found on the Step 3 exam? How are they distinguished?

Name	Presenting Age	Vomit Description	Findings/Key Words
Intussusception	3 mo–2 yr	Bilious	Currant-jelly stools (blood and mucus), palpable sausage-shaped mass, "target sign" on ultrasound; treat with pneumatic or hydrostatic enema guided by fluoroscopy or ultrasound (diagnostic and therapeutic)
Necrotizing enterocolitis	0–2 mo	Bilious	Premature baby, fever, rectal bleeding, air in bowel wall (pneumatosis intestinalis). Treat with NPO, orogastric tube, IV fluids, and antibiotics
Meconium ileus	0–1 wk	Feculent, late	Cystic fibrosis manifestation (as is rectal prolapse)
Midgut volvulus	0–2 yr	Bilious	Sudden onset of pain, distention, rectal bleeding, peritonitis, "bird's beak" on abdominal radiograph; treat with surgery
Meckel diverticulum	0–2 yr	Varies	Rule of 2s*; gastrointestinal ulceration/bleeding; use Meckel scan to detect; treat with surgery
Strangulated hernia	Any age	Bilious	Physical exam detects bowel loops in inguinal canal

IV, Intravenous; *NPO*, nothing by mouth (no feedings).
*Rule of 2s for Meckel diverticulum: 2% of population affected (most common GI tract abnormality; remnant of omphalomesenteric duct), 2 inches long, within 2 feet of ileocolic junction, presents in the first 2 years of life. Meckel diverticulum can cause intussusception, obstruction, or volvulus.

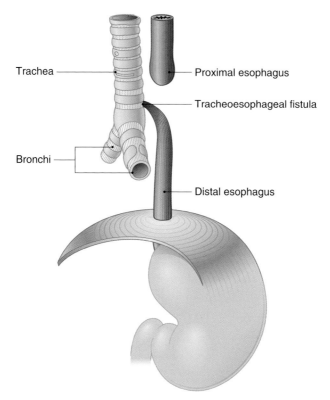

Fig. 5.1 Tracheoesophageal fistula. Diagram of the most common type of esophageal atresia and tracheoesophageal fistula. (From Gilbert-Barness E. *Potter's Pathology of the Fetus, Infant and Child.* 2nd ed. Philadelphia: Mosby; 2007 [fig. 25.6].)

3. How are omphalocele and gastroschisis differentiated?

An **omphalocele**, associated with other congenital anomalies, is located in the midline; the sac contains multiple abdominal organs, the umbilical ring is absent, and other anomalies are common. **Gastroschisis** is to the right of the midline, only small bowel is exposed (no true hernia sac), the umbilical ring is present, and other anomalies are rare. An omphalocele is covered in peritoneum, whereas gastroschisis is not.

4. List and differentiate the three common types of groin hernias.

- **Indirect hernias** are the most common type in both sexes and all age groups. The hernia sac travels through the inner and outer inguinal rings (protrusion begins lateral to the inferior epigastric vessels) and into the scrotum or labia because of a patent processus vaginalis (congenital defect).
- **Direct hernias** (no sac) protrude medial to the inferior epigastric vessels because of weakness in the abdominal musculature of Hesselbach triangle. They are less likely to become incarcerated than indirect hernias. They are also uncommon in women.
- **Femoral hernias** are more common than direct or indirect hernias in women (though they are still more common in men). The hernia (no sac) goes through the femoral ring onto the anterior thigh (located below the inguinal ring).

   Of the three types, femoral hernias are the most susceptible to incarceration and strangulation. All three types are treated with elective surgical repair if symptomatic.

5. Define incarcerated and strangulated hernias.

Incarceration occurs when a herniated organ is trapped and becomes swollen and edematous. Incarcerated hernias are the most common cause of small bowel obstruction in patients who have had no previous abdominal surgery and the second most common cause in patients who have had previous abdominal surgery. Treatment is prompt surgery.

Strangulation occurs after incarceration when the entrapment becomes so severe that the blood supply is cut off. Strangulation can lead to necrosis and is a surgical emergency. Patients may present with symptoms of small bowel obstruction and shock.

6. How do you manage a patient with blunt abdominal trauma?

In patients with blunt abdominal trauma, the initial findings determine the appropriate course of action. If the patient is awake and stable and your examination is "benign," observe the patient and repeat the abdominal exam later. You can also do a FAST (focused assessment by sonography in trauma) scan to check for free fluid in the abdomen and pelvis. Meanwhile, perform a CT scan of the abdomen and pelvis with oral and intravenous contrast.

If the patient is hemodynamically unstable (hypotension and/or shock that does not respond to fluid challenge), proceed directly to laparotomy.

If the patient has a positive FAST scan (i.e., there is free fluid, presumably blood, in the abdomen), proceed to laparotomy.

If the patient has altered mental status, the abdomen cannot be examined, or an obvious source of blood loss explains the hemodynamic instability, order a CT scan of the abdomen and pelvis with oral and intravenous contrast (also get a CT scan of the head and cervical spine if altered mental status is present). Diagnostic peritoneal lavage is no longer used because it is nonspecific and less sensitive than CT; it can also alter CT scan results.

7. How is penetrating abdominal trauma managed?

In patients with penetrating abdominal trauma (e.g., gunshot, stab wound), the type of injury and the initial findings determine the course of action. With any gunshot wound that may have violated the peritoneal cavity, proceed directly to laparotomy. With a wound from a sharp instrument, management is more controversial. Either proceed directly to laparotomy (your best choice if the patient is unstable) or perform CT scan if the patient is stable. With nonoperative management, perform serial abdominal exams.

8. What should you always remember when a question mentions that a child was given aspirin?

Reye syndrome, which causes encephalopathy and/or liver failure. This usually occurs after aspirin is given for influenza or varicella infection. Use acetaminophen in children to avoid this rare (but often tested) condition.

CHAPTER 6

BEHAVIORAL AND EMOTIONAL DISORDERS

1. What is the difference between objective and subjective psychological tests?
   Objective tests are generally multiple-choice tests that are scored by a computer; the classic example is the IQ test. **Subjective tests** have no "right" answers and are scored by the test-giver (the classic example is the Rorschach test).

2. Characterize each of the following psychological tests as objective or subjective, and briefly describe its use.

Name of Test	Description
Stanford-Binet	Objective IQ test for adults
Wechsler Intelligence Scale for Children	Objective IQ test for children (4–17 yr old)
Rorschach test	Subjective test in which patients describe what they see in an inkblot
Thematic Apperception Test	Subjective test in which the patient describes what is going on in a cartoon drawing of people
Beck Depression Inventory	Objective test to look for depression
Minnesota Multiphasic Personality Inventory	Objective test to measure personality type
Halstead-Reitan Battery	Objective test used to determine the location and effects of specific brain lesions
Luria-Nebraska Neuropsychological Battery	Objective test that assesses many cognitive functions as well as cerebral dominance (left or right)

Note: Psychologic tests can be used to aid in a difficult diagnosis; they are not used or needed for a straightforward case.

PSYCHOTIC DISORDERS

1. What are the differential diagnoses to consider in a patient presenting with psychosis?
   There are primary and secondary etiologies to consider when evaluating a patient exhibiting psychotic behavior. Primary causes include psychiatric illnesses such as acute psychotic disorder, schizophrenia, schizoaffective disorder, schizophreniform disorder, or a mood disorder with psychotic symptoms. Secondary causes include substance-induced psychosis (e.g., prescription or illicit drug use) or comorbid medical conditions (e.g., hepatic encephalopathy, uremic encephalopathy, electrolyte abnormalities, infection, or endocrine disturbances). Secondary causes should be ruled out before pursuing a primary cause.

2. How do you distinguish schizoaffective disorder from a mood disorder with psychotic symptoms?
   Schizoaffective disorder and mood disorder with psychotic features each have a mix of schizophrenic features and mood disturbance (either major depressive or bipolar). The difference is that schizoaffective disorder has *consistent* schizophrenic features with *occasional* mood disturbances, while mood disorder with psychotic features has *consistent* mood disturbances with *occasional* schizophrenic features. Patients with schizoaffective disorder will never show signs of the mood disturbance outside of the context of their schizophrenic features; conversely, patients with a mood disorder with psychotic symptoms will never display purely schizophrenic symptoms without features of the underlying mood disturbance (either major depressive or bipolar).

3. Psychosis and mania may present with similar features, including erratic behavior, speech disturbances, agitation, and grandiosity. How do you distinguish between the two?
   The erratic behavior in mania is fundamentally goal oriented, whereas psychosis is not. Hallucinations typical of psychosis will not be present in mania.

4. Why is the duration of symptoms important with psychosis?
   The time frame is important because given the exact same symptoms, a patient is given one of three different diagnoses based only on their duration:
   • Less than 1 month: acute psychotic disorder
   • 1–6 months: schizophreniform disorder
   • More than 6 months: schizophrenia

5. What are the five main diagnostic criteria for schizophrenia?

According to the fifth edition of the *Diagnostic and Statistical Manual of Mental Disorders* (DSM-V), the five main diagnostic symptoms of schizophrenia are:

1. Delusions
2. Hallucinations
3. Disorganized speech
4. Grossly disorganized or catatonic behavior
5. Negative symptoms (i.e., flat affect, avolition)

A minimum of two must be present, one of which must be either a delusion, hallucination, or disorganized speech pattern. The impairment must last for a minimum of 6 months to establish this diagnosis.

6. List the positive symptoms of schizophrenia.

- Delusions (e.g., severe paranoia, grandiosity)
- Hallucinations (auditory is the most common; visual is second most common)
- Disorganized speech patterns (e.g., tangentiality, circumstantiality, clanging)
- Abnormal psychomotor behavior

Positive symptoms are extreme distortions or severe exaggerations of normal behavior. Positive symptoms respond well to all currently used antipsychotics.

7. List the negative symptoms of schizophrenia.

- Flat affect
- Anhedonia (lack of pleasure)
- Alogia (no speech)
- Poor attention
- Avolition (apathy)
- Asociality

Negative symptoms are symptoms for which patients have lost some form of normal behavior; they no longer exhibit behaviors that normal individuals typically have. Negative symptoms respond poorly to typical antipsychotics (e.g., haloperidol) but may respond to atypical antipsychotics such as risperidone, olanzapine, aripiprazole, paliperidone, quetiapine, or ziprasidone. Note that the atypical antipsychotic clozapine is not used as a first-line treatment for schizophrenia due to its side effect profile that includes the risk of agranulocytosis. Strict additional criteria must be met to consider using clozapine in treatment-resistant schizophrenia.

8. What features of schizophrenia suggest a poor prognosis?

- Poor premorbid functioning (most important)
- Family history of schizophrenia
- Early onset
- Negative symptoms
- No precipitating factors
- Poor support system
- Single, divorced, or widowed status

9. What features of schizophrenia suggest a good prognosis?

- Good premorbid functioning (most important)
- Family history of mood disorders
- Late onset
- Positive symptoms
- Obvious precipitating factors
- Good support system
- Married status

10. What is the difference in age of onset for schizophrenia in males and females?

The typical age of onset is 15 to 25 years for males (look for someone going to college and deteriorating) and 25 to 35 years for females.

11. Roughly what percentage of patients with schizophrenia commit suicide?

In the United States, roughly 10% of patients with schizophrenia eventually commit suicide (a past attempt is the best predictor of eventual success)

12. True or False: Psychosocial treatment has been shown to improve outcomes in schizophrenia.

True. Antipsychotic medications are the mainstay of therapy, but psychosocial treatment has been shown to improve outcomes. Medications are needed first, but the best treatment (as in most psychiatric illnesses) is medications plus therapy.

13. Differentiate among the classes of antipsychotics drugs.

	High-Potency Typical Agents	Low-Potency Typical Agents	Atypical Agents*
Prototype drug	Haloperidol	Chlorpromazine	Cariprazine, risperidone, olanzapine, aripiprazole, paliperidone, quetiapine, ziprasidone
EPS side effects	High incidence	Low incidence	Low incidence
ANS side effects[†]	Low incidence	High incidence	Medium incidence
Positive symptoms	Works well	Works well	Works well
Negative symptoms	Works poorly	Works poorly	Works fairly well

ANS, Autonomic nervous system; *EPS*, extrapyramidal system.

*Atypical antipsychotics are generally first-line treatment and maintenance therapy due to reduced extrapyramidal side effects and efficacy with negative symptoms. Choose them over older agents. A 2017 study showed cariprazine to be the most effica-cious agent against negative symptoms. Remember that although it is an atypical antipsychotic, clozapine is *not* used first line due to the low but possible risk of agranulocytosis.

[†]ANS side effects include anticholinergic effects (dry mouth, urinary retention, blurry vision, mydriasis), alpha$_1$-blockade (ortho-static hypotension), and antihistamine effects (sedation).

14. What are the four commonly tested extrapyramidal side effects of antipsychotics?
Acute dystonia, akathisia, parkinsonism, and tardive dyskinesia.

15. Define acute dystonia. How is it treated?
Acute dystonia is an extrapyramidal movement disorder that occurs in the first few hours or days of treatment. Patients develop prolonged muscle spasms or stiffness such as torticollis (disfiguring neck muscle spasms; liter-ally "twisted column"), trismus (lockjaw), tongue protrusions and twisting, opisthotonos (back muscle spasm causing extension of the head, neck, and spine), and/or oculogyric crisis (forced sustained deviation of the head and eyes). Acute dystonia is most common in young men. Treat with antihistamines such as diphenhydramine or anticholinergics such as benztropine.

16. Define akathisia. How is it treated?
Akathisia occurs in the first few days to weeks of treatment. The patient has a subjective feeling of restlessness and may pace constantly, alternate sitting and standing, and be unable to sit still. Beta-blockers such as propran-olol are first-line treatment, with benztropine used as second line.

ANXIETY DISORDERS

1. How do you recognize and treat panic disorder?
Panic disorder classically affects patients age 20 to 40 years who have an abrupt surge of intense fear or discom-fort that reaches its peak within a few minutes. Patients often think that they are dying or having a heart attack, although in fact they are healthy and have a negative workup for organic disease. Females are more likely to have panic disorder in a 2:1 ratio. Patients often hyperventilate and are extremely anxious. They may experience tin-gling of the extremities, palpitations, sweating, trembling, sensation of shortness of breath, feelings of choking, chest pain, nausea, and fear of dying. Remember the association between panic disorder and agoraphobia (fear of leaving the house). Treat with selective serotonin reuptake inhibitors (SSRIs; e.g., fluoxetine), which are favored over benzodiazepines.

2. What is generalized anxiety disorder? How is it treated?
Patients with generalized anxiety disorder worry about everything (e.g., career, family, future, relationships, and money) at the same time. Symptoms are not as dramatic as in panic disorder; the patient is simply a severe wor-rier. Patients have difficulty controlling their worries and can have restlessness, fatigue, difficulty concentrating, irritability, muscle tension, and sleep disturbances. Treat with cognitive behavioral therapy and medications: SSRIs (especially if depressive symptoms coexist), buspirone (agonist of 5-hydroxytryptamine 1A serotonin receptor; nonaddictive, nonsedating but slow onset of action), or benzodiazepines (addictive, sedating).

3. Give the classic examples of simple phobias. How are they treated?
Classic examples of simple phobias include fear of needles, blood products, animals, and heights. Treat with be-havioral therapy, including flooding (sudden, intense exposure to the feared object without chance for escape), systematic desensitization (gradual increase in intensity and type of exposure until the person is comfortable with intense exposure to the feared object), and biofeedback (learning to control autonomic variables such as heart rate during anxiety-inducing maneuvers).

4. What is social anxiety disorder?
Social anxiety disorder, also known as social phobia, is a specific type of simple phobia (fear of social situations) that is best treated with behavioral therapy. To reduce symptoms, beta-blockers may be used before a public appearance that cannot be avoided, and SSRIs are increasingly being used as a primary treatment. Serotonin-norepinephrine reuptake inhibitors (SNRIs) and benzodiazepines may also be used.

5. Define obsessive-compulsive disorder (OCD). How is it treated?

OCD is marked by recurrent intrusive thoughts (obsessions) that lead to impulsive recurrent behaviors (compulsions) to such a degree that it causes dysfunction in the occupational or interpersonal life of the patient. Look for washing rituals (e.g., washing the hands 30 times per day) or checking rituals (checking to see if the door is locked 40 times per day). Patients may be aware that their behavior is abnormal but are unable to stop themselves. Onset is usually in adolescence or early adulthood. Treat with SSRIs (especially fluvoxamine) or clomipramine (a serotonin-specific tricyclic antidepressant). Therapies such as cognitive behavioral therapy and flooding also may be effective.

6. How do you recognize and treat posttraumatic stress disorder (PTSD)? How do you distinguish PTSD from acute stress disorder?

Look for someone who has been through a life-threatening event (e.g., war, severe accident, rape), repeatedly experiences the event (nightmares, flashbacks), exhibits hypervigilant behavior, and cannot stop thinking about the event. Patients may also have dissociative amnesia of the event, irritability, reckless or self-destructive behavior, depression, and poor concentration. Treat with peer group therapy; if you have to choose a medication, use an antidepressant, usually an SSRI. Use the alpha$_1$-antagonist prazosin to treat the sleep disturbance and nightmares. Note that symptoms of PTSD must be present for at least 1 month. Symptoms that have persisted for less than 1 month indicate acute stress disorder.

MOOD DISORDERS

1. Define depression.

Depression, or major depressive disorder as it is technically called, is defined as a depressed mood or a loss of interest or pleasure in daily activities for 2 weeks or longer. There is impaired function in social, occupational, or educational roles. A depressed mood, decreased interest, or lack of pleasure, along with at least five of the following symptoms, are required to diagnose major depressive disorder. The symptoms can be remembered by the mnemonic **SIGECAPS**:

Sleep disturbance
Interest loss
Guilt, worthless, or hopeless feelings
Energy loss
Concentration difficulty
Appetite disturbance
Psychomotor agitation or retardation
Suicidality

You can remember that five of the SIGECAPS criteria must be present by mentally replacing the letter *S* with the number 5 (i.e., 5IGECAPS).

2. Is depression more common in males or females?

Depression is more common in females.

3. True or False: Patients with depression often do not complain about it directly.

True. Patients often do not come out and say, "I'm depressed." You must watch for the clues by recognizing SIGECAPS or vague somatic complaints. The history may or may not reveal obvious precipitating factors such as loss of loved one, divorce or separation, unemployment or retirement, or chronic or debilitating disease.

4. How do you treat depression?

As with most psychiatric illnesses, the ideal treatment plan includes both medications (antidepressants) and psychotherapy. The addition of psychotherapy is more effective than medications alone. SSRIs are usually the preferred first-line agents. Other options include SNRIs and the tricyclic antidepressants. Bupropion and mirtazapine have unique modes of action and are more commonly used in treatment-resistant depression than as first-line agents. Be careful when prescribing bupropion as it is known to lower the seizure threshold.

5. Describe electroconvulsive therapy (ECT). What are the main side effects of ECT? When is ECT used?

ECT is performed by inducing a generalized cerebral seizure under general anesthesia and neuromuscular blockade. Primary side effects of ECT include headache, temporary cognitive impairment, and possible memory loss. ECT is typically used in major depressive disorder that is refractory to antidepressant therapy but may also be used in refractory bipolar disorder or urgent clinical situations such as acute suicidality, severe psychosis, malignant catatonia, or malnutrition due to a depressive state.

6. What is an adjustment disorder with depressed mood?

A diagnosis that you must be able to distinguish from major depressive disorder. In adjustment disorder, a patient goes through a normal life experience (e.g., relationship breakup, failing grade, job loss) but does not handle it well. There is marked distress that is in excess of what would be expected from exposure to the stressor or that causes significant impairment in social or occupational functioning. Although patients may have a depressed mood, they do not meet the criteria for full-blown major depressive disorder, and symptoms do not last longer than 6 months. An example is a woman who divorces her husband, seems to cry a lot for the next few weeks, and leaves work early on most days. Another example is a high school boy who doesn't make the basketball team and mopes around the house, crying, and not wanting to go to school or out with his friends for a few weeks.

7. True or False: Antidepressants can trigger mania or hypomania.
True—especially in bipolar patients. Remember to ask about any history of manic episodes when considering treatment for depression.

8. How do SSRIs work? Why are they preferred over tricyclics?
SSRIs (e.g., fluoxetine, citalopram, paroxetine, sertraline, fluvoxamine, escitalopram) prevent reuptake of serotonin only. They have less serious side effects (insomnia, anorexia, jitteriness, headache, sexual dysfunction) and are not dangerous with overdose compared to tricyclics.

9. How do SNRIs work?
SNRIs (e.g., venlafaxine, duloxetine, desvenlafaxine) prevent reuptake of serotonin and norepinephrine. The side effects of SNRIs are similar to those of SSRIs but also include noradrenergic symptoms such as sweating, dizziness, increased blood pressure, and sedation.

10. How do tricyclic antidepressants work? What are their side effects?
Tricyclic antidepressants (e.g., nortriptyline, amitriptyline) prevent reuptake of norepinephrine and serotonin, similar to SNRIs. They also block alpha-adrenergic receptors (which may cause orthostatic hypotension, dizziness, or falls), muscarinic receptors (watch for anticholinergic effects, such as dry mouth, blurred vision, constipation, and urinary retention), histamine receptors (causing sedation), and lower the seizure threshold. Tricyclic antidepressants are dangerous in overdose primarily because of **cardiac arrhythmias,** which may respond to bicarbonate. Remember the three *C*s of tricyclic antidepressant overdose: **c**oma, **c**onvulsions, and **c**ardiotoxicity.

11. What are monoamine oxidase (MAO) inhibitors? Describe their side effects.
MAO inhibitors (e.g., selegiline, phenelzine, tranylcypromine) are older medications that are not used as first-line agents for treatment of depression. They may be good for atypical depression (look for hypersomnia and hyperphagia—the opposite of classic depression) that fails to respond to other agents. When patients taking MAO inhibitors eat tyramine-containing foods (especially wine and cheese), they may get a hypertensive crisis. Be sure to discontinue other serotonin-related medications at least 2 weeks before starting an MAO inhibitor due to the risk of serotonin syndrome. Because of its longer half-life, the SSRI fluoxetine must be discontinued at leave 5 weeks before starting an MAO inhibitor.

12. What is the most notorious side effect of trazodone?
Priapism (persistent, painful erection in the absence of sexual desire that may lead to permanent impotence or tissue necrosis if not treated). Consult urology and consider an intracavernosal injection of phenylephrine along with detumescence if it does not resolve after 4 hours.

13. True or False: Children with depression frequently exhibit an irritable rather than a depressed mood.
True.

14. Define bipolar I disorder. What are the classic symptoms?
Mania is the only criterion required for a diagnosis of bipolar disorder, but a history of depression is commonly present as well. Remember the mnemonic **DIG FAST** for classic symptoms of mania: **d**istractibility, **i**nsomnia and **i**mpulsivity, **g**randiosity and **g**oal-directed activity, **f**light of ideas, **a**gitation, **s**pending sprees and **s**exual promiscuity, and **t**alking with pressured speech. Look for initial onset between the ages of 16 and 30 years.

15. Psychosis and mania may present with similar features, including erratic behavior, speech disturbances, agitation, and grandiosity. How do you distinguish between the two?
The erratic behavior in mania is fundamentally goal oriented, whereas psychosis is not. Hallucinations typical of psychosis will not be present in mania.

16. How is bipolar I disorder treated?
Both lithium and valproic acid are mood stabilizers and first-line agents. Typical antipsychotics (haloperidol), atypical antipsychotics (risperidone, quetiapine, clozapine, ziprasidone, and aripiprazole), carbamazepine, and gabapentin are second-line agents. Antipsychotics or antidepressants may be needed if the patient becomes psychotic or depressed; use at the same time as the mood stabilizer.

17. Define bipolar II disorder.
Bipolar II disorder is hypomania (mild mania without psychosis that does not cause occupational dysfunction) plus major depression. Note that major depression is not required to diagnose bipolar I disorder but *is* required to diagnose bipolar II disorder.

18. Define persistent depressive disorder (dysthymia) and cyclothymia. What features distinguish one from the other?

Both disorders involve a moderate mood disturbance that persists for at least 2 years. Persistent depressive disorder (dysthymia) is a depressed mood on most days for more than 2 years without episodes of major depression, mania/hypomania, or psychosis, while cyclothymia involves at least 2 years of hypomania alternating with depressed mood with *no* full-blown episodes of mania or major depression.

19. List the major risk factors for suicide.
- Age greater than 45 years
- Prior psychiatric history
- Alcohol or substance abuse
- Depression
- History of rage or violence
- Recent loss or separation
- Prior suicide attempts
- Loss of health
- Male gender (men commit suicide three times more often than women, but women attempt it four times more often than men)
- Unemployed or retired status
- Single, widowed, or divorced status
- Access to weapons
- Organized plan

20. What is the strongest predictor of a future suicide attempt?

A past attempt.

21. True or False: Some psychiatric patients can be hospitalized against their will.

True. Patients can be hospitalized against their will if they are a danger to themselves (suicidal or unable to take care of themselves) or others (homicidal).

22. True or False: Be careful in asking about suicide because you may plant the idea in the patient's head.

False. Always ask patients about suicidal thoughts; it does not make them more likely to commit suicide. If necessary, you should temporarily hospitalize acutely suicidal patients against their will.

23. True or False: When patients are just emerging from a deep depression, they are at an increased risk of suicide.

True. When the antidepressant begins to work, the patient gets a little more energy—possibly just enough to carry out a suicide plan.

24. True or False: The highest suicide rates are in people aged 15 to 24 years.

False. Suicide rates are rising most rapidly in 15- to 24-year-olds, but the highest absolute suicide rate is in people older than 65 years.

25. How do you distinguish between postpartum blues, postpartum depression, and postpartum psychosis? How is each condition managed?

The main way to distinguish postpartum blues from postpartum depression is the severity and duration of symptoms. Postpartum blues is milder, typically developing within a few days after delivery and resolving within 2 weeks, while postpartum depression lasts longer than 2 weeks and meets the diagnostic criteria for clinical depression (e.g., at least five SIGECAPS symptoms). Postpartum blues should be managed conservatively with reassurance and a scheduled follow-up appointment 2 weeks after delivery, while cognitive-behavioral therapy or antidepressant medical therapy may be used for postpartum depression. Postpartum psychosis is recognized clinically by the rapid onset of delusions, hallucinations, disorganized thought, or other bizarre behavior following delivery. These patients may threaten harm to themselves or their baby. Postpartum psychosis is a medical emergency and typically involves hospitalization.

SOMATOFORM DISORDERS

1. Explain the concept of somatic symptom disorders (previously called somatoform disorders).

A patient with somatic symptom disorder experiences psychiatric stress and expresses it through physical symptoms. Patients do not do so on purpose.

2. Describe the four major somatic symptom disorders.

Somatization disorder: the patient has multiple different complaints in multiple different organ systems over many years and has had extensive workups in the past. Mnemonic: Patients with **soma**tization disorder have **so ma**ny physical complaints.

Conversion disorder: the patient has an obvious precipitating factor (e.g., fight with boyfriend), then develops unexplainable neurologic symptoms (e.g., blindness, stocking-glove numbness). This is thought to be a physical manifestation of emotional distress. Think of it as the patient has subconsciously *converted* the emotional distress into this physical manifestation. The patient is not malingering and truly believes the symptom is real. However, clinical evidence is incompatible with symptomatology.

Hypochondriasis: the patient continues to believe in the presence of a disease despite extensive negative workup. These patients tend to be excessively worried about a minor symptom and are not reassured by multiple negative workups.

Body dysmorphic disorder: the patient is preoccupied with an imagined physical defect (e.g., a teenager who expresses having a big nose when it is normal in size).

3. How are somatic symptom disorders treated?
Treat all somatic symptom disorders with frequent return visits to the clinic and/or psychotherapy. Screen for and treat any coexisting depression.

4. Distinguish among somatic symptom disorders, factitious disorders, and malingering.
In **somatic symptom disorders,** the patient does not intentionally create symptoms (it is an unconscious process). In **factitious disorders,** patients intentionally create an illness or symptoms (e.g., they inject insulin to create hypoglycemia) and subject themselves to procedures in order to assume the role of a patient (no financial or other secondary gain). In **malingering,** patients intentionally create their illness for secondary gain (e.g., money, release from work or jail). Think of it as patients with **f**actitious disorders want to **f**eel like a patient, while patients who are **m**alingering want **m**oney or a similar external motivation.

5. How do you recognize dissociative fugue (also called psychogenic fugue or fugue state)?
Dissociative fugue is a reversible amnesia for personal identity, including the memories, personality, and other identifying characteristics of individuality. It usually involves unplanned travel or wandering. There is complete amnesia for the fugue episode. The classic patient develops amnesia, travels, and assumes a new identity, but does not remember the event upon returning.

EATING DISORDERS AND OTHER IMPULSE-CONTROL DISORDERS

1. How do you recognize anorexia?
The classic patient is a female adolescent who is a good athlete or student with a perfectionistic personality. According to DSM-V, the diagnostic criteria include restriction of energy intake leading to a significant low body weight, intense fear of gaining weight or becoming fat, and disturbance in the way one's body weight or shape is experienced. Patients often have a body mass index (BMI) of 18 or lower. Roughly 10% to 15% of patients die from complications of starvation or coexisting bulimia (electrolyte imbalances, cardiac arrhythmias, infections). Although more positive therapies are preferred, patients sometimes need to be hospitalized against their will for intravenous nutrition. Patients with anorexia may be of a restrictive type (severely restricted caloric intake) or a binge-purge type (self-induced vomiting or laxative abuse).

2. Define bulimia. What are the classic findings of the mouth and fingers?
Bulimic patients have binge-eating episodes, during which they feel a lack of control and then engage in purging behavior (vomiting, laxatives, exercise, fasting). Those affected are typically normal weight or overweight adolescent females. If these patients ever meet criteria for anorexia, they are diagnosed with the binge-purge type of anorexia (i.e., the anorexia diagnosis trumps the bulimia diagnosis). Patients may require hospitalization for electrolyte disturbances. Classic findings include eroded tooth enamel caused by frequent vomiting and eroded skin over the knuckles from putting the fingers into the throat to induce vomiting.

DISORDERS ORIGINATING IN INFANCY, CHILDHOOD, OR ADOLESCENCE

1. Define conduct disorder. With what adult disorder is it associated?
Conduct disorder is the pediatric form of **antisocial personality disorder.** Look for fire setting, cruelty to animals, lying, stealing, and/or fighting. As adults, patients often have antisocial disorder. **Note:** Evidence of conduct disorder as a child is required for a diagnosis of antisocial personality disorder in adults.

2. Describe the behavior of a child who has oppositional-defiant disorder. How is it distinguished from conduct disorder?
The child displays negative, hostile, and defiant behavior toward authority figures (e.g., parents, teachers). The child exhibits such behavior around adults but behaves normally around peers and is *not* a cruel, lying criminal (unlike patients with conduct disorder).

3. Give the classic description of children with separation anxiety disorder.
Affected children refuse to go to school because they think that something will happen to them or their parents if they separate. They will do anything to avoid separation (e.g., feign stomachache, headache, temper tantrum).

4. Define attention-deficit/hyperactivity disorder (ADHD).
As the name implies, patients are hyperactive and have short attention spans. ADHD is more common in males than in females. Look for a fidgety child who is impulsive and cannot pay attention but is not cruel. These symptoms must be present in two different settings (e.g., at home and school). Treat with stimulants (paradoxic calming effect) such as methylphenidate (Ritalin), an amphetamine, or atomoxetine. Stimulants and amphetamines may cause insomnia, abdominal pain, anorexia, weight loss, and growth suppression. Atomoxetine is an SNRI and alternative to stimulant therapy, but it has serious potential side effects, including cardiovascular events and suicidal thoughts.

5. What is a learning disorder?
Learning disorders describe isolated impairment in math, reading, writing, speech, language, or coordination. All other skills are normal; no intellectual disability is present (e.g., "Johnny just can't do math").

6. How do you recognize and diagnose autism spectrum disorder?
Autism symptoms start at a very young age, beginning as early as 6 months and becoming well established by age 2 or 3 years. Look for impaired social interaction (isolative, unaware of surroundings), impaired verbal and nonverbal communication (strange words, babbling, repetition), and restricted activities and interests (head banging, strange movements). Autism is a spectrum of disorders in which patients may range from very highly functioning (previously called Asperger syndrome) to severely intellectually disabled. Most individuals with autism manifest some degree of intellectual disability that is typically moderate in severity.

No single cause has been identified for the development of autism. Genetic origins are suspected on the basis of twin studies and a higher incidence among siblings. Possible contributing factors include fetal alcohol exposure, infections (congenital rubella infection), other perinatal factors, and immunologic causes.

PERSONALITY DISORDERS

1. Define personality disorders.
Personality disorders are lifelong maladaptive traits that affect the way a person interacts with the world. Look for a history dating back to childhood or teenage years. No real treatment is available, although psychotherapy may be attempted.

2. Give a one- or two-sentence description of each of the following 10 personality disorders.
Cluster A (**A**wkward disorders)
- **Paranoid:** patients are paranoid and think that everyone (friends, too) is out to get them; they often initiate lawsuits.
- **Schizoid:** patients are classic loners who have no friends and no interest in having friends. They also have a restricted range of emotions.
- **Schizotypal:** patients have bizarre beliefs (cults, superstition) and a bizarre manner of speaking but no psychosis.
Cluster B (**B**ad company: dramatic, emotional, or erratic disorders)
- **Histrionic:** patients are overly dramatic, attention seeking, and inappropriately seductive; they constantly seek the center of attention.
- **Narcissistic:** patients are egocentric, lack empathy, are often envious of others or believe that others are envious of them, and manipulate others for their own gain; they have a sense of entitlement and perceive any criticism as a personal insult.
- **Antisocial:** these patients are *anti-society*. Patients have long criminal records and may have tortured animals or set fires as children. A history of pediatric conduct disorder is required for this diagnosis. Patients are aggressive and do not pay their bills or support their children. They are liars and have no remorse or conscience. Antisocial personality disorder has a strong association with alcoholism, drug abuse, and somatization disorder. Most antisocial patients are male.
- **Borderline:** patients have unstable moods, behaviors, relationships, and self-image. Look for splitting; that is, these patients consider other individuals to be either all good or all bad and may frequently change categories. Other clues include threats of self-harm, micropsychotic episodes (2 minutes of psychosis), impulsiveness, and constant crisis.
Cluster C (**C**owardly, **c**lingy, and **c**ompulsive)
- **Avoidant:** patients have no friends but want them; they avoid others out of fear of criticism and rejection (inferiority complex). This is distinguished from schizoid personality disorder, in which the patient is isolated but has no desire for social contact.
- **Dependent:** patients cannot be or do anything alone. Generally, they have low self-esteem. A wife may stay with her abusive husband despite continued abuse.
- **Obsessive-compulsive:** patients are obsessed with rules, perfection, and organization. They may seem anal retentive and stubborn. Rules are more important than objectives, and affect is restricted. Money is a frequent concern and is often hoarded. This is distinct from OCD, as patients with this personality type do not find their obsessions distressful.

PSYCHOSOCIAL PROBLEMS

1. **Distinguish between normal grief and pathologic grief (i.e., depression).**
   Initial grief after a loss (e.g., death of a loved one) may include a state of shock, a feeling of numbness or bewilderment, distress, crying, sleep disturbances, decreased appetite, difficulty in concentrating, weight loss, and guilt (survivor guilt) for up to 1 year—in other words, the same symptoms as depression. It is normal to have an illusion or hallucination about the deceased, but a normal grieving person knows that it is an illusion, whereas a depressed person believes that it is real. Intense yearning (even years after the death) and even searching for the deceased are normal. Feelings of worthlessness, psychomotor retardation, and suicidal ideation are not signs of normal grief; they are signs of depression.

2. **Discuss the epidemiology of alcohol use disorder.**
   Roughly 10% to 15% of the population abuses alcohol. Alcohol use disorder is more common in men. The genetic component is passed most easily from father to son.

3. **What diseases and conditions may be caused by chronic alcohol intake?**
   - Gastritis
   - Fatty change in the liver
   - Hepatitis
   - Mallory-Weiss tears
   - Cirrhosis
   - Pancreatitis (acute or chronic)
   - Peripheral neuropathy (via thiamine deficiency and a direct effect)
   - Wernicke or Korsakoff syndrome
   - Cerebellar degeneration (ataxia, past-pointing)
   - Dilated cardiomyopathy
   - Rhabdomyolysis (acute or chronic)

4. **With which cancers is alcohol intake associated?**
   Cancers of the oral cavity, larynx, pharynx, esophagus, liver, and lung. It also may be associated with gastric, colon, pancreatic, and breast cancer.

5. **True or False: Alcohol withdrawal can be fatal.**
   True. Alcohol withdrawal needs to be treated on an inpatient basis because it can result in death (mortality rate of 1%–5% with delirium tremens).

6. **How is alcohol withdrawal treated?**
   With benzodiazepines (or, in rare cases, barbiturates). The dose is tapered gradually over several days until symptoms have resolved.

7. **What are the stages of alcohol withdrawal?**
   Minor withdrawal (6–36 hours after the last drink): tremors, mild anxiety, sweating, gastrointestinal (GI) upset, headache, and normal mental status.
   Seizures (6–48 hours after the last drink): single or brief generalized tonic-clonic seizures. Status epilepticus is rare.
   Alcoholic hallucinosis (12–24 hours after last drink): visual, auditory, or tactile hallucinations without autonomic signs (stable vital signs).
   Delirium tremens (48–72 days after last drink, possibly longer): hallucinations, confusion, insomnia, and autonomic lability (sweating, increased pulse and temperature). Fatality is usually associated with this stage.
   Of course, these stages may overlap. Delirium tremens may occur several days after the last drink. The classic example is a patient who develops delirium on postoperative day 2 but was fine before the surgery. The patient could have undisclosed alcohol use disorder, assuming other causes for delirium have been ruled out.

8. **What is the best treatment for alcohol use disorder?**
   Alcoholics Anonymous or other peer-based support groups have had the best success rates. Disulfiram (an aldehyde dehydrogenase enzyme inhibitor that makes people sick when they drink) can be used in some patients. Be sure to warn patients that metronidazole and certain cephalosporins have a similar effect on those who drink alcohol.

9. **Describe the effects of marijuana on users.**
   Effects of marijuana include amotivational syndrome (chronic use results in laziness and lack of motivation), time distortion, impaired judgment, conjunctival injection, paranoia, and the so-called munchies (eating binges during intoxication). No physical symptoms have been reported for withdrawal, but psychological cravings may be present. Marijuana is not dangerous in overdose (although patients may experience temporary dysphoria) and is a controversial teratogen (evidence is weak).

10. What is the basic rule of thumb about the difference in symptoms between intoxication and withdrawal for the same drug?
The symptoms are usually the opposite of each other. For example, stimulants (e.g., cocaine, amphetamines) cause insomnia with intoxication and hypersomnolence in withdrawal, whereas depressants (e.g., alcohol, benzodiazepines, and barbiturates) cause sedation with intoxication and insomnia in withdrawal.

11. Describe the effects of opioids. How are opioid overdoses treated?
Heroin and other opioids cause euphoria, analgesia, drowsiness, miosis, constipation, and central nervous system (CNS) depression. Overdoses can be fatal because of respiratory depression, which should be treated with **naloxone.** Because the drug is often taken intravenously, associated morbidity and mortality include endocarditis, human immunodeficiency virus (HIV) infection, hepatitis, cellulitis, and talc damage.

12. True or false: Benzodiazepines and barbiturates can be fatal in overdose but not in withdrawal.
False. Both can be fatal in overdose and withdrawal.

13. Describe the signs and symptoms of benzodiazepine or barbiturate intoxication.
Benzodiazepines and barbiturates cause sedation and drowsiness, as well as disinhibition and reduced anxiety. They can be fatal in overdose as a result of respiratory depression; treat acute overdoses of a benzodiazepine with **flumazenil** (although this may precipitate seizures). In withdrawal, death may result from seizures and/or cardiovascular collapse. Treat withdrawal on an inpatient basis with a long-acting benzodiazepine, and gradually taper off the dose over several days. Benzodiazepines and barbiturates are especially dangerous when mixed with alcohol because all three are CNS depressants.

14. What symptoms are associated with cocaine intoxication? Cocaine withdrawal?
Cocaine causes sympathetic stimulation (insomnia, tachycardia, mydriasis, hypertension, sweating) with hyperalertness and possible paranoia, aggressiveness, delirium, psychosis, or formications (so-called cocaine bugs—a type of tactile hallucination in which patients think bugs are crawling on them). Overdose can be fatal as a result of arrhythmia, myocardial infarction, seizure, or stroke. During withdrawal, the patient is sleepy, hungry (vs anorexic with intoxication), and irritable with possible severe depression. Cocaine withdrawal is not dangerous, but psychologic cravings are usually severe. Cocaine is teratogenic, causing vascular disruptions in the fetus.

15. Describe the symptoms of amphetamine intoxication.
Amphetamines are longer acting and associated more commonly with psychotic symptoms (patients may appear to be full-blown schizophrenics), but basically their effects are similar to those of cocaine.

16. How do you recognize intoxication with lysergic acid diethylamide (LSD) or hallucinogenic mushrooms?
Symptoms of intoxication with LSD or mushrooms include hallucinations (usually visual, unlike the auditory hallucinations common in schizophrenia), mydriasis, tachycardia, hypertension, diaphoresis, and perception and mood disturbances. Neither is dangerous in overdose—unless patients put themselves in physical danger because of their hallucination (e.g., thinking they can fly, then jumping out a window). No withdrawal symptoms or teratogenic effects have been reported. Users may experience flashbacks (brief feelings of being on the drug again even though none was taken) months to years later or a "bad trip" (acute panic reaction or dysphoria), which should be treated with reassurance, a benzodiazepine, or an antipsychotic, if needed.

17. What about phencyclidine (PCP) intoxication?
PCP intoxication causes LSD/mushroom symptoms plus confusion, agitation, and aggressive behavior. Also look for vertical and/or horizontal nystagmus, possible schizophrenic-like symptoms (e.g., paranoia, auditory hallucinations, disorganized behavior and speech), and combative behavior. Overdose can be fatal because of convulsions, coma, and respiratory arrest. Treat with supportive care and urine acidification to hasten elimination. No withdrawal symptoms have been reported.

18. Describe the signs and symptoms of inhalant intoxication. Who is likely to abuse inhalants?
Inhalant intoxication (e.g., gasoline, glue, varnish remover) causes rapid euphoria, dizziness, slurred speech, a feeling of floating, ataxia, and a sense of heightened power. It is usually seen in younger teenagers (11–15 years old) because these substances are cheap, legal to buy, and readily available. Inhalants can be fatal in overdose as a result of respiratory depression, cardiac arrhythmias, or asphyxiation and may cause severe permanent sequelae (CNS, liver or kidney toxicity, peripheral neuropathy). Chronic abuse may also cause methemoglobinemia, lead toxicity, anemia, muscle weakness, and carbon monoxide poisoning. There is no known withdrawal syndrome associated with inhalants.

19. What are the symptoms of caffeine withdrawal?
Headaches and fatigue.

TOXIC EFFECTS

1. What are the signs and symptoms of serotonin syndrome? Which medications may interact with SSRIs to precipitate serotonin syndrome? How is serotonin syndrome treated?
   Serotonin syndrome may present with a combination of GI upset, hyperreflexia, clonus, flushing of the skin, hyperthermia, or diaphoresis. Be careful when prescribing SSRIs to patients taking other antidepressants, including SNRIs, MAO inhibitors, and tricyclics. Less obvious medications that may also interact with SSRIs to cause serotonin syndrome include linezolid, ondansetron, tramadol, triptans, dextromethorphan, meperidine, and nonprescription drugs such as MDMA (ecstasy) or St. John wort. Serotonin syndrome is treated with cyproheptadine, a 5-HT receptor antagonist.

2. List the atypical antipsychotics associated with each of the side effects listed in the table.

Side Effect	Associated Atypical Antipsychotic(S)
Agranulocytosis	Clozapine
Increased prolactin	Risperidone
Weight gain	Olanzapine, quetiapine, clozapine
Extrapyramidal symptoms	Paliperidone, aripiprazole
QT prolongation	Ziprasidone, paliperidone, risperidone
Sedation	Olanzapine, quetiapine, clozapine
Orthostatic hypotension	Olanzapine, quetiapine, clozapine
Dry mouth	Olanzapine, quetiapine
Constipation	Clozapine, aripiprazole
Nausea	Ziprasidone, aripiprazole
Weakness	Ziprasidone

3. Describe the relationship between antipsychotics and parkinsonism. How is secondary parkinsonism treated?
   Parkinsonism usually occurs in patients taking antipsychotics within the first few days to months of treatment. It is thought that parkinsonism develops because of dopamine depletion, but that psychosis develops because of too much dopamine in the brain (a gross oversimplification). Thus antipsychotics create an iatrogenic decrease in effective dopamine in the brain by blocking dopamine receptors. The patient develops classic parkinsonian symptoms such as stiffness, cogwheel rigidity, a shuffling gait, masklike facies, and resting tremor. It is most common in older women. Treat with benztropine or consider the dopamine agonist amantadine if the patient cannot tolerate benztropine.

4. Define tardive dyskinesia. When does it occur?
   Tardive dyskinesia appears after years of treatment with antipsychotics. Most commonly, the patient develops painless perioral movements (darting, protruding movements of the tongue, chewing, grimacing, and puckering). The patient may also have involuntary, choreoathetoid movements of the head, limbs, and trunk. There is no known treatment for tardive dyskinesia. If you are asked to make a choice when the patient develops tardive dyskinesia, discontinue the current antipsychotic and consider switching to a second-generation antipsychotic such as clozapine or quetiapine. Anticholinergic medications or decreasing the antipsychotic may initially worsen the tardive dyskinesia.

5. What is neuroleptic malignant syndrome? How do you recognize and treat it?
   Neuroleptic malignant syndrome is a life-threatening condition that can occur at any time during antipsychotic treatment. Patients classically develop lead-pipe rigidity, tachycardia, profuse diaphoresis, mutism, obtundation, agitation, high fever (up to 107°F), very **high levels of creatine phosphokinase** (more than four times the normal upper limit), and myoglobinuria. Treat first by discontinuing the antipsychotic; then give supportive care for fever and potential renal failure caused by myoglobinuria (primarily intravenous fluids). Lastly, consider dantrolene (just as in malignant hyperthermia, which is thought to be a similar condition).

6. Describe the relationship between antipsychotics and prolactin levels.
   Dopamine blockade increases serum prolactin levels because dopamine is a prolactin-inhibiting factor in the tuberoinfundibular tract of the brain. The end result may be high serum prolactin levels, resulting in **galactorrhea** and impotence, menstrual dysfunction, and/or decreased libido.

7. What are the classic side effects of the low-potency typical antipsychotics thioridazine and chlorpromazine?
   - Thioridazine: retinal pigment deposits
   - Chlorpromazine: jaundice and photosensitivity

8. List the atypical antipsychotics associated with each of the side effects listed in the table.

Side Effect	Associated Atypical Antipsychotic(S)
Agranulocytosis	Clozapine
Increased prolactin	Risperidone
Weight gain	Olanzapine, quetiapine, clozapine
Extrapyramidal symptoms	Paliperidone, aripiprazole
QT prolongation	Ziprasidone, paliperidone, risperidone
Sedation	Olanzapine, quetiapine, clozapine
Orthostatic hypotension	Olanzapine, quetiapine, clozapine
Dry mouth	Olanzapine, quetiapine
Constipation	Clozapine, aripiprazole
Nausea	Ziprasidone, aripiprazole
Weakness	Ziprasidone

9. What are the side effects of lithium, valproic acid, and carbamazepine?
   - Lithium: thyroid dysfunction, diabetes insipidus, tremor (unintentional movements; lithium, get it?), and CNS effects at toxic levels. Lithium exposure is also teratogenic and is associated with the Ebstein anomaly if used during pregnancy.
   - Valproic acid: liver dysfunction, tremor, and GI distress. It is contraindicated in pregnancy due to its association with neural tube defects.
   - Carbamazepine: bone marrow suppression, diplopia, ataxia, agranulocytosis, aplastic anemia, syndrome of inappropriate antidiuretic hormone, Stevens-Johnson syndrome.

CHAPTER 7

DISORDERS OF THE MUSCULOSKELETAL SYSTEM

DEGENERATIVE/METABOLIC DISORDERS

1. What is the most common form of arthritis?

   Osteoarthritis (OA; at least 75% of cases), which is also called degenerative joint disease.

2. If the cause of arthritis is in doubt, what should you do?

   When in doubt, or if you suspect something other than OA, perform an x-ray of and aspirate fluid from the affected joint. Examine the fluid for cell count and differential, glucose, bacteria (Gram stain and culture), and crystals.

3. How do you distinguish among the common causes of arthritis?

	OA	RA	Gout	Pseudogout	Septic
Usual age/sex	Older adults	Women 20–45 yr	Older men	Older adults	Any age
Classic joints	DIP, PIP, hip, knee	PIP, MCP, wrist	Big toe	Knees, elbows	Knee
Joint fluid WBC	<2000	>2000	>2000	>2000	>50,000
% Neutrophils	<25%	>50%	>50%	>50%	>75%
Appearance	Transparent	Translucent or opaque	Translucent or opaque	Translucent or opaque	Opaque

   DIP, Distal interphalangeal joints; *MCP,* metacarpophalangeal joints; *OA,* osteoarthritis; *PIP,* proximal interphalangeal joints; *RA,* rheumatoid arthritis; *WBC,* white blood cells.

4. What other clues point to a diagnosis of osteoarthritis?

   OA typically occurs in those over the age of 40 and has few signs of inflammation on exam; thus the joints are not hot, red, or tender like rheumatoid arthritis (RA), gout, pseudogout, or septic arthritis. Look for Heberden nodes (visible and palpable distal interphalangeal [DIP] joint osteophytes) and Bouchard nodes (proximal interphalangeal [PIP] joint osteophytes), worsening of symptoms after use and in the evening, bony spurs, and increasing incidence with age. Imaging will show loss of joint space associated with cartilage degeneration and possibly osteophyte formation. Treat with weight reduction, physical therapy/activity, and as-needed nonsteroidal antiinflammatory drugs (NSAIDs) or acetaminophen, corticosteroid injections, and orthopedic referral for joint replacement surgery if severe and not responsive to conservative measures.

5. What clues point to a diagnosis of gout?

   Gout classically begins with podagra (gout in the big toe). Also look for high uric acid levels (not always present and tend to be lower in an acute attack), tophi (subcutaneous uric acid deposits that look like punched-out lesions on bone radiographs), **needle-shaped monosodium urate crystals with negative birefringence** in the joint fluid, and male gender (more commonly affected than female gender). Alcohol and protein-rich foods (e.g., shellfish, red meats) may precipitate an attack. Colchicine or NSAIDs (but *not* aspirin, which causes decreased excretion of uric acid by the kidney) are used for acute attacks. For scenarios in which colchicine or NSAIDs are contraindicated, steroids can be considered so long as septic arthritis is ruled out. For maintenance therapy, high fluid intake, alkalinization of the urine, and/or allopurinol or probenecid (neither drug is for acute attacks) may be used.

6. What causes pseudogout? How is it diagnosed?

   Pseudogout is caused by deposition of calcium pyrophosphate crystals into joints. Look for **rhomboid crystals** with **weakly positive birefringence** (vs negative birefringence with gout crystals in the joint fluid). Radiographs of affected joints can demonstrate chondrocalcinosis. Risk factors include OA, hyperparathyroidism, hemochromatosis, and renal diseases causing hypomagnesemia (Gitelman and Bartter syndromes). Acute attacks can be treated with corticosteroid injections, NSAIDs, or colchicine.

7. Name some other causes of arthritis.

   - Prior trauma (posttraumatic arthritis)
   - Lupus and other collagen vascular diseases (e.g., scleroderma)
   - Psoriasis

- Inflammatory bowel disease
- Lyme disease
- Ankylosing spondylitis
- Reactive arthritis
- Hemophilia
- Paget disease
- Hemochromatosis, Wilson disease
- Neuropathy (i.e., Charcot joint)

8. **Why do patients with hemophilia get arthritis?**
   Recurrent hemarthroses (bleeding into the joints) can cause a debilitating arthritis. Treatment is with acetaminophen. Avoid aspirin and other NSAIDs due to bleeding concern.

9. **Why do patients with sickle cell disease often have arthritis?**
   Patients frequently experience arthralgias (pain) from ischemic sickle crises, but the classic cause of arthritis is avascular necrosis (e.g., hip arthritis from avascular necrosis of the femoral head).

10. **How do hemochromatosis and Wilson disease cause arthritis? How are these diseases radiographically similar to pseudogout?**
    Via deposition of excessive iron (hemochromatosis) or copper (Wilson disease) into the joints. Radiographically, hemochromatosis and Wilson disease may be notable for chondrocalcinosis (calcium deposition within articular cartilage), which is most commonly associated with pseudogout.

11. **True or False: One of the major Jones criteria for the diagnosis of rheumatic fever is arthritis.**
    True. Migratory polyarthritis is one of the major Jones criteria. Look for a history of strep throat. The other major criteria are carditis, chorea, erythema marginatum, and subcutaneous nodules.

12. **What is avascular necrosis (AVN), and what are the risk factors? What is the best test to make the diagnosis?**
    AVN describes interruption of blood supply with subsequent bone ischemia and necrosis of cancellous bone and marrow. Patients present with pain in the affected area. There are many potential risk factors, including:
    - Trauma (usually in the setting of a fracture)
    - Corticosteroid excess (endogenous or iatrogenic)
    - Sickle cell disease or other hemoglobinopathy
    - Alcohol abuse
    - Lupus and other connective tissue disorders
    - Decompression sickness
    - Slipped capital femoral epiphysis
    - Pancreatitis

    The best test to make the diagnosis is magnetic resonance imaging (MRI), which becomes positive before regular x-rays.

13. **What are the most common locations of intervertebral disc herniations? What symptoms do they cause?**
    Lumbar disc herniation is a common, often correctable cause of low back pain. The most common location is the L5-S1 disc, which affects the S1 nerve root. Symptoms include low back pain, buttock pain, and leg pain (worse with sitting and improved by standing). On exam, look for decreased ankle jerk, weakness of plantar flexors in the foot, pain from the midgluteal area to the posterior calf, and a positive straight leg-raise test. The second most common location for herniation is the L4-L5 disc, which affects the L5 nerve root. Look for decreased biceps femoris reflex, weakness of foot extensors, and pain in the hip or groin.

    After the lumbar area, the second most common location is the cervical spine. The classic symptom of cervical disc disease is neck pain. Herniation is most common at the C6-C7 disc, which affects the C7 nerve root. Look for decreased triceps reflex and weakness of the triceps and wrist flexion.

14. **How is intervertebral disc herniation diagnosed and treated?**
    Diagnosis is made with an MRI scan (preferred) or by a computed tomography (CT) scan (use myelography if the patient has contraindications to MRI). Conservative treatment, including bed rest and analgesics, is usually tried first, as roughly 75% of cases will resolve with conservative management. Epidural steroid injection may help. Surgery (discectomy) may be required if conservative treatment fails or significant neurologic deficit is present (to prevent permanent nerve damage).

INFLAMMATORY OR IMMUNOLOGIC DISORDERS

1. **What generalized systemic signs of inflammation may suggest an autoimmune disorder?**
   Systemic signs and symptoms of inflammation include elevations in erythrocyte sedimentation rate and C-reactive protein, fever, anemia of chronic disease, fatigue, and weight loss. If these symptoms are present (especially in a woman of reproductive age), you should consider the possibility of an autoimmune disease.

2. Describe the hallmarks of ankylosing spondylitis.

Ankylosing spondylitis is associated with HLA-B27. Most often a 20- to 40-year-old man with a positive family history presents with back pain and morning stiffness. Patients may assume a bent-over posture. The sacroiliac joints are primarily affected, and radiographs may reveal a **"bamboo" spine**. Patients have other autoimmune-type symptoms, such as fever, elevations in erythrocyte sedimentation rate and C-reactive protein, and anemia. Some develop uveitis. Treat with NSAIDs, methotrexate, sulfasalazine, or tumor necrosis factor (TNF) antagonists (etanercept, infliximab, adalimumab).

3. What clues point to a diagnosis of rheumatoid arthritis?

RA often causes systemic symptoms (fever, malaise, subcutaneous nodules, pericarditis, pleural effusion, uveitis), prolonged morning stiffness, swan neck and boutonnière deformities, and atlantoaxial instability requiring cervical spine radiographs prior to surgery. The diagnosis is often made by an elevated sedimentation rate or C-reactive protein and positive rheumatoid factor, which is present in most adults but often negative in children. Anticyclic citrullinated peptide antibody (anti-CCP) is more specific for RA. Radiographs and magnetic resonance imaging can also support the diagnosis. General treatment strategies reflect the fact that the destruction of affected joints due to inflammation occurs early in the course of RA. The patient should be offered treatment with disease-modifying antirheumatic drugs (DMARDs) as soon as possible after the onset of disease. Escalate the intensity of treatment until synovitis and inflammation have improved.

4. How is rheumatoid arthritis treated?

There are five general classes of medications used for the treatment of RA, with DMARDs forming the backbone of treatment. Treatment options include the following: analgesics (from acetaminophen to narcotics), NSAIDs, glucocorticoids, nonbiologic DMARDs (methotrexate, sulfasalazine, leflunomide, hydroxychloroquine, and minocycline), and biologic DMARDs. Biologic DMARDs include TNF inhibitors (etanercept, infliximab, adalimumab), an interleukin-1 receptor antagonist (anakinra), a CD20 inhibitor (rituximab), and biologic response modifiers (abatacept).

5. If a pediatric patient has uveitis and an inflammatory arthritis, but the rheumatoid factor is negative, what disease should you suspect?

RA. The rheumatoid factor is often negative in the pauciarticular variant. Affected patients commonly develop uveitis.

6. True or False: Psoriasis can cause an arthritis that resembles osteoarthritis.

False. The arthritis more closely resembles RA. On the Step 3 exam, look for psoriatic skin lesions to make an easy diagnosis. The arthritis usually affects the hands and feet, and though it resembles RA, the rheumatoid factor is negative (seronegative spondyloarthropathy). Along with ankylosing spondylitis, inflammatory bowel disease, and reactive arthritis, psoriatic arthritis is associated with the human leukocyte antigen B27 (HLA-B27) serotype.

7. How is psoriatic arthritis treated?

NSAIDs are first-line therapy. Other treatments include nonbiologic DMARDS (methotrexate, psoralen and ultraviolet light A [PUVA], retinoic acid derivatives, and cyclosporine) and biologic DMARDS, including TNF inhibitors (etanercept, infliximab, adalimumab, golimumab).

8. What is tenosynovitis? How does it occur? What are the presenting symptoms?

Tenosynovitis is inflammation of a tendon and its synovial sheath; the cause is usually an infection. Infections can result from trauma with direct inoculation (e.g., puncture wound or bite), direct spread from adjacent soft tissues, or hematogenous spread. Many organisms can cause tenosynovitis, but skin flora such as *Staphylococcus* and streptococcal species are most common. Look for tenderness along the course of a tendon and enlargement and slight flexion of the affected digit. Ultrasound or an MRI scan may be helpful in confirming the diagnosis. Treat with surgery and antibiotic therapy.

9. Describe the presentation of the various inflammatory myopathies.

There are multiple subtypes of inflammatory myopathies, including dermatomyositis, polymyositis, inclusion body myositis, and overlap syndromes that occur with another rheumatic disease. All subtypes feature immune-mediated muscle injury. For dermatomyositis and polymyositis, look for elevated muscle enzymes (creatine kinase, lactate dehydrogenase, aldolase, alanine aminotransferase, and aspartate aminotransferase), positive autoantibodies such as antinuclear antibodies, and elevated serum and urine myoglobin. Electromyography abnormalities are common, but muscle biopsy is most useful in making a diagnosis and distinguishing the subtypes.

Dermatomyositis typically involves symmetric proximal muscle weakness that gradually worsens, as well as characteristic skin findings such as heliotrope eruption (an erythematous to violaceous eruption on the upper eyelids, sometimes with eyelid edema) and Gottron papules (erythematous to violaceous papules over the dorsal aspects of the metacarpophalangeal and interphalangeal joints). There are other, less common skin eruptions that are unlikely to be tested on the Step 3 USMLE. There is an increased risk of malignancy with dermatomyositis.

The presentation for polymyositis is similar but without the characteristic skin eruptions, which is a key distinguishing factor. Interstitial lung disease may occur with both polymyositis and dermatomyositis.

Inclusion body myositis and overlap syndromes (which occur with diseases such as systemic lupus erythematosus and systemic sclerosis) are unlikely to appear on the Step 3 USMLE.

HEREDITARY DEVELOPMENTAL DISORDERS

1. Describe genu valgum and genu varum. What is the appropriate management for each?
Genu varum, or bow-leg, is when the ankles come together but the knees do not. Genu valgum, or knock-knee, is when the knees come together but the ankles do not. Bow-leg is normal in infants and toddlers, and it generally resolves by age 4 years. Knock-knee is generally normal within the 2- to 8-year-old range. They are more likely to be pathologic if they are asymmetric. Both can be a sign of rickets, Blount disease, physeal deformity, or other bone conditions.

   Pathologic causes of genu valgum include trauma, neoplasms, rickets, and skeletal dysplasia. Clues to pathologic causes include severe valgus deformity, asymmetric valgus deformity, progressive deformity after the age of 4 years, and short stature. X-rays and orthopedic consultation are indicated for suspected pathologic valgus deformity.

   Clues to pathologic causes of genu varum include severe bowing, progressive or persistent bowing after 3 years of age, asymmetric bowing, and short stature. Management is the same as for genu valgum.

2. Specify age at presentation, epidemiology, signs and symptoms, and treatment for the three classically tested pediatric hip disorders.

Name	Age	Epidemiology	Symptoms/Signs	Treatment
DDH	At birth	Female, first-borns, breech delivery	Barlow and Ortolani signs	Observation, abduction splint, or open or closed reduction
LCPD	4–8 yr	Short male with delayed bone age	Knee, thigh, groin pain, limp	Orthoses
SCFE	9–13 yr	Overweight male adolescent	Knee, thigh, groin pain, limp	Surgical pinning

DDH, Developmental dysplasia of the hip; *LCPD,* Legg-Calvé-Perthes disease; *SCFE,* slipped capital femoral epiphysis.
Note: All of these conditions may present in an adult as arthritis of the hip.

3. If you forget everything else about differentiating the three pediatric hip disorders, what historical point will help you the most on the USMLE?
Age at onset of symptoms.

4. How do you check for scoliosis? Who is usually affected? What is the treatment?
Check for scoliosis by having patients touch their toes while you look at the spine. If scoliosis is present, you will see an abnormal lateral curvature of the spine. An imaginary straight line should run from C7 through the gluteal cleft. Scoliosis usually affects prepubertal girls and is idiopathic. Treat with a brace for anything other than very minor (<15 degrees) curvature. If the deformity is severe (e.g., respiratory compromise, rapid progression), surgery should be considered.

5. What is the most common type of muscular dystrophy? How is it inherited? What are the classic findings?
The most common type is Duchenne muscular dystrophy, an X-linked recessive disorder of dystrophin that usually presents in boys between the ages of 3 and 7 years. Look for muscle weakness, markedly elevated levels of creatine phosphokinase, pseudohypertrophy of the calves (due to fatty and fibrous infiltration of the degenerating muscle), and often a lower-than-normal IQ. Gower sign is also classic: The patient "walks" his hands and feet toward each other to rise from a prone position. Muscle biopsy establishes the diagnosis. Treatment is supportive. Most patients die by age 20 years.

6. List the five less common types of muscular dystrophies.
   1. Becker muscular dystrophy: also an X-linked recessive dystrophin disorder but milder.
   2. Fascioscapulohumeral dystrophy: an autosomal dominant disorder that affects the areas in the name (face, shoulder girdle). Symptoms begin between the age of 7 and 20 years. Life expectancy is normal.
   3. Limb-girdle dystrophy: affects pelvic and shoulder muscles; begins in adulthood.
   4. Mitochondrial myopathies: of interest because they are inherited mitochondrial defects (passed only from mother to offspring; cannot be transmitted by men). The key phrase is "ragged red fibers" on biopsy specimen. Ophthalmoplegia is usually present.
   5. Myotonic dystrophy: an autosomal dominant disorder that presents between the ages of 20 and 30 years. Myotonia (inability to relax muscles) classically presents as an **inability to relax the grip or release a handshake.** Look for coexisting mental retardation, baldness, and testicular or ovarian atrophy. Treatment is supportive, including genetic counseling. The diagnosis is clinical.

7. What class of inherited metabolic disorders affects muscle and may resemble muscular dystrophy?
The rare glycogen storage diseases (autosomal recessive inheritance) can cause muscular weakness, especially **McArdle disease,** a deficiency in glycogen phosphorylase that is relatively mild and presents with weakness and cramping after exercise due to lactic acid buildup.

NEOPLASMS

1. What is the most common type of bone tumor?
   Metastatic (especially from breast, lung, or prostate cancer).

2. What is a pathologic fracture? What is the most common cause of a pathologic fracture?
   A pathologic fracture is one that occurs in bone previously weakened by another disease. Osteoporosis (especially in elderly, thin women) is the most common cause, but you should always think about the possibility of malignancy.

3. What is a unicameral bone cyst? Who gets it? Describe the classic presentation.
   A unicameral bone cyst is an expansile, lytic, well-demarcated benign lesion in the proximal portion of the humerus in children and adolescents (Fig. 7.1). Although benign, it may weaken the bone enough to cause a pathologic fracture of the humerus (the classic presentation).

4. Give the basic facts of Paget disease. How is it linked with cancer?
   In Paget disease, bone is broken down and regenerated, often simultaneously. It is usually seen in persons over 40 years old and is more common in men. It is often discovered in an asymptomatic patient through a radiograph. Classic cases involve the pelvis and skull; watch for a person who has had to buy larger-sized hats. Patients may complain of bone pain, arthritis, or hearing loss. **Alkaline phosphatase** is markedly elevated in the presence of normal calcium and phosphorus levels. The risk of osteosarcoma is increased in affected bones. The main treatment is the antiresorptive agents (e.g., zoledronic acid, alendronate, risedronate, pamidronate).

5. What do you need to know about osteosarcomas for the Step 3 exam?
   Osteosarcomas are most commonly seen around the knee in 10- to 30-year-old patients. The classic x-ray finding is a sunburst periosteal reaction (Fig. 7.2) in the distal femur or proximal tibia in association with a mass. In older adults, the risk is increased in bones with long-standing Paget disease or osteomyelitis.

INFECTIONS

1. Which bacteria are the most common cause of septic arthritis? In what scenario should you think of another cause?
   Septic arthritis is most commonly due to *Staphylococcus aureus,* but in sexually active adults (especially when young and/or promiscuous), suspect *Neisseria gonorrhoeae.* In immunocompromised, elderly, or neonatal patients, also consider gram-negative organisms. Aspirate the joint, and order a Gram stain, culture, and cell count with differential if infection is suspected.

2. What clues point to Lyme disease as the cause of arthritis?
   Look for a history of a tick bite or hiking in the woods, **erythema chronicum migrans** rash (Fig. 7.3), and migratory arthritis (later). Treat *Borrelia burgdorferi,* the causative bacteria of Lyme disease, with doxycycline, amoxicillin, or cefuroxime. Avoid doxycycline in children under the age of 8 years and in pregnant or lactating women.

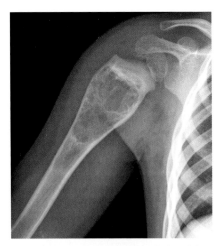

Fig. 7.1 Plain film of unicameral bone cyst manifesting as a large, expansile, completely cystic intramedullary lesion that has well-defined focally sclerotic borders. (From Gilbert-Barness E. *Potter's Pathology of the Fetus, Infant and Child.* 2nd ed. Philadelphia: Mosby; 2007.)

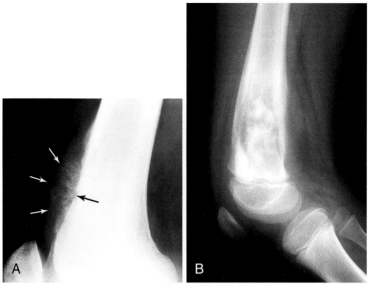

Fig. 7.2 Osteogenic sarcoma of the knee. (A) A lateral view of the knee in a 19-year-old man shows a sunburst-type periosteal reaction *(arrows)*. Knowing that the distal femur is the most common site of osteogenic sarcoma, that periosteal reaction is a feature, and that this patient is a teenager should make osteogenic sarcoma very high on your differential diagnostic list. (B) A destructive central lesion is seen here in the distal femur of an 8-year-old girl. (From Mettler F. *Essentials of Radiology*. 2nd ed. Philadelphia: Saunders; 2004.)

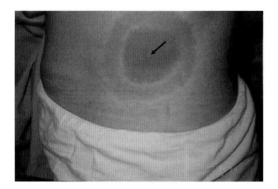

Fig. 7.3 Erythema migrans rash of Lyme disease. Bull's-eye lesion with central punctum. (From Dandache P, Nadelman RB. Erythema migrans. *Infect Dis Clin North Am.* 2008;22[2]:235-260.)

3. How do you recognize reactive arthritis as the cause of arthritis?
Reactive arthritis is also associated with HLA-B27. The classic triad of symptoms consists of **urethritis** (due to chlamydial infection), **conjunctivitis,** and **arthritis** ("can't pee, can't see, can't climb a tree"). Reactive arthritis may also follow enteric bacterial infections. Superficial oral and penile ulcers are common. Diagnose and treat the sexually transmitted disease, and use NSAIDs for arthritis. Also treat the patient's sexual partners.

4. What is the most common bacterial cause of osteomyelitis? In what clinical scenarios should you think of other causes?
Osteomyelitis is caused most commonly by *S. aureus.* Think of gram-negative bacteria in immunocompromised patients or intravenous drug abusers. *Salmonella* sp. is the most likely cause in patients with sickle cell disease. Think *Pseudomonas aeruginosa* if there is a puncture wound through a tennis shoe. Diabetic patients who develop a "diabetic foot" with subsequent osteomyelitis usually have a polymicrobial infection. The gold standard for selecting antibiotic therapy is aspiration or biopsy of the affected joint or bone, respectively. Order a Gram stain, culture, and cell count of the fluid or tissue if osteomyelitis is suspected. Check a serum white blood cell (WBC) and erythrocyte sedimentation rate (ESR) or C-reactive protein.

TRAUMATIC INJURIES

1. What are the common findings with ligament injuries of the knee? How do you distinguish injuries of the anterior cruciate, posterior cruciate, medial collateral, and lateral collateral ligaments on physical exam?

   Ligament injuries in the knee commonly cause pain, joint effusions, instability of the joint, and history of the joint popping, buckling, or locking up.

   - **Anterior cruciate ligament (ACL)** tears are the most common. Watch for the *anterior* drawer test. With the patient supine, the knee is placed in 90 degrees of flexion, and the tibia is pulled forward (like opening a drawer). If the tibia pulls forward more than normal (e.g., more than the unaffected side), the test is positive, and the patient has an ACL tear. Alternatively, use the Lachman test.
   - **Posterior cruciate ligament (PCL)** tears can be diagnosed with the *posterior* drawer test. Push the tibia back with the knee in 90 degrees of flexion. If the tibia pushes back more than the unaffected side, the test is positive, and a PCL tear is present.
   - **Medial collateral ligament (MCL)** tears are suggested during the *abduction* or *valgus* stress test. With the patient supine and the knee in 30 degrees of flexion, place a hand on the lateral knee and push the lower leg laterally at the ankle. If the knee joint abducts to an abnormal degree, the test is positive, and a medial compartment injury is present.
   - **Lateral collateral ligament (LCL)** tears are suggested during the *adduction* or *varus* stress test. This is the opposite of valgus stress. With the patient supine and the knee in 30 degrees of flexion, place a hand on the medial knee, and push the lower leg medially at the ankle. If the knee joint adducts to an abnormal degree, the test is positive, and a lateral compartment injury is present.

     MRI and/or arthroscopy can be used to confirm suspected tears and look for other injuries.

2. What type of radiographs should you order if you suspect a fracture?

   For any suspected fracture, order at least two views (usually anteroposterior and lateral) of the site, and consider radiographs of the joints above and below the fracture site.

3. How should you treat a patient with severe pain after trauma and negative x-rays?

   Rule out compartment syndrome. Treat the patient conservatively. Assume that there is a fracture and have the patient rest the injured area. Splinting may be appropriate for distal extremity injuries. Obtain follow-up radiographs 7 to 14 days after the injury if symptoms persist; many occult fractures will become visible at this time. The exception to waiting is a suspected hip fracture in an elderly person—proceed to CT or MRI of the hip to allow earlier diagnosis and treatment, which decrease operative morbidity and length of hospital stay compared with delayed diagnosis and treatment. In the pediatric population, x-rays may not always reveal fractures (because the growth plate is cartilaginous rather than bone so it isn't radiopaque), so if a child has pain over a growth plate, consider this a fracture (Salter-Harris type I) and immobilize.

4. What fracture is usually diagnosed in trauma patients with pain in the anatomic snuffbox? Why is it concerning?

   Scaphoid bone fracture (Fig. 7.4), classically after a fall onto an outstretched hand ("FOOSH"). The scaphoid is the most commonly fractured carpal bone. X-rays may not show a fracture initially, so if the patient has a fall onto an

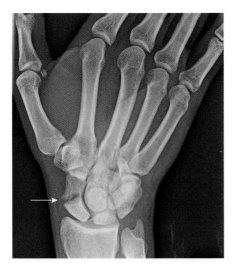

Fig. 7.4 Scaphoid fracture. Scaphoid view x-ray (anteroposterior [AP] view with ulnar deviation) is important to obtain in addition to standard wrist views (AP, lateral, and oblique) when scaphoid fracture is suspected. This scaphoid fracture was not seen on the x-rays on the day of the injury. The patient continued to have wrist pain and then presented 10 weeks later and x-rays were obtained demonstrating the scaphoid fracture. (From Bope E, Kellerman R. *Conn's Current Therapy.* Philadelphia: Elsevier; 2017:829-873.)

outstretched hand and has pain in the anatomic snuffbox, treat these injuries as a fracture. Repeat x-rays can be performed 1 to 2 weeks later. Complications include nonunion of the fracture, chronic arthritis, and avascular necrosis due to its unidirectional blood supply.

5. What orthopedic fractures are associated with the highest mortality rate?
   Pelvic fractures, because patients can bleed to death. If the patient is unstable, consider heroic measures such as military antishock trousers (MAST) and an external fixator.

6. Why should areas distal to the fracture site be assessed by physical examination?
   Areas distal to the fracture site should be assessed for neurologic and vascular compromise, either of which may be an emergency.

7. Distinguish between an open and a closed fracture.
   With an open (compound) fracture, the skin is broken over the fracture site. Suspect an open fracture with any overlying wound; the fractured bone does not have to be obviously exposed. In closed fractures, the skin is intact over the fracture site.

8. Explain the difference in management of open and closed fractures.
   With closed fractures, closed reduction (setting the bone without surgery) and casting can generally be done. With open fractures, prophylactic antibiotics are chosen based upon the size of the wound, contamination, type of fracture, and vascular injury. Cefazolin is appropriate for lower-risk fractures; vancomycin if the patient is at risk for methicillin-resistant *S. aureus* (MRSA); ceftriaxone plus gentamicin for higher-risk fractures with the addition of metronidazole if there has been soil contamination. Do surgical debridement, give a tetanus vaccine booster, lavage fresh wounds (if <8 hours old), and perform **open reduction and internal fixation** (ORIF). The main risk in open fractures is infection, which is usually not a problem with closed fractures because the skin is intact.

9. What are the indications for open reduction other than an open fracture?
   - Intraarticular fractures or articular surface malalignment
   - Nonunion or failed closed reduction
   - Neurovascular compromise
   - Multiple trauma (to allow mobilization at the earliest possible point)
   - Need for perfect reduction to optimize extremity function (e.g., professional athletes)

10. Define compartment syndrome. What is the cause?
    Compartment syndrome is a problem of muscle compartments, which are limited by the fascia in which they are contained. It is seen in the extremities (most commonly in the calf) when edema or hemorrhage causes swelling inside a muscle compartment. Rising pressure inside the fascial compartment can lead to decreased perfusion that can result in permanent muscle and nerve damage.
    The three common clinical scenarios in which compartment syndrome is seen are fractures (classically midshaft tibial fractures or supracondylar fractures of the humerus in children), burns (especially electrical and circumferential burns), and vascular compromise (or after vascular surgery procedures due to reperfusion injury).

11. What are the signs and symptoms of compartment syndrome? How is it treated?
    The seven *P*s (**p**ain, **p**aresthesia, **p**allow, **p**alpable swelling, **p**aralysis, absent **p**ulses, elevated **p**ressure):
    - Pain (especially pain on passive movement that is out of proportion to the injury)
    - Paresthesias, hypoesthesia, and numbness (decreased sensation and two-point discrimination)
    - Cyanosis or pallor
    - Palpable swelling and firm-feeling muscle compartment
    - Paralysis (late, ominous sign)
    - Absent peripheral pulses (late, ominous sign)
    - Elevated compartment pressure (>30–40 mm Hg)
    On the USMLE, the diagnosis of compartment syndrome often has to be made clinically without a pressure reading. Although pulses may be slightly decreased, they are usually palpable (or detectable with Doppler ultrasound) with compartment syndrome. Lack of palpable pulses is an ominous, late sign. Compartment syndrome is an emergency, and quick action can save an otherwise doomed limb. Treatment is immediate fasciotomy; incising the fascial compartment relieves the pressure.

12. Define Charcot joint. What causes it? How is it managed?
    Charcot joints (neuropathic joints) are seen in patients with diabetes mellitus or other conditions causing peripheral neuropathy (e.g., tertiary syphilis). Due to decreased sensation, joints are subject to repetitive microtrauma, causing gradual arthritis or arthropathy and joint deformity. Patients should get radiographs for any (even minor) trauma because they may not feel even a severe fracture.

13. What is complex regional pain syndrome (CRPS)? What symptoms do patients have? How is the diagnosis made?
    CRPS describes an array of painful conditions characterized by a continuing regional pain that is seemingly disproportionate in time or degree to the usual course of any known trauma or other lesion. The pain is not in a specific

nerve territory or dermatome. Patients have pain, swelling, limited range of motion, vasomotor instability, skin changes, and patchy bone demineralization. It frequently begins following a fracture, soft tissue injury, or surgery. Two subtypes of CRPS are recognized:

- Type I (formerly known as reflex sympathetic dystrophy) has no evidence of peripheral nerve injury and represents approximately 90% of clinical presentations
- Type II refers to cases in which peripheral nerve injury is present.

Diagnosis is based on clinical features, including symptoms developing after limb trauma, usually within 4 to 6 weeks; symptoms are no longer fully explained by the initial trauma; and symptoms affect the distal limb, go beyond the region involved in the trauma, or extend beyond the territory innervated by a single nerve or nerve root. There is no gold standard test for confirming the diagnosis. Three-phase bone scintigraphy may show increased radiotracer uptake in joints distant from the trauma site.

14. **True or False: There is a high incidence of vascular injury with posterior knee dislocations.**
True. Posterior displacement of the tibia is associated with popliteal artery injury. Order an angiogram if pulses are asymmetric (i.e., weaker or absent on the affected side) to check for injury.

15. **To what site is pain from hip inflammation or dislocation/fracture classically referred?**
The knee (especially in children).

16. **Define Osgood-Schlatter disease. How is it recognized and treated?**
Osgood-Schlatter disease is osteochondritis (aseptic ischemic necrosis) of the tibial tubercle. It is often bilateral and usually presents in boys between 10 and 15 years of age. It is mainly caused by overuse of the quadriceps muscles, leading to excess strain of the patellar ligament on the tibial tuberosity, resulting in traction apophysitis at the bony attachment. Signs and symptoms include pain, swelling, and tenderness in the knee (remember, the above-mentioned pediatric hip problems have referred pain in the knee but no knee swelling or tenderness upon palpation of the knee). Treat with rest, activity restriction, and NSAIDs. Most cases resolve on their own.

CHAPTER 8

DISORDERS OF THE SKIN AND SUBCUTANEOUS TISSUE

1. Cover the two right-hand columns in the following table and define the common terms used in dermatology to describe skin findings.

Term	Definition	Examples
Macule	Flat spot <1 cm (nonpalpable, just visible)	Freckles, tattoos
Patch	Same as macule but >1 cm	Port-wine birthmarks
Papule	Solid, elevated lesion <1 cm (palpable)	Wart, acne, lichen planus
Plaque	Same as papule but >1 cm and flat topped	Psoriasis
Nodule	Palpable, solid lesion >1 cm and not flat topped	Small lipoma, erythema nodosum
Vesicle	Elevated, circumscribed lesion <5 mm containing clear fluid (small blister)	Chickenpox, genital herpes
Bulla	Same as vesicle but >5 mm (large blister)	Contact dermatitis, pemphigus
Wheal	Itchy, transiently edematous area	Allergic reaction

SKIN ERUPTIONS

1. Define vitiligo. With what diseases is it associated? What is the treatment?
   Vitiligo is characterized by well-demarcated macules or patches of skin depigmentation due to autoimmune destruction of melanocytes of unknown etiology. It is an acquired condition that is associated with autoimmune diseases such as pernicious anemia, hypothyroidism, Addison disease, and type 1 diabetes. Patients often have antibodies to melanin, parietal cells, thyroid, or other factors. Vitiligo can be treated with topical corticosteroids, topical calcineurin inhibitors (e.g., tacrolimus, pimecrolimus), and phototherapy.

2. Name several conditions to think about on the Step 3 exam in patients with pruritis.
   Think of serious conditions first, such as obstructive biliary disease, uremia, and polycythemia rubra vera (classically seen after a warm shower or bath due to mast cell degranulation). Pruritis may also be caused by contact or atopic dermatitis, scabies, and lichen planus.

3. Define contact dermatitis. How do you recognize it? What are the classic culprits?
   Contact dermatitis is usually due to a type IV hypersensitivity reaction, although it may also be due to an irritating or toxic substance. Look for a new exposure to a classic offending agent, such as poison ivy, nickel earrings, or deodorant. Allergic contact dermatitis requires a previous sensitizing event as opposed to irritant contact dermatitis, which does not. The rash is well circumscribed and occurs only in the area of exposure. The skin is red and itchy and often has vesicles or bullae (Fig. 8.1). Avoidance of the agent is required. Patch testing can be done, if needed, to determine the antigen.

4. Define atopic dermatitis. What history points to this diagnosis? What is the treatment?
   Atopic dermatitis, also known as eczema, is a chronic allergic-type condition that begins in the first year of life with red, itchy, weeping skin on the head, upper extremities on extensor surfaces, and sometimes around the diaper area. In children and adults, it usually develops on the flexor surfaces. The clue to diagnosis is a family and/or personal history of allergies (e.g., hay fever) and asthma. The biggest problem is scratching of affected skin, which leads to skin breaks and possible bacterial infection. Treatment involves avoidance of drying soaps and use of antihistamines, moisturizing creams, topical steroids, and immune modulating agents (topical pimecrolimus or tacrolimus).

5. What is diaper dermatitis? Name the main causes.
   Diaper dermatitis is the term used for any inflammatory skin eruption that occurs in the diaper-covered region. Diaper-associated causes include irritant dermatitis, *Candida* dermatitis, and allergic dermatitis. Non–diaper-associated causes include seborrhea, atopic dermatitis, bacterial causes (impetigo and group A streptococcal infection), herpes simplex virus, psoriasis, scabies, and congenital syphilis. Child abuse must always be considered.

6. How are the most common causes of diaper dermatitis treated?
   Irritant dermatitis can be treated by avoiding skin contact with the diaper, such as allowing some time without the diaper on. Topical barriers such as petrolatum and zinc oxide can also be helpful. Candidal dermatitis can be treated with topical nystatin, clotrimazole, or miconazole. Classically, irritant dermatitis is present on the convex

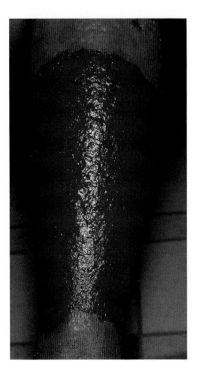

Fig. 8.1 Allergic contact dermatitis of the leg caused by an elastic wrap. Notice the well-marginated distribution that differentiates it from cellulitis. (From Auerbach PS. *Wilderness Medicine.* 6th ed. Philadelphia: Mosby; 2011 [fig. 82-46].)

surfaces of the skin, with the intertriginous (skin fold) areas spared because the irritant does not get into the folds. This is in contrast to candidal dermatitis, which prefers the moist areas in skin folds.

7. **Define rosacea. In what age group is it seen? How do you treat it?**
Rosacea often looks like acne but begins in middle age. There are several different subtypes (papulopustular, erythematotelangiectasia, ocular) of rosacea. The most common is the papulopustular subtype. Typically, patients present with facial erythema and flushing (Fig. 8.2). There are numerous triggers for rosacea, including sun exposure, emotional stress, alcohol consumption, spicy foods, and hot weather. Also look for **rhinophyma** (bulbous red nose) and coexisting blepharitis. Treat the papulopustular subtype with topical metronidazole or oral tetracycline. Treat the erythematotelangiectasia subtype with topical brimonidine. The pathogenesis is incompletely understood.

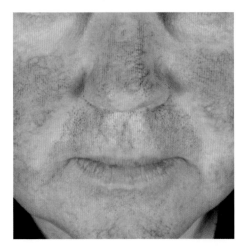

Fig. 8.2 Rosacea. Telangiectasias and erythema due to chronic actinic damage. (From Bolognia J, Schaffer J. *Dermatology Essentials.* Philadelphia: Saunders; 2014:261-267.)

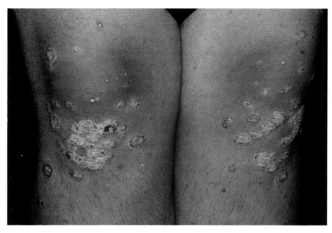

Fig. 8.3 Typical plaques of psoriasis with thick scale overlying erythema. (From Paller AS, Mancini AJ. *Hurwitz Clinical Pediatric Dermatology, A Textbook of Skin Disorders of Childhood and Adolescence.* 5th ed. Philadelphia: Elsevier; 2016.)

8. Describe the classic psoriatic lesion.

Psoriatic lesions are classically described as dry, well-circumscribed, erythematous, silvery, scaling papules and plaques that are *not* pruritic (Fig. 8.3). Classic lesions are found on the scalp, lumbosacral region, intergluteal clefts, and extensor surfaces of the elbows and knees. Look for Auspitz sign, which is a small amount of bleeding when a psoriatic scale is scraped away. It is caused by abnormal proliferation of keratinocytes.

9. What other historical points and physical findings may be seen with psoriasis? How is it diagnosed and treated?

A family history of psoriasis is often present, and the disease mostly occurs in whites with onset in early adulthood. Affected patients may have pitting of the nails and an arthritis that resembles rheumatoid arthritis but is rheumatoid factor negative. Diagnosis of psoriasis can often be made by appearance alone, but a biopsy can be used in doubtful cases. Certain types of psoriasis are associated with infectious causes. For example, diffuse, sudden-onset psoriasis is associated with human immunodeficiency virus (HIV) infection. Guttate psoriasis (scaly, droplike plaques/papules) typically occurs after a streptococcal infection. Treatment is complex but involves exposure to ultraviolet light, lubricants, topical corticosteroids, calcipotriene, and keratolytics (e.g., coal tar, salicylic acid, anthralin). Oral therapies may include immunosuppressive and immunomodulating drugs such as methotrexate, cyclosporine, and biologic agents.

10. What are the four *P*s that clinch a diagnosis of lichen planus?

Pruritic, **p**urple, **p**olygonal **p**apules (or plaques) classically on the wrists, lower legs, or genitalia, usually of adults (Fig. 8.4). Oral mucosal lesions with a whitish, lacelike pattern (Wickham striae) may also be present. These oral lesions must be monitored as they may increase the risk for oral cancer. It is associated with hepatitis C virus (HCV) infection.

11. Describe the classic lesion of erythema multiforme. What drugs classically cause it?

Look for the classic target (iris) lesions (Fig. 8.5). The classic cause is sulfa drugs or penicillins, but herpes infections may also cause erythema multiforme, and some cases are idiopathic. Erythema multiforme exists on a spectrum. As it becomes more severe and widespread, it is known as **Stevens-Johnson syndrome (SJS),** which

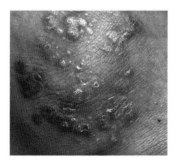

Fig. 8.4 Lichen planus. Flat-topped, purple polygonal papules of lichen planus. (From Kliegman RM. *Nelson Textbook of Pediatrics.* 19th ed. Philadelphia: Saunders; 2011 [fig. 649-10].)

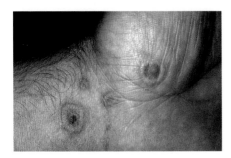

Fig. 8.5 Erythema multiforme. Bull's-eye annular lesions with central vesicles and bullae. (From Goldman L, Schafer AI. *Goldman's Cecil Medicine.* 24th ed. Philadelphia: Saunders; 2011 [fig. 447-10].)

is often fatal. SJS encompasses less than 10% of skin. Patients with SJS are treated supportively with therapy similar to what a burn victim would receive (wound care, fluid and electrolyte management, pain control, nutritional support, and monitoring for and treatment of superinfections). If greater than 30% of skin is involved, it is classified as toxic epidermal necrolysis.

12. **Define and describe pemphigus vulgaris. How is it different from bullous pemphigoid?**
    Pemphigus vulgaris is a potentially life-threatening autoimmune disease of middle-aged and elderly patients. It presents with multiple flaccid bullae, starting in the oral mucosa and spreading to the skin of the rest of the body. These bullae rupture easily. Look for Nikolsky sign, which is sloughing and ulcerations that occur when minor pressure is applied to the skin. Biopsy can be stained for antibody (an immunoglobulin G [IgG] antibody to desmoglein III, which is associated with desmosomes) and shows a lacelike or fishnet-like immunofluorescence pattern. Tombstone-like cells are seen on histology. Treat with oral corticosteroids.

    Bullous pemphigoid is a similar but milder condition that often presents as multiple tense bullae all over the body. Biopsy reveals a linear immunofluorescence pattern (different antibody), and this condition is also treated with oral corticosteroids (Fig. 8.6). Nikolsky sign is not present with bullous pemphigoid. Bullous pemphigoid is due to antibodies directed against the hemidesmosome. It is associated with certain neurologic diseases (Parkinson disease, multiple sclerosis) and malignancy. Treat with topical corticosteroids.

13. **What skin disease is associated with celiac disease (gluten intolerance or sensitivity)? How is it treated?**
    Dermatitis herpetiformis is associated with celiac disease. Patients have intensely pruritic vesicles, papules, and wheals on the extensor aspects of the elbows and knees and possibly on the face or neck (Fig. 8.7). Look for diarrhea and weight loss (due to gluten sensitivity). On biopsy, the skin has IgA deposits even in unaffected areas. Test for celiac disease, and treat both conditions with a gluten-free diet. Additionally, dapsone can be used for acute treatment.

14. **What are decubitus ulcers? What is the best method of prevention?**
    Decubitus ulcers (bedsores or pressure sores) are skin ulcers caused by prolonged pressure against the skin. The best treatment is prophylaxis. Periodic turning of paralyzed, bedridden, or debilitated patients (the populations in

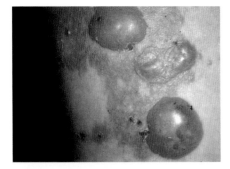

Fig. 8.6 Bullous pemphigoid. Tense subepidermal bullae on an erythematous base. (From Goldman L, Schafer AI. *Goldman's Cecil Medicine.* 24th ed. Philadelphia: Saunders; 2011 [fig. 447-6].)

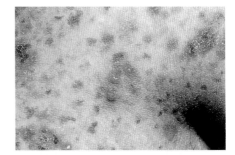

Fig. 8.7 Dermatitis herpetiformis is characterized by pruritis, urticarial papules, and small vesicles. (From Feldman M, Friedman LS, Brandt LJ. *Sleisenger and Fordtran's Gastrointestinal and Liver Disease.* 9th ed. Philadelphia: Saunders; 2010 [fig. 22-26]. Courtesy Dr. Timothy Berger, San Francisco, CA.)

which they are most common) and use of special air mattresses prevents bedsores. Cleanliness and dryness also help to prevent decubitus ulcers. Periodic skin inspection makes sure that the problem is recognized early. When missed, the lesions can ulcerate down to the bone and become infected, possibly leading to sepsis and death. Treat major skin breaks with aggressive surgical debridement; if signs of infection are present, administer antibiotics.

15. How are decubitus ulcers staged?
    Stage 1 is intact skin with nonblanchable redness of a localized area. Stage 2 is partial-thickness loss of the dermis presenting as a shallow open ulcer. These may also present as an intact or ruptured blister. Stage 3 is full-thickness tissue loss. Subcutaneous fat may be visible, but bone, tendon, or muscle is not exposed. Stage 4 is full-thickness skin loss with exposed bone, tendon, or muscle. An unstageable ulcer has full-thickness loss in which the base of the ulcer is covered with slough or eschar. The true depth of the ulcer cannot be determined until the slough or eschar is removed.

DISORDERS OF NAILS/HAIR/SWEAT GLANDS

1. How is acne described in medical terms? What bacteria may be partially involved in its pathogenesis?
   Acne vulgaris can be broken down into various subtypes, including comedonal, inflammatory, and nodular (cystic) acne. Comedonal acne presents with closed (whitehead) or open (blackhead) comedones primarily on the forehead, nose, and chin. Inflammatory acne presents with small (<5 mm), erythematous papules and pustules. Nodular (cystic) acne presents with large (>5 mm) nodules that may merge to form sinus tracts and subsequent scarring. *Propionibacterium acnes* is thought to be partially involved in pathogenesis, as is blockage of pilosebaceous glands.

2. What are the treatment options for acne?
   Treatment options are multiple. Start with topical retinoids and salicylic or azelaic acids; then try topical benzoyl peroxide, topical clindamycin, or erythromycin, either with or without an oral antibiotic (typically a tetracycline or erythromycin for *P. acnes* eradication). Oral isotretinoin is the last resort. Although highly effective, isotretinoin is teratogenic; pregnancy testing in women before and during therapy as well as contraceptive use is mandatory. Women of childbearing age must be on two forms of contraception. In addition, it may cause dry skin and mucosae, muscle and joint pain, and liver function test abnormalities.

3. Define seborrheic dermatitis. What part of the body does it involve? How is it treated?
   Seborrheic dermatitis causes the common conditions known as cradle cap and dandruff as well as blepharitis (eyelid inflammation). Look for scaling skin with or without erythema on the hairy areas of the head (scalp, eyebrows, eyelashes, mustache, beard) as well as on the forehead, nasolabial folds, external ear canals, and postauricular creases. Treat with dandruff shampoo (e.g., selenium sulfide or tar shampoo), topical corticosteroids, and/or ketoconazole cream.

4. What should you think about if hirsutism is described in the Step 3 exam?
   Hirsutism is most commonly idiopathic, but other signs of virilization (e.g., deepening voice, clitoromegaly, frontal balding) suggest an androgen-secreting ovarian tumor. In the absence of virilization, consider Cushing syndrome, polycystic ovary syndrome, and drugs (minoxidil, corticosteroids, and phenytoin).

5. What are the common pathologic causes of baldness?
   Watch out for trichotillomania (a psychiatric disorder in which patients pull out their hair; baldness is patchy and irregular) and alopecia areata (idiopathic but associated with antimicrosomal and other autoantibodies), and telogen effluvium (caused by stress). Baldness may also be seen in patients with lupus erythematosus or syphilis and after cancer chemotherapy.

6. What causes ordinary male pattern baldness?
   Although the exact pathophysiology is still not clear, male pattern baldness is considered a genetic disorder that requires androgens for expression.

7. What is hyperhidrosis? What causes it? How is it treated?
   Hyperhidrosis is sweating in amounts greater than what is required for thermoregulation. It typically occurs both awake and while sleeping, is bilateral, and affects the face, palms, soles, or axillae. Hyperhidrosis can have significant social and emotional consequences. Most cases are chronic and idiopathic, but consider medical conditions (e.g., hyperthyroidism, tuberculosis, HIV, malignancy, endocarditis) and medications (e.g., hypoglycemic agents, antidepressants, hormonal agents, sympathomimetics) as possible causes. Treatment typically starts with 20% aluminum chloride in ethanol (Drysol) topically. Beta-blockers or benzodiazepines can be considered for cases of hyperhidrosis attributed to stress. Anticholinergic agents and clonidine may help but are limited by side effects. Axillary hyperhidrosis can be treated with botulinum toxin. Palmar hyperhidrosis that is refractory to topical and systemic therapies can be treated with endoscopic thoracic sympathectomy.

LUMPS/TUMORS OF THE SKIN

1. Describe the classic lesion of erythema nodosum. With what diseases is it commonly associated? What should the workup include?

   Erythema nodosum (Fig. 8.8) is an inflammation of the subcutaneous tissue and skin, classically over the shins (pretibial). Look for tender, red, elevated nodules. Sarcoidosis, coccidioidomycosis, or ulcerative colitis classically accompany this condition on the USMLE, though multiple other infections (e.g., streptococcal, tuberculosis) and drugs (e.g., sulfonamides) can also result in this finding. The most common vasculitis associated with it is Behçet syndrome. Treat the underlying disease, and provide symptomatic therapies such as nonsteroidal antiinflammatory drugs, leg elevation, and compressive bandages. The workup should include basic laboratory testing, tuberculosis skin testing, antistreptolysin-O antibodies, and a chest x-ray to look for sarcoidosis and tuberculosis.

2. True or False: Most melanomas start out as simple moles.

   True. Moles are common and benign, but malignant transformation is possible (Fig. 8.9). **ABCDE characteristics of a mole** that should make you suspicious of malignant transformation are **a**symmetry, **b**orders (irregular), **c**olor (change in color or multiple colors), **d**iameter (the bigger the lesion, the more likely that it is malignant), and **e**volution over time. Excise any mole if it enlarges suddenly (or do a biopsy if the lesion is very large), develops irregular borders, darkens or becomes inflamed, changes color (even if only one small area of the mole changes color), begins to bleed, begins to itch, or becomes painful.

3. To what parameter is the prognosis of a malignant melanoma most closely related?

   The Breslow thickness (or depth) of the tumor. The 10-year survival rate decreases as the thickness of the tumor increases. Tumors less than 1 mm thick have the best prognosis.

4. What type of melanoma do black patients tend to develop? How do you recognize it?

   Although uncommon in blacks, melanoma tends to be of the acral lentiginous type. Look for black dots on the palms or soles or under the fingernail (Fig. 8.10) that start to change in appearance or cause symptoms.

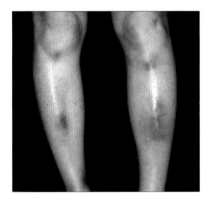

Fig. 8.8 Erythema nodosum on the legs of a young woman. (From Hochberg MA, Silman AJ, Smolen JS, et al. *Rheumatology.* 5th ed. Philadelphia: Mosby; 2010 [fig. 159-13].)

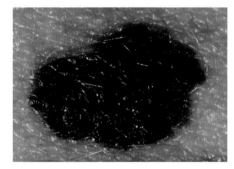

Fig. 8.9 Melanoma (superficial spreading type). (From Goldman L, Schafer AI. *Goldman's Cecil Medicine.* 24th ed. Philadelphia: Saunders; 2011 [fig. 210-3].)

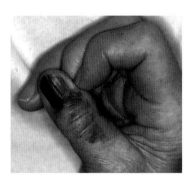

Fig. 8.10 Nailbed melanoma. (From Dartmouth University, Dermnet Weekly Clinic. 2001[July 30].)

5. Define dysplastic nevi syndrome. How is it managed?

Dysplastic nevus syndrome is a genetic condition with multiple dysplastic-appearing nevi (usually >100 moles). Also look for a family history of melanoma. Treat with careful and regular follow-up, excision or biopsy of any suspicious lesions, avoidance of sun exposure, and sunscreen use.

6. Why is keratoacanthoma of note?

Keratoacanthoma can mimic skin cancer (especially squamous cell cancer). Look for a flesh-colored lesion with a central crater that contains keratinous material, classically on the face (Fig. 8.11). Keratoacanthoma has a very rapid onset and grows to its full size in 1 to 2 months (which almost never happens with squamous cell cancer). The lesion involutes spontaneously in a few months and requires no treatment. If unsure, the best step is a biopsy, but choose observation as the answer in patients with a classic history of keratoacanthoma.

7. Describe the classic lesion of basal cell cancer. What should you do if you suspect it?

Basal cell cancer classically begins as a shiny papule on a skin-exposed area (the head is classic) and slowly enlarges and develops an umbilicated center with pearly borders (and later may ulcerate and bleed easily) with peripheral telangiectasias (Fig. 8.12). Like all skin cancers, sunlight exposure increases the risk. It is more common in elderly, light-skinned people. Treat with excision. Biopsy any suspicious skin lesions in the elderly. It is the most common type of skin cancer.

8. True or False: Basal cell skin cancer almost never develops metastases.

True. However, it may be locally invasive and destructive.

9. From what lesion does squamous cell cancer classically develop? What is Bowen disease?

Squamous cell cancer (Fig. 8.13) often develops in areas with preexisting actinic keratoses (hard, sharp, red, often scaly lesions in sun-exposed areas) (Fig. 8.14) or burn scars. The lesions become nodular, warty, or ulcerated; do a biopsy if such transformation occurs. Squamous cell cancer in situ is known as Bowen disease, and lesions are

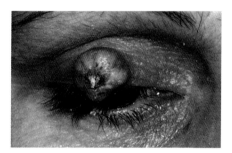

Fig. 8.11 Keratoacanthoma on the right upper lid. Lesions are solitary, smooth, dome-shaped red papules or nodules with a central keratin plug. (From Albert DM, Miller JW. *Albert and Jakobiec's Principles and Practice of Ophthalmology.* 3rd ed. Philadelphia: Saunders; 2008 [fig. 250-3].)

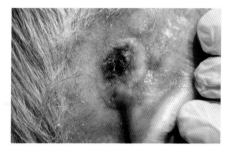

Fig. 8.12 An ulcerated basal cell carcinoma with rolled borders on the posterior ear. (From Abeloff MD, Armitage JO, Niederhuber JE, et al. *Abeloff's Clinical Oncology,* 4th ed. Philadelphia: Churchill Livingstone; 2008 [fig. 74-2].)

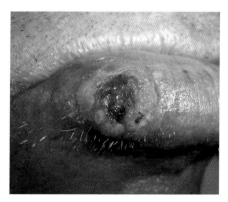

Fig. 8.13 Squamous cell carcinoma on the lower lip. (From Rakel D, Rakel RE. *Textbook of Family Medicine.* 8th ed. Philadelphia: Saunders; 2011 [fig. 33-85]. Copyright Richard P. Usatine.)

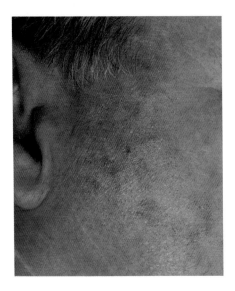

Fig. 8.14 Multiple actinic keratoses visible as thin, red, scaly lesions. (From Goldberg D. *Procedures in Cosmetic Dermatology: Lasers and Lights* [vol. 1]. 2nd ed. Philadelphia: Saunders; 2008 [fig. 5-2].)

typically well demarcated. Although metastases are rare in squamous cell cancer, they occur more frequently than in basal cell cancer. They can also cause numbness/paresthesias due to early perineural invasion.

10. **Describe Paget disease of the breast. What is its significance?**
    Paget disease of the breast presents as a unilateral, red, oozing or crusting nipple in an adult woman that fails to respond to typical dermatology treatments (Fig. 8.15). Though rare (roughly 1%–2% of breast cancers), it signifies an underlying breast cancer (usually invasive ductal carcinoma or ductal carcinoma in situ) with extension to the skin.

11. **What is the classic clinical manifestation of Kaposi sarcoma?**
    A rash that does not respond to multiple treatments in a HIV-positive patient. Kaposi sarcoma is a vascular skin tumor that commonly begins as a papule or plaque on the upper body or in the oral cavity (Fig. 8.16). It is highly associated with herpesvirus (human herpesvirus 8 [HHV-8]) infection.

12. **What is the main risk factor for skin cancer?**
    Ultraviolet light exposure.

13. **Describe the clinical findings in tuberous sclerosis.**
    The findings for this autosomal dominant disorder are hypopigmented skin macules (ash leaf spots), seizures, intellectual disability, and central nervous system hamartomas (tubers). There is an increased risk of cardiac

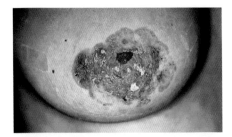

Fig. 8.15 Paget disease of the nipple. Note the erythematous plaques around the nipple. (From Bolognia JL, Jorizzo JL, Rapini RP. *Dermatology.* 1st ed. Edinburgh: Mosby; 2003 [fig. 53-8].)

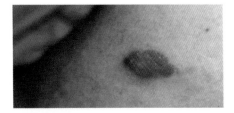

Fig. 8.16 Kaposi sarcoma. (From Hoffman R. *Hematology: Basic Principles and Practice.* 5th ed. Philadelphia: Churchill Livingstone; 2008 [fig. 121-35].)

rhabdomyomas and renal tumors known as angiomyolipomas (because they comprise vascular, muscle, and fatty tissue). Look for a positive family history, although most cases are new mutations.

14. **How are capillary hemangiomas treated?**
    Capillary hemangiomas (also known as strawberry hemangiomas) are benign vascular tumors that are often first noticed a few days after birth. They tend to increase in size after birth (sometimes becoming quite large) and gradually resolve within the first 2 years of life (Fig. 8.17). The best treatment is to do nothing but observe and follow. Laser therapy can be considered in cases in which a capillary hemangioma is causing impairment (such as covering an eye or the mouth).

15. **Describe the skin lesions of neurofibromatosis type 1 (NF1). What else do you need to know about NF1?**
    Café-au-lait macules (Fig. 8.18) and cutaneous neurofibromas are the hallmark lesions of NF1. There is increased risk of mental retardation with NF1. There is also an increased lifetime risk of malignancy in patients with NF1 (5%–10% of patients will develop peripheral nerve-sheath tumors; also look for malignancies such as pheochromocytoma and leukemia). Most patients with NF1 have macrocephaly, and many have short stature. Scoliosis is common. Hypertension may result from renovascular disease, coarctation of the aorta, or tumors that secrete vasoactive substances. Gastrointestinal neurofibromas can cause obstruction or anemia from bleeding. Seizures may result from intracranial tumors.

INFECTIONS

1. **Name the various dermatologic fungal infections.**
   Known as dermatophytosis, tinea, and ringworm. Fungal infections include the following:

   Tinea corporis (body/trunk): look for red ring-shaped lesions with raised borders that tend to clear centrally while they expand peripherally (Fig. 8.19).

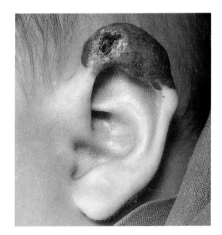

Fig. 8.17 Infantile hemangioma. These lesions grow rapidly during the first few months of life once they appear (20% at birth), but they are asymptomatic unless they bleed, become infected, or obstruct a vital structure. Complete resolution is typical before the age of 7 years, and no treatment is usually required. (From du Vivier A. *Atlas of Clinical Dermatology.* 3rd ed. New York: Churchill Livingstone; 2002 [fig. 8-28].)

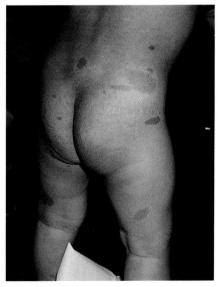

Fig. 8.18 Multiple café-au-lait macules on a child with neurofibromatosis type 1. (From Eichenfield LF, Frieden IJ, Esterly NB. *Neonatal Dermatology.* 2nd ed. Philadelphia: Saunders; 2007 [fig. 22-2].)

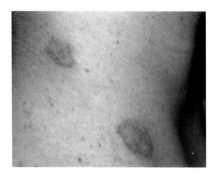

Fig. 8.19 Tinea corporis. Red ring-shaped lesions with scaling and some central clearing. (From Kliegman RM. *Nelson Textbook of Pediatrics.* 19th ed. Philadelphia: Saunders; 2011 [fig. 658-8].)

Tinea pedis (athlete's foot): look for macerated, scaling web spaces between the toes that often itch and may be associated with thickened, distorted toenails (onychomycosis). It may be acquired from using locker rooms or swimming pools. Treatment includes good foot hygiene and disposal of old footwear (or treatment with antifungal powder).

Tinea unguium (onychomycosis): thickened, distorted, and discolored nails with debris under the nail edges.

Tinea capitis (scalp): mainly affects children (highly contagious), who have scaly patches of hair loss with residual "black dots" in the affected area and may have an inflamed, boggy granuloma of the scalp (known as a kerion) that usually resolves on its own.

Tinea cruris (jock itch): more common in obese males; is usually found in the crural folds of the upper, inner thighs. Increased prevalence in patients with diabetes or other immunodeficiency.

2. **What organisms cause fungal infections?**
   Most fungal infections are due to *Trichophyton* sp. In tinea capitis, if the hair fluoresces green under the Wood lamp, *Microsporum* sp. is the cause; if not, it is likely *Trichophyton.*

3. **How are fungal infections diagnosed and treated?**
   Formal diagnosis of any fungal infection can be made by scraping the lesion and doing a potassium hydroxide (KOH) preparation to visualize the fungus via a microscope or by doing a culture. Because they are so common clinically, empiric treatment without a formal diagnosis is common, but for the USMLE, get a formal diagnosis before treating. Oral antifungals (e.g., griseofulvin) must be used to treat tinea capitis and onychomycosis; the others can be treated with topical antifungals (imidazoles such as miconazole, clotrimazole, and ketoconazole or allylamines such as terbinafine) or oral griseofulvin, which is better for severe or persistent infections.

4. **True or False: Candidiasis is often a normal finding in some women and children.**
   True. Oral thrush (creamy white patches on the tongue or buccal mucosa that can be scraped off) is seen in normal children, and *Candida* vulvovaginitis is seen in normal women, especially during pregnancy or after taking antibiotics. However, at other time periods and in different patients, candidal infections may be a sign of diabetes or immunodeficiency (e.g., thrush in a man should make you think about the possibility of acquired immunodeficiency syndrome [AIDS], and recurrent vulvovaginal candidiasis should prompt screening for diabetes).

5. **How is candidiasis diagnosed and treated?**
   Diagnose with KOH prep and look for pseudohyphae. Treat with local/topical nystatin or imidazoles (e.g., miconazole, clotrimazole). Oral therapy (nystatin or ketoconazole) is used for extensive or resistant disease.

6. **How do you recognize and treat the rash of impetigo? What causes it?**
   Impetigo is a superinfection of a break in the skin (e.g., previous chickenpox, insect bite, scabies, cut). Impetigo is caused by *Streptococcus* and *Staphylococcus* spp. The rash starts as thin-walled vesicles that rupture and form yellowish crusts (Fig. 8.20). The skin classically is described as "weeping." Typical lesions appear on the face and

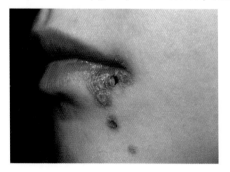

Fig. 8.20 Impetigo. Multiple crusted and oozing lesions. (From Kliegman RM. *Nelson Textbook of Pediatrics.* 19th ed. Philadelphia: Saunders; 2011 [fig. 657-1].)

tend to be localized. The rash is infectious; look for a history of sick contacts. Treat with dicloxacillin, cephalexin, or clindamycin to cover both *Streptococcus* and *Staphylococcus* spp. Topical mupirocin also may be used.

7. **Distinguish between impetigo and erysipelas.**
Both are superficial skin infections due to streptococci or *Staphylococcus aureus* and often occur after a break in the skin (e.g., trauma, scabies, insect bite). **Impetigo** classically changes first from maculopapules to vesicopustules and bullae and then to honey-colored, crusted lesions. Staphylococci are a more frequent cause than streptococci. Definitely think of staphylococci if a furuncle or carbuncle is present; think of streptococci if glomerulonephritis develops. Impetigo is contagious; watch for sick contacts. If there are a limited number of lesions without bullae, topical mupirocin may be used. If there are bullous or many lesions, treat with dicloxacillin, cephalexin, or clindamycin. **Erysipelas** (Fig. 8.21) is a superficial cellulitis (it involves the upper dermis and superficial lymphatics) that appears red, shiny, and swollen; it is tender and may be associated with vesicles and bullae, fever, and lymphadenopathy. Erysipelas typically has well-demarcated and raised borders. Treat with penicillin or amoxicillin, though erysipelas may require parenteral therapy with a cephalosporin (ceftriaxone or cefazolin) if systemic symptoms such as fever and chills are present.

8. **What organisms typically cause cellulitis? What special circumstances should make you think of atypical causes?**
Streptococci and staphylococci cause most cases. Think of *Pseudomonas* sp. with burns or severe trauma, of *Pasteurella multocida* after dog or cat bites (treat with ampicillin), of *Vibrio vulnificus* in fishermen or other patients exposed to saltwater (treat with tetracycline). Diabetic patients with foot ulcers tend to have polymicrobial infections and need powerful broad-spectrum antibiotic coverage.

9. **Describe the physical findings of cellulitis.**
In patients with cellulitis, the involved overlying skin is red, hot, and frequently tender. It looks like erysipelas but involves deeper dermis and subcutaneous fat. Antibiotic selection depends on whether the cellulitis is purulent or nonpurulent. These are newer terms and are designations within the 2011 Infectious Diseases Society of America clinical practice guidelines for methicillin-resistant *S. aureus* (MRSA). The idea is that a purulent infection may be caused by *S. aureus*. Oral treatment options for purulent cellulitis are trimethoprim-sulfamethoxazole, doxycycline, clindamycin, and linezolid. Oral treatment options for nonpurulent cellulitis are dicloxacillin, cephalexin, and clindamycin.

10. **Define necrotizing fasciitis. How is it treated?**
Necrotizing fasciitis is defined as the progression of cellulitis to necrosis and gangrene, which can quickly become limb and life threatening. Watch for crepitus and signs of systemic toxicity (e.g., tachycardia, fever, and hypotension). Often multiple organisms are involved (aerobes and anaerobes). Treat with intravenous fluids, aggressive surgical debridement, and broad-spectrum antibiotics. This includes a carbapenem (imipenem or meropenem) plus clindamycin plus vancomycin.

11. **What is folliculitis? What is a carbuncle? What is a furuncle?**
Folliculitis is a superficial bacterial infection of the hair follicles with purulent material in the epidermis but not the deeper soft tissue. A carbuncle is a coalescence of several inflamed follicles into one mass with purulent drainage from multiple follicles. A furuncle is an infection of the hair follicle with purulent material extending into the subcutaneous tissue and forming a small abscess.

12. **What pathogen usually causes folliculitis? What less common pathogen do you need to remember?**
Folliculitis is most commonly caused by *S. aureus*. Think *Pseudomonas* in the setting of inadequately chlorinated hot tubs or swimming pools. *Candida* folliculitis can occur in immunocompromised patients or after broad-spectrum antibiotic use.

13. **How is folliculitis treated?**
Most cases of folliculitis resolve on their own. Advise patients to use warm compresses and avoid shaving in the affected area. For persistent cases, prescribe topical mupirocin. Systemic antibiotics are not usually warranted.

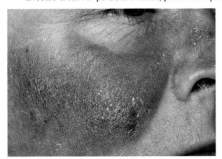

Fig. 8.21 Sharply defined erythema and edema characteristic of erysipelas. (From Zaoutis LB, Chiang VW. *Comprehensive Pediatric Hospital Medicine.* 1st ed. Philadelphia: Mosby; 2007 [fig. 156-2].)

14. **What is an abscess? What is the most common pathogen? How is an abscess treated?**
An abscess is a collection of pus within the dermis and deeper skin tissues. *S. aureus*, particularly MRSA, is the most common cause. Incision and drainage (I&D) is the main treatment modality. The data are unclear as to whether antibiotics provide any additional benefit following I&D.

15. **What causes scabies? How do you recognize it?**
Scabies is caused by the mite *Sarcoptes scabiei*, which tunnels into the skin and leaves visible burrows on the skin, classically in the finger web spaces and flexor surface of the wrists (Fig. 8.22). You should know what these burrows look like. Facial involvement is sometimes seen in infants. Patients also have severe pruritis, and scratching can lead to secondary bacterial infection. Crusted or Norwegian scabies typically occurs in patients who are immunocompromised, elderly, or living in institutions. In this form of scabies, there are hundreds to thousands of mites in the skin (as opposed to 15–20 with regular scabies), leading to a scaly rash or plaque, which may resemble psoriasis.

16. **How do you diagnose and treat scabies?**
Diagnosis is made by scraping a mite out of a burrow and viewing it under a microscope, though it is often a clinical diagnosis. Treat scabies with 5% permethrin cream applied to the whole body. Remember to treat all contacts (e.g., the whole family). Do *not* use lindane unless permethrin is not an option. Lindane used to be the treatment of choice but can cause neurotoxicity, especially in young children. Oral ivermectin can also be used. Close contacts may also require treatment. The patient's clothing, bedding, and towels must be cleaned or placed in a plastic bag for longer than 3 days (mites can only live for 2–3 days away from human skin) to prevent reinfection.

17. **How do you recognize and treat tinea versicolor?**
Tinea versicolor (also known as pityriasis versicolor) is usually caused by the *Malassezia globosa* fungus, presenting most commonly with multiple patches of various size and color (brown, tan, and white) on the torso of young adults (Fig. 8.23). It often becomes noticeable in the summer because the affected areas fail to tan and look white. Diagnose from lesion scrapings (KOH preparation yields septated hyphae and yeast in a "spaghetti and meatball" pattern). Treat with selenium sulfide shampoo or topical imidazoles.

18. **What causes lice? How is lice treated?**
Lice (pediculosis) can involve the hair of the head (caused by *Pediculus capitis;* common in school-aged children), body (caused by *Pediculus corporis;* unusual in people with good hygiene), or pubic area (crabs, caused by

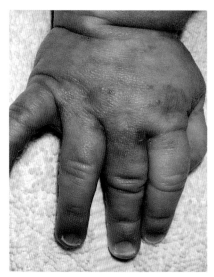

Fig. 8.22 Scabies. Itchy papules and pustules on the web spaces of the hand. (From Paige D, Wakelin S. *Kumar and Clark's Clinical Medicine.* Elsevier; 2017:1337-1386.)

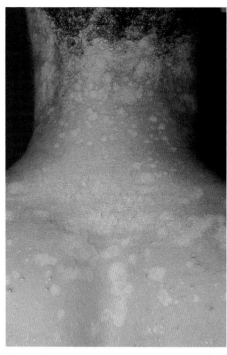

Fig. 8.23 Tinea versicolor. Hypopigmented macules and patches of seborrheic areas of the trunk. (From Paller AS, Mancini AJ. *Hurwitz Clinical Pediatric Dermatology, A Textbook of Skin Disorders of Childhood and Adolescence.* 5th ed. Elsevier; 2016.)

Pthirus pubis and transmitted sexually). Infected areas tend to itch. Diagnosis is made by seeing the lice (live mites or nits) on hair shafts. Treat with permethrin cream (preferred over lindane, which is neurotoxic), and decontaminate sources of reinfection (wash or sterilize combs, hats, bed sheets, clothing).

19. What causes warts? How are they treated?

Warts are caused by the human papillomavirus (HPV). They are infectious and are most commonly seen in older children, classically on the hands. They are spread by skin-to-skin contact. The most common serotypes are 6 and 11. Multiple treatments are available, including salicylic acid, liquid nitrogen, curettage, cytostatic treatment (5-fluorouracil, trichloroacetic acid), and immune response modifiers (imiquimod and interferon-alpha). Genital warts are also caused by HPV. Approximately 15 of the HPV serotypes are considered high-risk types for the development of cervical cancer; serotypes 16 and 18 are associated with most cases of cervical cancer.

20. Define molluscum contagiosum. How do you recognize it? How is it treated?

Molluscum contagiosum is a poxvirus infection that is common in children but may also be sexually transmitted. Diagnosis is made by the characteristic appearance of the lesions (skin-colored, smooth, waxy, dome-shaped papules with a central depression [umbilicated] that are roughly 0.5 cm) or by looking at contents of the lesion, which include cells with characteristic inclusion bodies (Fig. 8.24). The usual treatment is freezing or curettage. Consider immunodeficiency if the lesions are giant or very diffuse.

21. True or False: A child with genital molluscum is probably a victim of sexual abuse.

False. A child who has genital molluscum may or may not have contracted the disease from sexual contact. The more common mechanism is autoinoculation, in which the child has a lesion on the hand that spreads to the genital area from scratching. Do *not* automatically assume child abuse, although it must be ruled out.

22. Give the classic description and natural course of pityriasis rosea.

Pityriasis rosea is typically seen in young adults. Look for a herald patch (slightly erythematous, scaly, ring-shaped or oval patch classically seen on the trunk), followed 1 week later by many similar lesions that tend to itch (Fig. 8.25). Look for lesions on the back with a long axis that parallels the Langerhans skin cleavage lines,

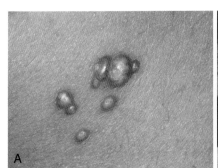 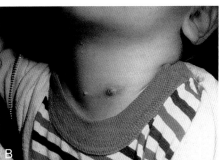

Fig. 8.24 Molluscum contagiosum. (A) Multiple papules of molluscum contagiosum demonstrating a characteristic central keratotic core. (B) Inflammatory molluscum contagiosum in a young child demonstrating both small, waxy, umbilicated papules and an inflammatory lesion simulating a furuncle. (From Nguyn N, Reed R. *Dermatology Secrets Plus.* Elsevier; 2016:229-234. A, Courtesy James E. Fitzpatrick MD; B, courtesy Fitzsimons Army Medical Center teaching files.)

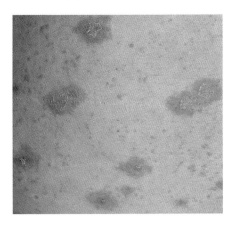

Fig. 8.25 Pityriasis rosea. Both small oval plaques and multiple small papules are present. (From Habif TP. *Clinical Dermatology.* 5th ed. Philadelphia: Mosby; 2009 [fig. 8-44].)

typically in a Christmas tree–like pattern. The condition usually remits spontaneously in about 1 month. The etiology is unknown, but some think it is related to HHV-6 and HHV-7. Think about syphilis (which presents with a maculopapular rash in the secondary form) in the differential diagnosis. Treat with reassurance.

23. **How do you recognize measles (rubeola) infection in a child?**
Pathognomonic Koplik spots (tiny white spots on buccal mucosa) are seen 3 days after high fever, cough, runny nose, and conjunctivitis with or without photophobia. On the next day, a maculopapular rash begins on the head and neck and spreads downward to cover the trunk (cephalocaudal progression). Look for a history of lack of immunization. Treat supportively. Patients are contagious until several days after the rash first appears. Don't forget to contact the health department regarding cases of measles.

24. **Describe the complications of measles.**
Complications include giant cell pneumonia, especially in very young and immunocompromised patients; otitis media; and encephalitis, either acute or late (**subacute sclerosing panencephalitis,** which usually occurs years later).

25. **How do you recognize a rubella infection in children? What are the complications?**
Rubella is milder than measles. Signs and symptoms include low-grade fever, malaise, and tender swelling of the suboccipital and postauricular nodes; arthralgias are common. After a 2- to 3-day prodrome, a faint maculopapular rash appears on the face and neck and spreads to the trunk (cephalocaudal progression), just as in measles. Complications include encephalitis and otitis media.

26. **Why is rubella infection an important disease?**
Infection in pregnant mothers can cause severe birth defects in the fetus. Screen all women of reproductive age, and immunize those without evidence of rubella antibodies before pregnancy to avoid this complication. Remember, however, that the vaccine is contraindicated in pregnant women.

27. **How do you recognize roseola infantum (exanthem subitum)? What causes it?**
Roseola infantum is often easy to recognize because of the progression: high fever (may be higher than 40°C) with no apparent cause for 4 days, which may result in febrile seizures, followed by an abrupt return to normal temperature just as a diffuse macular/maculopapular rash appears on the chest and abdomen. It may be associated with lymphadenopathy, erythematous tympanic membranes, and sterile pyuria. It is caused by HHV-6 (a DNA herpes family virus). The diagnosis is clinical, and treatment is supportive. The disease is rare in children older than 3 years.

28. **How do you recognize erythema infectiosum (fifth disease) in children? What causes it?**
Look for the classic "slapped-cheek" rash (Fig. 8.26) (i.e., confluent erythema over the cheeks looks like someone slapped the child across the face) accompanied by mild constitutional symptoms (e.g., low fever, malaise). One day later, a maculopapular rash appears on the arms, legs, and trunk. The disease is caused by parvovirus B19, the same virus that causes aplastic crisis in sickle cell disease. Parvovirus can have serious consequences during pregnancy, including fetal demise via hydrops fetalis (high output heart failure and anasarca).

29. **How do you recognize chickenpox? What causes it?**
The description and progression of the rash should lead you to the diagnosis: discrete, intensely pruritic macules (usually on the trunk) turn into papules, which turn into vesicles that rupture and crust over. Such changes occur within 1 day. Because the lesions appear in successive crops, the rash will be in different stages of progression in different areas. It is caused by the varicella-zoster virus.

30. **How can you make a definitive diagnosis of chickenpox? At what point is a patient with chickenpox no longer infectious?**
A Tzanck smear of tissue from the base of a vesicle shows multinucleated giant cells. A presumptive diagnosis can be made if the rash is classic. Infectivity ceases only when the last lesion crusts over. The virus, however, remains dormant in the dorsal root ganglion for possible future reactivation.

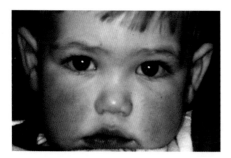

Fig. 8.26 Slapped-cheek appearance of erythema infectiosum. (From Baren JM, Rothrock SG, Brennan J, et al. *Pediatric Emergency Medicine.* 1st ed. Philadelphia: Saunders; 2007 [fig. 123-5].)

31. What are the complications of chickenpox?
A complication is infection of the lesions with streptococci or staphylococci, which can cause impetigo, erysipelas, cellulitis, and/or sepsis. The patient should be instructed to keep clean to avoid infection. Other complications include pneumonia (especially in very young children, adults, and immunocompromised patients), encephalitis, and **Reye syndrome.** Do not give aspirin to a child with a fever unless you have a diagnosis that requires its use (e.g., Kawasaki disease). The varicella-zoster virus can reactivate years later from its dormant state to cause herpes zoster (also known as shingles) (Fig. 8.27), a painful vesicular rash that develops in a dermatomal distribution, often with preceding pain and paresthesias. A child who has not been immunized or exposed to chickenpox can catch the disease from someone with shingles.

32. Describe the treatment and prophylaxis for chickenpox.
No treatment other than supportive care (e.g., acetaminophen, fluids, avoidance of infecting others) is needed in most cases. Acyclovir can be used in severe cases. Routine vaccination with the varicella vaccine is now recommended for all children in the United States. Varicella zoster immune globulin is available for prophylaxis in patients with debilitating illness (e.g., leukemia, AIDS) if you see them within 4 days of exposure and for newborns of mothers with chickenpox. Intravenous immunoglobulin can be given if varicella zoster immune globulin is not available.

33. What is scarlet fever? What causes it? How is it recognized and treated?
Scarlet fever is a febrile illness with a rash caused by certain *Streptococcus* spp. Look for a history of untreated streptococcal pharyngitis. Note that only streptococcal species that produce erythrogenic toxin can cause scarlet fever. Pharyngitis is followed by a sandpaper-like rash on the abdomen and trunk with classic circumoral pallor and strawberry tongue. The rash tends to desquamate once the fever subsides. Oral penicillin V is the treatment of choice for streptococcal pharyngitis to prevent rheumatic fever. Alternative therapies include amoxicillin, cephalosporins, macrolides, or clindamycin.

34. What are the diagnostic criteria for Kawasaki disease (mucocutaneous lymph node syndrome)?
Fever for more than 5 days (mandatory for diagnosis); bilateral conjunctival injection; changes in the lips, tongue, or oral mucosa (e.g., strawberry tongue, fissuring, injection); changes in the extremities (e.g., skin desquamation, edema, erythema); polymorphous truncal rash, which usually begins 1 day after the fever starts; and cervical lymphadenopathy. Also look for arthralgia or arthritis. This is a rare disease seen in patients under 5 years old.

35. What is the most feared complication of Kawasaki disease? How do you prevent it?
Complications involving the heart (coronary artery aneurysms, congestive heart failure, arrhythmias, myocarditis, and even myocardial infarction [MI]). Follow the child with echocardiography to detect heart involvement. Include Kawasaki disease in the differential diagnosis of any child who has an MI. If Kawasaki disease is suspected, give aspirin and intravenous immunoglobulins. Both have been proven to reduce cardiac morbidity. Kawasaki disease is one of the few indications for aspirin in a child.

TRAUMA AND TOXIC EFFECTS

1. List the classic drugs that cause photosensitivity of the skin.
Tetracyclines, phenothiazines, and birth control pills. Other drugs include furosemide, hydrochlorothiazide, antipsychotics (chlorpromazine, prochlorperazine), fluoroquinolones, amiodarone, and promethazine.

2. When and where are keloids seen?
Keloids are overgrowths of scar tissue after an injury and extend beyond the margins of the original wound. They are seen most frequently in blacks. They are usually slightly pink and classically appear on the upper back, chest, and deltoid area. Also look for keloids to develop after ear piercing (Fig. 8.28). Do not excise these lesions because it may worsen scarring.

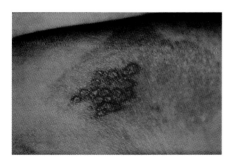

Fig. 8.27 Herpes zoster. Grouped vesicopustules on an erythematous base. (From Marx J, Hockberger R, Walls R. *Rosen's Emergency Medicine: Concepts and Clinical Practice.* 7th ed. Philadelphia: Mosby; 2009 [fig. 118-28]. Courtesy David Effron MD).

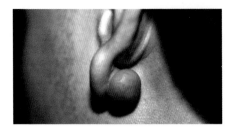

Fig. 8.28 Keloid scar on the earlobe after piercing. (From Kliegman RM. *Nelson Textbook of Pediatrics.* 19th ed. Philadelphia: Saunders; 2011 [fig. 651-1].)

3. **What are the three types of burns? How should all burns be managed initially? What is the Parkland formula?**
The three types of burns may be thermal, chemical, and electrical. Initial management of all burns should begin with management of the ABCs—**a**irway, **b**reathing, and **c**irculation—with a low threshold for intubation. Remove all clothing and other smoldering/exposed items on the body to ensure you can see the full breadth of the patient's injuries. For fire-related thermal burns, give 100% oxygen until carbon monoxide poisoning from smoke inhalation can be ruled out. Remember that burn patients are at an increased risk of dehydration, so administer plenty of intravenous fluids (lactated Ringer solution is first line, with normal saline as second line) and follow the **Parkland formula** (Fig. 8.29) to administer the appropriate amount of fluids over the first 24 hours: **4 × body weight (kg) × body surface area (BSA),** with half administered over the first 8 hours and the remaining half administered over the ensuing 16 hours. BSA is estimated using the rule of 9s. (Remember that only superficial partial-thickness burns or worse are included when using the rule of 9s.)

4. **How is burn severity classified? Describe the management of each class.**
Burn depth terminology no longer includes the use of first-, second-, and third-degree burn classifications. Burn severity is now organized into four categories:

Superficial burns are erythematous *without* blister formation. They involve only the epidermis and are locally painful.
Superficial partial-thickness burns are painful, warm, and moist *with* blister formation. They penetrate through the epidermis and superficial papillary dermis.
Deep partial-thickness burns are *painless* and present with mottled, waxy, or whitened skin. Blisters may be present. Pressure sensation is intact.
Full-thickness burns involve both the epidermis and dermis, have a white to gray, leathery, charred, or translucent appearance, and *do not blanch* with pressure. Pinprick sensation is absent.

5. **What are the important sequelae of electrical burns?**
Because most of the tissue destruction due to electrical burns is internal, sequelae include muscle necrosis, rhabdomyolysis, compartment syndrome, dislocations (e.g., posterior shoulder dislocation), acidosis, and renal failure. Use large amounts of intravenous hydration to prevent renal shutdown. The immediate life-threatening concern with an electrical burn is a cardiac arrhythmia, so order an electrocardiogram and monitor for seizures.

6. **How are chemical burns managed? Which is worse, acid or alkali burns?**
All chemical burns should be treated with copious irrigation from the nearest source (e.g., tap water), because the sooner you dilute the chemical, the less damage will be done. Do not delay irrigation while searching for sterile

PARKLAND FORMULA

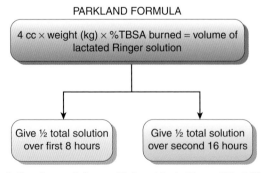

4 cc × weight (kg) × %TBSA burned = volume of lactated Ringer solution

Give ½ total solution over first 8 hours

Give ½ total solution over second 16 hours

Fig. 8.29 Parkland formula. (From Cameron JL, Cameron AM. *Current Surgical Therapy.* 12th ed. Philadelphia: Elsevier; 2017.)

saline for irrigation. Alkali burns are considered worse than acidic burns, as they cause liquefactive necrosis. Compare this to the coagulative necrosis caused by acidic burns—the eschar that forms due to the coagulative necrosis will prevent the deeper substance penetration that occurs due to liquefactive necrosis in alkali burns.

7. Besides dehydration, what additional complication is burned skin prone to develop?
Burned skin is much more prone to infection, usually by *S. aureus* or *Pseudomonas aeruginosa.* With pseudomonal infection, look for a fruity odor and/or blue-green appearance. If given, prophylactic antibiotics should only be administered topically. Irrigation and debridement are vitally important to infection prevention. Consider a tetanus booster shot if the patient has received fewer than three lifetime doses of the tetanus vaccine or if the patient's most recent booster shot was received more than 10 years ago.

8. Distinguish between frostnip and frostbite. How are they managed?
Frostnip, a mild form of cold injury, occurs when there is partial skin freezing resulting in cold and painful skin. In **frostbite,** a more severe form of cold injury, the skin is cold and numb. Treat both with analgesia and slow warming of the affected areas using lukewarm or tepid water (not scalding hot, as this will cause greater tissue damage) combined with local wound care and generalized warming (e.g., blankets).

CHAPTER 9

DISORDERS OF THE ENDOCRINE SYSTEM

1. **What is the difference between a primary and a secondary endocrine disorder?**
   In **primary disorders,** the problem is in the gland; the hypothalamic-pituitary axis is functioning appropriately. In primary hypothyroidism, for example, the thyroid gland does not function properly for whatever reason, but the pituitary and hypothalamus respond appropriately. Therefore thyroid hormone is low (as in all cases of hypothyroidism), but thyroid-stimulating hormone (TSH) and thyroid-releasing hormone (TRH) are high (the appropriate response from the pituitary and hypothalamus to low levels of thyroid hormone).
   In **secondary disorders,** the true dysfunction is outside the gland itself. For example, in secondary hypothyroidism, thyroid hormone is low, but TSH and/or TRH is also low (inappropriate in the setting of low thyroid hormone). If the pituitary is destroyed or surgically removed, secondary hypothyroidism results from low TSH; the thyroid gland functions well, but no TSH is available to stimulate it. To confuse the picture, the dysfunction may also be completely outside the endocrine axis (e.g., heart failure that causes secondary hyperaldosteronism).
   This concept in endocrine gland dysfunction is quite important. Simple blood tests can localize the problem. You may be able to answer a USMLE question simply by reading through the various values for hormones and hormone-releasing factors and figuring out where in the hypothalamus-pituitary-target gland axis the problem lies.

THYROID DISORDERS

1. **What physical and laboratory findings suggest thyroid cancer? What is the most common type of thyroid cancer? What historical point is of concern with thyroid cancer?**
   Patients often have a single, stony-hard nodule or mass in the thyroid gland, which may be rapidly enlarging. The nodule is cold on a nuclear scan (i.e., it fails to take up radioactive tracer). The most common type is papillary thyroid cancer. Other worrisome findings are hoarseness, which indicates recurrent laryngeal nerve invasion, and increased calcitonin level, which indicates the rare medullary thyroid cancer. Patients with medullary thyroid cancer may have a multiple endocrine neoplasia (MEN) syndrome. Historically, irradiation to the head or neck is of concern due to its association with thyroid cancer.

2. **How should you evaluate a thyroid mass for possible malignancy?**
   To evaluate a nodule in the thyroid, order thyroid function tests and a thyroid ultrasound. TSH is the best screening test; toxic or functional nodules are unlikely to be cancer. If the TSH is normal/elevated or the ultrasound has suspicious findings, obtain a fine-needle aspiration of the mass. If the TSH is decreased, then order a nuclear scan. A cold nodule or area of decreased uptake is more suspicious than a nodule with normal or increased uptake (i.e., hot nodule). Fine-needle aspiration and biopsy should be performed for almost all thyroid nodules.

3. **What are the common signs and symptoms of hyperthyroidism?**
   Signs: enlarged thyroid gland, warm skin, thyroid stare/lid lag, exophthalmos, proptosis, ophthalmoplegia (Graves disease), pretibial myxedema (Graves disease), tremor, tachycardia, and atrial fibrillation. Check TSH when patients present with new-onset atrial fibrillation.
   Symptoms: nervousness, anxiety, irritability, insomnia, heat intolerance, sweating, palpitations, tremors, weight loss with increased appetite, fatigue, weakness, hair loss, emotional lability, amenorrhea, and diarrhea.

4. **What are the most common causes of hyperthyroidism?**
   The most common cause is **Graves disease,** which is characterized by a diffusely enlarged thyroid gland, the presence of thyrotropin receptor antibodies (TRAb), exophthalmos, proptosis, ophthalmoplegia, and pretibial myxedema. In elderly patients, look for toxic multinodular goiter (individual lumps instead of diffuse enlargement of the gland and hot nodules on thyroid nuclear scan). Other causes include adenoma (single lump that is hot on nuclear scan), multinodular goiter (multiple lumbs that are hot on nuclear scan), subacute thyroiditis (viral infection with **tender, painful** thyroid gland), painless thyroiditis, and factitious hyperthyroidism (in which the patient takes thyroid hormone). Rare, exotic causes include amiodarone (which can cause hypo- or hyperthyroidism), TSH-producing pituitary tumor, thyroid carcinoma, and struma ovarii (an ovarian teratoma that secretes thyroid hormone).

5. **Describe the classic laboratory pattern of primary hyperthyroidism.**
   The TSH level is low (unless the patient has a TSH-secreting tumor), whereas triiodothyronine (T3) and thyroxine (T4) are increased.

6. **How is hyperthyroidism treated?**

   Short-term (stabilizing) treatment: Propylthiouracil (PTU) and methimazole/carbimazole can be used as suppressive agents (in pregnancy, PTU is recommended in the first trimester with transition to methimazole at the start of the second trimester). Beta-blockers are used in the setting of thyroid storm (severe hyperthyroid state—an emergency) for control of adrenergic symptoms. Iodine can also suppress the thyroid gland through negative feedback but can only be given after administering antithyroid medication and steroids (to reduce conversion of T4 to T3) during thyroid storm.

   Definitive (curative) treatment: Radioactive iodine ablation of the thyroid gland is typically used. In patients with Graves ophthalmoplegia, glucocorticoids can be used to prevent the worsening of the ophthalmopathy when radioactive iodine is administered. Surgery is preferred in pregnant patients. Hypothyroidism may result from either treatment; if so, it is treated with thyroid hormone replacement (for life).

7. **What are the signs and symptoms of hypothyroidism?**

   Signs: bradycardia; dry, coarse, cold, and pale skin; periorbital and peripheral edema; coarse, thin hair; thick tongue; slow speech; decreased and delayed reflexes; hypertension; carpal tunnel syndrome and paresthesias; vitiligo, pernicious anemia, and diabetes (remember the autoimmune association between these three conditions and Hashimoto disease); and coma (severe disease).

   Symptoms: weakness, lethargy, fatigue, cold intolerance, weight gain with anorexia, constipation, loss of hair, hoarseness, menstrual irregularity (menorrhagia is classic), myalgias and arthralgias, memory impairment, and dementia. Always rule out hypothyroidism as a cause of dementia.

   In children, congenital hypothyroidism may occur (mental, motor, and growth retardation).

8. **What are the common causes of hypothyroidism?**

   The most common known cause is Hashimoto thyroiditis (chronic autoimmune thyroiditis). Women of reproductive age outnumber men by 8:1. Histology reveals lymphocytes in the thyroid gland as well as antithyroid peroxidase, antithyroglobulin, and antimicrosomal antibodies. Other autoimmune diseases may coexist. The associated goiter is nontender. The second most common cause is iatrogenic after treatment of hyperthyroidism. Other, less common causes include iodine deficiency, amiodarone, lithium, and secondary hypothyroidism due to pituitary or hypothalamic failure (look for decreased TSH), such as with Sheehan syndrome (hypopituitarism caused by pituitary necrosis from blood loss and hypovolemic shock during and after childbirth).

9. **Describe the laboratory findings in primary hypothyroidism.**

   Elevated TSH (unless due to secondary causes), decreased T3 and T4, antithyroid and antimicrosomal antibodies (if due to Hashimoto thyroiditis), hypercholesterolemia, and anemia (which may be due to chronic disease or coexisting pernicious anemia).

10. **Why is free T4 (or free T4 index) better than total T4 for measuring thyroid hormone activity?**

    Free T4 (free T4 index) measures the active form of thyroid hormone. Many conditions cause a change in the amount of thyroid-binding globulin (TBG), thus changing total T4 levels in the absence of hypo- or hyperthyroidism. Common examples include pregnancy, estrogen therapy, and oral contraceptive pills, all of which increase TBG. Nephrotic syndrome, cirrhosis, and corticosteroid treatment all decrease TBG. T3 resin uptake is an older test that is not worth the effort to learn for Step 3, but if you are asked, it should rise or fall in the same way as free T4. Although an oversimplification, this principle should serve you well on the exam.

11. **How is hypothyroidism treated?**

    With T4 or thyroxine. T3 should not be used. In elderly patients, it is important to "start low and go slow" because overtreatment can be dangerous.

12. **What is nonthyroidal illness (formerly euthyroid sick syndrome)?**

    Any patient with any illness may have temporary derangements in thyroid function tests that resemble hypothyroidism. Thyroid function should not be assessed in seriously ill patients unless there is a strong suspicion of thyroid dysfunction. TSH ranges from normal to mildly elevated, serum T4 ranges from normal to mildly decreased, and T3 levels are low. Clinical circumstances and physical findings are the best guides to whether the patient has true hypothyroidism. In patients with nonthyroidal illness, simply treat the underlying illness. If the diagnosis is in doubt, either remeasure thyroid tests after the patient recovers (preferred) or try an empiric dose of levothyroxine (if the patient does not respond to treatment of the underlying illness).

13. **What are the different types of thyroiditis? What are the presenting symptoms?**

    Thyroiditis can present as an acute illness with significant thyroid pain (e.g., subacute thyroiditis and infectious thyroiditis) or as a condition with no evidence of thyroid inflammation in which there is only thyroid dysfunction or goiter.

    Subacute thyroiditis manifests in the hyperthyroid phase as neck pain, a tender goiter, and elevated T4 and/ or T3 levels. Patients typically go from a hyperthyroid to a hypothyroid state to recovery.

    Infectious thyroiditis may be acute or chronic. Acute infections are most commonly caused by *Staphylococcus* and *Streptococcus* and frequently involve abscess formation. Acute infections present with fever, rapid-onset neck pain, and tenderness that usually is unilateral. Thyroid ultrasound can differentiate subacute thyroiditis from infectious thyroiditis. Treat with intravenous antibiotics. Chronic infections are often bilateral, usually have less thyroid pain and tenderness than acute infections, and are typically caused by organisms such as mycobacteria, fungi, and *Pneumocystis*. Needle aspiration is required to identify the causative organism.

Other causes of thyroiditis that are unlikely to appear in the USMLE include painless thyroiditis (painless but with transient hyperthyroidism then sometimes hypothyroidism before recovery), postpartum thyroiditis (similar to painless thyroiditis but within 1 year of childbirth), drug-induced thyroiditis (look for lithium, amiodarone, or interferon-alpha), radiation thyroiditis, and fibrous thyroiditis.

DIABETES MELLITUS

1. Outline the current recommendations for diabetes mellitus screening.
   Universal screening is not generally recommended. Screening is more accepted, but not universal, in patients who are obese, people over 45 years of age, people with a family history of diabetes, and members of certain minority groups (blacks, Hispanics, Pima Indians). Screening in pregnancy is mandatory!

2. Define diabetes.
   Diabetes is defined as (1) a glucose level greater than or equal to 126 mg/dL after an overnight (or 8-hour) fast on two separate occasions or (2) a random glucose level greater than 200 mg/dL or (3) a hemoglobin A1c (HbA_{1c}) level greater than or equal to 6.5% on two separate occasions. If the patient has classic symptoms of diabetes (see later), one test is sufficient to make the diagnosis. In an asymptomatic patient it is best to repeat the test. An oral glucose tolerance test is common in pregnancy, otherwise it is rarely used because of poor reproducibility and patient compliance. With a glucose tolerance test, diabetes is diagnosed when glucose levels in the blood reach or exceed 200 mg/dL within 2 hours of receiving a 75-g oral dose of glucose.

3. What are the classic presenting symptoms of new-onset diabetes?
   Polyuria, polydipsia, and polyphagia ("pee a lot, drink a lot, and eat a lot"). You also should be suspicious if patients present with candidal infections (e.g., thrush or vaginal yeast infection), weight loss (as a result of excessive urination), or blurry vision. Prolonged hyperglycemia causes the lenses in the eyes to swell, and the patient may become myopic. Older patients may even claim that they no longer need their reading glasses (i.e., presbyopia is temporarily corrected by lens swelling).

4. What are the classic differences between type 1 and type 2 diabetes?

	Type 1 (10% of Cases)	Type 2 (90% of Cases)
Age at onset	Most commonly <30 yr	Most commonly >30 yr
Associated body habitus	Thin	Obese
Development of ketoacidosis	Yes	No
Development of hyperosmolar state	No	Yes
Level of endogenous insulin	Low to none	Normal to high (insulin resistance)
Twin concordance	<50%	>50%
HLA association	Yes	No
Response to oral hypoglycemics	No	Yes
Antibodies to insulin	Yes (at diagnosis)	No
Risk for diabetic complications	Yes	Yes
Islet cell pathology	Insulitis (loss of most B cells)	Normal number, but with amyloid deposits

Remember, however, that these findings may overlap.

5. What is the most important risk factor for developing type 2 diabetes?
   Genetic predisposition is the **most important** risk factor for developing type 2 diabetes (think high rate of twin concordance). Other risk factors include age, obesity, and physical activity. There is also increased prevalence among minority populations due to a combination of genetic and environmental factors.

6. What are the goals of treatment in terms of glucose levels?
   The goals are to keep postprandial glucose levels less than 180 mg/dL and fasting glucose levels 70 to 130 mg/dL. Attempts at stricter control may result in hypoglycemia; watch for symptoms of sympathetic nervous system activation and mental status changes.

7. What is a good measure of long-term diabetes control?
   HbA_{1c} measures the average control of blood glucose level over the prior 2 to 3 months. The current recommendation is to keep the HbA_{1c} level below 7 in most patients. Less stringent HbA_{1c} goals (such as <8%) may be appropriate for patients with a history of severe hypoglycemia, limited life expectancy, advanced microvascular or macrovascular complications, and extensive comorbid conditions.

The HbA_{1c} is a good way to catch patients with nocturnal hyperglycemia or less than honest patients who falsely record low glucose test readings. A rough rule of thumb is that HbA_{1c} times 20 equals the average blood glucose level.

8. **When a nondiabetic patient has hypoglycemia, how can you distinguish between a factitious disorder (exogenous insulin) and an insulinoma (endogenous insulin)?**
Measure the **C-peptide level.** C-peptide is produced when the body makes insulin, but it is absent in prescription insulin preparations. Therefore C-peptide is high for an insulinoma and low for factitious disorder. This is a classic USMLE question. Endogenous insulin has C-peptide, so overdoses of sulfonylurea medications will also cause increased C-peptide levels; investigate this possibility with a urine sulfonylurea screen.

9. **What should you remember before giving intravenous iodinated contrast material to a patient with diabetes or a patient with renal insufficiency?**
Patients with diabetes and patients with renal insufficiency are prone to acute kidney injury from the intravenously administered iodinated contrast agents used for intravenous pyelography (IVP), conventional angiography, and computed tomography (CT). You need to carefully weigh the risk-to-benefit ratio of using intravenous contrast agents. If you choose to give contrast, first hydrate the patient well with intravenous fluids to avoid renal shutdown. Acetylcysteine and bicarbonate may decrease the risk of contrast nephropathy in patients at high risk. The concerns about intravenous iodinated contrast do not apply to oral contrast agents (e.g., barium).
Patients on metformin are at risk for development of lactic acidosis if acute kidney injury were to occur after administration of intravenous contrast. Patients with advanced chronic kidney disease, those with acute kidney injury, or those who are undergoing a procedure that may result in emboli to the kidney, and those who require studies with intravenous contrast, should have their metformin held before the procedure and for 48 hours afterward. Metformin should be restarted only after kidney function has been reevaluated and no injury is identified.

10. **What is diabetic ketoacidosis (DKA)? How is it treated?**
All patients with type 1 will die without insulin. DKA is what happens before they die. Clinically, look for Kussmaul breathing (deep, rapid respirations), dehydration, hyperglycemia, acidosis (due to excessive ketone formation), and increased ketones in the serum (often associated with a fruity odor of the breath) and urine.
Treatment involves intravenous fluids, insulin, and replacement of electrolytes (especially potassium and phosphate). For the boards, do not use bicarbonate to correct acidosis. Remember to search for the cause of DKA, which most commonly is noncompliance with insulin therapy. The second most common cause is an infection. The mortality rate of DKA with current treatment efforts is less than 10%.

11. **What is nonketotic hyperglycemic hyperosmolar state? How is it treated?**
Nonketotic hyperglycemic hyperosmolar state is what happens to patients with type 2 diabetes who go without adequate treatment before they die. Hyperglycemia and increased serum osmolarity are present in the absence of ketones and acidosis. Most patients are severely dehydrated; the first three treatments are thus "fluids, fluids, and fluids" (i.e., intravenous hydration with normal saline). Insulin and electrolyte replacement is also required. The mortality rate can approach 50% if mental status changes are present at the time of diagnosis.

12. **What are the common long-term complications of diabetes mellitus?**
- **Atherosclerosis, coronary artery disease, myocardial infarction**. Patients with diabetes often have "silent" heart attacks (no chest pain because of autonomic neuropathy).
- **Retinopathy**. Diabetes is the leading cause of blindness in the United States for persons under the age of 50 years.
- **Nephropathy** Diabetes is the number-one cause of end-stage renal disease requiring hemodialysis (roughly 30% of cases; hypertension is a close second).
- **Peripheral vascular disease**. Diabetes is a leading cause of limb amputation and may lead to claudication, strokes, and impotence.
- **Peripheral neuropathy**. This complication causes "silent" heart attacks, numbness in the feet, and other findings (see later).
- **Increased risk of infection**. White blood cells do not function as well in a hyperglycemic environment. Couple this dysfunction with an inability to sense pain and clogged arteries that cannot deliver white cells to the site of an early infection, and you have a recipe for disaster.
All of these complications can be delayed or even prevented by good glucose control.

13. **What problems may result from diabetic peripheral neuropathy?**
- **Gastroparesis.** Because the stomach does not empty well, patients experience early satiety and vomiting. Treat with motility enhancers such as metoclopramide.
- **Charcot joints.** Joints in the foot and ankle are deformed secondary to lack of sensation. Patients may break a bone and not feel it.
- **Impotence.** The causes are neuropathy and atherosclerosis.
- **Cranial nerve palsies** (especially of cranial nerves III, IV, and VI). Patients present with diplopia and extraocular muscle paralysis, which should resolve within 8 weeks without treatment.
- **Orthostatic hypotension.** This problem occurs even when the patient is well hydrated because the arteries do not clamp down when the patient stands up, and the heart rate fails to increase appropriately.

- **Pressure ulcers in the feet.** As with Charcot joints, lack of sensation leads to overuse or failure to rest an injured or tired foot because it is numb and the patient is unaware. All patients with diabetes with foot numbness should wear socks and comfortably fitting shoes and inspect their feet regularly. Most cases of foot gangrene in patients with diabetes begin as a simple callus or blister.

14. Describe the treatment for diabetic retinopathy.

If the retinopathy is proliferative (neovascularization or new, irregular vessel formation), the treatment is **panretinal laser photocoagulation.** A laser beam is used to burn tiny spots around the periphery of the retina, sparing the central retina, to prevent progression to blindness. Focal (limited) laser photocoagulation is generally done for nonproliferative retinopathy only if symptoms are present (from macular edema). All patients with diabetes should be seen annually by an ophthalmologist to monitor retinal changes.

15. Describe the onset, peak, and duration of action of each of the insulin preparations.

Insulin Preparation	Onset (HR)	Peak (HR)	Duration (HR)
Ultrarapid Acting			
Insulin aspart	<0.25	1–3	3–5
Insulin lispro	0.25–0.5	0.5–2.5	3–5
Insulin glulisine	0.2–0.5	1.5–2.5	3–4
Rapid Acting			
Regular insulin	0.5–1	2–4	5–8
Intermediate to Long Acting			
NPH insulin	2–3	4–12	12–20
Long Acting			
Insulin glargine	1.5–4	None	24+
Insulin detemir	3–4	3–9	Dose dependent; 6–23 hr

NPH, Neutral protamine Hagedorn.

16. How do you adjust the dosage of neutral protamine Hagedorn (NPH) or regular insulin for high glucose levels?

Regular insulin starts to work in 45 minutes; its action peaks around 3 to 4 hours after injection, and the duration of action is 6 to 8 hours. NPH insulin takes 1 to 1.5 hours until onset of action; its action peaks at 6 to 8 hours, and the total duration of action is about 12 to 20 hours. For insulin adjustments, the following guidelines therefore apply:

- If the patient has high (low) glucose at 7 am, increase (decrease) NPH insulin at dinner the night before.
- If the patient has high (low) noon glucose, increase (decrease) the morning dose of regular insulin.
- If the patient has high (low) glucose at 5 pm, increase (decrease) the morning dose of NPH insulin.
- If the patient has high (low) glucose at 9 pm, increase (decrease) the dinnertime dose of regular insulin.

17. Define the Somogyi effect and the dawn phenomenon.

The **Somogyi effect** is the body's reaction to hypoglycemia. If too much NPH insulin is given at dinnertime, the glucose level at 3 am on the next morning will be low (hypoglycemia). The body reacts to hypoglycemia by releasing stress hormones, which cause a high glucose level at 7 am. The treatment is to decrease evening (NPH) insulin. The **dawn phenomenon** is hyperglycemia caused by normal secretion of growth hormone (GH) early in the morning. The glucose level is high at 7 am and normal or high at 3 am (no hypoglycemia). The treatment is to increase evening (NPH) insulin.

18. How do you manage patients with diabetes who are not allowed to eat because they are scheduled for surgery?

Generally, one-third to one-half of the normal dose of insulin is given. Glucose is monitored closely intra- and postoperatively by the anesthesiologist. Regular intravenous insulin can be given to control glucose levels based on blood glucose measurements.

19. What is the deal with beta-blockers, hypoglycemia, and diabetes?

If you give a beta-blocker to a patient with diabetes, you may mask the classic symptoms of hypoglycemia (tachycardia, diaphoresis), which are caused by catecholamine release. You must weigh the risk-to-benefit ratio of using beta-blockers in patients with diabetes (as in all patients). If a patient with diabetes is having or has had a previous myocardial infarction, the benefits outweigh the risks of treatment.

20. What are the best oral agents to use in type 1 diabetes?

None. Patients with type 1 diabetes require insulin. Currently available oral agents do not work for patients with type 1 diabetes.

21. What is the first treatment for type 2 diabetes?

Weight loss because it may reduce glucose levels by reducing insulin resistance. However, medications are usually needed, and oral agents are tried first, typically beginning with metformin. Other agents include insulin secretagogues (glipizide, glimepiride, nateglinide, glyburide, repaglinide), thiazolidinediones (rosiglitazone, piogli-tazone), alpha-glucosidase inhibitors (acarbose, miglitol), GLP-1 agonists (exenatide, liraglutide), DPP-IV inhibitors (saxagliptin, sitagliptin, linagliptin), and amylin analogues (pramlintide). The thiazolidinediones are falling out of favor because of the risk of fluid retention and congestive heart failure (CHF) exacerbation (rosiglitazone and pio-glitazone), the risk of myocardial infarction (rosiglitazone), and the risk of bladder cancer (pioglitazone).

Many patients with type 2 diabetes eventually require insulin, and insulin may be required early if the blood glucose or HbA$_{1c}$ levels are significantly elevated. In fact, current guidelines suggest using a basal insulin early in therapy (generally after one or two oral agents have been started) to get the blood glucose and HbA$_{1c}$ under control as early as possible.

ADRENAL DISORDERS

1. What is the significance of adrenal tumors?
Most are benign, but they may be functional and cause primary hyperaldosteronism (Conn syndrome) or hypercor-tisolism (Cushing syndrome). Another possibility is pheochromocytoma, which is associated with intermittent, severe hypertension, mental status changes, headaches, and diaphoresis.

2. How can you differentiate a Wilms tumor from a neuroblastoma?
Both present as flank masses in children (peak age: around 2 years). Neuroblastomas most commonly arise from the adrenal gland and often contain calcifications, whereas Wilms tumors arise from the kidney and rarely calcify, thus imaging (CT scan) can usually distinguish the two. In addition, neuroblastomas can cross the midline, whereas Wilms tumors are always unilateral. In rare cases, neuroblastomas regress spontaneously (for unknown reasons).

3. What do you need to know about neuroblastoma for the USMLE?
Neuroblastomas are a heterogeneous group of tumors that arise from neural crest cells. They can arise anywhere throughout the sympathetic nervous system, with the adrenal gland and abdomen being the two most common sites, in that order. Neuroblastoma metastasizes widely, including to lymph nodes, bone marrow, liver, and skin. Presenting symptoms depend on the location of the tumor and sites of metastases. In the USMLE, look for symptoms and signs such as abdominal pain, an abdominal mass (hepatic or retroperitoneal), anorexia, weight loss, back pain, bone pain, secretory diarrhea, hypertension, and leg edema.

Laboratory findings may include elevated ferritin and lactate dehydrogenase (LDH). A complete blood count, serum chemistries, and liver and renal function tests should be ordered. Urine or serum catecholamine levels (vanillylmandelic acid [VMA] and homovanillic acid [HVA]) assist in diagnosis. Bone marrow biopsy, bone radio-graphs, bone scan, abdominal CT scan or magnetic resonance imaging (MRI), chest x-ray, and head CT scans are used for diagnosis and staging. Tissue biopsy is required for definitive diagnosis.

Neuroblastomas are treated with surgery, but they may also require chemotherapy and sometimes radiation therapy. Infants younger than 1 year have a better prognosis than older children.

4. What are the signs and symptoms of primary hyperaldosteronism (Conn syndrome)? What are the causes?
Signs: hypertension, hypokalemia, hypernatremia, and edema.
Symptoms: weakness and edema.
Conn syndrome is caused by an aldosterone-secreting adrenal neoplasm. Because it is a primary disease, renin levels are low; the rest of the endocrine axis responds appropriately to gland dysfunction. Conn syndrome can be determined by measuring a plasma aldosterone concentration (PAC) and plasma renin activity (PRA). The PAC:PRA ratio should be greater than 20 with decreased PRA and PAC of 15 or more. Next order a CT of the abdomen to look for an adrenal mass. The treatment is surgical removal of the tumor. Conn syndrome can also be caused by unilateral or bilateral adrenal hyperplasia; in these cases, treat with mineralocorticoid receptor antagonists (spironolactone or eplerenone).

5. What causes secondary hyperaldosteronism?
Secondary hyperaldosteronism is much more common than primary disease. It is due to low perfusion of the kidney, as in CHF, renal artery stenosis (bruit), dehydration, nephrotic syndrome, and cirrhosis. Other causes include diuretics, renin-secreting tumors, and coarctation of the aorta. The key mechanism is that the kidney senses hypoperfusion and secretes renin, therefore the renin level is high. In secondary hyperaldosteronism, both PAC and PRA are elevated with the PAC:PRA ratio approximately equal to 10. Treatment of the underlying disorder (if possible) resolves the hyperaldosteronism. Potassium levels may be normal or even high. Of note, hyperkalemia may be the cause of increased aldosterone release just as hypocalcemia causes increased release of parathyroid hormone (PTH). Both are normal physiologic responses.

6. What are the signs and symptoms of Cushing syndrome (hypercortisolism)?
Signs: buffalo hump, truncal and central obesity with wasting of extremities, round plethoric facies (moon facies), purplish skin striae, acne, hirsutism, weakness (especially of the proximal muscles), hypertension, depression, psychosis, peripheral edema, poor wound healing, glucose intolerance or diabetes, osteoporosis, and hypokalemic metabolic alkalosis (due to mineralocorticoid effects of certain corticosteroids). Growth may be stunted in children.

Symptoms: weight gain, changes in appearance, easy bruising, acne, hirsutism, emotional lability, depression, psychosis, weakness, menstrual changes, sexual dysfunction, insomnia, and memory loss.

7. What causes Cushing syndrome?

The most common cause is iatrogenic, since steroids are frequently prescribed. The second most common cause is Cushing disease (a pituitary adenoma that secretes adrenocorticotropic hormone [ACTH]), which causes roughly 60% of noniatrogenic cases. Women of reproductive age outnumber men by 5:1. Other causes include ectopic ACTH production (classically by small cell lung cancer, which is more common in men) and adrenal adenomas or carcinomas (more common in children).

8. How is Cushing syndrome diagnosed?

Initial testing is with two of the following first-line tests: a 24-hour measurement of free cortisol in urine (free cortisol levels are abnormally elevated), late-night salivary cortisol, or an overnight low-dose (1 mg) dexamethasone suppression test (cortisol levels are not appropriately suppressed after administration of dexamethasone). Random cortisol level is an inappropriate test because of wide inter- and intrapatient as well as circadian variations.

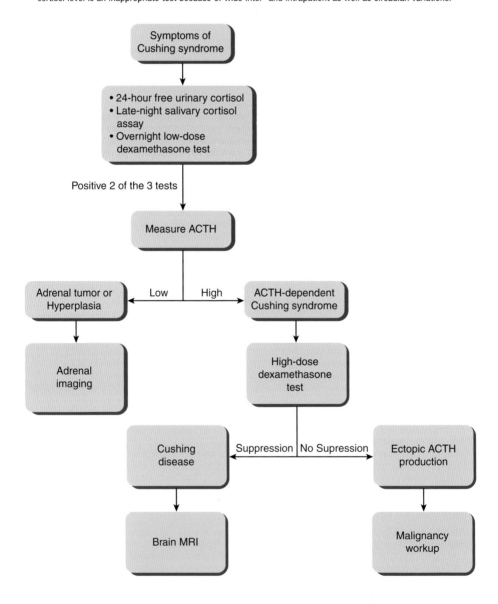

Remember that ACTH is elevated in Cushing disease but decreased with an adrenal adenoma. If ACTH is increased, a high-dose (8 mg) dexamethasone test should be ordered. A high-dose dexamethasone suppression test is not used to make a diagnosis of Cushing syndrome but is used to distinguish Cushing disease (suppresses) from ectopic ACTH production such as adrenal adenoma (does not suppress). Alternatively, a corticotropin-releasing hormone (CRH) test can be used. A positive response indicates Cushing disease, whereas no response indicates an ectopic source of ACTH. If Cushing disease is suspected, MRI of the brain should be obtained to look for a pituitary adenoma. Primary cancer is usually obvious when ectopic ACTH is the cause (e.g., weight loss, hemoptysis with lung mass on chest radiograph in patients with small cell lung cancer). If ACTH is decreased and the patient has no history of taking steroids, an abdominal CT scan or MRI should be obtained to look for an adrenal tumor. Primary cancer is usually obvious when ectopic ACTH is the cause (e.g., weight loss, hemoptysis with lung mass on chest radiograph in patients with small cell lung cancer). Treatment is based on the cause and usually involves surgery.

9. **Define hirsutism. What causes it?**
Hirsutism is a male pattern hair growth in women or prepubescent children. The most common cause is familial, genetic, or idiopathic hirsutism, but on the boards watch for **polycystic ovary syndrome** (Stein-Leventhal syndrome), Cushing syndrome, and drugs (minoxidil, phenytoin, cyclosporine). These disorders do not produce virilization. If virilization (clitoral enlargement, deepening of the voice, temporal balding) accompanies the hirsutism, an androgen-secreting ovarian tumor (e.g., Sertoli-Leydig cell tumor or arrhenoblastoma) or adrenal source (congenital adrenal hyperplasia, Cushing syndrome, or adrenal tumor) is likely.

10. **What causes virilization in children?**
In female neonates, congenital adrenal hyperplasia is a likely cause of virilization. The classic example is a female infant born with ambiguous genitalia. However, the patient may also be a male child with precocious puberty. At least 90% of cases are due to **21-hydroxylase deficiency.** Because 21-hydroxylase is involved in the production of both aldosterone and cortisol, children develop signs of hypoadrenalism, with salt wasting, hypotension, hyperkalemia, hyponatremia, hypoglycemia, acidosis, and nausea and vomiting. Abnormally high levels of serum 17-hydroxyprogesterone or urinary 17-ketosteroids (dehydroepiandrosterone [DHEA], DHEA sulfate, and androsterone), along with decreased free cortisol in the serum, clinch the diagnosis. Give corticosteroids to prevent death. In older children with virilization, worry about a testosterone-secreting gonadal neoplasm such as a Sertoli-Leydig tumor. Additionally, children with a 5-alpha reductase deficiency can present with virilization during puberty. These patients are phenotypically female as dihydrotestosterone, which is converted from testosterone by 5-alpha reductase, is needed for external male genitalia development. Increased testosterone levels at puberty will cause clitoromegaly, voice deepening, and increased muscle mass in these patients.

11. **What is the classic cause of ambiguous genitalia in the Step 3 exam?**
Adrenogenital syndrome, also known as congenital adrenal hyperplasia. Ninety percent of cases are caused by **21-hydroxylase deficiency.** Patients are female because affected males experience precocious sexual development. Patients with 21-hydroxylase deficiency have salt wasting (low sodium), hyperkalemia, hypotension, and elevated 17-hydroxyprogesterone. Treat with steroids and intravenous fluids immediately to prevent death.

12. **What should you tell the parents of a child with ambiguous genitalia?**
Tell the parents the truth: You do not know the child's gender. No patient with ambiguous genitalia should be assigned a sex until the workup is complete. Karyotyping must be performed.

13. **What are the signs and symptoms of adrenal insufficiency (hypoadrenalism)?**
Signs: hypotension, hyperkalemia, hyponatremia, hyperpigmentation (only if the pituitary is functioning because of melanocyte stimulating hormone), nausea and vomiting, diarrhea, abdominal pain, mild fever, hypoglycemia, acidosis, eosinophilia, orthostatic hypotension, and shock.
Symptoms: anorexia, weight loss, weakness, dizziness, apathy.

14. **What is the most common type of adrenal insufficiency?**
Tertiary (iatrogenic) adrenal insufficiency due to steroid treatment in which exogenous steroids inhibit the secretion of CRH by the hypothalamus. People who are removed abruptly from long-term steroid therapy may be unable to secrete an appropriate amount of corticosteroids in response to stress for up to 1 year. Watch out for the classic postoperative patient who crashes (with hypotension, shock, and hyperkalemia) shortly after surgery and has a history of a disease requiring steroid therapy within the past year. You may assess ACTH (inappropriately low) and cortisol levels (inappropriately low) to help make the diagnosis, but do not wait for the results to give steroids. The patient may die. Give prophylactic stress doses of corticosteroids in the setting of an illness, operation, or other stressor to prevent an adrenal crisis.

15. **What are the other causes of adrenal insufficiency?**
The most common primary (noniatrogenic) cause is autoimmune (idiopathic) disease in the developed world, and tuberculosis is the most common cause in the developing world. Patients may have other autoimmune diseases,

such as hypothyroidism, pernicious anemia, vitiligo, diabetes, or hypoparathyroidism. Secondary adrenal insufficiency can be caused by a pituitary adenoma, which decreases ACTH production, or Sheehan syndrome. Other causes include metastatic cancer (especially lung cancer), infection (tuberculosis, fungal infections, opportunistic infections in acquired immunodeficiency syndrome and other immunosuppressed states), ketoconazole, and pituitary/hypothalamic failure.

16. How is adrenal insufficiency diagnosed?
    Measurement of morning cortisol soon after wakening can suggest the diagnosis of adrenal insufficiency. A high-dose ACTH stimulation (cosyntropin) test is the most accurate way to establish the diagnosis. Plasma cortisol is measured, ACTH is administered intravenously or intramuscularly, and cortisol is measured again at either 30 minutes or 30 and 60 minutes postinjection. If adrenal function is normal, the cortisol level should rise appropriately (18–20 mcg/dL for intravenous cosyntropin or 16 mcg/dL for intramuscular cosyntropin) and indicates a secondary or tertiary adrenal insufficiency. An inappropriate response to ACTH indicates primary adrenal insufficiency. Do not withhold treatment to make a diagnosis if the patient is crashing.

PARATHYROID/PITUITARY DISORDERS

1. What are the signs and symptoms of hyperparathyroidism?
   Since PTH serves to increase serum calcium, the symptoms of hyperparathyroidism are the same as those for hypercalcemia ("bones, stones, groans, thrones, and psychiatric overtones"; see question 5). In primary cases, serum calcium is high, phosphorus is normal to low, and PTH is increased. In secondary cases, calcium is low.

2. What causes hyperparathyroidism?
   Ninety percent of primary cases are due to a parathyroid adenoma, which can usually be confirmed with a nuclear medicine scan. Other causes include parathyroid hyperplasia and, rarely, parathyroid carcinoma. Secondary cases include low calcium levels (e.g., from renal failure), to which an increase in PTH is a normal physiologic response. Tertiary hyperparathyroidism occurs when PTH has been elevated for too long (secondary to longstanding hypocalcemia) and continues to be oversecreted via parathyroid hyperplasia even when calcium is normalized with treatment. Translation: Put all patients with renal failure on calcium supplements to prevent this complication.

3. What are the signs and symptoms of hypoparathyroidism?
   The same as those for hypocalcemia (tetany, prolonged QT interval on electrocardiogram (ECG); see question 8). Calcium is low, phosphorus is high, and PTH is low.

4. What causes hypoparathyroidism?
   The most common cause is accidental removal or damage during thyroid surgery. Watch for tetany after thyroid surgery. Rare causes are genetic. Watch for **DiGeorge syndrome** (22q11.2 deletion syndrome) in children with congenital absence of parathyroid glands, tetany in the first 48 hours of life, absent thymus gland, immunodeficiency, cardiac anomalies, and midline facial defects.

5. What are the signs and symptoms of hypercalcemia?
   Signs: shortened QT interval on ECG, weakness, polyuria, bone changes and kidney stones on radiograph, and renal failure.
   Symptoms: "bones, stones, groans, thrones, and psychiatric overtones." In other words: bone resorption with osteomalacia and osteitis fibrosa cystica (a condition where calcified portions of bone are replaced by fibrosis, and cystlike brown tumors, which are masses of fibrosis, form); kidney stones; abdominal pain secondary to nausea and vomiting, ileus, nephrolithiasis, peptic ulcer disease, constipation, or pancreatitis (all increased with hypercalcemia); increased urination; and emotional lability, delirium, depression, and/or psychosis.

6. What causes hypercalcemia?
   In outpatients, the most common cause is hyperparathyroidism. In hospitalized patients, the most common cause is malignancy. The first test to order is PTH, which helps differentiate hyperparathyroidism (high PTH) from other causes of hypercalcemia such as malignancy, vitamin D intoxication, or thiazide diuretic use (low PTH). Multiple types of cancers can cause hypercalcemia, but the classic board question involves either multiple myeloma or paraneoplastic secretion of PTH-related hormone (PTHrP) by a squamous cell carcinoma, especially in the lung. Familial hypocalciuric hypercalcemia is characterized by hypercalcemia with low calcium levels in the urine (opposite of other hypercalcemias). Other causes include vitamin A or D intoxication, sarcoidosis or other granulomatous diseases, and excessive calcium intake (milk-alkali syndrome).

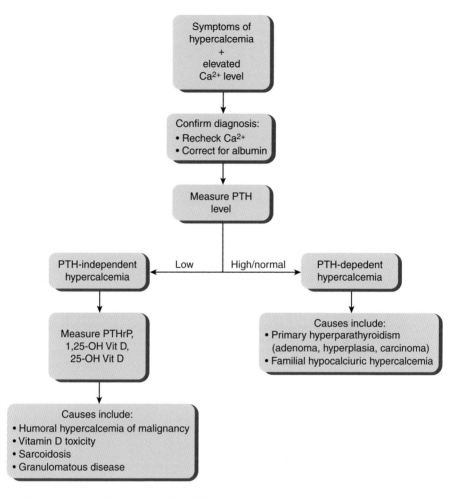

7. What is the treatment for hypercalcemia?

If the hypercalcemia is asymptomatic or mildly symptomatic with a calcium level of less than 12 mg/dL, immediate treatment is not required. Such patients should be advised to avoid factors that can cause hypercalcemia (e.g., thiazide diuretics, calcium supplements, high-calcium diet, volume depletion).

Severe hypercalcemia (>14 mg/dL) or symptomatic hypercalcemia should be treated with **fluids** as first-line therapy. Calcitonin and bisphosphonates (zoledronic acid or pamidronate) can also be used.

8. What are the signs and symptoms of hypocalcemia?

Signs: prolonged QT interval on ECG, tetany, **Chvostek sign** (tetany elicited by tapping on the facial nerve to cause facial muscle contraction), **Trousseau sign** (carpopedal spasm caused by inflation of a blood pressure cuff or application of a tourniquet), dementia, depression, psychosis, seizures, and papilledema.

Symptoms: paresthesias (the classic pattern is perioral or distal extremities), muscle aches, dementia, depression, and psychosis.

9. What causes hypocalcemia?

- Hypoparathyroidism (usually after thyroid gland surgery)
- Pseudohypoparathyroidism (genetic end-organ unresponsiveness to PTH with normal PTH levels, shortened metacarpal bones, short stature, and intellectual disability)
- DiGeorge syndrome (22q11.2 deletion syndrome)
- Vitamin D deficiency (osteomalacia, rickets)
- Renal failure of any cause and certain renal tubular problems
- Acute pancreatitis (one of the Ranson criteria)
- Secondary to hypomagnesemia

Hypoproteinemia of any cause may lead to low levels of total serum calcium, but levels of ionized calcium (the active form) are normal. In any patient with low serum calcium, the first step is to determine whether the serum albumin level is decreased. If it is, no treatment is required, and no symptoms will develop.

10. **How does a prolactinoma typically present?**
Look for the manifestations of elevated prolactin levels:
- Infertility, amenorrhea, or galactorrhea in premenopausal women.
- Postmenopausal women are already amenorrheic and usually do not get galactorrhea. A prolactinoma in postmenopausal women usually becomes large and causes headache or visual changes.
- Men may develop decreased libido, impotence, infertility, or gynecomastia.

Measure the prolactin level if prolactinoma is suspected. If the prolactin level is elevated, an MRI scan of the brain should be performed. Treatment is with a dopamine agonist such as cabergoline or bromocriptine. If medical management is unsuccessful or if the prolactinoma is large, transsphenoidal surgery and radiation therapy are indicated.

11. **What is acromegaly and how it is diagnosed and treated?**
Acromegaly is caused by excessive secretion of GH and presents with large hands/feet/brow/jaw, enlarged organs, and glucose intolerance. Additionally, acromegaly leads to concentric myocardial cardiomyopathy, which results in heart failure. It is most commonly caused by a GH-secreting pituitary adenoma. It is first screened with a serum insulin-like growth factor-1 level (elevated) and confirmed with a glucose suppression test, in which glucose fails to suppress GH secretion. Treatment is usually resection, but acromegaly can be medically managed with octreotide (a somatostatin analogue).

12. **Give the classic clinical description of a pheochromocytoma. How is it diagnosed?**
Look for wild swings in blood pressure (with some measurements dangerously high), tachycardia, postural hypotension, headaches, sweating, flushing, dizziness, mental status changes, and/or a feeling of impending doom (like a panic attack). A memory aid to remember the common symptoms of a pheochromocytoma is the five paroxysmal Ps: pressure, pain, pallor, palpitations, perspiration. The screening test is a 24-hour urine collection for metanephrines, HVA, and/or VMA (catecholamine breakdown products that are abnormally elevated in the urine). An alternative screening test is a plasma fractionated metanephrine assay. If levels are high, order an abdominal CT scan to look for an adrenal mass. Surgical tumor removal is the treatment of choice after stabilization with first alpha-blockers (e.g., phenoxybenzamine) and then beta-blockers.

13. **Define diabetes insipidus (DI). What are the two types?**
DI is a lack of antidiuretic hormone (ADH or vasopressin) effect in the body. Patients with DI secrete inappropriately dilute urine because of a lack of ADH effect and may urinate up to 25 L of urine per day resulting in dehydration and hypernatremia. Plasma osmolality is often greater than 295 mOsm/kg. Such patients die rapidly if they are unable to drink water. Normally, when the body is dehydrated, ADH causes urine to become highly concentrated through retention of free water. In DI, the urine remains dilute even though the serum osmolarity is quite high as a result of dehydration. The two types are **central** and **nephrogenic.**

14. **What causes central DI?**
Central DI is caused by a lack of ADH production by the posterior pituitary. Although it is often idiopathic, look for trauma, neoplasm, sarcoid/granulomatous disease, or ischemic encephalopathy as the cause. Order a CT scan or MRI of the head, if indicated.

15. **What causes nephrogenic DI?**
Nephrogenic DI is due to kidney unresponsiveness to ADH. Look for medications (e.g., lithium and demeclocycline), hypercalcemia, or hereditary mutations as the cause.

16. **What diagnostic test can reveal whether DI is central or nephrogenic? How are these conditions treated?**
Give the patient a dose of ADH or desmopressin, then measure urine osmolarity. If central DI is the cause, urine osmolarity increases with ADH challenge. In nephrogenic DI, the urine remains inappropriately dilute after the patient is given ADH. Additionally, serum Na^+ can help differentiate between the two. Patients with central DI tend to be hypernatremic, whereas patients with nephrogenic DI are euvolemic. This is because in nephrogenic DI, patients have an intact thirst mechanism, so they have adequate water intake to compensate for the renal loss of water. Treatment for central DI is ADH replacement (desmopressin, given orally or as a nasal spray). Treatment for nephrogenic DI involves stopping any offending drug and giving a thiazide diuretic; ADH does not help. Although giving a diuretic to a patient with DI seems counterintuitive, it has the paradoxic effect of decreasing urine output.

TRAUMA AND TOXIC EFFECTS

1. **Define hyperthermia. What causes it? How is it managed?**
Hyperthermia is defined as a body temperature greater than 104°F (40°C). The three primary causes are infections, medications, and heat stroke. If heat stroke is the cause, look for a history of prolonged heat exposure and a high

temperature (>104°F [40°C]) without clues to other culprits. Treat with immediate cooling (e.g., wet blankets, ice, cold water). The immediate threats to life are convulsions (treat with diazepam) and cardiovascular collapse. Always rule out infection and medications (especially those with anticholinergic activity such as antihistamines, antipsychotics, and antidepressants) as the cause.

2. What are the two classic examples of hyperthermia caused by medication?

Malignant hyperthermia is a rare idiosyncratic, genetically related reaction to medications, usually caused by inhaled anesthetics (e.g., halothane) or succinylcholine exposure. Treat with dantrolene.

Neuroleptic malignant syndrome is thought to be related to malignant hyperthermia and is an idiosyncratic, genetically related reaction to an antipsychotic agent. Look for extremely high levels of creatine phosphokinase and mental status changes in a patient taking antipsychotic agents. The first step is to stop the medication. The second step is supportive treatment, especially with lots of intravenous fluids to prevent renal shutdown caused by rhabdomyolysis. The third step, if necessary, is to treat with dantrolene.

Drug fevers are idiosyncratic reactions to a medication that was typically started within the previous week. They rarely cause fever above 104°F (40°C).

3. True or False: Alcohol can precipitate hypoglycemia.

True. But give thiamine first, then glucose in patients with alcohol use disorder.

4. Define hypothermia. How is it managed? What are the complications?

Hypothermia is defined as a body temperature of less than 95°F (35°C), usually accompanied by mental status changes and generalized neurologic deficits. If the patient is conscious, you can rewarm the individual slowly with blankets. If the patient is unconscious, consider gastric and bladder lavage with warm water as well as warm intravenous fluids.

Monitor the ECG for arrhythmias, which are common in hypothermic patients. You may see the classic **J wave**—a small, positive deflection following the QRS complex. Also monitor electrolytes, renal function, and acid-base status.

5. True or False: You should not give up resuscitation efforts until the patient is fully warmed in the setting of hypothermic cardiac arrest.

True. According to an old saying in medicine, the patient is not considered dead "until warm and dead." Hypothermia can slow body function to a remarkable degree, and there are case reports of resuscitation hours after initial attempts in the field once the body was warmed.

CHAPTER 10

RENAL AND URINARY DISORDERS

LOWER URINARY TRACT

1. **What is nocturnal enuresis? When can it be diagnosed? What are the treatment options?**
Enuresis is discrete episodes of urinary incontinence during sleep in children who are at least 5 years of age. This is a common issue in children at rates that decrease with age, but prevalence is 5% even at age 10 years. Evaluate with a thorough history and physical examination, as well as urinalysis to rule out conditions such as urinary tract infection (UTI) and diabetes. Advise on the use of a voiding diary. Ultrasound is helpful if there is a history of UTIs or if structural urologic abnormalities are suspected. Estimation of bladder capacity and postvoid residual volume can also be helpful. First-line treatment involves education about the natural course of enuresis, with bladder training, voiding before bedtime, and limiting fluids before bedtime. Enuresis alarms can be used if these behavioral modifications do not work. Desmopressin can be used and is effective in the short term but has high rates of relapse.

2. **What are the presenting symptoms of bladder obstruction? What are the causes? What is the treatment?**
Look for abdominal pain, a decrease in urine output, and a mass in the lower abdomen (from a distended bladder). Urinalysis is generally benign but may show hematuria. Serum creatinine may be increased. The most common causes are prostatic enlargement, posterior urethral valves, and neurogenic bladder. In women, consider cervical, uterine, and ovarian cancers. (Also be aware that urinary obstruction can occur above the level of the bladder because of conditions such as kidney stones, transitional cell carcinoma, and external compression by tumors.) Diagnosis is typically made with ultrasound, although a noncontrast computed tomography (CT) scan is preferred if an obstructing stone is suspected. Treat with bladder decompression using a urethral catheter (unless the patient has had recent urologic surgery). The evidence is mixed on when the catheter can be removed, but about a week is typical. Consider medication such as an alpha-blocker (e.g., tamsulosin) or a 5-alpha reductase inhibitor (e.g., finasteride) if benign prostatic hyperplasia (BPH) is the cause of the obstruction.

3. **What is neurogenic bladder? What are the causes?**
Patients with neurogenic bladder have difficulty with bladder control and passing urine because of brain, spinal cord, or peripheral nerve issues. Medications such as oxybutynin may help, but patients often require intermittent catheterization several times per day or may even require an indwelling catheter. Look for a history of spinal cord disease such as spinal cord injury, multiple sclerosis, spina bifida, or syringomyelia, but also consider a brain tumor or peripheral nerve diseases (such as from diabetes) as the cause. Neurogenic bladder may also result as a complication of pelvic surgery. Watch for UTIs as a result of having neurogenic bladder.

4. **What clinical vignette is suspicious for bladder cancer?**
Persistent, painless hematuria, especially in patients older than 40 years who smoke or work in the rubber or dye industry (exposure to aniline dye). CT scan to evaluate the upper urinary tract and cystoscopy should be performed to evaluate for potential bladder cancer (as well as other causes of hematuria, including renal cell carcinoma).

UPPER URINARY TRACT

1. **How do you recognize glomerulonephritis? How do you evaluate a possible case of glomerulonephritis?**
Look for new-onset hypertension, edema, hematuria, and decreased urine output. If glomerulonephritis is suspected, order urinalysis and measurement of serum creatinine, serum albumin, and the urinary protein-to-creatinine ratio to estimate protein excretion in the urine.

There are many causes of glomerulonephritis (e.g., postinfectious glomerulonephritis, immunoglobulin A [IgA] nephropathy, membranoproliferative glomerulonephritis, rapidly progressive glomerulonephritis [RPGN], lupus nephritis), but you do not need to be able to differentiate all of them for the Step 3 exam. However, it is helpful to be able to differentiate them into patterns. The findings on urinalysis can point to whether you are dealing with a nephrotic or a nephritic pattern. The nephrotic pattern typically has proteinuria of greater than 3.5 g/day and lipids in the urine but few cells or casts. The nephritic pattern is characterized by red cells, occasionally white cells, and either the presence or absence of red cell or mixed cellular casts. Serologic testing (e.g., complement levels, antineutrophil cytoplasmic antibody [ANCA], hepatitis B virus [HBV], hepatitis C virus [HCV], antistreptolysin O, cryoglobulin, antiglomerular basement membrane antibodies) may be helpful, but renal biopsy is usually necessary to confirm a diagnosis.

2. Define nephrotic syndrome. What causes it? How is it diagnosed?

Nephrotic syndrome is defined by proteinuria (>3.5 g/day), hypoalbuminemia, edema (the classic pattern is morning periorbital edema), and hyperlipidemia with lipiduria. In children it is usually due to minimal change disease (podocytes with missing "feet" on electron microscopy), which is most commonly idiopathic but also follows infections or is associated with underlying malignancy. Measure 24-hour urine protein or spot urine protein-to-creatinine ratio to confirm the diagnosis. Treat with steroids. Causes in adults include membranous nephropathy, diabetes, hepatitis B and C, human immunodeficiency virus (HIV), amyloidosis, lupus erythematosus, and drugs (e.g., penicillamine, captopril).

3. Define nephritic syndrome. What is the classic cause? How is it treated?

Nephritic syndrome is generally defined as oliguria, azotemia (rising blood urea nitrogen [BUN] and creatinine), hypertension, and hematuria. The patient may have some degree of proteinuria but not in the nephrotic range. The classic cause is poststreptococcal glomerulonephritis (PSGN). Treatment is supportive and includes control of hypertension and maintenance of urine output with intravenous (IV) fluids and diuretics.

4. How do you recognize poststreptococcal glomerulonephritis? How is it treated?

PSGN occurs most commonly after a streptococcal skin infection but may also occur after pharyngitis. Patients are usually children (although older age is a predictor of poorer outcomes) and generally have a history of infection with a nephritogenic strain of *Streptococcus* sp. 1 to 3 weeks previously and abrupt onset of edema (especially periorbital), hypertension, proteinuria (mild, not in the nephrotic range), hematuria (red blood cell casts), and elevated BUN and creatinine. *Red blood cell casts* on urinalysis confirm the diagnosis of nephritic syndrome. Laboratory tests that support a PSGN diagnosis include proof of recent streptococcal infection (e.g., antistreptolysin O and antiDNAse B titers) and evidence of complement-mediated glomerular inflammation (low C3 and C4 levels).

Treat supportively. Control blood pressure and use diuretics for severe edema. Unlike rheumatic fever, treatment of the initial streptococcal infection does not reduce the incidence of PSGN. Nonetheless, any residual infection should be treated with antibiotics. Another nephritic condition, IgA nephropathy (Berger syndrome), can occur within 1 to 2 days of an upper respiratory tract infection or viral pharyngitis and is hence termed *synpharyngitic*. The differentiation on the USMLE would be the delay of only a few days from pharyngitis to nephritic syndrome in IgA nephropathy versus the delay of a few weeks for PSGN.

5. Define Goodpasture syndrome. How does it present?

Goodpasture syndrome (a cause of RPGN) is due to the presence of measurable antiglomerular basement membrane antibodies, which cause a linear immunofluorescence pattern on renal biopsy. These antibodies react with and damage the kidneys and the lungs. Look for a young man with hemoptysis, dyspnea, and renal failure. Treat with steroids and cyclophosphamide.

6. Define granulomatosis with polyangiitis. How does it present?

Granulomatosis with polyangiitis is a vasculitis that also affects the lungs and kidneys. Look for nasal involvement (bloody nose, nasal perforation, saddle nose deformity) or hemoptysis and pleurisy as presenting symptoms, along with renal disease. Patients test positive for **antineutrophil cytoplasmic antibody** titers (specifically, c-ANCA/PR3-ANCA). Treat with cyclophosphamide and glucocorticoids. Methotrexate is an alternative.

7. What else should you watch for as a cause of glomerulonephritis?

Watch for lupus erythematosus as a cause of glomerulonephritis. Renal failure is a major cause of morbidity and mortality in patients with lupus.

8. What are the signs and symptoms of acute kidney injury (AKI)?

Signs: increased BUN and creatinine levels, metabolic acidosis, hyperkalemia, tachypnea (caused by acidosis and hypervolemia), and hypervolemia (bilateral rales on lung examination, elevated jugular venous pressure, dilutional hyponatremia).

Symptoms: fatigue, nausea and vomiting, anorexia, shortness of breath, mental status changes, oliguria.

9. What are the three broad categories of acute kidney injury?

Prerenal, intrinsic/intrarenal, and postrenal.

10. Define prerenal acute kidney injury. What are the causes? How do you recognize it?

In prerenal failure, the kidney is not adequately perfused. The most common cause is hypovolemia (dehydration, hemorrhage). Look for a BUN-to-creatinine ratio greater than 20 and signs of hypovolemia (e.g., tachycardia, weak pulse, depressed fontanelle). Fractional excretion of sodium (FeNa) will be less than 1% (as the body tries to retain sodium). Give IV fluids and/or blood. Other common prerenal causes are sepsis (treat the sepsis and give IV fluids), heart failure (give inotropes and diuretics), liver failure (hepatorenal syndrome; trial an albumin challenge followed by octreotide/midodrine to maintain renal perfusion), and renal artery stenosis.

11. Define postrenal acute kidney injury. What causes it?

In postrenal failure, urine is blocked from being excreted at some point beyond the kidneys (ureters, prostate, urethra). The most common cause is benign prostatic hyperplasia (BPH). Patients are men over age 50 with BPH symptoms (e.g., hesitancy, dribbling, weak stream, nocturia); ultrasound demonstrates bilateral hydronephrosis.

Additional scenarios may include females with complicated gynecologic history (e.g., recent cesarean section with ureter transection). Treat with catheterization (suprapubic, if necessary) or urologic intervention (e.g., nephrostomy tube) to relieve the obstruction and prevent further renal damage. Alpha-blockers (e.g., terazosin) or a 5-alpha reductase inhibitor (e.g., finasteride) can improve the symptoms, and surgery should be considered (transurethral resection of the prostate). Other causes are nephrolithiasis (but remember that stones generally have to be bilateral to cause renal failure), retroperitoneal fibrosis (watch for a history of radiation therapy or methysergide, bromocriptine, methyldopa, or hydralazine use), and pelvic/intraabdominal malignancies.

12. What is the most common cause of intrinsic acute kidney injury?
Intrinsic failure, which results from a problem within the kidney itself, is most commonly due to **acute tubular necrosis** from various causes.

13. What do you need to know about intravenous contrast and acute kidney injury?
IV contrast can precipitate AKI, usually in patients with preexisting renal disease. Avoid contrast in such patients if possible. If you must give IV contrast, administer IV hydration before and after the contrast is given, and avoid the use of nonsteroidal antiinflammatory drugs (NSAIDs) to decrease the chance of renal failure. The data on the use of acetylcysteine are conflicting.

14. True or False: Muscle breakdown can cause renal failure.
True. Myoglobinuria or rhabdomyolysis due to strenuous exercise (e.g., running marathons), alcohol, burns, muscle trauma, muscle compression (e.g., prolonged immobilization after a fall), seizure activity, heat stroke, and neuroleptic malignant syndrome may cause renal failure. The cellular debris that results from muscle breakdown plugs the renal filtration system, and myoglobin breakdown products are directly nephrotoxic. Look for very high levels of creatine phosphokinase (CPK). Urinalysis may reveal red urine that is positive for blood on dipstick (caused by the heme contained in myoglobin) but has no red blood cells. Treat with aggressive hydration. Alkalinization of the urine (with bicarbonate) may be helpful in severe cases. Diuretics may be helpful if the patient develops volume overload but have not been shown to be useful in preventing AKI. Monitor calcium and potassium levels carefully during treatment of rhabdomyolysis.

15. What medications commonly cause renal insufficiency or failure?
Chronic use of NSAIDs may cause acute tubular necrosis, acute interstitial nephritis, or papillary necrosis; additionally, consider cyclosporine, aminoglycosides, and methicillin.

16. What are the indications for dialysis in patients with renal failure?
When renal failure is present, first try to determine the cause and fix it, if possible, to correct the renal failure. Indications for acute dialysis are remembered by the mnemonic **AEIOU**: **a**cidosis (severe metabolic, roughly a pH <7.2), **e**lectrolytes (hyperkalemia, typically >6.5 mEq/L or rapidly rising potassium levels), **i**ngestion of a dialyzable drug or toxin, **o**verload, and **u**remia (includes uremic pericarditis or encephalopathy).

17. What causes chronic kidney disease (CKD)?
Any of the causes of acute renal failure can cause CKD if the insult is severe or prolonged. Most cases of CKD are due to diabetes mellitus (leading cause) or hypertension (second most common cause). A popular cause on the USMLE exam is polycystic kidney disease (PKD). Watch for multiple cysts in the kidney; look for a positive family history (usually autosomal dominant; the autosomal recessive form presents in children), hypertension, hematuria, palpable renal masses, berry aneurysms in the circle of Willis, and cysts in liver.

18. What metabolic derangements are seen in end-stage renal disease (ESRD)?
- Azotemia (high levels of BUN and creatinine)
- Metabolic acidosis
- Hyperkalemia
- Fluid retention (may cause hypertension, edema, congestive heart failure, and pulmonary edema)
- Hypocalcemia and hyperphosphatemia (impaired vitamin D production with secondary hyperparathyroidism; bone loss leads to renal osteodystrophy); treat with phosphorus binders (sevelamer), vitamin D repletion (calcitriol), and parathyroid hormone–lowering therapy (cinacalcet)
- Anemia (due to lack of erythropoietin; give synthetic erythropoietin to correct)
- Anorexia, nausea, vomiting (from buildup of toxins)
- Central nervous system disturbances (mental status changes and even convulsions or coma from toxin buildup; dialysis disequilibrium syndrome with seizures can occur from rapid correction of BUN during hemodialysis)
- Bleeding (due to uremic platelet dysfunction)
- Uremic pericarditis (friction rub may be heard)
- Skin pigmentation and pruritus (skin turns yellowish-brown and itches because of metabolic by-products)
- Increased susceptibility to infection (due to decreased cellular immunity)

19. How is end-stage renal disease treated?
Treat renal failure with regular hemodialysis (usually three times/week), water-soluble vitamins (which are removed during dialysis), phosphate restriction and binders (calcium carbonate, calcium acetate, or sevelamer), erythropoietin as needed, and hypertension control. The only cure is renal transplant.

20. **When is kidney transplantation considered for patients with renal disease?**
    Kidney transplant is an option for patients with ESRD (glomerular filtration rate <10–15 mg/min), unless they have active infections or other life-threatening conditions (e.g., acquired immunodeficiency syndrome [AIDS], malignancy). Lupus erythematosus and diabetes are not contraindications to transplantation.

21. **Who makes the best donor for patients who need a kidney transplant?**
    Living, related donors are best (siblings or parents), especially when human leukocyte antigens (HLA) are similar, but cadaveric kidneys are more commonly used because of availability. Before transplant, perform ABO blood typing and lymphocytotoxic (HLA) cross-matching to ensure a reasonable chance at success.

22. **Describe unacceptable kidney donors.**
    Unacceptable kidney donors include newborns (most centers set an age <18 years as an exclusion criterion) and patients with a history of generalized or intraabdominal sepsis, malignancy, or any disease with possible renal involvement (e.g., diabetes, hypertension, lupus erythematosus).

23. **Where is the transplanted kidney placed? What happens to the native kidneys?**
    A transplanted kidney is placed in the iliac fossa or pelvis (for easy biopsy access in case of later problems as well as for technical reasons). Usually the recipient's kidneys are left in place to reduce the morbidity of the surgery.

24. **What are the three basic types of rejection after kidney transplantation?**
    Hyperacute, acute, and chronic.

25. **What causes hyperacute rejection? What is the classic clinical description?**
    Hyperacute rejection is due to preformed cytotoxic antibodies against the donor kidney; it occurs with ABO blood-type mismatch as well as other preformed antibodies. In the classic clinical description, the surgery is completed, the vascular clamps are released to allow blood flow, and the transplanted kidney quickly turns bluish black. Treat by removing the kidney.

26. **What causes acute rejection? How does it present? How is it treated?**
    Acute rejection is T-cell mediated. It presents *days to weeks* after the transplant with fever, oliguria, weight gain, tenderness and enlargement of the graft, hypertension, and/or laboratory derangements. Increases in creatinine are more reliable than increases in BUN. Treatment involves pulse corticosteroids, anti–T-cell antibody therapies (polyclonal antibodies, OKT3), other antibody therapies (basiliximab, daclizumab), and other immunosuppressants (tacrolimus, mycophenolate, cyclosporine). **Accelerated rejection** occurs over the *first few days* and is thought to reflect reactivation of previously sensitized T cells.

27. **What causes chronic rejection? How does it present? How is it treated?**
    Chronic rejection can be T-cell or antibody mediated. This late cause (months to years after transplant) of renal deterioration presents with gradual decline in kidney function, proteinuria, and hypertension. Treatment is supportive and not effective, but the graft may last several years before it gives out completely. A new kidney can be transplanted if this occurs.

28. **How do you distinguish the nephrotoxicity of cyclosporine from rejection?**
    Cyclosporine is a well-known cause of nephrotoxicity that can be difficult to clinically distinguish from graft rejection. When in doubt, a percutaneous needle biopsy of the graft should be performed if the patient is taking cyclosporine because in most cases the two can be distinguished histologically. Renal ultrasound also helps. In a practical context, if you increase the immunosuppressive dose, acute rejection should decrease, whereas cyclosporine toxicity stays the same or worsens.

29. **What else do you need to know about polycystic kidney disease?**
    There are two types: autosomal dominant PKD (ADPKD) and autosomal recessive PKD (ARPKD); the latter is less common because most patients die in utero or shortly after birth because of severe oligohydramnios and associated problems. PKD is characterized by the presence of multiple cysts, usually in both kidneys, which leads to massive enlargement of the kidneys. Extrarenal manifestations include cerebral aneurysms, pancreatic cysts, hepatic cysts, cardiac valvular disease, and aortic root dilatation. ADPKD is responsible for approximately 10% of all cases of ESRD.

30. **How do you differentiate among the common pediatric hematologic disorders that affect the kidney?**

	HUS	*HSP*	*TTP*	*ITP*
Most common age	Children	Children	Young adults	Children or adults
Previous infection	Diarrhea (*Escherichia coli*)	URI	None	Viral (especially in children)
Red blood cell count	Low	Normal	Low	Normal
Platelet count	Low	Normal	Low	Low

Continued on following page

	HUS	HSP	TTP	ITP
Peripheral smear	Hemolysis	Normal	Hemolysis	Normal
Kidney effects	AKI, hematuria	Hematuria	AKI, proteinuria	None
Treatment	Supportive*	Supportive*	Plasmapheresis, NSAIDs; no platelets‡	Steroids,† splenectomy if drugs fail
Key differential points	Age, diarrhea	Rash, abdominal pain, arthritis, melena	CNS changes, age	Antiplatelet antibodies

AKI, Acute kidney injury; *CNS,* central nervous system; *HSP,* Henoch-Schönlein purpura; *HUS,* hemolytic uremic syndrome; *ITP,* idiopathic thrombocytopenia; *NSAIDs,* nonsteroidal antiinflammatory drugs; *TTP,* thrombotic thrombocytopenic purpura; *URI,* upper respiratory infection

*In HUS and HSP, patients may need dialysis and transfusions.

†Give steroids only if the patient is bleeding or platelet counts are very low (<20,000–30,000/μL).

‡Do not give platelet transfusions to patients with TTP; clots may form.

31. Which is more likely to be seen on a plain abdominal radiograph: kidney stones or gallbladder stones?

Kidney stones (85%), which more commonly calcify, are more likely to be seen than gallstones (15%).

32. What are the signs and symptoms of renal stones? How are they diagnosed and treated?

Kidney stones (nephrolithiasis) generally present with severe, intermittent, unilateral flank and/or groin pain when the stone dislodges and gets stuck in the ureter (ureterolithiasis). Most stones can be seen on abdominal radiographs and are composed of calcium. Renal ultrasound or CT scan can be used to detect a stone if clinical suspicion is high but plain abdominal radiographs are negative. Symptomatic urolithiasis should be treated with lots of hydration and pain control (to see if the stone will pass). Most stones less than 5 mm will pass on their own. If the stone does not pass, it needs to be removed surgically (preferably endoscopically) or by lithotripsy.

33. What causes kidney stones?

Nephrolithiasis is often idiopathic, but on the Step 3 exam watch for one of the following underlying disorders that predispose to the development of kidney stones:

Hypercalcemia: due to hyperparathyroidism or malignancy (calcium stones).

Infection: from ammonia-producing bugs (*Proteus* spp., staphylococci). Look for **staghorn calculi** (large stones composed of magnesium, ammonia, and phosphate [struvite] that fill the renal calyceal system).

Hyperuricemia: uric acid stones due to gout or leukemia treatment (allopurinol and IV hydration are given before leukemia chemotherapy to prevent this complication).

Cystinuria/aminoaciduria: should be suspected if the stone is made of cystine or you are presented with a repetitive stone-forming patient.

Note: Send any recovered stones to the lab for stone analysis to determine the type of stone.

34. How is renal cell carcinoma diagnosed and treated?

Painless hematuria (gross or microscopic) is the most typical presenting sign. Patients rarely have the classic triad of hematuria, flank pain, and a palpable flank mass. A CT scan (preferred over IV pyelography) is a good initial diagnostic test. The treatment for disease confined to the kidney or with extension limited to renal vein invasion (classic) is surgical resection. For other organ invasion or distant metastatic disease (usually to the lung or bone), immunotherapy (e.g., interleukin-2) is the preferred treatment.

35. What are the signs and symptoms of renal stones? How are they diagnosed and treated?

Kidney stones (nephrolithiasis) generally present with severe, intermittent, unilateral flank and/or groin pain when the stone dislodges and gets stuck in the ureter (ureterolithiasis). Most stones can be seen on abdominal radiographs and are composed of calcium. Renal ultrasound or CT scan can be used to detect a stone if clinical suspicion is high but plain abdominal radiographs are negative. Symptomatic urolithiasis should be treated with lots of hydration and pain control (to see if the stone will pass). Most stones less than 5 mm will pass on their own. If the stone does not pass, it needs to be removed surgically (preferably endoscopically) or by lithotripsy.

36. What are the different types of stones? What causes them?

Roughly 75% to 85% of stones contain calcium. Look for hypercalcemia (usually due to hyperparathyroidism) or small bowel bypass, which increases oxalate absorption and thus calcium stone (envelope-shaped crystals) formation. Roughly 10% to 15% of stones are struvite (magnesium-ammonium-phosphate) stones (coffin-lid crystal), which are caused by urinary tract infection (usually with *Proteus* sp.). The classic example is the staghorn calculus (a stone that fills the entire calyceal system). About 5% to 10% of stones are uric acid (rhomboid crystal). Look for gout or leukemia. The remaining 1% to 3% are cystine stones (hexagonal crystal), which suggest hereditary cystinuria.

37. How is nephrolithiasis treated?

The cornerstones of nephrolithiasis treatment are large amounts of fluid hydration, narcotics for pain, an alpha-blocker (tamsulosin) to reduce ureteral spasm, and observation because most stones pass spontaneously. Most stones less than or equal to 4 mm in diameter pass spontaneously. Stones 4 to 10 mm in diameter may or may not pass. Spontaneous passage is unlikely with stones greater than or equal to 10 mm in diameter. If a stone does not pass, treat with lithotripsy, ureteroscopy with stone retrieval, or open surgery (last resort).

FLUID, ELECTROLYTE, AND ACID-BASE DISORDERS

1. **How do you analyze arterial blood gas values?**
   Remember three points:
   1. The pH tells you whether the primary process is an acidemia or an alkalemia. The body will compensate as much as it can (secondary process) but will never perfectly compensate or overcompensate.
   2. If the carbon dioxide (CO_2) is high, the patient either has respiratory acidosis (pH <7.4) or is compensating for a metabolic alkalosis (pH >7.4). If CO_2 is low, the patient either has a respiratory alkalosis (pH >7.4) or is compensating for a metabolic acidosis (pH <7.4).
   3. If the bicarbonate (HCO_3) is high, the patient either has a metabolic alkalosis (pH >7.4) or is compensating for a respiratory acidosis (pH <7.4). If bicarbonate is low, the patient either has a metabolic acidosis (pH <7.4) or is compensating for a respiratory alkalosis (pH >7.4).

2. **True or False: The body does not compensate beyond a normal pH.**
   True. For example, a patient with metabolic acidosis will eliminate CO_2 (the body will increase the respiratory rate to help "blow off" CO_2) to help restore a normal pH, and a compensatory respiratory alkalosis will develop. However, the compensatory alkalosis will not correct the pH to greater than 7.4. Overcorrection does not occur.

3. **List the common causes of acidosis.**
   Respiratory acidosis: hypoventilation, chronic obstructive pulmonary disease [COPD], asthma, drugs (e.g., opioids, benzodiazepines, barbiturates, alcohol, other respiratory depressants), chest wall and neuromuscular problems (paralysis, pain), and sleep apnea.
   Metabolic acidosis: ethanol, diabetic ketoacidosis, uremia, lactic acidosis (e.g., sepsis, shock, bowel ischemia), methanol/ethylene glycol, aspirin/salicylate overdose, isoniazid, diarrhea, and carbonic anhydrase inhibitors.

4. **What is the anion gap? Why is it useful?**
   The anion gap is the calculated difference between the major cations and anions in the blood. The formula used to determine it is $[Na^+] - ([HCO_3^-] + [Cl^-])$. The normal value of the anion gap is 8 to 12 mEq/L. The anion gap is a useful measure to know when evaluating a metabolic acidosis because differential diagnoses can be included based on the value.

5. **What is the differential diagnosis for a high anion gap metabolic acidosis? What is the differential diagnosis for a normal anion gap metabolic acidosis?**
   An anion gap greater than 12 mEq/L is considered high and occurs in several disease states. The **MUDPILES** mnemonic can be used to remember the offending diseases: **m**ethanol toxicity, **u**remia, **d**iabetic ketoacidosis, **p**ropylene glycol toxicity, **i**ron or **i**soniazid toxicity, **l**actic acidosis, **e**thylene glycol toxicity, and **s**alicylate toxicity (late).
   The **HARDASS** mnemonic can be used to remember the disorders that cause a normal anion gap metabolic acidosis: **h**yperalimentation, **A**ddison disease, **r**enal tubal acidosis, **d**iarrhea, **a**cetazolamide, **s**pironolactone, and **s**aline infusion.

6. **List the common causes of alkalosis.**
   Respiratory alkalosis: anxiety/hyperventilation and aspirin/salicylate overdose.
   Metabolic alkalosis: diuretics (except carbonic anhydrase inhibitors), vomiting, volume contraction, antacid abuse/milk-alkali syndrome, and hyperaldosteronism.

7. **What effect do serum acidosis and serum alkalosis have on potassium and calcium levels?**
   Alkalosis may cause hypokalemia and symptoms of hypocalcemia (perioral numbness, tetany) caused by cellular shift, whereas acidosis may cause hyperkalemia via the same mechanism. Correction of acid-base status will correct the potassium and calcium derangements.

8. **What type of acid-base disturbance does aspirin overdose cause?**
   Respiratory alkalosis and anion gap metabolic acidosis (two different primary disturbances). Look for coexisting tinnitus, hypoglycemia, vomiting, and a history of "swallowing several pills." Anion gap will be elevated. Alkalinization of the urine with bicarbonate speeds excretion. Consider dialysis if a patient has a pH less than 7.1, altered mental status, pulmonary edema, initial salicylate level greater than 100, renal failure, or if acidosis is refractory to medical management.

9. **What happens to the blood gas of patients with chronic lung conditions?**
   Many people with chronic lung disease (e.g., COPD) develop a chronic respiratory acidosis because of CO_2 retention. During an exacerbation of a respiratory disorder, the respiratory acidosis worsens, and a compensatory metabolic alkalosis develops. As the respiratory acidosis improves with treatment of the exacerbation, the metabolic alkalosis is no longer a compensatory mechanism and becomes a primary disturbance. However, in certain people with chronic lung conditions (especially those with sleep apnea), pH may be alkaline during the day because breathing improves when awake. As a side note, remember that sleep apnea, like other chronic lung diseases, can cause right-sided heart failure (cor pulmonale) by causing pulmonary hypertension.

10. **List the signs and symptoms of hyponatremia.**
    - Lethargy
    - Seizures
    - Mental status changes or confusion
    - Cramps
    - Anorexia
    - Coma

11. **How do you determine the cause of hyponatremia?**
    The first step in determining the cause is to assess the patient's volume status:

	Hypovolemic	*Euvolemic*	*Hypervolemic*
Think of	Dehydration, diuretics, diabetes, Addison disease/hypoaldosteronism (high potassium)	SIADH, psychogenic polydipsia, oxytocin use, hypothyroidism	Heart failure, nephrotic syndrome, cirrhosis, toxemia, renal failure

    SIADH, Syndrome of inappropriate antidiuretic hormone secretion.

12. **Define the syndrome of inappropriate antidiuretic hormone secretion (SIADH). How is it diagnosed?**
    The name says it all: ADH is released inappropriately. SIADH is a consideration in patients with hyponatremia and normal volume status (euvolemic). In SIADH, serum osmolality is low, but urine osmolarity is high (inappropriate urine concentration). Look for the values of all electrolytes and lab tests to be low (the classic example is uric acid) because of dilution of the serum with free water secondary to inappropriate ADH.

13. **What causes syndrome of inappropriate antidiuretic hormone secretion?**
    Central nervous system causes: stroke, hemorrhage, infection, trauma.
    Medications: narcotics, oxytocin (watch for pregnant patients), chlorpropamide, antiepileptic agents, selective serotonin reuptake inhibitors (SSRIs).
    Trauma: Pain is a powerful stimulus for ADH. Watch for the postoperative patient who is receiving fluids (and often narcotics) and has pain to develop SIADH.
    Lung problems: simple pneumonia or ADH-secreting small cell cancer of the lung.

14. **How is hyponatremia treated?**
    For hypovolemic hyponatremia, the treatment for Step 3 purposes is normal saline to restore the intravascular volume. Euvolemic and hypervolemic hyponatremia are treated with water/fluid restriction; diuretics may be needed for hypervolemic hyponatremia.

15. **How is syndrome of inappropriate antidiuretic hormone secretion treated?**
    Treat with water restriction. Stop IV fluids (as normal saline will worsen hyponatremia due to increased free water retention) and restrict oral fluid intake. For Step 3 purposes, do not give hypertonic saline unless the patient has active seizures before your eyes. You may cause osmotic demyelination syndrome (ODS; formerly central pontine myelinolysis) from too rapid correction of sodium level (memory aid: "from low to high [sodium], the pons will die"). **Demeclocycline** is sometimes used to treat SIADH if water restriction fails because it induces nephrogenic diabetes insipidus, which allows the patient to get rid of free water.

16. **What happens if hyponatremia is corrected too quickly?**
    You may cause ODS, which can result in irreversible or only partially reversible neurologic symptoms such as dysarthria, paresis, behavioral disturbances, lethargy, confusion, and coma (remember the saying "from low to high [Na^+], the pons will die"). Hypertonic saline is used only when a patient has seizures from severe hyponatremia (usually Na <120 mEq/L)—and even then, only briefly and cautiously. Normal saline is a better choice 99% of the time for board purposes. In chronic severe symptomatic hyponatremia, the rate of correction should not exceed 0.5 to 1 mEq/L/hr.

17. **What causes spurious (false) hyponatremia?**
    - Hyperglycemia (once glucose is >200 mg/dL, sodium decreases by 1.6 mEq/L for each rise of 100 mg/dL in glucose). Make sure you know how to make this correction.
    - Hyperproteinemia
    - Hyperlipidemia
    - Mannitol
      In these instances, the lab value is low, but the total body sodium is normal. Do not give the patient extra salt or saline.

18. **What causes hyponatremia in postoperative patients?**
    The most common cause is the combination of pain and narcotics (causing SIADH) with overaggressive administration of IV fluids. A rare cause that you may see on Step 3 is adrenal insufficiency, particularly in a patient who is on chronic steroids and had medications stopped before surgery. In this instance, potassium is high, and the blood pressure is low.

19. **What is the classic cause of hyponatremia in pregnant patients about to deliver?**
Oxytocin, which has an ADH-like effect.

20. **What are the signs and symptoms of hypernatremia?**
Basically, the same as the signs and symptoms of hyponatremia:
- Mental status changes or confusion
- Seizures
- Hyperreflexia
- Coma

21. **What causes hypernatremia?**
The most common cause is dehydration (free water loss) due to inadequate fluid intake relative to bodily needs. Watch for diuretics, diabetes insipidus, diarrhea, and renal disease as well as iatrogenic causes (administration of too much hypertonic IV fluid). Sickle cell disease, which may lead to renal damage and isosthenuria (inability to concentrate urine), is a rare cause of hypernatremia, as are hypokalemia and hypercalcemia, which also impair the kidney's concentrating ability. Cushing syndrome and primary hyperaldosteronism are potential endocrine causes of hypernatremia.

22. **How is hypernatremia treated?**
Treatment involves water replacement, but the patient is often severely dehydrated; therefore normal saline is used most frequently. Once hemodynamically stable, the patient is often switched to dextrose 5% (D5) one-half normal saline; D5 in water (D5W) should not be used for hypernatremia, since dextrose is not an effective osmole and would just worsen hypernatremia.

23. **What do you need to know about diabetes insipidus?**
Think of diabetes insipidus as the opposite of SIADH. There is a lack of ADH (vasopressin) effect in the body. Diabetes insipidus may lead to dehydration and hypernatremia. There are two types: central and nephrogenic. See Chapter 9 on endocrinology for a more in-depth discussion.

24. **What are the signs and symptoms of hypokalemia?**
Hypokalemia causes muscular weakness, which can lead to paralysis and ventilatory failure. When smooth muscles are also affected, patients may develop ileus and/or hypotension. Best known and most tested, however, is the effect of hypokalemia on the heart. Electrocardiogram (ECG) findings include loss of the T wave or T-wave flattening, ST depressions, the presence of U waves, premature ventricular and atrial complexes, and ventricular and atrial tachyarrhythmias.

25. **What is the effect of pH on serum potassium?**
Changes in pH cause changes in serum potassium as a result of cellular shift. Alkalosis causes hypokalemia, whereas acidosis causes hyperkalemia. For this reason, bicarbonate is given to severely hyperkalemic patients. If the pH is deranged, normalization will most likely correct the potassium derangement automatically without the need to give or restrict potassium.

26. **Describe the interaction between digoxin and potassium.**
The heart is particularly sensitive to hypokalemia in patients taking digoxin. This is because digoxin binds to the K^+ site on the Na^+/K^+ ATPase, so hypokalemia leads to increased binding. Potassium levels should be monitored carefully in all patients taking digoxin, especially if they are also taking diuretics (a common occurrence).

27. **How should potassium be replaced?**
Like all electrolyte abnormalities, hypokalemia should be corrected slowly. Oral replacement is preferred, but if the potassium must be given intravenously for severe derangement, do not give more than 20 mEq/hr. Put the patient on an ECG monitor when giving IV potassium because potentially fatal arrhythmias may develop.

28. **When hypokalemia persists even after administration of significant amounts of potassium, what should you do?**
Check the magnesium level. When magnesium is low, the body cannot retain potassium effectively. Correction of a low magnesium level allows the potassium level to return to normal.

29. **What are the signs and symptoms of hyperkalemia?**
Weakness and paralysis may occur, but the cardiac effects are the most tested. ECG changes (in order of increasing potassium value) include **tall, peaked T waves**, widening of QRS, prolongation of the PR interval, loss of P waves, and a sine-wave pattern ECG. Arrhythmias include asystole and ventricular fibrillation.

30. **What causes hyperkalemia?**
- Renal failure (acute or chronic)
- Severe tissue destruction such as rhabdomyolysis or hemolysis (because potassium has a high intracellular concentration)
- Hypoaldosteronism (watch for hyporeninemic hypoaldosteronism in diabetes)
- Medications (stop potassium-sparing diuretics, beta-blockers, NSAIDs, angiotensin-converting enzyme inhibitors, angiotensin receptor blockers, trimethoprim-sulfamethoxazole, cyclosporine, digoxin, and succinylcholine)

- Adrenal insufficiency (also associated with low sodium and low blood pressure)
- Insulin deficiency

31. **What should you suspect if an asymptomatic patient has hyperkalemia?**

With hyperkalemia, the first consideration (especially if the patient is asymptomatic and the ECG is normal) is whether the lab specimen is hemolyzed. Hemolysis causes a false hyperkalemia due to high intracellular potassium concentrations. Repeat the test.

32. **The specimen was not hemolyzed. What is the first treatment?**

Get an ECG first to look for cardiotoxicity. In general, the best therapy for hyperkalemia is decreased potassium intake and administration of a gastrointestinal cation exchange (e.g., patiromer or zirconium cyclosilicate). The oral sodium polystyrene resin Kayexalate is only used in rare instances due to increased risk of bowel necrosis. But if the potassium level is greater than 6.5 or cardiac toxicity is apparent (more than peaked T waves), immediate IV therapy is needed. First give **calcium gluconate** (which is cardioprotective, although it does not change potassium levels); then give **sodium bicarbonate** (alkalosis causes potassium to shift inside cells) and **glucose with insulin** (insulin also forces potassium inside cells, and glucose prevents hypoglycemia). Beta$_2$-agonists also drive potassium into cells and can be given if the other choices are not listed on the test. If the patient has renal failure (high creatinine) or initial treatment is ineffective, prepare to institute dialysis emergently.

33. **What are the signs and symptoms of hypocalcemia?**

Hypocalcemia produces neurologic findings, the most tested of which is tetany. Tapping on the facial nerve at the angle of the jaw elicits contraction of the facial muscles (**Chvostek sign**), and inflation of a tourniquet or blood pressure cuff elicits hand and foot muscle (carpopedal) spasms (**Trousseau sign**). Other signs and symptoms are perioral tingling, hyperreflexia, depression, encephalopathy, dementia, laryngospasm, and convulsions/seizures. The classic ECG finding is QT-interval prolongation.

34. **What causes hypocalcemia?**

- DiGeorge syndrome (tetany 24–48 hours after birth, absent thymic shadow on x-ray, cardiofacial abnormalities)
- Renal failure (remember the kidney's role in vitamin D metabolism)
- Hypoparathyroidism (watch for a postthyroidectomy patient; all four parathyroids may have been accidentally removed)
- Vitamin D deficiency
- Pseudohypoparathyroidism (short fingers, short stature, intellectual disability, and elevated parathyroid hormone level with end-organ unresponsiveness to parathyroid hormone)
- Acute pancreatitis
- Renal tubular acidosis

35. **What should you do if the calcium level is low?**

Check the albumin and correct the calcium as necessary to account for hypoalbuminemia. Remember that hypoproteinemia (i.e., low albumin) of any etiology can cause hypocalcemia because the protein-bound fraction of calcium is decreased. In this instance, however, the patient is asymptomatic because the ionized (unbound, physiologically active) fraction of calcium is unchanged. Thus you should first check the albumin level and/or the ionized or free calcium level to make sure "true" hypocalcemia is present. For every 1-g/dL decrease in albumin below 4 g/dL, correct the calcium by adding 0.8 mg/dL to the given calcium value.

36. **Describe the relationship between low calcium and low magnesium.**

It is difficult to correct hypocalcemia until hypomagnesemia (of any cause) is also corrected, as magnesium is needed to produce parathyroid hormone.

37. **How does pH affect calcium levels?**

Alkalosis can cause symptoms similar to hypocalcemia through effects on the ionized fraction of calcium (alkalosis causes calcium to shift intracellularly or because alkalosis induces the dissociation of hydrogen ions from albumin, allowing free Ca^{2+} to bind, which lowers ionized Ca^{2+}). Clinically, this scenario is most common with hyperventilation/anxiety syndromes, in which the patient eliminates too much CO_2, becomes alkalotic, and develops perioral and extremity tingling. Treat by correcting the pH. Treat anxiety if hyperventilation is the cause.

38. **Describe the relationship between calcium and phosphorus.**

Phosphorus and calcium levels usually go in opposite directions (when one goes up, the other goes down), and derangements in one can cause problems with the other. This relationship becomes clinically important in patients with chronic renal failure, in whom you must not only try to raise calcium levels (with vitamin D and calcium supplements) but also restrict/reduce phosphorus.

39. **What are the signs and symptoms of hypercalcemia?**

Hypercalcemia is often asymptomatic and discovered by routine lab tests. When symptoms are present, recall the following rhyme:

Bones (bone changes such as osteopenia, pathologic fractures, and osteitis fibrosa cystica)

Stones (kidney stones and polyuria)

Groans (abdominal pain, anorexia, constipation, ileus, nausea, vomiting)
Psychiatric overtones (depression/anxiety, psychosis, delirium/confusion)
  Abdominal pain may also be due to peptic ulcer disease and/or pancreatitis, both of which have an increased incidence with hypercalcemia. The ECG classically shows QT-interval shortening when hypercalcemia is present.

40. **What causes hypercalcemia?**
Primary hyperparathyroidism is the most common cause of hypercalcemia in outpatients. In inpatients, the most common cause is malignancy. Check the parathyroid hormone level to differentiate hyperparathyroidism from other causes.
  Other causes include vitamin A or D intoxication, sarcoidosis, thiazide diuretics, familial hypocalciuric hypercalcemia (look for low urinary calcium, which is rare with hypercalcemia), and immobilization. Hyperproteinemia (e.g., high albumin) of any etiology can cause hypercalcemia because of an increase in the protein-bound fraction of calcium, but the patient is asymptomatic because the ionized (unbound) fraction is unchanged.

41. **Why is asymptomatic hypercalcemia usually treated?**
Prolonged hypercalcemia can cause nephrocalcinosis, urolithiasis, and renal failure due to calcium salt deposits in the kidney and may result in bone disease secondary to loss of calcium.

42. **How is hypercalcemia treated?**
First, give IV fluids. Then, once the patient is well hydrated, give furosemide (a loop diuretic) to cause calcium diuresis. Thiazides are contraindicated because they increase serum calcium levels. Other treatments include phosphorus administration (use oral phosphorus; IV administration can be dangerous), calcitonin, bisphosphonates (e.g., etidronate, which is often used in Paget disease), plicamycin, or prednisone (especially for malignancy-induced hypercalcemia). Correction of the underlying cause of hypercalcemia is the ultimate goal. The previous measures are all temporary until definitive treatment can be given. For hyperparathyroidism, surgery is the treatment of choice.

43. **In what clinical scenario is hypomagnesemia usually seen?**
Alcoholism. Magnesium is wasted through the kidneys.

44. **What are the signs and symptoms of hypomagnesemia?**
Signs and symptoms are similar to those of hypocalcemia (prolonged QT interval on ECG and possibly tetany).

45. **In what clinical scenario is hypermagnesemia seen?**
Hypermagnesemia is classically iatrogenic in pregnant patients who are treated for preeclampsia with magnesium sulfate. It also commonly occurs in patients with renal failure. Patients who receive magnesium sulfate should be monitored carefully because the physical findings of hypermagnesemia are progressive. The initial sign is a decrease in deep tendon reflexes; then hypotension and respiratory failure occur sequentially.

46. **How is hypermagnesemia treated?**
First, stop any magnesium infusion! Remember the ABCs (**a**irway, **b**reathing, **c**irculation), and intubate the patient if respiratory failure is pending. If the patient is stable, start IV fluids. Furosemide can be given next, if needed, to cause a magnesium diuresis. The last resort is dialysis.

47. **In what clinical scenarios is hypophosphatemia seen? What are the signs and symptoms?**
Uncontrolled diabetes (especially diabetic ketoacidosis) and alcoholism. Signs and symptoms of hypophosphatemia include neuromuscular disturbances (encephalopathy, weakness), rhabdomyolysis (especially in alcoholics), anemia, and white blood cell and platelet dysfunction.

48. **What is the intravenous fluid of choice in hypovolemic patients?**
Normal saline or lactated Ringer solution (regardless of other electrolyte problems). First, fill the tank; then correct the imbalances that the kidney cannot sort out on its own.

49. **What is the maintenance fluid of choice for patients who are not eating?**
One-half normal saline with D5 in adults. Typically, one-fourth normal saline with D5 in children under 10 kg; one-third or one-half normal saline with D5 in children over 10 kg.

50. **Should anything be added to the IV fluid for patients who are not eating?**
Potassium chloride, 10 or 20 mEq, is usually added to a liter of IV fluid each day to prevent hypokalemia (assuming that the baseline potassium level is normal).

INFECTIONS

1. **What are the signs and symptoms of urinary tract infection (UTI)? What are the most likely organisms?**
Signs and symptoms include urgency, dysuria, suprapubic and/or low back pain, and low-grade fever. UTIs are usually caused by *Escherichia coli* (75%–85% of cases) but may also be caused by *Staphylococcus saprophyticus*

or *Proteus, Pseudomonas, Klebsiella, Enterobacter,* and/or *Enterococcus* spp. (or other enteric organisms). Patients who acquire UTIs in the hospital or from a chronic indwelling Foley catheter are more likely to have organisms other than *E. coli.* While rare, if urinary cultures grow *S. aureus*, the patient should receive repeat urinary cultures as well as assessment for bacteremia/endocarditis with blood cultures and transthoracic echocardiography.

2. What factors increase the likelihood of UTIs?
Female gender and conditions that promote urinary stasis (BPH, pregnancy, stones, neurogenic bladder, vesicoureteral reflux) or bacterial colonization (indwelling catheter, fecal incontinence, surgical instrumentation) predispose to UTI.

3. How do you diagnose and treat UTIs?
The gold standard for diagnosis is a positive urine culture with at least 100,000 colony-forming units (measure of bacterial load) of specific bacteria. At the least, get a midstream sample; the best method is a catheterized sample or suprapubic tap. Urinalysis shows white blood cells, bacteria (on Gram stain of the urine), positive leukocyte esterase, and/or positive nitrite.
    Empiric treatment is usually based on symptoms and urinalysis while awaiting culture results. Commonly used antibiotics include trimethoprim-sulfamethoxazole, amoxicillin, nitrofurantoin, ciprofloxacin, or a first-generation cephalosporin for about 5 days.

4. Why are UTIs in children and males of special concern?
In children, a UTI is cause for concern because it may be the presenting symptom of a genitourinary malformation. The most common examples are vesicoureteral reflux and posterior urethral valves. Urine culture should be obtained. Order an ultrasound and either a voiding cystourethrogram (VCUG) or radionuclide cystogram (RNC) to evaluate the urinary tract in any child 2 months to 2 years with a first UTI. Recommendations for imaging in older children are less clear-cut.
    If a male has symptoms and a urinalysis suggestive of a UTI, consider the possibility of prostatitis (the prostate may be tender and boggy on exam). Bacterial prostatitis requires 6 weeks of antibiotics to ensure eradication.

5. True or False: You should treat asymptomatic bacteriuria in most patients.
False. The exception is the pregnant patient, in whom asymptomatic bacteriuria is treated because of the high risk of progression to pyelonephritis. Use antibiotics that are safe in pregnancy, such as penicillins. Patients undergoing urologic procedures should also be treated to avoid translocation of bacteria from mucosal damage.

6. How does pyelonephritis usually occur? What are the signs and symptoms? How is it treated?
Pyelonephritis is most often due to an ascending UTI caused by *E. coli* (>80% of cases). Patients present with high fever, shaking chills, costovertebral angle tenderness, flank pain, and/or UTI symptoms. Order urinalysis and urine and blood cultures to establish the diagnosis. If the patient cannot tolerate oral antibiotics, the patient should be admitted for IV antibiotics, typically IV ceftriaxone or fluoroquinolones. Outpatient management in uncomplicated pyelonephritis typically consists of an oral fluoroquinolone. Always choose an antibiotic regimen with good *E. coli* coverage. If the patient continues to have fevers, leukocytosis, or hemodynamic instability while being treated over 48 to 72 hours, consider imaging evaluation for a perinephric abscess.

TRAUMA AND TOXIC EFFECTS

1. What are the important renal sequelae of electrical burns?
Because most of the tissue destruction due to electrical burns is internal, sequelae include muscle necrosis, myoglobinuria, acidosis, and renal failure. Use large amounts of IV hydration to prevent renal shutdown. The immediate life-threatening risk with electricity exposure and burns (including lightning and a child who puts a finger in an electrical outlet) is cardiac arrhythmia. Perform ECG.

DISEASES AND DISORDERS OF THE FEMALE REPRODUCTIVE SYSTEM

CHAPTER 11

BREAST

1. **When a woman presents with a nipple discharge, what key pieces of patient history may suggest the underlying etiology?**
A history of using oral contraceptive pills, hormone therapies, antipsychotic medications (which elevate prolactin), or symptoms suggestive of hypothyroidism all may cause nipple discharge. The color of the discharge and whether the discharge is unilateral or bilateral is also very important. For example, if nipple discharge is bilateral and nonbloody, it is likely galactorrhea due to a prolactinoma (check prolactin level) or endocrine disorder (check a thyroid-stimulating hormone [TSH] level). Alternatively, when nipple discharge is unilateral and bloody, it may represent an underlying ductal papilloma (benign) or carcinoma (malignant). Perform a core needle biopsy of any breast mass that is discovered on physical exam.

2. **What are the most likely causes of a breast mass in a woman under the age of 35 years?**
Fibrocystic disease: bilateral, multiple cystic lesions that are tender to the touch, especially premenstrually. This is the most common of all breast diseases. Generally this is secondary to prior breast trauma, and no workup is needed other than routine follow-up. Oral contraceptive pills, progesterone, or danazol may help to relieve symptoms.
Fibroadenoma: a painless, discrete, sharply circumscribed, unilateral, rubbery mobile mass. This is the most common benign tumor of the female breast. Patients may be observed for one or more menstrual cycles to see if it regresses spontaneously. Because tumors are estrogen dependent, estrogen-containing oral contraceptive pills may stimulate growth, whereas menopause causes regression. Excision is curative but not required except for cosmetic reasons.
Mastitis/abscess: typically in the first few months postpartum, lactating women may develop a painful, swollen, erythematous breast(s). The nipple may be cracked or fissured. Patients with this presentation *plus a fever* have either mastitis or abscess: to distinguish these two, check for *fluctuance* of the area. If fluctuance is absent, the diagnosis is mastitis. If fluctuance is present, it is an abscess.

3. **How does the management of mastitis differ from the management of a breast abscess?**
The patient with mastitis should be treated with analgesics (e.g., acetaminophen, ibuprofen), antibiotics, and instructed to continue breastfeeding with the affected breast(s) even though it is painful. Use a breast pump to empty the breast if needed to prevent further milk duct blockage and potential abscess formation. An antistaphylococcal antibiotic (e.g., dicloxacillin or cephalexin) should be given for more than mild symptoms. If there is risk for methicillin-resistant *Staphylococcus aureus* (MRSA) or if MRSA is cultured, use trimethoprim-sulfamethoxazole or clindamycin. If a fluctuant mass develops or there is no response to antibiotics within a few days, an abscess is likely present and must be drained.

4. **What are the risk factors for breast cancer?**
   - Personal history of breast cancer (major risk factor)
   - Female sex
   - Family history in first-degree relatives
   - Age greater than 40 (rare before age 30, incidence steadily increases with age)
   - Early menarche or late menopause (longer estrogen exposure)
   - Late first pregnancy or nulliparity (more menstrual cycles = higher risk)
   - Atypical hyperplasia of the breast
   - Radiation exposure before age 30 years
   - Inherited gene mutations (e.g., *BRCA1* and *BRCA2*)
   - Dense breast tissue
   - High-fat diet
   - Diethylstilbestrol (DES) exposure
   - Recent oral contraceptive use
   - Combined postmenopausal hormone replacement therapy
   - Excessive alcohol consumption
   - Obesity

5. **What classic signs and symptoms suggest that a breast mass is cancer?**
   - Fixation of the breast mass to the chest wall or overlying skin
   - Satellite nodules or ulcers on the skin
   - Lymphedema (peau d'orange)
   - Matted or fixed axillary lymph nodes
   - Inflammatory skin changes (peau d'orange or red, hot thickened skin with enlargement of the breast due to inflammatory carcinoma)
   - Prolonged unilateral scaling erosion of the nipple with or without discharge (may be Paget disease of the nipple)
   - Microcalcifications on mammography
   - **Any new breast mass in a postmenopausal woman**

6. **What is the conservative approach to ensure that you do not miss a breast cancer?**
   When in doubt, biopsy every palpable breast mass in women over age 35 years that is not clearly a cyst (ultrasound is needed make the determination), especially if the patient has any of the risk factors mentioned in the previous question. If the Step 3 question does not want you to biopsy the mass, it will give clues that the mass is not a cancer (e.g., bilateral lumpy breasts that become symptomatic with every menses and have no dominant mass, patient age <30 years).

7. **What should you do with a breast mass in a woman under age 30 years?**
   In women under age 30 years, breast cancer is rare. With a discrete breast mass in this age group, you should think of fibroadenoma. Consider ultrasound of the breast and observe the patient over a few menstrual cycles before considering biopsy unless the ultrasound is suspicious (e.g., solid mass or complex cyst). Fibroadenomas are usually roundish, rubbery feeling, and mobile.

8. **What is the most common histologic type of breast cancer?**
   Invasive (infiltrating) ductal carcinoma accounts for about 70% of breast cancer.

9. **What is the role of mammography in deciding whether to biopsy a breast mass?**
   When a palpable breast mass is detected, the decision to biopsy is made on *clinical* grounds. A mammogram that looks benign should not deter you from doing a biopsy if you are clinically suspicious. On the other hand, a lesion that is detected on mammography and looks suspicious should be biopsied even if it is not palpable. Needle localization biopsy can be used.

10. **True or False: A mammogram should not be done in women under age 30 years.**
    True in most cases. The breast tissue in women under age 30 is too dense for mammogram to be of value. First-line imaging in women under age 30 years is breast ultrasound.

11. **What are the adjuvant therapies for breast cancer? How does each type of therapy work?**
    Tamoxifen is a selective estrogen-receptor modulator (SERM) that improves outcomes in premenopausal women with estrogen receptor–positive breast cancer. Tamoxifen has also been shown to decrease the risk of breast cancer in women at high risk of developing the disease.
    Aromatase inhibitors block the peripheral conversion of androgens to estrogens. Examples include anastrozole, exemestane, and letrozole.
    Ovarian suppression (with a gonadotropin-releasing hormone [GnRH] agonist such as goserelin) or ablation inhibits endogenous estrogen production from the ovaries.

12. **How are the adjuvant therapies used in nonmetastatic, hormone receptor–positive breast cancer?**
    The endocrine options for treatment depend on whether a woman is in menopause. A premenopausal woman at high risk of recurrence is usually treated with ovarian suppression and exemestane. A premenopausal woman not at high risk of recurrence is usually treated with tamoxifen, which avoids the toxicities of ovarian suppression and endocrine therapy.
    A postmenopausal woman is usually treated with an aromatase inhibitor (no ovarian suppression is needed because estrogen is not being produced by the ovaries).

13. **How is human epidermal growth factor receptor 2 (Her-2/neu) breast cancer treated?**
    HER-2/neu breast cancer is treated with chemotherapy (usually doxorubicin and cyclophosphamide) with trastuzumab as adjuvant therapy. Trastuzumab targets the HER-2 protein.

14. **What is the recommended treatment for women at high risk of developing breast cancer who have not yet developed breast cancer?**
    For women at high risk of developing breast cancer, endocrine therapy is generally preferred over observation. Postmenopausal women can be treated with a SERM (tamoxifen or raloxifene) or an aromatase inhibitor (anastrozole or exemestane). Premenopausal women at high risk are usually treated with tamoxifen.

15. **True or False: Mastectomy and breast-conserving surgery with radiation are considered equal in efficacy.**
    True. In either case, do an axillary node dissection (or a sentinel node biopsy) to determine spread to the nodes. If nodes are positive, chemotherapy is warranted.

UTERUS

1. **What are fibroids? How common are they? How often do they become malignant?**
   Fibroids (i.e., leiomyomas) are benign uterine tumors. They are the most common tumors in women and the most common indication for hysterectomy (when they grow too large or cause symptoms). Up to 40% of women have fibroids by age 40 years. Malignant transformation is quite rare (<1%).

2. **Explain the relationship between uterine leiomyomas and hormones. How do leiomyomas present? What is the treatment?**
   Leiomyomas of the uterus are estrogen dependent, therefore you may see rapid growth during pregnancy or the use of estrogen-containing oral contraceptive pills and regression after menopause. Leiomyomas may cause infertility, pain, and menorrhagia or metrorrhagia. Anemia due to leiomyoma is an indication for hysterectomy. Rarely, patients may present with a polyp protruding through the cervix. Dilation and curettage are needed to rule out endometrial cancer in women who present after age 35 years.
   The treatment for leiomyoma is usually surgical (the levonorgestrel-releasing intrauterine device [IUD] is seeing more widespread use, though randomized trials are lacking). Myomectomy can sometimes maintain or even restore fertility. For those no longer desiring pregnancy, total abdominal hysterectomy may be performed.

3. **Define endometriosis. What are the signs and symptoms?**
   Endometriosis is defined as endometrial glands outside the uterus (ectopic). Patients are usually nulliparous and over age 30 years with the following symptoms: **dysmenorrhea** (painful menstruation), **dyspareunia** (painful intercourse), **dyschezia** (painful defecation), and/or perimenstrual spotting. The most common site for the ectopic endometrial glands is the ovaries (chocolate cyst appearance); look for tender adnexa in an afebrile patient. Other sites include the broad (uterosacral) ligament and peritoneal surface. Nodularities on the broad ligament are classic findings on physical exam; the classic sequela is a retroverted uterus.

4. **How is endometriosis diagnosed and treated?**
   The gold standard of diagnosis is laparoscopy with visualization of the ectopic tissue showing classic powder-burn lesions. Manage medically with birth control pills (if acceptable to the patient) or second-line agents danazol and GnRH agonists (e.g., leuprolide). Surgery with electrocauterization will definitively destroy the ectopic glands and often improves fertility. In an older patient, consider hysterectomy and bilateral salpingoophorectomy for severe symptoms.

5. **What is the most likely cause of infertility in a menstruating woman over age 30 years without a history of pelvic inflammatory disease (PID)?**
   Endometriosis.

6. **Define adenomyosis. How does it classically present? What is the treatment?**
   Adenomyosis is defined as endometrial glands within the uterine musculature. Patients are usually over age 40 years with dysmenorrhea and menorrhagia. Look for descriptions of a "large, boggy uterus" on physical exam. Be sure to obtain an endometrial biopsy sample to rule out endometrial cancer. Total abdominal hysterectomy would definitively relieve the symptoms; consider trialing GnRH agonists (e.g., leuprolide) to medically manage symptoms.

7. **What is the rule of thumb for postmenopausal vaginal bleeding?**
   Postmenopausal vaginal bleeding is cancer until proven otherwise. Endometrial cancer is the most common type to present in this fashion; it is also the fourth most common cancer overall in women. Do an endometrial biopsy (generally preferred) or a transvaginal ultrasound for any woman with postmenopausal bleeding (as well as a Papanicolaou [Pap] smear).

8. **List the main risk factors for endometrial cancer.**
   - Obesity
   - Nulliparity
   - Late menopause
   - Diabetes, hypertension, and gallbladder disease (probably related to obesity)
   - Chronic, unopposed estrogen stimulation (e.g., polycystic ovary syndrome [PCOS], estrogen-secreting neoplasm [granulosa-theca cell tumor], and estrogen replacement therapy without progesterone)

9. **What is the most common type of endometrial cancer? How is it treated?**
   Most uterine cancers are adenocarcinomas and spread by direct extension. Treat with surgery and radiation.

OVARY, FALLOPIAN TUBE, AND BROAD LIGAMENT

1. **What are the presenting symptoms for torsion of the ovary and fallopian tube?**
   The classic presentation for ovarian torsion is acute pelvic pain in a woman with an adnexal mass, either with or without nausea and vomiting. However, the presenting signs and symptoms can be nonspecific (e.g., abdominal pain, fever, abnormal genital tract bleeding), so maintaining a high index of suspicion is important. Ovarian torsion is one of the most common gynecologic emergencies and may affect both adult and pediatric patients, although it occurs most commonly in the reproductive years.

2. **What are the risk factors for ovarian torsion? How is it diagnosed?**
The main risk factor for torsion is an ovarian mass, but pregnancy also increases the risk, and torsion may occur with a normal ovary. Prompt diagnosis is important to preserve ovarian/tubal function. Order a pregnancy test, complete blood count (CBC), and electrolyte panel. Pelvic ultrasound is the imaging modality of choice when torsion is suspected.

3. **How is ovarian torsion managed?**
With prompt surgery to preserve ovarian function and prevent other adverse events such as hemorrhage and peritonitis.

4. **What are the various causes of ovarian and fallopian tube masses?**
Ovarian masses may be caused by physiologic cysts (i.e., follicular cyst or corpus luteum cyst), benign neoplasms (e.g., dermoid cyst), ovarian cancer, or metastatic disease. Fallopian tube masses may be an ectopic pregnancy, fallopian tube malignancy, or hydrosalpinx.

5. **What should you think about when evaluating an adnexal mass?**
Adnexal masses are common, and the goal of evaluation is to determine the most likely cause. The likelihood of different types of adnexal mass depends on the anatomic location and the age and reproductive status of the patient. In children, ovarian torsion and ovarian malignancy are the most likely causes of an adnexal mass. In premenopausal women, most masses are benign and are associated with the menstrual cycle (e.g., follicular cysts), but always consider ectopic pregnancy. In postmenopausal women, malignancy must be ruled out.

6. **How is an adnexal mass evaluated?**
After taking a history and performing a physical examination, order a pregnancy test, CBC, and pelvic ultrasound. Most diagnoses can be established on the basis of these studies. If there is a clinical suspicion of malignancy (based on the ultrasound, age/menopausal status, risk factors, and laboratory results), surgical exploration is needed to make a definitive diagnosis.

7. **What is premature ovarian failure? What are the presenting symptoms?**
Premature ovarian failure, also called premature menopause or, more recently, 46,XX primary ovarian insufficiency, is a spectrum disorder with a continuum of impaired ovarian function. The condition involves the development of hypergonadotropic hypogonadism before 40 years of age in a woman with a normal karyotype. Premature ovarian failure is characterized by oligomenorrhea and/or amenorrhea, elevated serum gonadotropin, and low serum estradiol concentrations. Symptoms of estrogen deficiency are typically present (e.g., hot flashes and vaginal dryness). Ovarian function occurs intermittently in many of these women, so pregnancy can occur. Additional information about the evaluation of secondary amenorrhea is discussed in more detail later in the chapter.

CERVIX

1. **What is the best available screening method to reduce the incidence and mortality of cervical cancer?**
Pap smears. Perform a Pap smear on all female patients if they are due, even if they present for a totally unrelated complaint. Screening should start at age 21 years regardless of sexual activity. The frequency of screening depends on whether human papillomavirus (HPV) testing is also being used as well as the patient's age and results of previous Pap smears. See Chapter 1 for additional details.

2. **What should you do if a Pap smear is abnormal?**
The follow-up for an abnormal Pap smear depends on the cervical cytologic results. Lower-grade lesions may be evaluated with HPV testing and colposcopy/endocervical curettage, if needed. Higher-grade lesions require colposcopy with biopsy and/or loop electrosurgical excision procedure (LEEP). Invasive cancer requires surgery (at least a hysterectomy) and includes radiation plus cisplatin-based chemotherapy.

3. **List the main risk factors for cervical cancer.**
   - HPV infection
   - Early onset of sexual activity
   - Multiple sexual partners
   - A high-risk sexual partner (e.g., partner with multiple sexual partners or known HPV infection)
   - Smoking
   - History of sexually transmitted infection
   - Immunosuppression
   - Low socioeconomic status

4. **Where does cervical cancer begin? How does it present? How is it treated?**
Invasive cervical cancer begins in the transformation zone and usually presents with vaginal bleeding or discharge (postcoital bleeding, intermenstrual spotting, or abnormal menstrual bleeding). Treat with surgery and/or radiation.

5. What do you need to know about diethylstilbestrol (DES) and cancer?
Maternal exposure to DES during pregnancy increases a daughter's risk of developing clear cell cancer of the cervix and/or vagina.

VAGINA/VULVA

1. What tumor resembles "a bunch of grapes" coming out of the vagina?
Sarcoma botryoides, a type of embryonal rhabdomyosarcoma usually seen in children.

2. What causes vaginitis or discharge in prepubescent girls?
Most cases are nonspecific or physiologic, but look for a vaginal foreign body (most common cause of prepubertal vaginal bleeding), sexual abuse (especially if a sexually transmitted disease is present), or *Candida* fungal infection. A candidal infection may be a presentation of diabetes; check the serum glucose level and/or the urine for glycosuria.

3. How do you recognize and treat an imperforate hymen?
Imperforate hymen classically presents at menarchal age with primary amenorrhea and hematocolpos (blood in the vagina) that cannot escape, thus the hymen bulges outward. Treatment is surgical opening of the hymen.

MENSTRUAL DISORDERS

1. What is dysmenorrhea? How is it diagnosed? How is it treated?
Dysmenorrhea is pain that precedes and/or occurs during menstruation and interferes with daily activities. The pain can be sharp, dull, throbbing, burning, or shooting. Dysmenorrhea is a clinical diagnosis that requires a thorough history, physical examination, and sometimes additional tests (e.g., Pap test, pelvic ultrasound, testing for gonorrhea/chlamydia). Nonsteroidal antiinflammatory drugs (NSAIDs) help in many cases of dysmenorrhea. Hormonal contraceptives are also helpful.

2. What is premenstrual dysphoric disorder (PMDD)? How is it treated?
PMDD is a severe form of premenstrual syndrome (PMS) occurring in a predictable, cyclic pattern just before menstruation and resolving shortly after menstruation. Mood symptoms predominate and include feelings of sadness or despair, irritability, anxiety, anhedonia, trouble concentrating, fatigue, and difficulty in sleeping. Other signs and symptoms may include food cravings, bloating, breast swelling/tenderness, and headaches. Selective serotonin reuptake inhibitors are the first-line treatment for PMDD. Fluoxetine, sertraline, paroxetine, and escitalopram are approved by the Food and Drug Administration (FDA) for this indication. Oral contraceptive pills containing drospirenone and ethinylestradiol are FDA approved to treat PMDD.

3. What is the first test to order in any woman of reproductive age with abnormal uterine bleeding (AUB)?
A pregnancy test.

4. Define abnormal uterine bleeding. What does the PALM-COEIN classification stand for?
AUB is defined as menstrual flow outside of the normal frequency, duration, volume, or regularity in nonpregnant women of reproductive age. PALM-COEIN classifies abnormal bleeding into the most common causes of AUB as structural causes (PALM: **p**olyp, **a**denomyosis, **l**eiomyoma, **m**alignancy and hyperplasia) and nonstructural causes (COEIN: **c**oagulopathy, **o**vulatory dysfunction, **e**ndometrial dysfunction, **i**atrogenic, **n**ot yet classified).
More than 70% of cases are associated with anovulatory cycles (e.g., unopposed estrogen stimulates continued endometrial proliferation until the tissue finally outgrows its blood supply and randomly begins to slough off). The age of the patient is important because immediately following menarche and immediately before menopause, AUB is common. In fact, AUB during these two transitional times is considered physiologic. Most other women experiencing AUB have PCOS, the most common nonphysiologic cause of AUB.

5. Why is endometrial biopsy recommended in women over age 35 years with abnormal uterine bleeding? What other test should be ordered in all women with abnormal uterine bleeding (regardless of age)?
Endometrial biopsy in this age range is to rule out endometrial cancer. Hemoglobin and hematocrit (or CBC) should be ordered on all women with AUB to make sure that the patient is not anemic from excessive blood loss.

6. How is abnormal uterine bleeding treated?
Estrogen-progestin oral contraceptive pills are first-line management for many women with AUB. The levonorgestrel IUD is a highly effective option for treatment of heavy menstrual bleeding (HMB) in women who do not desire pregnancy. Depot medroxyprogesterone acetate (DMPA) may be used for women with AUB who have contraindications to or prefer to avoid estrogen or if they prefer this method of contraception. High-dose oral prestins may be used to treat AUB in women who have contraindications to or prefer to avoid estrogen or women who are trying to become pregnant. Tranexamic acid is an option for women with HMB who do not desire or should not use hormonal treatment. NSAIDs are a nonhormonal, noncontraceptive option for treatment of HMB and reduce the volume of menstrual blood loss by causing a decline in the rate of prostaglandin synthesis in the endometrium, leading to

vasoconstriction and reduced bleeding agent for menorrhagia and AUB if the patient does not desire pregnancy and menstrual cycles are irregular. Monotherapy with progesterone is used for severe bleeding.

7. **Distinguish between primary and secondary amenorrhea.**
A patient with primary amenorrhea has never experienced menarche, whereas a patient with secondary amenorrhea has a history of normal menstruation, which has now stopped.

8. **Until proven otherwise, what is the cause of secondary amenorrhea in a previously menstruating woman of reproductive age?**
Pregnancy. Always order a urine pregnancy test to measure human chorionic gonadotropin (hCG) to rule out pregnancy as the first step in your evaluation of secondary amenorrhea.

9. **True or False: Excessive exercise may cause amenorrhea.**
True. It is not uncommon to find amenorrhea (or hypomenorrhea) in hard-training athletes. It results from an exercise-induced depression of GnRH, which reduces the entire hypothalamic-pituitary-gonadal axis.

10. **What are other common causes of secondary amenorrhea?**
Additional causes of secondary amenorrhea include:
- PCOS
- Hypothyroidism
- Anorexia nervosa
- Endocrine disorders (headaches, galactorrhea, and visual field defects may indicate a prolactin-secreting pituitary tumor)
- Primary ovarian insufficiency
- Antipsychotic medications (due to increased prolactin)
- History of chemotherapy (causes premature ovarian failure and menopause)
   Although not considered secondary amenorrhea, **menopause** should be kept in mind as a cause for cessation of menstruation in patients beginning at age 45 years.

11. **After ruling out pregnancy, if the cause of secondary amenorrhea is not obvious from the history and physical exam, what is the next step in your evaluation?**
Administer progesterone to assess the patient's estrogen status. If vaginal bleeding develops within 2 weeks of completing the progesterone challenge, the patient has sufficient estrogen. In this case, check the luteinizing hormone (LH) level. If it is high, consider PCOS. If it is low or normal, check the levels of prolactin and TSH. The high TSH level in hypothyroidism causes high prolactin levels. If the prolactin is high with a normal TSH level, order magnetic resonance imaging (MRI) of the brain to rule out pituitary prolactinoma. If the prolactin level is normal, look for low levels of GnRH, which may be induced by drugs, stress, or exercise. In these patients, clomiphene or leuprolide can be used in an attempt to facilitate pregnancy.

12. **What if the patient fails to have vaginal bleeding after the progesterone challenge test?**
If the patient has no vaginal bleeding, estrogen levels are inadequate. Check the follicle-stimulating hormone (FSH) level next. If it is elevated, premature ovarian failure is the problem; check for autoimmune disorders, karyotype abnormalities (e.g., Turner syndrome), and a history of chemotherapy. If the FSH level is low or normal, the problem may be a brain tumor (e.g., craniopharyngioma). Order an MRI of the brain. Clomiphene would be ineffective in these patients.

13. **At what age can primary amenorrhea be diagnosed? What is the first step in evaluation?**
Primary amenorrhea is defined as the absence of menses at age 15 years in the presence of normal growth and secondary sexual characteristics (e.g., breast development, axillary and pubic hair). If no menses have occurred by age 13 years and there is a complete absence of secondary sexual characteristics such as breast development, evaluation for primary amenorrhea should begin. The first step is to rule out pregnancy.

14. **In a patient older than age 13 years with no secondary sexual characteristics or thelarche, what is the most likely cause of amenorrhea?**
The most likely cause in this setting is a congenital problem. In a phenotypically female patient with normal breast development but no axillary or pubic hair, think of **androgen insensitivity syndrome.** In such patients, the internal female genitalia (e.g., uterus, fallopian tubes, and upper third of the vaginal canal) will be absent. Contrast this against a patient with no breast development and no axillary or pubic hair; these patients most likely have **5-alpha reductase deficiency**.
   In the presence of normal breast development and internal female genitalia, the next step is to measure the serum prolactin level to rule out pituitary adenoma. If the prolactin level is high, order an MRI of the head. If serum prolactin is normal, administer progesterone and follow the same procedure as in the evaluation of secondary amenorrhea.

15. **When in doubt, what is the best way to evaluate any type of amenorrhea?**
First, order a pregnancy test. If it is negative, attempt a progesterone challenge test. Further testing depends on whether the progesterone challenge induces withdrawal bleeding or not. Measuring serum levels of TSH and/or prolactin should also be performed.

MENOPAUSE

1. **When does menopause occur? What are the signs and symptoms?**
   The average age of menopause is around 51 years. Patients have irregular cycles or amenorrhea, hot flashes and mood swings, and an elevated FSH level. Amenorrhea for 1 year signals the completion of menopause. Patients also may complain of dysuria, dyspareunia, incontinence, and/or vaginal itching, burning, or soreness. Vaginal symptoms are often due to atrophic vaginitis; expect the vaginal mucosa to be thin, dry, and atrophic with in- creased parabasal cells on cytology. Topical estrogen improves vaginal symptoms, but other symptoms (e.g., hot flashes) require oral therapy.

2. **Describe the current state of hormone replacement therapy.**
   Hormone replacement therapy is currently recommended for short-term management of moderate to severe va- somotor flushing. Long-term use for the prevention of disease (such as osteoporosis or cardiovascular disease) is no longer recommended due to increased risk of venous thromboembolism (VTE) and risk of endometrial cancer.

3. **Which women are candidates for hormone replacement therapy?**
   Hormone replacement therapy (i.e., estrogen with or without progesterone) is now controversial and probably best used only as a means of menopause-related symptom relief. Observation during therapy is necessary be- cause estrogen and progesterone are not harmless. Every woman should make the decision on her own after weighing the risks and benefits.

4. **What are the known benefits of estrogen therapy?**
   Known benefits of estrogen therapy include:
   - Decreased osteoporosis and decreased fractures
   - Reduced hot flashes and genitourinary symptoms of menopause (dryness, urgency, atrophy-induced inconti- nence, frequency)
   - Decreased risk of colorectal cancer (according to the Women's Health Initiative, when combined estrogen and progesterone therapy is used)

5. **What are the known risks of estrogen therapy?**
   Known risks of estrogen therapy include:
   - Increased risk of endometrial cancer (eliminated by coadministration of progesterone)
   - Small increase in risk of coronary heart disease with combined estrogen and progesterone therapy, though the risk is not increased in women who are less than 10 years postmenopausal or 50 to 59 years of age
   - Increased risk of VTE
   - Increased risk of breast cancer (according to the Women's Health Initiative when combined estrogen and pro- gesterone therapy is used. There was a slightly decreased risk of breast cancer with estrogen only, though this decrease was not statistically significant.)
   - Increased risk of stroke (according to the Women's Health Initiative, with either estrogen only or combined estrogen and progesterone therapy)
   - Increased risk of gallbladder disease

6. **What are the most common side effects of estrogen therapy?**
   Common side effects of estrogen therapy include:
   - Endometrial bleeding
   - Bloating
   - Breast tenderness
   - Headache
   - Nausea

7. **What are the absolute contraindications to estrogen therapy?**
   Contraindications to estrogen therapy include:
   - Unexplained vaginal bleeding
   - Active liver disease
   - History of thromboembolism or stroke
   - Coronary artery disease
   - History of endometrial or breast cancer
   - Pregnancy

8. **What are the relative contraindications to estrogen therapy?**
   Relative contraindications to estrogen therapy include:
   - Seizure disorder
   - Hypertension
   - Uterine leiomyomas
   - Familial hyperlipidemia
   - Migraine headache with aura
   - Thrombophlebitis

- Endometriosis
- Gallbladder disease

9. **What study is often done before starting estrogen therapy?**
Women classically get an endometrial biopsy, ultrasound, or dilation and curettage at the onset of treatment to rule out endometrial hyperplasia and/or cancer and an evaluation of any unexplained bleeding, even while on therapy, unless they have had a normal evaluation within the past 6 months.

10. **What is postmenopausal vaginal bleeding? What do you need to do to evaluate postmenopausal vaginal bleeding?**
Vaginal bleeding starting 12 months or more after the cessation of menses or unscheduled bleeding in a postmenopausal woman who has been taking hormone replacement therapy for 12 months or more. All women with postmenopausal vaginal bleeding require evaluation for potential malignancy (i.e., endometrial cancer, premalignant atypical endometrial hyperplasia, and cervical cancer). Evaluation includes a Pap smear and either an endometrial biopsy or transvaginal ultrasound. If ultrasound is performed and the endometrial lining is thicker than 4 mm or is otherwise abnormal, endometrial biopsy is required.

11. **True or False: Women without a uterus do not need to take progesterone with estrogen.**
True. The main reason for giving progesterone with hormone replacement therapy is to eliminate the increased risk of endometrial cancer that accompanies unopposed estrogen therapy. If a woman has no uterus, then she has no need for progesterone.

PELVIC RELAXATION AND URINARY DISORDERS

1. **What causes pelvic relaxation or vaginal prolapse? What are the signs and symptoms?**
Pelvic relaxation is due to a weakening of pelvic supporting ligaments. Look for a history of several vaginal deliveries, a feeling of heaviness or fullness in the pelvis, urinary incontinence, backache, worsening of symptoms upon standing, and resolution of symptoms with lying down.

2. **What types of pelvic relaxation are seen clinically? How are they treated?**
Cystocele: the bladder bulges into the *upper anterior vaginal wall.* Common symptoms include urinary urgency, frequency, and/or incontinence.
Rectocele: the rectum bulges into the *lower posterior vaginal wall.* Watch for difficulty with defecation.
Enterocele: loops of bowel bulge into the *upper posterior vaginal wall.*
Urethrocele: the urethra bulges into the *lower anterior vaginal wall.* Common symptoms include urinary urgency, frequency, and/or incontinence.
Conservative treatment for all types of pelvic relaxation involves pelvic and detrusor muscle strengthening exercises and/or a pessary (artificial device to provide support). Surgery is used for refractory or severe cases or patient desire.

FEMALE FERTILITY/INFERTILITY

1. **Other than abstinence, what are the most effective forms of birth control (when used properly)?**
The most effective forms of birth control, in order of efficacy, are sterilization (e.g., tubal ligation or vasectomy), implants (etonogestrel implant) or an IUD, injectable hormone depot preparations (progesterone), and birth control pills/patch or a hormonal vaginal ring.

2. **Which forms of birth control prevent most sexually transmitted illnesses?**
Abstinence and condoms.

3. **Do intrauterine devices increase the risk of ectopic pregnancy or pelvic inflammatory disease?**
An IUD does not increase a woman's risk of having an ectopic pregnancy; however, if a woman who has an IUD is found to be pregnant, it is more likely to be an ectopic pregnancy than if she didn't have the IUD.
Similarly, IUDs do not increase the risk of PID. If a woman has an IUD in place and is diagnosed with PID, do not remove the IUD unless the organism is *Actinomyces israelii.* Treat with antibiotics with the IUD in place. *Actinomyces* should be treated with penicillin when present.

4. **What are the absolute contraindications to combined oral contraceptive pills?**
Contraindications to combined oral contraceptive pills include:
- Acute deep vein thrombosis/pulmonary embolism (DVT/PE)
- History of DVT/PE, not on anticoagulant therapy
- Known thrombogenic mutations
- VTE, current or past (DVT/PE)
- History of stroke

- Ischemic heart disease
- Moderately or severely impaired cardiac function
- Vascular disease
- Complicated valvular heart disease
- Diabetes with complications (can be a relative contraindication if the complications are not severe)
- Current breast cancer
- Pregnancy
- Decompensated cirrhosis
- Liver tumors (hepatocellular adenoma or hepatoma)
- Migraine with aura at any age or migraine without aura and age greater than or equal to 35 years
- Major surgery with prolonged immobilization
- Age greater than 35 years and smoking 15 or more cigarettes per day
- Hypertension (blood pressure >160/100 mm Hg or with concomitant vascular disease)
- Complicated solid organ transplantation

5. **What are the relative contraindications to combined oral contraceptive pills?**
   Relative contraindications to combined oral contraceptive pills include:
   - Less than 21 days since delivery
   - Breastfeeding sooner than 1 month postpartum
   - Undiagnosed vaginal or uterine bleeding
   - History of breast cancer but no recurrence in past 5 years
   - History of DVT/PE with lower risk for recurrence
   - Peripartum cardiomyopathy greater than or equal to 6 months
   - History of breast cancer with no evidence of current disease for 5 years
   - Interacting drugs (certain anticonvulsants, rifampin, ritonavir-boosted protease inhibitors)
   - Gallbladder disease (unless asymptomatic or history of cholecystectomy)
   - Migraine without aura, and age greater than or equal to 35 years
   - Hypertension (well controlled or blood pressure 140–159/90–99 mm Hg)
   - Multiple risk factors for arterial cardiovascular disease
   - Acute viral hepatitis

6. **What is the relationship between oral contraceptive pills and hypertension?**
   Oral contraceptive pills are one of the most common causes of secondary hypertension. Any patient taking birth control pills who is noted to have an increased blood pressure should discontinue the pills and have her blood pressure rechecked at a later date.

7. **What do you need to know about oral contraceptive pills and surgery?**
   Because of the risks of thromboembolism, oral contraceptive pills should be stopped 1 month before elective surgery and not restarted until 1 month after surgery.

8. **What are the side effects of oral contraceptive pills?**
   The side effects include glucose intolerance (check for diabetes mellitus annually in women at high risk), depression, edema (bloating), cholelithiasis, **benign liver adenomas,** melasma ("the mask of pregnancy"), nausea, vomiting, headache, hypertension, and drug interactions. Drugs such as rifampin and antiepileptics may induce metabolism of oral contraceptive pills and reduce their effectiveness.

9. **What is the relationship between oral contraceptive pills and breast and cervical cancer?**
   Oral contraceptive pills have little if any effect on the risk of developing breast cancer. Cervical neoplasia may be increased in users of birth control pills.

10. **What is the relationship between oral contraceptive pills and ovarian and endometrial cancer?**
    Oral contraceptive pills have been shown to reduce the incidence of ovarian cancer by 50%; they also reduce the incidence of endometrial cancer.

11. **What are the other beneficial effects of oral contraceptive pills?**
    They decrease the incidence of menorrhagia, dysmenorrhea, benign breast disease, functional ovarian cysts, premenstrual tension, iron-deficiency anemia, ectopic pregnancy, and salpingitis.

12. **True or False: Women who smoke should not take birth control pills.**
    True—if the woman is over the age of 35 years and smokes or is younger than 35 and smokes 15 or more cigarettes per day. The risk of thromboembolism is increased sharply in women who smoke and take birth control pills. Postmenopausal women, however, can take estrogen therapy regardless of smoking status.

13. **What is the most common cause of preventable infertility in the United States?**
    Pelvic inflammatory disease.

14. **What is the most likely cause for infertility in a woman under age 30 years with abnormal menstruation?**
Polycystic ovarian syndrome.

15. **Define polycystic ovarian syndrome. How do you recognize it?**
PCOS is an endocrine imbalance characterized by an excess of androgens in a female patient, often suggested in a clinical vignette by a LH:FSH ratio greater than 3:1. On physical exam, look for a combination of hirsutism, significant acne, AUB, and/or infertility in an overweight female. Patients also frequently develop enlarged ovaries with multiple peripherally oriented cysts, which can be seen on ultrasound. However, an ultrasound is not required to make a diagnosis of PCOS. On the Step 3 exam, watch for an overweight woman who has acne, hirsutism, amenorrhea, and/or infertility.

16. **How is polycystic ovarian syndrome managed? With what risk is this syndrome associated?**
Manage the dysmenorrhea with oral contraceptive pills or cyclic progesterone. If the patient desires pregnancy, you can use **letrozole** to induce ovulation. Chronic unopposed estrogen (i.e., not enough progesterone, hence infrequent menses) increases the risk of **endometrial cancer** in patients with PCOS. **Spironolactone** can be used to treat the hirsutism associated with PCOS. Metformin is sometimes used to treat the insulin resistance associated with PCOS and may help restore ovulation. However, metformin is not FDA approved for this use, and oral contraceptive pills or cyclic progesterone is the preferred agent for endometrial protection.

17. **Is infertility usually a male or a female problem?**
Two-thirds of cases are due to a female problem, one-third to a male problem.

18. **Assuming that the history and physical exam offer no clues, what is the first step in evaluating a couple for infertility?**
Investigate the male first by performing semen analysis, as it is cheap, easy, and noninvasive.

19. **What is the next step to workup infertility if semen evaluation returns normal results?**
Documentation of ovulation. The history may suggest an ovulatory problem (irregular menstrual cycle length, duration, or amount of flow; lack of PMS symptoms). Monitoring basal body temperature, luteal phase progesterone levels, and/or obtaining an endometrial biopsy during the luteal phase can all be done to check for ovulation.

20. **What radiologic test is commonly used to investigate the fallopian tubes and uterine anatomy? What points in the history may lead you to suspect a uterine or tube problem?**
A hysterosalpingogram is commonly used to investigate the anatomy of the uterus and fallopian tubes. Clues in the patient's history may suggest a tubal problem (e.g., PID, previous ectopic pregnancy) or a uterine problem (e.g., previous dilation and curettage resulting in intrauterine synechiae; history of fibroids; or symptoms of endometriosis; uterine anomalies such as septate, bicornuate, and didelphys).

21. **What study is the last resort in the workup for infertility?**
Laparoscopy may be performed as a last resort or with a history suggestive of endometriosis. Lysis of adhesions and destruction of endometriosis lesions often restore fertility.

22. **Which two medications can be used to try to restore female fertility? In what situations are they effective?**
Medical therapy usually consists of clomiphene citrate to induce ovulation, but this approach requires adequate endogenous production of estrogen. If the woman is hypoestrogenic, use human menopausal gonadotropin (hMG), which is a **combination of FSH and LH**, to increase estrogen production. If medications fail, in vitro fertilization can be attempted.

23. **What is the main risk associated with medical induction of ovulation?**
Multiple-gestation pregnancies.

NEOPLASMS

1. **What do you need to know about breast cancer for the USMLE?**
Please see the earlier section on the breast.

2. **How does ovarian cancer classically present? How are ovarian masses evaluated?**
Ovarian cancer classically presents late with weight loss, pelvic mass, ascites, and/or bowel obstruction. Any ovarian enlargement in a postmenopausal female is cancer until proven otherwise. In women of reproductive age, most ovarian enlargements are benign. Ultrasound is the first-line test to evaluate an ovarian lesion.

3. **How is ovarian cancer treated? What is the cell of origin? What is the most common type of ovarian cancer?**
Ovarian cancer is usually treated with debulking surgery and chemotherapy. The prognosis is usually poor due to a late presentation. Most ovarian cancers arise from ovarian epithelium. Serous cystadenocarcinoma is the most

common type; histopathologic studies classically reveal psammoma bodies. Mucinous cystadenocarcinoma is also common. When clinicians use the term "ovarian cancer" without a qualifier, they are talking about epithelial malignancies (i.e., cystadenocarcinomas).

4. **List the three commonly tested germ cell tumors. What clues suggest their presence?**
   1. **Teratoma/dermoid cyst** (most common and most tested type). Look for a description of the tumor to include skin, hair, and/or teeth or bone; it may show up with calcifications on radiograph.
   2. **Sertoli-Leydig cell tumor,** which causes virilization (hirsutism, receding hairline, deepening voice, clitoromegaly).
   3. **Granulosa-theca cell tumors,** which cause feminization and precocious puberty.
      Female patients with germ cell tumors of the ovary are classically under the age of 30 years.

INFECTIONS

1. **What is pelvic inflammatory disease? How do you recognize it on the USMLE Step 3 exam?**
   PID is typically due to an ascending sexually transmitted infection of the upper female genital tract that may involve the endometrial cavity (endometritis), fallopian tubes (salpingitis), ovaries (oophoritis), parametrial tissues/ligaments (parametritis), and/or peritoneal cavity (peritonitis). Look for a sexually active female aged 13 to 35 years with the following symptoms: (1) abdominal pain, (2) adnexal tenderness, *and* (3) **cervical motion tenderness.** All three criteria must technically be present. In addition, one or more of the following should be present: elevated erythrocyte sedimentation rate (ESR) or C-reactive protein (CRP) level, leukocytosis, fever, or purulent cervical discharge.

2. **How is pelvic inflammatory disease treated? What are the common sequelae?**
   There are several different regimens recommended by the Centers for Disease Control and Prevention (CDC), but there is one main antibiotic combination used for outpatient PID and two commonly used combinations for inpatient PID. Ceftriaxone plus doxycycline is the typical outpatient combination. For inpatient treatment, consider either cefoxitin or cefotetan plus doxycycline; or consider clindamycin plus gentamicin. Remember these inpatient regimens with the mnemonics "*foxy doxy* (ce*fox*itin + *doxy*cycline)" or "*gently clean-da* uterus with *gent*amicin + *clinda*mycin."

   Common sequelae include chronic pelvic pain, increased risk of ectopic pregnancy, infertility due to scarring of the fallopian tubes, and progression to tubo-ovarian abscess. If suspected PID does not begin to improve after 48 hours, look for an abscess with an ultrasound or CT scan. Ruptured abscess will present with hemodynamic instability; manage this with emergent laparotomy and excision of the affected tube (for unilateral disease) or total abdominal hysterectomy and bilateral salpingoophorectomy (for bilateral disease).

3. **Cover the right-hand columns. Specify the findings and treatment for the following vaginal infections.**

Organism	Findings	Treatment
Candida sp.	"Cottage cheese," pseudohyphae on KOH preparation, history of diabetes, antibiotic treatment, or pregnancy	Topical or oral antifungal (e.g., fluconazole)
Trichomonas vaginalis	Pale yellow-green, frothy, watery discharge; "strawberry" cervix; motile organisms on microscopic inspection, vaginal pH >4.5	Metronidazole
Gardnerella vaginalis	Bacterial vaginosis; malodorous discharge; fishy smell on KOH preparation, clue cells; vaginal pH >4.5	Metronidazole
Human papillomavirus	Venereal warts; koilocytosis on Pap smear; postcoital bleeding	Many (acid, cryotherapy, laser, podophyllin)
Herpesvirus	Multiple shallow, painful ulcers; recurrence and resolution	Acyclovir, valacyclovir
Treponema pallidum (primary syphilis)	Painless chancre; occasional inguinal lymphadenopathy; spirochete on dark-field microscopy	Penicillin
Treponema pallidum (secondary syphilis)	Condyloma lata, maculopapular rash on palms, serology	Penicillin
Treponema pallidum (tertiary syphilis)	Tabes dorsalis, gummas, Argyll-Robertson pupils, CSF fluid examination	Penicillin
Chlamydia trachomatis	Most common STD; dysuria; positive culture and nucleic acid amplification tests (NAAT)	Doxycycline or azithromycin*
Neisseria gonorrhoeae	Mucopurulent cervicitis; growth on chocolate agar; positive NAAT	Ceftriaxone

Continued on following page

Organism	Findings	Treatment
Molluscum contagiosum	Characteristic appearance of dome-shaped lesions with central umbilication, intracellular inclusions	Curette, cryotherapy, or electrocauterization/ coagulation
Pediculosis	"Crabs"; pruritic; lice can be seen on pubic hairs	Permethrin cream (or malathion)

CSF, Cerebrospinal fluid; *KOH,* potassium hydroxide; *STD,* sexually transmitted disease.
*Chlamydia can be treated with erythromycin if the patient is pregnant. If compliance is a concern (e.g., history of nonadherence, substance abuse, or homelessness), give azithromycin 1 g orally in a single dose so that you can watch the patient take it. Patients with gonorrhea should always be treated for presumed chlamydial coinfection, but *if exclusive Chlamydial infection is confirmed by NAAT,* you do *not* have to treat for potential gonorrheal coinfection (e.g., do *not* give ceftriaxone along with the doxycycline or azithromycin). In clinical practice this distinction is not often made, but that doesn't stop it from appearing on licensing exams. If the NAAT results aren't back yet, treat empirically for both organisms.

4. True or False: With every infection listed in the previous table, you should seek out and treat the patient's sexual partners.
   False. *Candida* and *Gardnerella* spp. are not typically sexually transmitted diseases; they are usually caused by disturbances in the normal vaginal flora. You should treat the patient's sexual partners and give counseling (e.g., condoms) for the other infections, which are sexually transmitted.

5. True or False: Patients with gonorrhea should be treated for presumed chlamydial infection.
   True. The established treatment strategy for gonorrhea is to give both ceftriaxone (for gonorrhea) and doxycycline (for potential coinfection with chlamydia). However, *if exclusive Chlamydial infection is confirmed by NAAT,* the reverse is not true; do *not* automatically give gonorrhea treatment (e.g., ceftriaxone) to patients with confirmed chlamydial infection. If the NAAT results aren't back yet, treat empirically for both organisms. But if NAAT results show exclusively a chlamydial infection with results negative for gonorrhea, the patient should only receive chlamydial treatment (e.g., either doxycycline or azithromycin *without* ceftriaxone).

6. Which group of patients should always be screened for syphilis?
   Pregnant women. Early treatment can prevent birth defects.

7. True or False: Sexually active teenaged girls need screening for chlamydial infection and gonorrhea.
   True. There are high numbers of reported cases of chlamydia and gonorrhea in younger women. The CDC recommends annual screening for chlamydia for all sexually active females age 25 years and under. The CDC recommends screening high-risk sexually active females for gonorrhea.

CHAPTER 12

PREGNANCY, LABOR AND DELIVERY, THE FETUS, AND THE NEWBORN

PREGNANCY COMPLICATIONS

1. True or False: A high-normal blood urea nitrogen (BUN) or creatinine level during pregnancy often indicates renal disease.
   True. BUN and creatinine decrease significantly in pregnancy after the first trimester in women with normal renal function.

2. Define oligohydramnios. What causes it? Why is it worrisome?
   Oligohydramnios means a deficient amount of amniotic fluid is present (<500 mL or an amniotic fluid index <5). Causes include intrauterine growth restriction (IUGR), premature rupture of the membranes (PROM), postmaturity, and renal agenesis (Potter disease). Oligohydramnios is worrisome because it may cause fetal problems, including pulmonary hypoplasia, cutaneous or skeletal abnormalities due to compression (Potter sequence), and hypoxia due to cord compression.

3. Define polyhydramnios. What causes it? Why is it worrisome?
   Polyhydramnios means an overabundance of amniotic fluid is present (>2 L or an amniotic fluid index >25). Causes include maternal diabetes, multiple gestation, neural tube defects (e.g., anencephaly, spina bifida), gastrointestinal anomalies (e.g., omphalocele, esophageal atresia), chromosomal abnormalities (e.g., trisomy 18 and 21), and hydrops fetalis. Polyhydramnios is worrisome because it may cause maternal problems, including postpartum uterine atony (with resultant postpartum hemorrhage) and maternal dyspnea (an overdistended uterus compromises pulmonary function).

4. Define macrosomia. What is the likely cause?
   Macrosomia is defined as a fetus or newborn who weighs more than 4000 g (roughly 9 lb). The cause is maternal diabetes mellitus until proven otherwise.

5. What is a hydatidiform mole? What are the clues to its presence?
   A hydatidiform mole is one form of gestational trophoblastic neoplasia in which the products of conception essentially become a tumor. Look for the following clues:
   • Hyperemesis gravidarum
   • Very high human chorionic gonadotropin (hCG) levels during pregnancy and levels that do not return to zero after delivery (or abortion/miscarriage)
   • First- or second-trimester bleeding with possible expulsion of "grapes" from the vagina (grossly, the tumor looks like a bunch of grapes) and excessive nausea/hyperemesis
   • Uterine size/date discrepancy, with the uterus larger than expected for dates
   • Snowstorm-like pattern on ultrasound

6. Distinguish between complete and partial hydatidiform moles. How are hydatidiform moles treated?
   Complete moles have a karyotype of 46,XX or 46,XY (with all chromosomes from the father) and no fetal tissue. **Incomplete (partial) moles** usually have a karyotype of 69,XXY with fetal tissue in the tumor.
   Treat hydatidiform moles with uterine dilation and curettage and follow with serial measurements of hCG levels until they fall to zero. If the hCG level does not fall to zero or begins to rise, the patient either has an invasive mole or a choriocarcinoma. If a choriocarcinoma occurs, these increasingly aggressive forms of gestational trophoblastic neoplasia require chemotherapy (methotrexate or dactinomycin is most effective).

7. How is intrauterine growth restriction defined? List the possible etiologies of symmetric and asymmetric Intrauterine growth restriction.
   IUGR is defined as fetal size below the 10th percentile for gestational age. Symmetric IUGR (e.g., proportional decrease in all four biometric measurements) is typically caused by intrinsic maternal or fetal factors. Maternal factors may include TORCH infections, underlying medical conditions (e.g., hypertension, diabetes, chronic renal disease), or exposure to growth-restricting substances (e.g., alcohol, tobacco, cocaine, heroin and methadone, warfarin, antiepileptic medications, or antineoplastic medications), while fetal factors may include aneuploidy (e.g., trisomy 13 or 18) or structural anomalies (e.g., gastroschisis, cardiac malformation, renal agenesis).
   Asymmetric IUGR (typically seen as normal head measurements with abnormally low limb and abdomen measurements) is most often caused by extrinsic factors during the third trimester such as uteroplacental

dysfunction, causing inadequate nutrient delivery or inadequate waste and carbon dioxide removal. Other placental factors include preeclampsia, placental abruption, and twin-twin transfusion.

8. **List the teratogenic effects of maternal diabetes mellitus. What is the best way to reduce these complications?**
   Maternal diabetes may cause any of the following fetal defects:
   • Cardiovascular malformations
   • Cleft lip and/or palate
   • Caudal regression (lower half of the body is incompletely formed)
   • Neural tube defects
   • Left colon hypoplasia or immaturity
   • Macrosomia (most common and classic effect)
   • Microsomia (can occur if the mother has long-standing diabetes)
       Tight control of glucose during pregnancy, typically by a strict insulin regimen, dramatically reduces these complications.

9. **What other problems does maternal diabetes cause in pregnancy?**
   In the mother, diabetes can result in polyhydramnios and preeclampsia (as well as the complications of diabetes). Problems in infants born to a diabetic mother (other than birth defects) include an increased risk of respiratory distress syndrome (RDS), transposition of the great arteries, and postdelivery **hypoglycemia**. After birth, the infant is cut off from the mother's glucose and the hyperglycemia resolves, but the infant's islet cells still overproduce insulin and may cause hypoglycemia. The risk can be decreased before delivery with strict glucose control. After delivery, treat infant hypoglycemia with intravenous glucose.

10. **True or False: Oral hypoglycemic agents should not be used during pregnancy.**
    Historically this has been true, though some obstetricians are now using oral agents. Use insulin to treat diabetes if diet and exercise cannot control glucose levels. Oral hypoglycemics, unlike insulin, may cross the placenta and cause fetal hypoglycemia.

11. **True or False: In terms of surgery, the usual rule of thumb is to treat disease in a pregnant woman the same as you would treat it in a nonpregnant woman.**
    The answer to this question depends on the circumstances. It is definitely true in the case of an acute surgical emergency. Pregnant women can develop appendicitis, for which the presenting symptom may be right upper quadrant pain because of displacement of the appendix by the pregnant uterus. Just as in nonpregnant patients, laparotomy or laparoscopy is perfectly appropriate when the diagnosis is uncertain, and the patient has signs of peritoneal involvement.
        For semiurgent conditions (e.g., ovarian neoplasm), it is best to wait until the second trimester to perform surgery (when the pregnancy is most stable). Purely elective cases are avoided during pregnancy.

12. **What are the options for anesthesia in obstetric patients? Why?**
    Many women elect to manage the pain of labor with breathing and other relaxation techniques. Epidural anesthesia is the most common method in obstetric patients and is generally safe and effective. Spinal anesthesia can interfere with the mother's ability to push and is associated with a higher incidence of hypotension than epidural anesthesia but is commonly used for anesthesia during cesarean section deliveries. General anesthesia is the method of choice for emergent cesarean sections when time is of the essence, but it involves a higher risk of aspiration and resulting pneumonia because the gastroesophageal sphincter is relaxed in pregnancy, and patients usually have not refrained from eating before going into labor. There is also concern about the effect of general anesthetic agents on the fetus.

13. **What are the risk factors for developing an ectopic pregnancy?**
    The major risk factor for ectopic pregnancy is scarring of the fallopian tube. You might see this in a patient with previous history of pelvic inflammatory disease (PID), which increases the ectopic pregnancy rate 10-fold. Other risk factors include a previous ectopic pregnancy, history of tubal ligation or tuboplasty, and pregnancy that occurs with an intrauterine device in place.

14. **What are the classic signs and symptoms of a ruptured ectopic pregnancy?**
    A recent history of amenorrhea with current signs of peritonitis and acute, severe abdominal pain. Patients also have a positive hCG pregnancy test.

15. **What should you do if you suspect an ectopic pregnancy?**
    Order a transvaginal ultrasound to look for a gestational sac or fetus. When the diagnosis is in doubt and the patient is hemodynamically unstable (e.g., hypovolemia, shock, severe abdominal pain, rebound tenderness), perform laparoscopic exploration for definitive diagnosis and treatment.

16. **How is unruptured ectopic pregnancy managed?**
    An unruptured ectopic pregnancy is also definitively managed with surgery, but a different procedure is performed than in the case of a ruptured ectopic pregnancy. An unruptured tubal pregnancy, if stable and less than 3 cm in

diameter, can be treated with salpingostomy and removal of the products of conception. The tube is left open to heal on its own; this strategy retains normal tubal function and fertility. Methotrexate is an alternative medical treatment for small (<3 cm), unruptured tubal pregnancies. If the patient is unstable, the ectopic pregnancy has ruptured, or the fallopian tube has dilated to greater than 3 cm in diameter, a salpingectomy must be performed. In Rh-negative patients, give RhoGAM after treatment to prevent possible alloimmunization.

17. **What are the diagnostic signs and symptoms of preeclampsia? When does it occur?**
    Preeclampsia is new-onset **hypertension** after week 20, defined as two blood pressure readings greater than 140/90 mm Hg, separated by at least 4 hours, in a woman with previously normal blood pressure, or a greater than 30-point increase in systolic or a greater than 15-point increase in diastolic blood pressure over baseline in a woman with underlying hypertension. Other signs and symptoms include **proteinuria** (≥2+ protein on urinalysis, >0.3 on a spot urine protein/creatinine ratio, or >300 mg on a 24-hour urine collection), or end-organ damage such as oliguria, edema of the hands or face, headache, visual disturbances, or the HELLP syndrome (**h**emolysis, **e**levated **l**iver enzymes, **l**ow platelets, and right upper quadrant or epigastric **p**ain).

18. **What are the main risk factors for preeclampsia? How is it treated?**
    The risk factors (in decreasing order of importance) include preeclampsia in a prior pregnancy, chronic renal disease, chronic hypertension, family history of preeclampsia, multiple gestations, nulliparity, extremes of reproductive age, diabetes, and black race. The definitive treatment is delivery. This is the treatment of choice if the patient is at term (≥37 weeks). In a preterm patient with mild disease, the hypertension can be treated with hydralazine, labetalol, or methyldopa. Advise bed rest and observe. If the patient has severe disease (defined as oliguria, mental status changes, headache, blurred vision, pulmonary edema, cyanosis, HELLP syndrome, blood pressure >160/110 mm Hg, or progression to eclampsia [seizures]), deliver the infant once the mother is stabilized.

19. **Define the different types of hypertension in pregnancy.**
    Chronic hypertension: hypertension diagnosed before pregnancy, or elevated blood pressure of at least 140/90 mm Hg measured on two occasions, taken at least 4 hours apart, either before 20 weeks of gestation or persisting beyond 12 weeks postpartum.
    Gestational hypertension: new-onset hypertension after 20 weeks of gestation with *no proteinuria*. If a patient presents for care after 20 weeks of pregnancy, you may not be able to differentiate chronic hypertension from gestational hypertension.
    Preeclampsia: hypertension that begins after week 20, plus new-onset proteinuria. Proteinuria is considered positive if at least 300 mg of protein is collected in a 24-hour urine sample, or a urinary protein/creatinine ratio of 0.3 or greater is measured. A single severe feature representing end-organ damage in combination with hypertension is also sufficient for the diagnosis. The following are severe features of preeclampsia:
    • Elevated blood pressure (systolic ≥160 mm Hg, diastolic ≥110 mm Hg)
    • Elevated creatinine level (>1.1 mg/dL or ≥2 times baseline)
    • Hepatic dysfunction (transaminase levels ≥2 times upper limit of normal) or right upper quadrant or epigastric pain
    • New-onset headache or visual disturbances
    • Platelet count less than 100,000
    • Pulmonary edema

20. **What are the recommended gestational ages for delivery for chronic hypertension? Gestational hypertension? Preeclampsia?**
    Chronic hypertension: consider delivery at 38 weeks of gestation (depending on blood pressure control throughout pregnancy)
    Gestational hypertension: delivery at 37 weeks of gestation
    Preeclampsia with no severe features: delivery at 37 weeks of gestation
    Preeclampsia with severe features: timing is based on maternal factors and fetal considerations, with delivery ideally occurring at 34 weeks of gestation. However, urgent delivery may be required earlier with the use of betamethasone to accelerate fetal lung maturity indicated between 24 and 34 weeks of gestation.

21. **What are the potential complications of chronic maternal hypertension in pregnancy?**
    Preexisting hypertension (present before conception) increases the risk for IUGR and preeclampsia.

22. **When is edema normal during pregnancy? When is it not?**
    Mild ankle edema is normal in pregnancy, but severe edema of the lower extremities or edema of the hands or face is likely to indicate preeclampsia.

23. **What should you consider if preeclampsia develops before the third trimester?**
    The possibility of gestational trophoblastic disease (i.e., the presence of hydatidiform mole or choriocarcinoma).

24. **Distinguish between preeclampsia and eclampsia. How can eclampsia be prevented?**
    Preeclampsia plus seizures equals eclampsia. Eclampsia can be prevented by regular prenatal care so that you catch the disease in the preeclamptic stage and treat appropriately.

25. **What should you use to treat seizures in eclampsia? What are the toxic effects?**
Use **magnesium sulfate** for eclamptic seizures; it also lowers blood pressure. Toxic effects include hyporeflexia (first sign of toxicity), respiratory depression, central nervous system depression, coma, and death. If toxicity occurs, the first step is to stop the magnesium infusion. Consider giving calcium gluconate to reverse magnesium toxicity.

26. **True or False: When eclampsia occurs, you must deliver the infant immediately, regardless of maternal status.**
False. Do *not* try to deliver the infant until the mother is stable (e.g., do not perform a cesarean section while the mother is actively seizing).

27. **True or False: Preeclampsia and eclampsia are risk factors for development of hypertension in the future.**
False, but they are risk factors for later cardiovascular disease.

28. **Why are preeclampsia and eclampsia so important?**
Preeclampsia and eclampsia cause uteroplacental insufficiency, IUGR, fetal demise, and increased maternal morbidity and mortality rates.

29. **What causes third trimester bleeding? How do you distinguish the four major causes from one another?**
The four most notable causes of third trimester bleeding include:
• Placenta previa (*painless* bleeding with *no* fetal bradycardia)
• Vas previa (*painless* bleeding *with* fetal bradycardia)
• Abruptio placentae (*painful* bleeding)
• Uterine rupture
    Other causes to consider include:
• Cervical or vaginal infections (e.g., herpes simplex virus, gonorrhea, chlamydial or candidal infection)
• Cervical or vaginal trauma (usually from sexual intercourse)
• Bleeding disorders (rare before delivery; more common after delivery)
• Cervical cancer (which may occur in pregnant patients)
• Bloody show

30. **Describe the initial management of third trimester bleeding.**
For all cases of third trimester bleeding, start intravenous fluids, give blood if needed, start the patient on oxygen, and start fetal and maternal monitoring. Then order a complete blood count (CBC), coagulation profiles, ultrasound, and a drug screen (if drug use is suspected because cocaine causes placental abruption). Give RhoGAM if the mother is Rh negative. A Kleihauer-Betke test can quantify fetal blood in the maternal circulation and can be used to calculate the dose of RhoGAM.

31. **True or False: Ultrasound must be performed before performing a pelvic exam when investigating the cause of third trimester bleeding?**
True. You may perform a history and partial physical exam before performing the ultrasound, but *always* do an ultrasound before you do a pelvic exam to better understand the patient's uterine anatomy and placental placement. In the case of placenta previa, for example, disturbing the placenta by performing a pelvic exam may make the bleeding worse and turn a worrisome case into an emergency.

32. **Define placenta previa. How does it present? How is it diagnosed and treated?**
True placenta previa occurs when the placenta implants and grows to cover the cervical opening (os). Predisposing factors include multiparity, increasing maternal age, multiple gestation, and a history of prior placenta previa. Placenta previa typically presents as painless third trimester bleeding, and the bleeding may be profuse. Because of this condition, you *always* do an ultrasound before a pelvic exam for third-trimester bleeding. Ultrasound is 95% to 100% accurate in diagnosis. The only delivery option for placenta previa is by cesarean section.

33. **Define placental abruption. How does it present? How is it managed?**
Placental abruption (or abruptio placentae) is premature detachment of a normally situated placenta. Predisposing factors include hypertension (with or without preeclampsia), trauma, polyhydramnios with rapid decompression after membrane rupture, cocaine or tobacco use, and preterm PROM. Patients can have this condition without visible vaginal bleeding; the blood may be contained behind the placenta. Usual symptoms include pain (which may be described as abdominal, pelvic, or back pain), uterine tenderness, increased uterine tone with a hyperactive contraction pattern, and fetal distress. Placental abruption may also cause disseminated intravascular coagulation if fetal products enter the maternal circulation. Ultrasound detects only a small percentage of cases. Treat with intravenous fluids (and blood if needed) and rapid delivery (vaginal preferred).

34. **What causes fetal bleeding to present as third trimester vaginal bleeding?**
Visible fetal bleeding usually is due to vasa previa or velamentous insertion of the cord, which occurs when umbilical vessels present in advance of the fetal head, usually traversing the membranes and crossing the cervical

os. The biggest predisposing risk factor is multiple gestation (the higher the number of fetuses, the higher the risk). Bleeding is painless, and the mother is typically stable, whereas the fetus shows worsening distress (tachycardia initially, then bradycardia as the fetus decompensates). An Apt test may be performed on vaginal blood, which will be positive for fetal blood if fetal bleeding is occurring. Treat with immediate cesarean section delivery.

35. **Define hyperemesis gravidarum. How do you recognize and treat it?**
Hyperemesis gravidarum is intractable nausea and vomiting leading to dehydration and possible electrolyte disturbances. It presents in the first trimester, usually in younger patients with their first pregnancy while experiencing underlying social stressors or psychiatric problems. Treat hyperemesis gravidarum with supportive care along with small, frequent meals and antiemetic medications such as pyridoxine-doxylamine, diphenhydramine, meclizine, dimenhydrinate, prochlorperazine, metoclopramide, or ondansetron. Hyperemesis gravidarum can be a sign of trophoblastic disease, so be sure to rule it out with ultrasound. Dehydrated patients need intravenous fluids, and electrolyte abnormalities must be corrected. Remember that hyperemesis gravidarum plus severely elevated hCG or a uterus greater than gestational age is suggestive of a hydatidiform molar pregnancy.

36. **Define cholestasis of pregnancy. How is it managed?**
Cholestasis of pregnancy presents with itching (often severe) and/or abnormal liver function tests, usually in the second and third trimesters. In rare cases, jaundice may coexist. It is dangerous because of the associated risk of fetal demise. Heightened fetal surveillance and induction of labor at 37 weeks is typically recommended. The only known definitive treatment is delivery, but ursodeoxycholic acid or cholestyramine may help with symptoms.

37. **What is acute fatty liver of pregnancy? How is it managed?**
Acute fatty liver of pregnancy is a more serious disorder than cholestasis. It presents in the third trimester or after delivery and usually progresses to hepatic coma. Treat with intravenous fluids, glucose, and fresh frozen plasma to correct coagulopathies. Vitamin K does not work because the liver is in temporary failure. If the patient survives with supportive care, liver dysfunction usually resolves on its own with time.

38. **What are the maternal and fetal complications of multiple gestations?**
Maternal complications include anemia, hypertension, premature labor, postpartum uterine atony, postpartum hemorrhage, and preeclampsia.
Fetal complications include polyhydramnios, malpresentation, placenta previa, abruptio placentae, velamentous cord insertion/vasa previa, PROM, prematurity, umbilical cord prolapse, IUGR, congenital anomalies, and increased perinatal morbidity and mortality.

39. **How are multiple gestations delivered?**
With vertex-vertex presentations of twins (both infants are headfirst), you can try vaginal delivery for both infants, but with any other twin presentation combination or more than two infants, perform cesarean section.

40. **List the top three causes of maternal mortality in the United States.**
- Pulmonary embolus
- Hypertension/pregnancy-induced hypertension (preeclampsia/eclampsia)
- Hemorrhage
  The maternal mortality rate increases with age and is higher among black women.

UNCOMPLICATED PREGNANCY

1. **Which vitamin should be recommended to all women of reproductive age? Why?**
All women of reproductive age should take vitamin B_9 (folate), dosed at 400 mcg/day, to prevent neural tube defects. Folate is essential to prevent neural tube defects, with its most critical window occurring early in the first trimester before many women may know they are pregnant. If an expectant mother waits to start folate until after pregnancy is confirmed, she still runs the risk of fetal neural tube defects.

2. **List the signs and symptoms of pregnancy.**
Symptoms of pregnancy include:
- Amenorrhea
- Nausea or morning sickness
- Breast enlargement or tenderness; possible darkening of the areola
- Fatigue
- Weight gain
Signs of pregnancy include:
- Hegar sign (softening and compressibility of the lower uterine segment)
- Chadwick sign (color change of the vulva, cervix, and vaginal walls; often darkening or becoming bluish)
- Suprapubic palpation/ballottement of uterine fundus
- Linea nigra (linear stripes of hyperpigmented skin across the abdomen)
- Melasma (also known as chloasma or the mask of pregnancy)

3. **What commonly used drugs are generally considered safe in pregnancy?**
   A short list of drugs that are generally safe in pregnancy includes acetaminophen, penicillins, cephalosporins, erythromycin, nitrofurantoin, histamine-2 receptor blockers, antacids, heparin, hydralazine, methyldopa, labetalol, insulin, and docusate.

4. **How is pregnancy diagnosed? At what gestational age will each method show a positive result?**
   There are four ways that pregnancy can be definitively diagnosed:
   - Detection of elevated beta-hCG (e.g., the beta subunit of human chorionic gonadotropin) in the patient's blood or serum
   - Detection of elevated beta-hCG in the patient's urine
   - Detection of a gestational sac, yolk sac, or fetal pole by transvaginal ultrasound (TVUS)
   - Detection of fetal cardiac activity on Doppler ultrasound

   While there is variability when measuring beta-hCG in real-life patients, for the purpose of your licensing exams, elevated beta-hCG may be detected in blood and serum samples as early as 3 weeks of gestation (i.e., 1 week after fertilization), while elevated beta-hCG is not detectable in urine until at least 4 weeks of gestation (i.e., at least 2 weeks after fertilization). TVUS can typically identify a gestational sac at 4.5 weeks, yolk sac at 5 weeks, and fetal pole with cardiac activity around 5.5 weeks. Due to the reduced image resolution of transabdominal ultrasound compared to the transvaginal approach, TVUS is preferred. Doppler ultrasound can first detect fetal cardiac activity between weeks 10 and 12.

5. **True or False: Levels of human chorionic gonadotropin roughly double every 2 days in the first trimester.**
   True. An hCG level that stays the same or increases only slowly on serial testing indicates a fetus in trouble (e.g., threatened abortion, ectopic pregnancy) or fetal demise. A rapidly increasing hCG level or one that does not decrease after delivery may indicate a hydatidiform mole or choriocarcinoma.

6. **Explain how to determine a patient's gestational age and how it differs from embryonic age. Which method is most commonly used in a clinical setting? Why?**
   Gestational age is measured in weeks since the first day of the patient's last menstrual period (LMP). Embryonic age (also called postconception age) is defined as the number of weeks since the ovulated egg was fertilized. Embryonic age is therefore approximately 2 weeks behind that patient's gestational age. Due to the varied length of each patient's follicular phase, it is difficult to identify an exact ovulation or fertilization date; the first day of most menstrual periods is fairly unambiguous, therefore gestational age is typically used to date pregnancies in most clinical settings. When a clinician says, "The patient is at X weeks," you can bet the clinician is talking about gestational age.

7. **Visualization of a gestational sac via transvaginal ultrasound typically correlates with what serum levels of beta-human chorionic gonadotropin?**
   1000 to 2000 mIU/mL.

8. **Visualization of a gestational sac via transabdominal ultrasound typically correlates with what serum levels of beta-human chorionic gonadotropin?**
   5000 to 6000 mIU/mL.

9. **Describe Nägele rule used to determine a patient's estimated due date (EDD).**
   A patient's EDD is the day she reaches a gestational age of exactly 40 weeks (i.e., 280 days since LMP). Nägele rule can be used to quickly estimate EDD by taking the date of the patient's LMP, subtracting 3 months, and adding 7 days. For example, a patient with LMP of April 15 would have an EDD of January 22 the following year, since January is 3 months before April, and April 22 is 7 days after April 15.

10. **What lab tests should be performed on all pregnant patients during the first prenatal visit?**
    According to the American College of Obstetrics and Gynecology (ACOG), the following tests are part of the first prenatal visit:
    - **Hemoglobin, hematocrit, and platelet count:** to establish baseline values as you monitor for anemia or thrombocytopenia during future visits.
    - **Blood type, rhesus (Rh) type, and Rh antibody screen:** to investigate possible isoimmunization.
    - **Venereal Disease Research Laboratory (VDRL)/rapid plasma reagin (RPR) test:** to assess for syphilis.
    - **Hepatitis B surface antigen (HBsAg) screen:** to prevent perinatal hepatitis B virus (HBV) transmission.
    - **Human immunodeficiency virus (HIV) test:** current ACOG guidelines recommend an opt-out approach rather than an opt-in approach to increase screening rates.
    - **Rubella antibody titer:** if the patient if found to be nonimmune, counsel her to get postpartum immunization. *No live vaccines* should be given during pregnancy.
    - **Urinalysis and culture:** to establish baseline protein content and screen for bacteriuria.

    There are additional supplemental lab tests that may be performed during the initial prenatal visit but only if indicated. These include:

- **Pap smear:** if the patient is due. Pregnancy does not change the frequency of screening.
- **Human papillomavirus (HPV) screen:** if indicated.
- **Chlamydia and gonorrhea screening:** typically in teenage patients or if clinical suspicion is high.
- **Varicella antibody titer:** as with rubella, vaccination can be offered postpartum for nonimmune patients, but a live vaccine should *not* be given during pregnancy.
- **Hemoglobin electrophoresis:** if high risk for sickle cell disease or thalassemia.
- **Tuberculosis test:** typically by purified protein derivative (PPD) if the patient is considered high risk.
- **Thyroid function:** maternal hypothyroidism may affect fetal neurologic development. Maternal hyperthyroidism can lead to fetal and maternal complications.
- **Down syndrome screening:** should be offered to all pregnant patients. There are multiple ways to screen.

11. **How often should a pregnant patient attend antenatal visits?**
Antenatal appointments should be scheduled every 4 weeks until week 28, then every 2 weeks until week 36, then weekly until week 40. If the patient has not delivered by week 40, schedule twice-weekly visits until week 42.

12. **On every prenatal visit, listen to fetal heart tones and measure fundal height. When can these two features first be noticed?**
As mentioned previously, **fetal heart tones** can be heard with Doppler ultrasound at 10 to 12 weeks and can be auscultated with a normal stethoscope around 16 to 20 weeks. **Fundal height** is measured as the distance in centimeters from the symphysis pubis to the top of the uterine fundus. The uterine fundus becomes palpable above the symphysis pubis around week 12 and reaches the umbilicus around week 20. In a patient with normal body habitus and uncomplicated singleton pregnancy, the fundal height should roughly equal the gestational age between weeks 16 and 36. After week 36, the fundal height may appear to decrease as the fetus begins to descend and engage with the lower pelvis in anticipation of labor.

13. **How is a size/date discrepancy identified? What is the next step?**
A discrepancy of more than 2 to 3 cm between the measured fundal height and the gestational age is considered a **size/date discrepancy.** This may have a benign explanation such as multiple gestations or an incorrectly estimated date of conception, or it may represent complications such as IUGR, molar pregnancy, or fetal demise. An ultrasound exam should be performed for further evaluation.

14. **When in pregnancy is ultrasound most accurate at estimating the fetal age? Which parameters are used to estimate gestational age during the first, second, and third trimesters?**
Dating by ultrasound is more accurate when done early in the pregnancy. The most accurate first-trimester estimation of gestational age is achieved by measuring the crown-rump length (CRL), which can be done as soon as a fetal pole can be identified (around 5.5 weeks) and continues to be the primary dating method until week 13+6 (i.e., the end of the first trimester). Starting week 14 and continuing into the third trimester, dating is usually done by a composite measurement of four fetal biometric characteristics: the fetal head circumference, biparietal diameter (BPD), abdominal circumference, and femur length. Of these, the BPD is generally considered the most reliable.

15. **How is fetal biparietal diameter measured? Which two landmarks must be visible to ensure an accurate measurement?**
Fetal BPD is measured as the distance between the outer edge of the proximal skull to the inner edge of the distal skull. The third ventricle and thalami must be visible to ensure an accurate BPD is measured.

16. **When is ultrasound most accurate at estimating fetal age?**
At 7 to 10 weeks the CRL is the most accurate measure for estimating fetal age. At 16 to 20 weeks the BPD (measured on ultrasound) gives the most accurate estimate.

17. **When should ultrasound be used to evaluate the fetus?**
The indications for ultrasound are now quite liberal. Order ultrasound for all patients who have a size/date discrepancy greater than 2 to 3 cm or risk factors for pregnancy-related problems (e.g., hypertension, diabetes, renal disease, lupus erythematosus, smoking, alcohol or drug use, and a history of previous pregnancy-related problems). Ultrasound is also used when fetal death, distress, or abortion or miscarriage is suspected (e.g., a baby that stops kicking, vaginal bleeding, or a slow fetal heartbeat on auscultation).

18. **What normal changes in laboratory results during pregnancy may be encountered on the Step 3 exam?**
- The erythrocyte sedimentation rate becomes markedly elevated; hence this test is essentially worthless in pregnancy.
- Total thyroxine (T4) and thyroid-binding globulin increase, but free T4 remains normal.
- Hemoglobin increases, but plasma volume increases even more; thus the net result is a decrease in hemoglobin and hematocrit.
- BUN and creatinine decrease because of an increase in the glomerular filtration rate. BUN and creatinine levels at the high end of the normal range indicate renal disease in pregnancy.

- Alkaline phosphatase increases markedly.
- Mild proteinuria and glycosuria are normal in pregnancy.
- Electrolytes and liver function tests remain normal.

19. **What cardiovascular and pulmonary changes occur in a normal pregnancy?**
Normal cardiovascular changes: blood pressure decreases slightly, the heart rate increases by 10 to 20 beats/min, the stroke volume increases, and cardiac output increases (by up to 50%).
Normal pulmonary changes: minute ventilation increases because of an increase in tidal volume, but the respiratory rate remains the same or increases only slightly; the residual volume and carbon dioxide decrease. Collectively these changes cause the physiologic hyperventilation/respiratory alkalosis of pregnancy.

20. **What is the average weight gain during pregnancy? What commonly causes weight gain to be greater or less than the average?**
The average weight gain in pregnancy is roughly 28 lb (12.5 kg). A greater weight gain may mean maternal diabetes. A smaller weight gain may indicate hyperemesis gravidarum or a psychiatric or major systemic disease.

21. **Explain Rh incompatibility. In what situations does it occur?**
Rh blood-type incompatibility is of concern because it can lead to hemolytic disease of the newborn. Rh incompatibility occurs when the mother is Rh negative and her infant is Rh positive. This is only possible if the father is Rh positive. If both the mother and the father are Rh negative, there is no possibility of producing an Rh-positive infant; if the mother is Rh positive, there is no possibility of her producing Rh antibodies.

22. **True or False: The first child is usually the most severely affected by Rh incompatibility.**
False. Previous maternal sensitization is required for disease to occur. In other words, if a nulliparous Rh-negative mother has never received blood products, her first Rh-positive infant will not be affected by hemolytic disease because the antibodies generated will be immunoglobulin M (IgM), which cannot cross the placenta. The second Rh-positive infant, however, will be affected because IgG antibodies that can cross the placenta will be generated. This is why, in Rh-negative mothers, you must administer RhoGAM at 28 weeks and within 72 hours after delivery during the first pregnancy to prevent the generation of anti-Rh antibodies that will affect the next Rh-positive fetus.

23. **When should RhoGAM be given?**
RhoGAM should only be given when the mother is Rh negative and antibody negative, and the father is Rh positive or his blood type is unknown. During routine prenatal care, check for Rh antibodies at the first visit. If the test is positive, do not give RhoGAM—you are too late, and the mother has already generated anti-Rh antibodies. Giving RhoGAM will not change this. Otherwise, give RhoGAM routinely in these patients at 28 weeks and immediately after delivery. Also give RhoGAM after an abortion, stillbirth, ectopic pregnancy, amniocentesis, chorionic villus sampling (CVS), and any other invasive procedure that may cause mixing of maternal and fetal blood during pregnancy.

24. **How do you recognize, monitor, and treat hemolytic disease of the newborn?**
Hemolytic disease of the newborn in its most severe form causes hydrops fetalis (edema, ascites, pleural and/or pericardial effusions) and death. Amniotic fluid spectrophotometry and ultrasound can help gauge the severity of fetal hemolysis. Treatment of hemolytic disease involves (1) delivery, if the fetus is mature (check lung maturity with a lecithin-to-sphingomyelin ratio); (2) intrauterine transfusion; and (3) phenobarbital, which helps the fetal liver break down bilirubin.

25. **True or False: ABO blood group incompatibility can cause hemolytic disease of the newborn.**
True. ABO blood group incompatibility can cause hemolytic disease of the newborn when the mother is type O and the infant is type A, B, or AB. *This condition does not require previous sensitization* because IgG antibodies with transplacental potential occur naturally in mothers with blood type O—but not in mothers with other blood types. The hemolytic disease is usually less severe than with Rh incompatibility, but treatment is the same.

26. **How do you treat gonorrheal and chlamydial genital infections during pregnancy?**
The treatment for gonorrhea remains unchanged because ceftriaxone is safe during pregnancy. For chlamydial infection, give azithromycin, amoxicillin, or erythromycin base instead of doxycycline or erythromycin estolate.

27. **What do you need to know about vaginal group B streptococcal (GBS) colonization during pregnancy?**
Pregnant women should be tested for vaginal GBS at 35 to 37 weeks of gestation. Women who are carriers should be treated during labor with intrapartum penicillin G or ampicillin. Earlier testing and treatment (e.g., second trimester) is ineffective because GBS frequently returns. The exception is for women with GBS bacteriuria (often detected on first trimester screening urine culture)—these women are not retested later but are instead treated empirically during labor, as they are assumed to be chronically colonized with GBS. The reason for treating asymptomatic carriers is to prevent neonatal sepsis and endometritis, both of which are commonly caused by GBS.

28. **What lab test is used to screen for neural tube defects, and at what time during pregnancy is it measured? Explain the significance of low or high levels in maternal serum.**
    Maternal alpha-fetoprotein (AFP) is most accurate when measured between 15 and 20 weeks of gestation. A low AFP may represent **Down syndrome,** fetal demise, or inaccurate dates. A high AFP may represent **neural tube defects** (e.g., anencephaly, spina bifida), **ventral wall defects** (e.g., omphalocele, gastroschisis), multiple gestation, or inaccurate dates.

29. **What should be done if the AFP is elevated?**
    Repeat the test. As many as 30% of elevated maternal serum AFP test results may be elevated but are normal upon repeat testing. The initial elevation is not associated with an increased risk of neural tube defects.

30. **What further testing should a patient undergo if the AFP remains elevated?**
    If the AFP remains elevated, the patient is advised first to undergo ultrasound to determine whether a neural tube defect or abdominal anomaly is present. The ultrasound is also used to confirm gestational age, number of fetuses, and fetal viability. Further evaluation with amniocentesis may be required if the ultrasound findings are uncertain or there is a concern for nonvisualized neural tube defects (via elevated AFP level in amniotic fluid or detection of acetylcholinesterase in amniotic fluid). There is a small risk of miscarriage after amniocentesis.

31. **What is the first trimester combined test? When is it performed?**
    The first trimester combined test is performed at 11 to 13 weeks of gestation. The test involves determination of nuchal translucency (NT) by ultrasound, combined with serum pregnancy-associated plasma protein-A (PAPP-A) and serum hCG. If positive, CVS is used to confirm the diagnosis. The combined test is most appropriate for women who place a higher value on identifying Down syndrome during the first trimester than on the risk of pregnancy loss from invasive diagnostic testing such as CVS.

32. **Describe the full-integrated and serum-integrated screening tests.**
    The full-integrated test includes an ultrasound measurement of NT at 10 to 13 weeks of gestation, serum PAPP-A at 10 to 13 weeks of gestation, and serum levels of AFP, unconjugated estradiol (uE3), hCG, and inhibin A measured at 15 to 18 weeks of gestation. No matter which results come back first, all results of the full-integrated test are withheld until the second trimester. The full-integrated test is most appropriate for women who place a higher value on minimizing the risk of pregnancy loss from invasive diagnostic testing than on first trimester identification of Down syndrome.
    The serum-integrated screening test measures the same lab markers as the full-integrated test, but it excludes the ultrasound evaluation of NT. This test is used in areas where expertise in the ultrasound measurement of NT is not available. Results of the serum-integrated test are not available until the second trimester.
    Stepwise sequential testing has been developed to provide a risk estimate during the first trimester. The first trimester portion of the integrated screen is performed. If the tests indicate a very high risk of having an affected fetus, CVS is offered. Those women whose results do not place them at very high risk of having an affected fetus go on to have the second trimester portion of the screening.
    Contingent testing has not yet been proven efficacious in a prospective clinical trial.

33. **What is the quadruple test? For whom is it typically used? When is it performed?**
    The quadruple test includes the serum markers AFP, uE3, hCG, and inhibin A. The quadruple test is the best available test for women who present for prenatal care in the second trimester but can be used for women who receive earlier prenatal care. It is typically performed around 15 to 18 weeks of gestation.

34. **What is a maternal plasma–based test?**
    This is the newest option that is just becoming widely available to screen for genetic aneuploidiec cuch as trisomy 21 (Down syndrome), trisomy 18, and trisomy 13. This test, also called cell-free fetal DNA (cfDNA) testing, detects fetal DNA in the maternal circulation. It has a detection rate greater than 98%, false-positive rate of 1%, and false-negative rate of 1.4% for Down syndrome (the detection rates are lower and the false-negative rate higher for trisomy 18 and trisomy 13). cfDNA testing is not yet validated in low-risk women and is not commonly used as a primary screening test in the United States. However, it can be used in higher-risk women (i.e., women who will be age >35 years at the time of delivery or those with sonographic findings associated with fetal aneuploidy, history of previous pregnancy with fetal trisomy, positive screening results on tests such as the first trimester combined test, the integrated test, or the quadruple test). As such, it is commonly used as a secondary screening test.

35. **What is the next step if a woman has a positive screening test for Down syndrome?**
    Offer fetal karyotype determination. This is done by CVS in the first trimester and by amniocentesis in the second trimester.

36. **Why is CVS done instead of amniocentesis in some cases?**
    CVS can be done at 9 to 12 weeks of gestation (earlier than amniocentesis) and is generally reserved for women with previously affected offspring or known genetic disease. It offers the advantage of a first-trimester abortion if the fetus is affected. CVS is associated with a slightly higher miscarriage rate than amniocentesis.

37. **True or False: Chorionic villus sampling can detect neural tube defects but not genetic disorders.**
False. CVS can detect genetic or chromosomal disorders but not neural tube defects.

38. **How is tuberculosis treated in pregnancy?**
Use isoniazid, rifampin, and ethambutol to treat tuberculosis in pregnancy if the risk of a drug-resistant organism is low. Pyrazinamide should be used with caution because of a lack of data on the risk of teratogenicity. However, pyrazinamide should be added if a drug-resistant organism is suspected. Streptomycin, which is a rarely used second-line agent, should be avoided. Give vitamin B_6 to pregnant patients treated with isoniazid to avoid a deficiency.

39. **How is fetal well-being evaluated?**
A **nonstress test** (NST) is the easiest initial screen for fetal well-being. A fetal heart rate tracing is obtained over the course of 20 minutes. A normal NST has at least two accelerations of heart rate during those 20 minutes. For gestational age of 32 weeks or more, each acceleration must be at least 15 beats per minute above baseline and last at least 15 seconds. For gestational age less than 32 weeks, each acceleration must be 10 beats per minute above baseline and last for 10 seconds each.

    A **biophysical profile** (BPP) is composed of NST plus **ultrasound** evaluation, scoring fetal (i) breathing, (ii) movement, (iii) muscle tone, (iv) heart rate, and (v) amniotic fluid index.

    If the fetus scores poorly on the biophysical profile, the next test is the **contraction stress test,** which looks for uteroplacental dysfunction. Oxytocin is given, and a fetal heart strip is monitored. If late decelerations are seen on the fetal heart strip with each contraction, the test is positive. In most cases of a positive contraction stress test, delivery is performed by cesarean section.

40. **True or False: A biophysical profile is often used in high-risk pregnancies despite the absence of obvious problems.**
True. For patients referred for antenatal testing, a NST or biophysical profile may be done once or twice a week from the start of the third trimester until delivery to monitor for potential problems.

41. **True or False: Aspirin should be avoided during pregnancy.**
False. Low-dose aspirin reduces the frequency of preeclampsia and related adverse pregnancy outcomes such as preterm birth and growth restriction when given to women at moderate to high risk of the disease. There is no consensus on the exact criteria that confer high risk, though the following are generally accepted:
- Previous pregnancy with preeclampsia
- Multifetal gestation
- Chronic hypertension
- Type 1 or type 2 diabetes mellitus
- Chronic kidney disease
- Autoimmune disease with potential vascular complications

    Further, it is reasonable to offer low-dose aspirin for preeclampsia prevention with two or more of the following moderate risk factors:
- Nulliparity
- Obesity
- Family history of preeclampsia in mother or sister
- Age 35 years and older
- Low socioeconomic status

42. **Define postterm pregnancy. Why is it a major concern? How is postterm pregnancy treated?**
Postterm pregnancy is defined as more than 42 weeks of gestation. Both prematurity and postmaturity increase perinatal morbidity and mortality rates. With postmaturity, **dystocia** (or difficult delivery) becomes more common because of the increased size of the infant. Placental insufficiency or meconium aspiration may also occur in postterm pregnancies.

    In general, if the gestational age is known to be accurate and the cervix is favorable, labor is induced (e.g., with oxytocin). If the cervix is not favorable or the dates are uncertain, twice-weekly biophysical profiles are done. At 41 weeks, most obstetricians advise induction of labor. A 2012 meta-analysis demonstrated that routine labor induction at greater than 41 weeks compared with expectant management resulted in **lower perinatal mortality** and a lower rate of meconium aspiration syndrome.

43. **What two rare disorders are associated with prolonged gestation?**
Anencephaly and placental sulfatase deficiency.

44. **True or False: Asymptomatic bacteriuria, detected on routine urinalysis, should be treated during pregnancy.**
True. Up to 20% of patients develop cystitis or pyelonephritis if untreated. This rate is much higher than in non-pregnant patients, who should not be treated for asymptomatic bacteriuria. In pregnancy, the gravid uterus can

compress the ureters, and increased progesterone can decrease the tone of the ureters, increasing urinary stasis and the risk of urinary tract infection. Treat with nitrofurantoin, cephalexin, or amoxicillin-clavulanate.

45. **Define abortion.**
Abortion is the termination (intentional or not) of a pregnancy at less than 20 weeks of gestation or when the fetus weighs less than 500 g. *Miscarriage* is the term used to describe a spontaneous abortion. After week 20, the term *fetal demise* is used.

46. **What are the different categories of spontaneous abortion?**
Threatened abortion: uterine bleeding *without* cervical dilation and no expulsion of tissue. Treat with pelvic rest.
Inevitable abortion: uterine bleeding *with* cervical dilation but no tissue expulsion.
Incomplete abortion: passage of some products of conception through the cervix.
Complete abortion: expulsion of *all* products of conception through the cervix, often without cervical dilation. Manage with serial testing of hCG level to make sure that it returns to zero.
Missed abortion: fetal death with no expulsion of tissue (in some cases not for several weeks). Treat with misoprostol or dilation and curettage, or consider induction termination if the pregnancy is a more advanced gestation.
 All the abovementioned terms apply only to patients who have not yet reached 20 weeks of gestation. If the mother has an Rh-negative blood type with a negative Rh-antibody screen, be sure to give her RhoGAM as well to avoid possible alloimmunization.

47. **Define induced and recurrent abortions. What do recurrent abortions suggest?**
Induced or therapeutic abortion is an elective termination of pregnancy at less than 20 weeks of gestation. Methotrexate is the most commonly used medication for this purpose.
Recurrent abortion is defined as two or more sequential, unplanned abortions. History and physical exam may suggest the cause:
   - Infection (*Listeria, Mycoplasma,* or *Toxoplasma* sp., syphilis)
   - Inherited thrombophilia (factor V Leiden, *G20210A* gene mutation, antithrombin deficiency, deficiency of protein C or protein S)
   - Substance use (alcohol, tobacco, drugs)
   - Diabetes mellitus
   - Hypothyroidism
   - Systemic lupus erythematosus (especially with positive antiphospholipid/lupus anticoagulant antibodies, sometimes an isolated syndrome without coexisting lupus)
   - Cervical insufficiency (watch for a history of cervical procedures [e.g., loop electrosurgical excision procedure or cold-knife cone procedure] or exposure to diethylstilbestrol [DES] in the patient's mother during pregnancy and/or a patient with recurrent painless second trimester abortions; treat future pregnancies with intramuscular or vaginal progesterone and cervical cerclage)
   - Congenital female tract abnormalities (if possible, correct to restore fertility)
   - Fibroids (remove them by performing a myomectomy)
   - Chromosomal abnormalities (e.g., maternal or paternal translocations)

48. **Explain the term bloody show. How is it diagnosed?**
With cervical effacement, a blood-tinged mucous plug may be released from the cervical canal and mark the onset of labor. This normal occurrence is a diagnosis of exclusion when investigating third trimester bleeding.

49. **Define quickening. When does it occur?**
Quickening is the term used to describe when the mother first detects fetal movements, usually between 18 and 20 weeks of gestation in a primigravida and 16 and 18 weeks of gestation in a multigravida.

LABOR, DELIVERY, AND THE POSTPARTUM PERIOD (INCLUDING PLACENTAL ABNORMALITIES)

1. **How do you manage fetal malpresentation?**
External cephalic version can be used to rotate the fetus from the breech to the cephalic position. Absolute contraindications to external cephalic version are placenta previa and history of classical (vertical) cesarean incision. Occiput posterior (OP) presentations can cause protraction of the second stage of labor. Most fetuses eventually rotate to occiput anterior (OA) presentations on their own or can be delivered OP, but providers may also attempt internal manual rotation. If this fails, the decision must be made whether to attempt vaginal delivery or do a cesarean section. Frank and complete breech presentations must be delivered by cesarean section, as should shoulder presentation or incomplete/footling breech. For face and brow presentations, watchful waiting is best because most cases convert to vertex presentations. Cesarean section must be performed if they do not.

2. **Distinguish between true labor and false labor.**
In true labor, normal contractions occur at least every 3 minutes, are fairly regular, and are associated with cervical changes (effacement and dilation). In false labor, known as Braxton-Hicks contractions, the patient experiences contractions that are irregular with no cervical changes.

3. Define preterm labor. How is it managed?

Preterm labor is true labor that begins between 20 and 37 weeks of gestation. Put the mother in the lateral decubitus position, order bed and pelvic rest, and give oral or intravenous fluids and oxygen. In some cases, these maneuvers stop the contractions. If they fail, you can give a tocolytic if no contraindications are present (e.g., heart disease, hypertension, diabetes, hemorrhage, ruptured membranes, cervix dilated >4 cm).

4. What are tocolytics? When is it not appropriate to give them?

Tocolytics are medications that slow or stop uterine contractions. Common examples are $beta_2$-agonists (terbutaline, ritodrine), indomethacin, and magnesium sulfate. Do not give tocolytics to the mother in the presence of preeclampsia, severe hemorrhage, chorioamnionitis, IUGR, fetal demise, or fetal anomalies incompatible with survival. Indomethacin cannot be used after 32 weeks of gestation because it risks premature closure of the ductus arteriosus.

5. Define premature rupture of membranes. How is it diagnosed?

PROM is rupture of the amniotic sac before the onset of labor. Diagnosis of rupture of membranes (whether premature or not) is based on history, sterile speculum exam, and/or a positive nitrazine test. The sterile speculum exam shows pooling of amniotic fluid and a ferning pattern when the fluid is placed on a microscopic slide. Nitrazine paper turns blue (indicating basicity) in the presence of amniotic fluid. Ultrasound should be done in cases of PROM to assess amniotic fluid volume as well as gestational age and any anomalies that may be present.

6. What usually follows membrane rupture? What should you do if it does not occur?

Spontaneous labor usually follows membrane rupture; for this reason, an amniotomy may be done in an attempt to induce labor if membranes do not rupture spontaneously. If labor does not occur within 18 hours of membrane rupture, and the mother is term, and if the cervix is favorable, labor should be induced. Labor is induced because the main risk of PROM is infection, which may occur in the mother (chorioamnionitis) and/or the infant (neonatal sepsis, pneumonia, meningitis).

7. Define preterm premature rupture of membranes (PPROM). How is it managed?

PPROM is the premature rupture of membranes that occurs during the preterm period (i.e., <37 weeks of gestation). The risk of infection increases with the duration of ruptured membranes, especially if 18 hours have elapsed since membrane rupture. Order a culture and Gram stain of the amniotic fluid. If it is negative, management for a hemodynamically stable patient with reassuring fetal heart tones simply involves pelvic rest with frequent follow-up. Hemodynamic instability or nonreassuring fetal testing could deteriorate quickly with expectant management and should instead be managed with delivery. If the culture is positive for GBS, treat the mother with penicillin G or ampicillin even if she is asymptomatic.

8. What is fetal fibronectin? When is a test for this substance useful? Is the test more helpful when positive or negative?

Fetal fibronectin is an extracellular matrix protein that helps attach the amniotic membranes to the uterine lining. It can be detected in the vaginal secretions of some women presenting with signs and symptoms of preterm labor. The test is most helpful when negative between 22 and 34 weeks of gestation because it indicates a very low likelihood of impending delivery over the next 2 weeks. Thus a more conservative observational approach can be used. When fetal fibronectin is positive in this setting, the woman is at a higher risk for delivery within the next 2 weeks, and a more aggressive approach to tocolysis and fetal lung maturity hastening is typically employed. In other words, fetal fibronectin has a high negative predictive value.

9. When should fetal lung maturity be evaluated?

Evaluation of fetal lung maturity is indicated before elective deliveries that are, or may be, less than 39 weeks of gestation. Testing is not necessary for well-documented pregnancies that are 39 or more weeks of gestation, pregnancies that are less than 32 weeks of gestation (because fetal lung maturity is unlikely), or when delaying delivery will place the mother or fetus at significant risk.

10. What tests can be used to assess fetal lung maturity?
- Lamellar body count
- Lecithin/sphingomyelin ratio
- Phosphatidylglycerol
- Surfactant/albumin ratio
- Optical density at 650 nm
- Foam stability index

    For the purposes of the USMLE exam, it is not necessary to know the details of these tests. No test performs better than another. All these tests are better at predicting the absence, rather than the presence, of respiratory distress.

11. What is the role of steroids in preterm labor?

Steroids (e.g., betamethasone) typically are given in the setting of preterm labor between 24 and 37 weeks of gestation to hasten fetal lung maturity and thus decrease the risk of RDS in the neonatal period.

12. What problems may be encountered when oxytocin is used to augment labor?
On the Step 3 exam, watch for uterine hyperstimulation (painful, overly frequent, and poorly coordinated uterine contractions), uterine rupture, fetal heart-rate decelerations, and water intoxication/hyponatremia (caused by the antidiuretic hormone effect of oxytocin). Treat all these complications first by discontinuing the oxytocin infusion, for which the half-life is less than 10 minutes.

13. What problems are associated with the use of intravaginal prostaglandin and amniotomy?
Prostaglandin E2 (dinoprostone) or misoprostol may be used locally to induce the cervix (a process sometimes called ripening) and is highly effective in combination with (or before) oxytocin. However, these uterotonics may also cause uterine hyperstimulation. **Amniotomy** (manual rupture of the amniotic membrane) also hastens labor but exposes the fetus and uterine cavity to possible infection if labor does not progress promptly.

14. What are the contraindications to labor induction or augmentation?
The list is almost the same as the list of contraindications to vaginal delivery: placenta or vasa previa, umbilical cord prolapse, prior classical (vertical) cesarean section, transverse fetal lie, active genital herpes, cephalopelvic disproportion, and cervical cancer.

15. What does a basic fetal heart trace show?
The fetal heart rate and the uterine contraction pattern over time.

16. In fetal heart monitoring, what is the difference between early decelerations, variable deceleration, and late decelerations?
In **early decelerations** (Fig. 12.1), the peaks are aligned (nadir of fetal heart deceleration and peak of uterine contraction). This pattern signifies **head compression** (probably a vagal response) and is not a concerning heart tracing.
   Variable decelerations (Fig. 12.2) are so called because the fetal heart rate deceleration does not appear to be related to uterine contractions—the timing of the decelerations is *variable*. Note that in variable decelerations, each deceleration lasts no more than 30 seconds. This is the most commonly encountered type of deceleration pattern and signifies **cord compression.** If variable decelerations are seen, place the mother in the lateral decubitus position, administer oxygen by face mask, stop any oxytocin infusion, and consider giving an intravenous fluid bolus to increase intravascular volume.
   Late decelerations (Fig. 12.3) occur when fetal heart rate deceleration begins after uterine contraction, with the nadir of each deceleration occurring after the peak of contraction and at regular intervals. This pattern signifies **uteroplacental insufficiency** and is the most worrisome fetal heart tracing. If it is seen, first place the mother in the lateral decubitus position; then give oxygen by face mask and stop oxytocin, if applicable. Next, give a tocolytic (often a beta$_2$-agonist such as ritodrine or magnesium sulfate) if the mother is not in active labor and intravenous fluids (if the mother is hypotensive). If the late decelerations persist, measure the fetal oxygen saturation or scalp pH and prepare for operative delivery.

17. What other patterns of fetal distress may be seen on a fetal heart tracing? What is a normal fetal heart rate?
Loss of variability may signify fetal acidemia. This may present as loss of short-term (beat-to-beat) or long-term (baseline changes in heart rate >1 minute) variability. Prolonged fetal tachycardia (>160 beats/min) can be an early sign of infection such as chorioamnionitis. The normal fetal heart rate is 110 to 160 beats/min.

18. What if the question gives you a value for fetal oxygen saturation or scalp pH?
Any fetal scalp pH less than 7.2 or significantly decreased oxygen saturation is an indication for immediate cesarean delivery. If the pH is greater than 7.2 or oxygenation is normal, immediate surgical intervention is not warranted.

19. Define the characteristics and duration of the normal stages of labor.

Stage	Characteristics	Nulligravida	Multigravida
First stage (latent + active phase)	Onset of true labor (contractions + cervical dilation) to full cervical dilation (10 cm)	Highly variable	Highly variable
Latent phase	From 0–6 cm cervical dilation (slow, irregular)	<20 hr	<14 hr
Active phase	From 6–10 cm dilation (rapid, regular)	>1.2 cm/hr dilation	>1.5 cm/hr dilation
Second stage	From full dilation to birth of baby	30 min–3 hr	5 min–2 hr
Third stage	Delivery of baby to delivery of placenta	0–30 min	0–30 min
Fourth stage	Placental delivery to maternal stabilization	Up to 48 hr	Up to 48 hr

20. List the order of fetal positions that occur during normal labor and delivery.
1. Descent
2. Flexion
3. Internal rotation

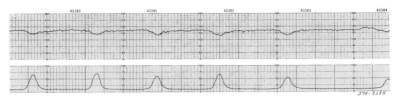

Fig. 12.1 Early decelerations are caused by compression of the fetal head. They are shallow, symmetric, uniform decelerations that begin early in the contraction, have a nadir coincident with the peak of the contraction, and return to the baseline by the time the contraction is over. (From Gabbe SG, Niebyl JR, Simpson JL. *Obstetrics: Normal and Problem Pregnancies.* 5th ed. Philadelphia: Churchill Livingstone; 2007 [fig. 15-13].)

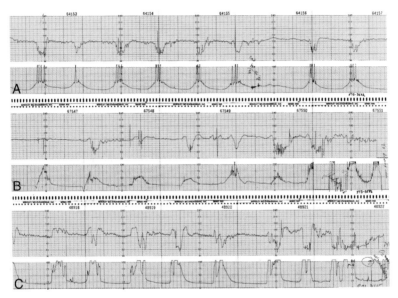

Fig. 12.2 Examples of typical variable decelerations. Variable decelerations are often recognized by the accelerations that precede and follow the decelerations. (From Gabbe SG, Niebyl JR, Simpson JL. *Obstetrics: Normal and Problem Pregnancies.* 5th ed. Philadelphia: Churchill Livingstone; 2007 [fig. 15-18].)

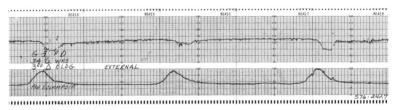

Fig. 12.3 Late decelerations in a case complicated by third-trimester bleeding. Note the presence of persistent late decelerations with only three contractions in 20 minutes, as well as the apparent loss of variability of the fetal heart rate. The rise in baseline tone of the uterine activity channel cannot be evaluated with the external system. (From Gabbe SG, Niebyl JR, Simpson JL. *Obstetrics: Normal and Problem Pregnancies.* 5th ed. Philadelphia: Churchill Livingstone; 2007 [fig. 15-14].)

4. Extension
5. External rotation
6. Expulsion

21. **In the fetal circulation, where are the highest and lowest oxygen concentrations?**
The highest oxygen concentration in the fetal circulation is in the umbilical vein (blood coming from the mother), and the lowest is in the umbilical arteries. Remember also that the oxygen concentration is higher in blood going to the upper extremities than in blood going to the lower extremities.

22. What changes occur in the circulation as an infant goes from intrauterine to extrauterine life?

The first breaths inflate the lungs and cause decreased pulmonary vascular resistance, which increases blood flow to the pulmonary arteries. This and the clamping of the cord increase left-sided heart pressure, causing functional closure of the foramen ovale. The increased oxygen concentration shuts off prostaglandin production in the ductus arteriosus, causing gradual closure.

23. Distinguish between a protraction disorder and an arrest disorder. What should you do when either occurs?

A **protraction disorder** occurs once true labor has begun if the mother takes longer than the table in Question 19 indicates, but labor nonetheless is progressing slowly. An **arrest disorder** (failure to progress) occurs once true labor has begun if no change in dilation is seen over 2 hours or no change in descent is seen over 1 hour.

In either situation, first rule out an abnormal position and cephalopelvic disproportion. If neither is present, the mother can be treated with labor augmentation (e.g., oxytocin, prostaglandin). If these steps fail, manage expectantly and perform a cesarean section at the first sign of trouble.

24. What is the most common cause of protraction or arrest disorder?

Cephalopelvic disproportion, which is a disparity between the size of the infant's head and the size of the mother's pelvis. Labor augmentation is contraindicated in this setting.

25. What should you do if shoulder dystocia or impaction occurs during vaginal delivery?

The first step is to try the McRoberts maneuver. Have the mother sharply flex her thighs against her abdomen, which may free the impacted shoulder. Other maneuvers include applying suprapubic pressure, performing the Woods screw maneuver (applying pressure to the anterior aspect of the fetus's posterior shoulder), the Rubin maneuver (applying pressure to the posterior aspect of the anterior shoulder), and delivery of the posterior arm. Some clinicians may intentionally fracture the clavicle by pulling the anterior clavicle outward, though this comes with its own set of complications and is not a universally practiced method of management. If these maneuvers fail, options are limited. Delivery by cesarean section is usually the procedure of choice and must be performed after performing the Zavanelli maneuver (pushing the infant's head back into the birth canal).

26. What are the signs of placental separation during the third stage of labor?

There are three primary signs of placental separation: a fresh show or "gush" of blood from the vagina, lengthening of the umbilical cord, and a rising fundus that becomes firm and globular. If placental separation does not occur within 30 minutes of delivery, retained placenta may be diagnosed.

27. True or False: After cesarean section, a patient may have a vaginal delivery in the future.

It depends on the type of cesarean. After a classic (vertical) uterine incision, patients must have cesarean sections for all future deliveries because of the increased rate of uterine rupture with vaginal delivery. After a low transverse (horizontal) uterine incision, a patient may deliver future pregnancies vaginally with only a slightly increased (i.e., acceptable) risk of uterine rupture.

28. How do you recognize an amniotic fluid embolism?

Look for a recently postpartum mother who develops sudden shortness of breath, tachypnea, and chest pain within minutes of delivery. Hypotension and disseminated intravascular coagulation may soon follow. Treatment is supportive.

29. What factors predispose to uterine rupture? How does it present? How is it managed?

Predisposing factors include previous uterine surgery (especially prior classic cesarean section with vertical incision), trauma, oxytocin, grand multiparity (several previous deliveries), excessive uterine distention (e.g., multiple gestation, polyhydramnios), abnormal fetal lie, cephalopelvic disproportion, and shoulder dystocia. Uterine rupture is very painful, has a sudden and dramatic onset with loss of fetal station, and often is accompanied by maternal hypotension or shock. Other classic signs are the ability to feel fetal body parts on abdominal exam and a sudden change in the abdominal contour. Maternal distress usually is more pronounced than fetal distress (unlike abruptio placentae, in which fetal distress is greater). Treat with immediate laparotomy and delivery. Hysterectomy is usually required after delivery.

30. Define postpartum hemorrhage. What are the most common causes?

Postpartum hemorrhage is blood loss greater than 500 mL during vaginal delivery or greater than 1 L during cesarean section. The most common cause is **uterine atony** (75%–80% of cases). Other causes include lacerations, retained placental tissue, coagulation disorders, low placental implantation, and uterine inversion. Retained placental tissue results from placenta accreta (penetration of the placenta through the endometrium into the myometrium), increta (deeper penetration of the placenta into the myometrium), or percreta (penetration of the placenta through the myometrium to the uterine serosa); in all three conditions, the placenta grows more deeply into the uterine wall than it should. The major risk factors for this condition include previous uterine surgery, multiparity, or prior cesarean section, and the typical treatment is a total abdominal hysterectomy.

31. **What causes uterine atony? How is it managed?**
Uterine atony is caused by overdistention of the uterus (due to multiple gestation, polyhydramnios, or macrosomia), prolonged labor, oxytocin usage, grand multiparity (a history of five or more deliveries), chorioamnionitis, and precipitous labor (too fast or $<$3 hours). Manage uterine atony with a dilute oxytocin infusion to tighten the uterus, and use bimanual compression to massage the uterus while the oxytocin infusion is running. If this approach fails, use ergonovine (contraindicated with maternal hypertension), prostaglandin f_2-alpha (contraindicated with maternal history of asthma), or misoprostol. If these strategies also fail, the patient may need a hysterectomy. Ligation of the uterine vessels may be attempted to preserve fertility if the patient desires.

32. **What is the treatment for retained products of conception?**
With retained products of conception, the most common cause of a *delayed* postpartum hemorrhage, remove the placenta manually to stop the bleeding. Next, perform dilation and curettage in the operating room under anesthesia. If placenta accreta, increta, or percreta is present, total abdominal hysterectomy is usually necessary to stop the bleeding.

33. **What causes uterine inversion? How is it treated?**
When the uterus inverts, it usually can be seen outside the vagina and will not be palpable in the suprapubic region. Uterine inversion is usually iatrogenic, a result of *pulling too hard on the umbilical cord.* If it occurs, immediately manually replace the uterus; if you wait too long, the uterus may become edematous or swollen and become ischemic. Anesthesia may be required for pain management. Once the uterus is back in place, give intravenous fluids and oxytocin to anchor the uterus in place.

34. **Define postpartum fever. What are the common causes?**
Postpartum fever is defined as a temperature greater than 100.4°F ($>$38°C) for at least 2 consecutive days following delivery. It is classically due to endometritis. However, do not forget typical postoperative causes of fever, such as a urinary tract infection or atelectasis/pneumonia. Pulmonary problems are especially common after a cesarean section.

35. **What should you do if a patient has postpartum fever?**
Look for clues in the history and physical examination. For example, for a patient with a history of PROM and a tender uterus on examination, endometritis is almost certainly the cause of the fever. Next, order cultures of the endometrium, vagina, blood, and urine. Start empiric antibiotic treatment if indicated. Clindamycin plus gentamicin is a good choice; add big-gun antibiotics if the patient is crashing.

36. **What should you do if postpartum fever does not improve with antibiotics?**
If a postpartum fever does not resolve with broad-spectrum antibiotics such as clindamycin plus gentamicin, there are two main etiologies to consider: progression to pelvic abscess or pelvic thrombophlebitis. Computed tomography (CT) scan will identify a pelvic abscess, which needs to be drained. Pelvic thrombophlebitis presents with persistent spiking fevers, lack of response to antibiotics, and no abscess on CT. Give heparin or low-molecular-weight heparin to manage this diagnosis of exclusion.

37. **What should you consider if a postpartum patient goes into shock without evident bleeding?**
    • Amniotic fluid embolism (minutes to hours postpartum)
    • Uterine inversion
    • Concealed hemorrhage (e.g., uterine rupture with bleeding into the peritoneal cavity)

38. **Define lochia. When is it a problem?**
For the first several days after delivery, some vaginal discharge (known as lochia) is normal. It is red for the first few days and gradually turns white or yellow-white by day 10. If the lochia is foul smelling, suspect endometritis.

39. **What treatment may be given to a woman who does not want to breastfeed?**
Because the breasts can be become engorged with milk and thus quite painful, you may prescribe tight-fitting bras, ice packs, and analgesia to reduce symptoms. Medications for the suppression of lactation (e.g., bromocriptine and estrogens or oral contraceptive pills) are generally no longer recommended due to risks of thromboembolism and stroke.

40. **List the common contraindications for breastfeeding.**
    • Use of alcohol or illicit drugs (with a few caveats that will not be tested on the USMLE)
    • HIV infection (though the World Health Organization [WHO] recommends breastfeeding in developing countries because of the risks of unsafe drinking water)
    • Some medications, including antineoplastic agents, antimetabolic agents (cyclophosphamide, mercaptopurine), some anticonvulsants (topiramate), amiodarone.
       Note that hepatitis C is *not* a breastfeeding contraindication—this fact happens to be a board exam favorite.

41. **When does mastitis occur? How do you recognize and treat it?**
Mastitis (inflammation of the breast) usually develops in the first 2 months postpartum. Breasts are red, indurated, and painful, and nipple cracks or fissuring may be seen. The patient with mastitis will be febrile, but there

will be no fluctuance; if fluctuance is present, it is an abscess. *Staphylococcus aureus* is the usual cause. Treat mastitis with analgesics (e.g., acetaminophen, ibuprofen), warm and/or cold compresses, and continued breast-feeding with the affected breast(s) even though it is painful. Advise the patient to use a breast pump to empty breasts, if needed. Despite the pain, continued breastfeeding is important to prevent further milk duct blockage and abscess formation. An antistaphylococcal antibiotic (e.g., cephalexin, dicloxacillin) is usually given.

42. What are the major causes of maternal mortality associated with childbirth?
In decreasing order: pulmonary embolism, pregnancy-induced hypertension (preeclampsia/ eclampsia), and hemorrhage.

FETUS AND NEWBORN

1. Define stillbirth.
A stillbirth (fetal death) is a prenatal or natal (during delivery) death after 20 weeks of gestation.

2. Name the major cause of neonatal mortality. What is the neonatal mortality rate in the United States?
The major cause of neonatal mortality is prematurity. The neonatal mortality rate in the United States is roughly 6 in 1000 births (higher in blacks).

3. List the top three causes of infant mortality in the United States.
   • Congenital abnormalities
   • Prematurity/low birthweight
   • Sudden infant death syndrome

4. What is an Apgar score? At which time points should an Apgar score be measured? Explain the scoring criteria for each Apgar category.
The Apgar score (developed by Virginia Apgar in 1952) is a general measure of newborn well-being, with five categories worth 2 points each for a total of 10 possible points. A score of 8 or above is considered acceptable. An Apgar score should be assessed at minutes 1 and 5 postpartum. Additional Apgar scores should be recorded every 5 minutes only if a score of 8 or higher has not been achieved. Use APGAR as a mnemonic to remember the five categories: **a**ppearance (skin color), **p**ulse (heart rate), **g**rimace (reflex irritability), **a**ctivity (muscle tone), and **r**espiratory effort (breathing).

NUMBER OF POINTS GIVEN

Category	0	1	2
Appearance (color)	Completely cyanotic	Acrocyanosis: body pink, extremities blue	Completely pink
Pulse (heart rate)	Absent	<100 beats/min	>100 beats/min
Grimace (reflex irritability)[a]	None	Excessive stimulation required	Grimace and strong cry, cough, and sneeze
Activity (muscle tone)	Flaccid limbs	Limbs are flexed but do *not resist* active extension	Active motion or able to partially resist active extension
Respiratory effort	Apneic	Irregular respirations or a slow, weak cry	Good, strong cry

[a]Reflex irritability usually is measured by the infant's response to stimulation of the sole of the foot or a catheter put into the nose.

5. True or False: The Apgar score may be used to predict long-term outcomes.
False. The Apgar score tells you what is happening *right now* but does not predict long-term outcomes.

6. What is the first task you must complete when assessing a newborn immediately after delivery?
Stimulate respirations. Suction the **m**outh then **n**ose (i.e., in alphabetical order) if secretions appear to be impairing respiration.

7. When should positive pressure ventilation (PPV) be initiated?
Begin PPV if the neonate's heart rate drops below 100 beats/min or if the neonate is experiencing respiratory difficulty (e.g., gasping, irregular breathing pattern).

8. When should you initiate cardiopulmonary resuscitation (CPR) on a newborn? What is the appropriate compression-to-ventilation ratio?
CPR should be initiated if the newborn's heart rate drops below 60 beats/min. Perform CPR at a ratio of 3:1 chest compressions to ventilations.

9. How can transient tachypnea of the newborn (TTN) be distinguished from respiratory distress syndrome?

Look at the gestational age when delivery occurred and look at the infant's chest x-ray. When TTN occurs, it is often in term or near-term infants delivered by cesarean section. When RDS occurs, it will be in a premature infant due to insufficient surfactant production. The chest x-ray of TTN will show *hyper*expanded lungs, possibly with pulmonary edema (caused by fluid retention); the chest x-ray of RDS will show *hypo*expanded lungs that may be described as having a ground-glass appearance (due to atelectasis and decreased alveolar recruitment).

10. How does the management of transient tachypnea of the newborn differ from managing respiratory distress syndrome?

TTN management is more conservative, typically resolving after simple oxygen administration and occasionally requiring PPV. RDS, on the other hand, may require intubation with positive end-expiratory pressure (PEEP). Giving antenatal steroids to the mother may help reduce the severity of RDS if premature delivery is anticipated.

11. What are the potential sequelae of extended oxygen delivery by PEEP in a premature neonate?

Retinopathy of prematurity (caused by neovascularization and treated by laser ablation), intraventricular hemorrhage, and bronchopulmonary dysplasia are the three main sequelae to watch for that may be caused by excessive PEEP.

12. How many blood vessels does a normal umbilical cord have? What disorder should be suspected if one of the vessels is absent?

The umbilical cord is checked at birth for the presence of **three** blood vessels: two arteries and one vein. If only one artery is present, investigate with ultrasound for congenital renal malformations (e.g., renal agenesis).

13. Which two shots should all newborns receive?

All newborns should receive intramuscular vitamin K and the hepatitis B vaccine within 24 hours following delivery. If the mother is positive for HBsAg, also give HBV immunoglobulin to the newborn. If the mother's HBV status is unknown, draw a serum HBsAg level to decide if the newborn needs immunoglobulin or if just giving the vaccine will be sufficient.

14. Why is a vitamin K injection given to the neonate immediately following delivery?

The neonate's gut flora is not yet mature enough to produce its own vitamin K. Giving an intramuscular injection of vitamin K is prophylactic against hemorrhagic disease of the newborn.

15. What are the commonly performed screening tests for metabolic and congenital disorders?

States vary widely in their policies regarding newborn screening, but there are a few nearly universal screens to know. All states screen for hypothyroidism and phenylketonuria at birth; these screens must be done within the first month of life. Most states also screen for galactosemia, cystic fibrosis, and hemoglobinopathies such as sickle cell disease. Less common screening tests that may still appear on the USMLE include homocystinuria, maple syrup urine disease, congenital adrenal hyperplasia, cystic fibrosis, biotinidase deficiency, tyrosinemia, and toxoplasmosis. Remember that screening tests are highly sensitive, so if any of these screens come back positive, your next step should be to order a confirmatory test with high *specificity* to rule out a false-positive result.

16. Which gastrointestinal malformation causes primarily respiratory problems?

Diaphragmatic hernia, which is more common in males. Ninety percent are on the left side. The main point to know is that bowel herniates into the thorax through the diaphragmatic defect, compressing the lung and impeding lung development (pulmonary hypoplasia develops). Patients present with respiratory distress and have bowel sounds in the chest and bowel loops in the thorax on chest radiographs. Treat with surgical correction of the diaphragm.

17. How do you recognize and diagnose a tracheoesophageal fistula? How is it treated?

The most common type (85% of cases) of tracheoesophageal fistula is an esophagus with a blind pouch proximally and a fistula between a bronchus/carina and the distal esophagus (Fig. 12.4). Look for a neonate with excessive oral secretions, coughing or cyanosis on attempted feeding, abdominal distention, and aspiration pneumonia. The diagnosis is made on the basis of an inability to insert a nasogastric tube; alternatively, an injection of air via a nasogastric tube under x-ray (i.e., fluoroscopy) guidance shows only the proximal esophagus. Treatment is early surgical correction.

18. Compare and contrast gastroschisis versus omphalocele. How do they present clinically? Which is enclosed in a membrane? What is the appropriate management for each condition?

Gastroschisis and omphalocele are two types of bowel extrusion that may be present at birth. Gast**r**oschisis is typically extruding to the **r**ight of the umbilicus and is *not* covered in membrane. O**m**phalocele typically extrudes directly through the umbilicus (i.e., **m**idline) and *is* covered by a **m**embrane. Both are managed the same way: wrapped in a saline-soaked sterile dressing and covered (also called siloed) to prevent infection or desiccation as the intestines slowly return where they belong. A nasogastric tube may be considered to decompress the bowel.

19. How is imperforate anus diagnosed?

Imperforate anus is diagnosed with an *upside-down* x-ray, to allow colonic gas to rise and show exactly how far the imperforate lesion is from the anus.

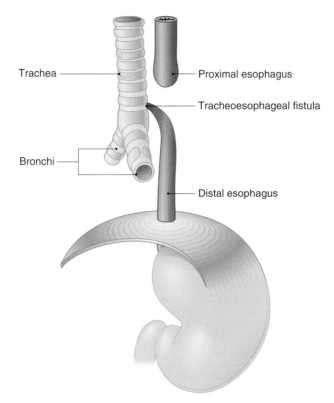

Trachea

Proximal esophagus

Tracheoesophageal fistula

Bronchi

Distal esophagus

Fig. 12.4 Tracheoesophageal fistula. Diagram of the most common type of esophageal atresia and tracheoesophageal fistula. (From Gilbert-Barness E. *Potter's Pathology of the Fetus, Infant and Child.* 2nd ed. Philadelphia: Mosby; 2007 [fig. 25-6].)

20. Once imperforate anus has been diagnosed, which studies do you order next? Why?
    Imperforate anus is associated with the VACTERL anomalies. VACTERL is an acronym for **v**ertebral anomalies, imperforate **a**nus, **c**ardiac malformations, **t**racheal-**e**sophageal malformation, **r**enal dysfunction, and **l**imb malformation (especially the thumbs). Order a spinal x-ray, fetal echocardiogram, renal ultrasound, and attempt to pass a nasogastric tube to work up each potential VACTERL complication before diving straight into management for imperforate anus.

21. How does the management of imperforate anus differ if the lesion is distal (e.g., closer to the anus) versus proximal (e.g., further from the anus)?
    After additional VACTERL complications have been ruled out, distal lesions can be corrected as soon as they are identified—either by dilation or minor surgery. Proximal lesions require further neonatal development before they can be corrected, so your management *right now* should be to place a colostomy and defer surgical correction for the future (but before the infant begins to toilet train).

22. A neonatal abdominal x-ray shows a double-bubble sign. What is on your differential? What clinical or imaging clues can be used to distinguish between these possibilities?
    A neonatal abdominal x-ray with a double-bubble sign is not as narrow of a differential diagnosis as you may think. The most testable diagnoses include malrotation, intestinal atresia, duodenal atresia, and annular pancreas. These can be distinguished by looking at what is going on with the air-fluid levels: a double-bubble sign with *normal air-fluid levels* suggests malrotation; a double-bubble sign with *multiple air-fluid levels* suggests intestinal atresia; a double-bubble sign with *no distal air-fluid levels* indicates either duodenal atresia or annular pancreas. In clinical practice it is difficult to tell duodenal atresia and annular pancreas from imaging alone, but on the USMLE look for mention of **D**own syndrome to indicate **d**uodenal atresia as the most likely etiology rather than annular pancreas.

23. How does Hirschsprung disease present? What is its pathophysiology?
    Hirschsprung disease presents as constipation in a newborn with explosive diarrhea on digital rectal exam (squirt sign). Less severe conditions may not present until the child is 2 to 3 years old. Hirschsprung disease is caused

by a lack of neural crest cell migration, resulting in no Meissner plexus or Auerbach plexus in the rectum. Because of this, the sphincter *cannot relax*, resulting in fecal retention. Hirschsprung disease is associated with trisomy 21 (Down syndrome).

24. **How is Hirschsprung disease worked up, diagnosed, and managed?**
    If suspected, Hirschsprung disease is worked up with anorectal manometry (which would show increased rectal tone). Diagnosis is made by suction biopsy, taking care to include the **submucosa,** which is where the absent neurons *should* be found. Hirschsprung disease is managed with surgical resection of the affected colon.

25. **What clinical presentation and physical exam findings would make you suspect pyloric stenosis in an infant? How is it managed once diagnosed?**
    Pyloric stenosis is characterized by nonbilious projectile vomiting with possibly visible peristaltic waves or a palpable olive-shaped mass in the infant's abdominal right upper quadrant. Surgically correct with pyloromyotomy; be sure to give intravenous fluids and electrolytes to reduce the risk of postoperative apnea.

26. **What three characteristic acid-base and electrolyte abnormalities are typically present in infants with pyloric stenosis? Explain why these occur.**
    Expect to see hypochloremic hypokalemic metabolic alkalosis in these infants. Pyloric stenosis causes projectile vomiting of gastric acid, meaning your patient is actively losing H^+, Cl^-, and fluid. The body acts to prevent fluid-related dehydration by releasing aldosterone, which exchanges K^+ for Na^+ to facilitate water retention. The ultimate result of this physiologic cascade is hypochloremic hypokalemic metabolic alkalosis.

27. **What is the leading diagnosis for a prematurely born infant now presenting with bloody stool? What is your next step?**
    A premature infant with bloody stool will almost always have necrotizing enterocolitis (NEC). If you see *pneumatosis intestinalis* (air in the bowel wall), you have confirmed NEC. This patient needs to become nil per os immediately, with feeding provided by total parenteral nutrition and intravenous fluids. Decompress the bowel with a nasogastric tube and start broad-spectrum antibiotics to prevent shock. Surgery is only necessary if clinical deterioration or perforation occurs; perforation will present as air under the diaphragm on imaging studies.

28. **How is infant colic defined and treated?**
    Infant colic is described as crying/fussing for no apparent reason lasting 3 or more hours/day for at least 3 days/week in a healthy infant younger than 3 months. Parents should be educated regarding feeding and soothing techniques and reassured that the condition is self-limited.

29. **What is the first step in evaluating neonatal jaundice? Why is jaundice of concern in a neonate?**
    The first step is to determine whether the jaundice is physiologic or pathologic. Measure total, direct, and indirect bilirubin. The main concern is bilirubin-induced neurologic dysfunction (BIND), which is due to high levels of unconjugated bilirubin with subsequent deposit in the basal ganglia. Kernicterus is the term for the chronic and permanent sequelae of BIND. Look for poor feeding, seizures, flaccidity, opisthotonos, and apnea in the setting of severe jaundice.

30. **What causes physiologic jaundice of the newborn? Who gets it?**
    Physiologic (nonpathologic) jaundice is caused by normal neonatal changes in bilirubin metabolism, which results in increased bilirubin production, decreased bilirubin clearance (low UDP-glucuronyl transferase activity), and increased enterohepatic circulation. These changes result in the low-risk unconjugated (indirect) bilirubinemia that occurs in most newborns and is even more prevalent in premature infants. Bilirubin is mostly unconjugated because of incomplete maturation of liver function. In full-term infants, bilirubin is less than 12 mg/dL, peaks at day 2 to 4, and returns to normal by 2 weeks. In premature infants, bilirubin is less than 15 mg/dL, peaks at day 3 to 5, and may be elevated for up to 3 weeks.

31. **What are the causes of neonatal jaundice?**
    Breastfeeding jaundice: occurs in 1 in 10 breastfed infants and is typically seen in the first week of life. This is essentially an exaggerated physiologic jaundice due to insufficient milk intake (usually due to inadequate maternal milk production), which leads to fluid and weight loss and an inadequate number of bowel movements to remove bilirubin from the body.
    Breast milk jaundice: typically presents after the first 3 to 5 days of life and has traditionally been defined as the persistence of physiologic jaundice beyond the first week of life. Breast milk jaundice results from a direct effect of breast milk itself, as human milk promotes an increase in intestinal absorption of bilirubin. In contrast to breastfeeding jaundice, breast milk jaundice does not present with signs of dehydration. Bilirubin levels peak within 2 weeks after birth and decline to normal levels by 12 weeks of age. Breastfeeding should continue as long as the hyperbilirubinemia remains in the safe zone.
    Illness: infection or sepsis, hypothyroidism, liver insult, cystic fibrosis, and other illnesses may prolong neonatal jaundice and lower the threshold for kernicterus. The youngest, sickest infants are at greatest risk for hyperbilirubinemia and kernicterus. Make sure to obtain blood cultures.

Hemolysis: from Rh incompatibility or congenital red cell diseases (e.g., hereditary spherocytosis, elliptocytosis, G6PD deficiency) that cause hemolysis in the neonatal period. ABO incompatibility may cause mild jaundice but usually is not clinically significant. Look for anemia, peripheral smear abnormalities, positive family history, and higher levels of unconjugated bilirubin.

Metabolic disorders: Crigler-Najjar syndrome causes severe unconjugated hyperbilirubinemia, whereas Gilbert syndrome causes a mild form. Both are due to problems with UDP-glucuronyl transferase. Rotor and Dubin-Johnson syndromes cause conjugated hyperbilirubinemia. These are due to decreased intrahepatic excretion.

Biliary atresia: full-term infants with clay- or gray-colored stools and high levels of conjugated bilirubin. Treat with surgery.

Medications: avoid sulfa drugs in neonates; they displace bilirubin from albumin and may precipitate kernicterus.

32. How is severe hyperbilirubinemia recognized?

Severe hyperbilirubinemia (sometimes called pathologic jaundice) is suggested by jaundice that is recognized in the first 24 hours of life, total bilirubin that is higher than the hour-specific 95th percentile, a rate of rise is greater than 0.2 mg/dL/hour, jaundice in a term newborn after 2 weeks of age, or a direct bilirubin concentration that is more than 20% of the total bilirubin.

33. How is severe hyperbilirubinemia treated?

Unconjugated hyperbilirubinemia that persists, rises above 15 mg/dL, or rises rapidly is treated with **phototherapy** to convert unconjugated bilirubin to a water-soluble form that can be excreted. A last resort is exchange transfusion, but don't even think about it unless the level of unconjugated bilirubin is greater than 20 mg/dL.

34. What should you do if an infant is born to a mother with active hepatitis B?

An infant born to a mother with active hepatitis B should receive the first immunization shot and hepatitis B immunoglobulin at birth.

35. Describe the effects of alcohol on pregnancy.

Alcohol is a teratogen and the most common cause of preventable mental retardation in the United States. You should be able to recognize the classic presentation of a child affected by fetal alcohol syndrome: intellectual disability, smooth philtrum, thin vermilion border, microcephaly, short palpebral fissures, and cardiac defects. No amount of alcohol consumption can be considered safe during pregnancy. Fetal alcohol syndrome rates vary but may affect as many as 1 in 1000 births in the United States.

36. What is the usual cause of vaginal bleeding in neonates? How is it treated?

Vaginal bleeding in neonates is usually physiologic and due to maternal estrogen withdrawal. No treatment is needed because the bleeding resolves on its own.

37. What causes DiGeorge syndrome? How do you recognize it?

DiGeorge syndrome is caused by a chromosomal deletion at 22q11.2. It causes hypoplasia of the third and fourth pharyngeal pouches. Look for hypocalcemia and tetany (from hypocalcemia caused by absent parathyroid glands) in the first 24 to 48 hours of life. The thymus may also be absent or hypoplastic, and congenital heart defects and typical facies are often present.

38. How do you recognize Down syndrome?

Down syndrome (trisomy 21) is the most common known cause of intellectual disability in the United States. The biggest risk factor is maternal age (1 in 1500 offspring of 16-year-old mothers and 1 in 25 offspring of 45-year-old mothers). At birth look for hypotonia, a transverse palmar crease, and characteristic facies (Fig. 12.5). Congenital cardiac defects (especially ventricular septal defects) are common, and affected individuals have an increased risk of leukemia, duodenal atresia, and early Alzheimer disease.

39. What is the second most common known cause of inherited intellectual disability?

Fragile X syndrome (X-linked recessive). Affected males often have an elongated face, large ears, and large testicles (macroorchidism).

40. How is neonatal hypoglycemia diagnosed and managed?

Serum glucose levels below 40 mg/dL are considered diagnostic for neonatal hypoglycemia. There are four management options for neonatal hypoglycemia, depending on the level of severity. *Asymptomatic* hypoglycemia is managed with simple oral feeding. *Symptomatic* hypoglycemia (e.g., lethargic, tremulous, excessively irritable infants) should be managed with a bolus of dextrose (typically D10W): 2 L/kg body weight. If that bolus does not resolve the hypoglycemia, *refractory* hypoglycemia should be treated with a dextrose infusion. In the most severe cases, where serum glucose is either unmeasurable or the infant appears obtunded, administer intramuscular glucagon.

41. What clinical signs suggest galactosemia?

Congenital cataracts and neonatal sepsis with vomiting after breastfeeding. Patients should avoid galactose- and lactose-containing foods.

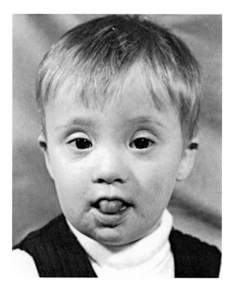

Fig. 12.5 Child with Down syndrome. Note the flat facial profile, flat nasal bridge, open mouth, protruding tongue, folded ears, and epicanthic folds. (From Kliegman RM. *Nelson Textbook of Pediatrics*. 19th ed. Philadelphia: Saunders; 2011 [fig. 76-8A].)

42. Cover the right-hand column, then specify the effects of the following classic teratogens on an exposed fetus.

Agent	Defect(S) Caused
Thalidomide	Phocomelia (absence of long bones, with flipperlike appearance of hands)
Antineoplastics	Many
Tetracycline	Yellow or brown teeth
Aminoglycosides	Deafness
Valproic acid	Spina bifida, hypospadias
Progesterone	Masculinization of female fetus
Cigarettes	Intrauterine growth restriction (IUGR), low birthweight, prematurity
Lithium	Cardiac (Ebstein) anomalies
Radiation	IUGR, central nervous system defects, eye defects, malignancy (e.g., leukemia)
Alcohol	Fetal alcohol syndrome
Phenytoin	Craniofacial, limb, and cerebrovascular defects; intellectual disability; fetal hydantoin syndrome
Warfarin	Craniofacial defects, IUGR, central nervous system malformation, stillbirth
Carbamazepine	Fingernail hypoplasia, craniofacial defects, fetal hydantoin syndrome
Isotretinoin*	Central nervous system, craniofacial, ear, and cardiovascular defects
Iodine	Goiter, neonatal hypothyroidism
Cocaine	Cerebral infarcts, intellectual disability
Diazepam	Cleft lip and/or palate
Diethylstilbestrol	Clear cell vaginal cancer, adenosis, cervical incompetence

*Vitamin A in general is considered teratogenic when recommended intake levels are exceeded.

43. Which vitamin is a known teratogen?

Vitamin A. Female patients taking one of the vitamin A analogs as treatment for acne must have a negative pregnancy test before the medication is started and should be counseled about the risks of teratogenicity. Some form of birth control should be used, and periodic pregnancy tests should be offered.

Isotretinoin is such a significant teratogen that access to this medication is very restricted. All patients and prescribers must be in a special program designed to eliminate fetal exposure to isotretinoin. There are strict qualification criteria, including monthly pregnancy testing, and two forms of contraception are recommended.

44. Distinguish between caput succedaneum and cephalohematoma. How are these conditions treated?

Both conditions are noted in newborns after vaginal delivery. **Caput succedaneum** defines diffuse swelling or edema of the scalp that crosses the midline, is benign, and requires no further investigation or treatment.

A **cephalohematoma** is a subperiosteal hemorrhage that does not cross suture lines and is usually benign and self-resolving but in rare cases may indicate an underlying skull fracture. Order a radiograph or CT scan of the head to rule out a fracture.

PERINATAL INFECTIONS

1. What are three common causes of neonatal conjunctivitis?
Chemical, *Neisseria gonorrhoeae*, and *Chlamydia trachomatis*.

2. What causes chemical conjunctivitis? How do you recognize it?
Silver nitrate (or erythromycin) drops, which are given to all newborns to prevent gonorrhea conjunctivitis, can cause chemical conjunctivitis. The drops may cause a chemical conjunctivitis (with no purulent discharge) that appears within 12 hours of instilling the drops and resolves within 48 hours. Chemical conjunctivitis is always the best guess if the conjunctivitis develops in the first 24 hours of life.

3. How can you distinguish gonorrheal from chlamydial conjunctivitis?
In cases of suspected **gonorrheal conjunctivitis,** look for symptoms of gonorrhea in the mother. The infant has an extremely purulent discharge starting between 2 and 5 days after birth. Infants who were given prophylactic drops should not develop gonorrheal conjunctivitis. Treatment involves systemic ceftriaxone or cefotaxime.

    In cases of **chlamydial (inclusion) conjunctivitis,** the mother often reports no symptoms. The infant has mild-to-severe conjunctivitis beginning between 5 and 14 days after birth. Oral erythromycin is recommended for chlamydial conjunctivitis or pneumonia; topical therapy for chlamydial conjunctivitis is not effective.

4. If you forget everything else about neonatal conjunctivitis, what point should you remember to help you distinguish among the three discussed causes?
The varying time frames during which they present.

5. What is the definition of neonatal sepsis? What pathogens typically cause neonatal sepsis? What are the risk factors?
Neonatal sepsis is a syndrome that manifests as systemic signs of infection and/or isolation of a bacterial pathogen in the bloodstream of an infant 28 days old or younger. Early-onset sepsis usually is due to vertical transmission from amniotic fluid or during vaginal delivery from bacteria colonizing or infecting the mother's lower genital tract. Late-onset sepsis comes either from maternal vertical transmission or from contact with care providers or environmental sources. GBS and *Escherichia coli* are the most common causes. *Listeria monocytogenes* is another cause of sepsis but is rare and is usually seen during outbreaks of listeriosis. *S. aureus* is an emerging pathogen; enterococci and other gram-negative rods can also cause neonatal sepsis.

6. What are the maternal and neonatal risk factors for neonatal sepsis?
Intrapartum maternal fever, delivery at less than 37 weeks of gestation, chorioamnionitis, a 5-minute Apgar score of 6 or less, evidence of fetal distress, maternal GBS colonization, and a duration of 18 hours or longer since membrane rupture.

7. What are the clinical manifestations of neonatal sepsis?
The signs and symptoms are subtle and nonspecific, so be careful. Look for temperature instability, jaundice, respiratory distress, hepatomegaly, anorexia, vomiting, lethargy, cyanosis, and apnea. Also look for abdominal distention, irritability, and diarrhea, although these are less common.

8. How do you evaluate an infant with suspected neonatal sepsis?
Blood culture, CBC, chest x-ray (if respiratory abnormalities are present), and lumbar puncture. Neutropenia is a fairly specific marker for neonatal sepsis. A urine culture should be ordered if the child is older than 6 days.

9. How do you treat neonatal sepsis?
Treat empirically with ampicillin and gentamicin for early-onset sepsis to cover GBS and *E. coli*. Empiric treatment for late-onset neonatal sepsis (infants age >7 days) is ampicillin and gentamicin if the infant is being admitted from the community. For an infant who has been hospitalized since birth, substitute vancomycin for ampicillin to cover antimicrobial-resistant organisms.

10. What do you need to know about vaginal group B streptococcal colonization during pregnancy?
Pregnant women should be tested for vaginal GBS at 35 to 37 weeks of gestation. Women who are carriers should be treated during labor with intrapartum penicillin G or ampicillin. Earlier testing and treatment (e.g., second trimester) is ineffective because GBS frequently returns. The exception is for women with GBS bacteriuria (often detected on first trimester screening urine culture)—these women are not retested later but are instead treated empirically during labor, as they are assumed to be chronically colonized with GBS. The reason for treating asymptomatic carriers is to prevent neonatal sepsis and endometritis, both of which are commonly caused by GBS.

11. What are the TORCH syndromes? What do they cause?

TORCH is an acronym for several maternal infections that can cross the placenta and cause devastating intrauterine fetal complications. Most TORCH infections can cause intellectual disability, microcephaly, hydrocephalus, hepatosplenomegaly, jaundice, anemia, low birthweight, and IUGR.

T = **T**oxoplasma gondii: look for exposure to cats. Specific defects include intracranial calcifications and chorioretinitis.

O = **O**ther: varicella-zoster causes limb hypoplasia and scarring of the skin. Syphilis causes rhinitis, saber shins, Hutchinson teeth, interstitial keratitis, and skin lesions.

R = **R**ubella: worst in the first trimester (some recommend abortion if the mother has rubella in the first trimester). Always check antibody status on the first visit in patients with a poor immunization history. Look for cardiovascular defects (e.g., patent ductus arteriosus), deafness, cataracts, and microphthalmia.

C = **C**ytomegalovirus: most common infection of the TORCH group. Look for deafness, intracerebral calcifications, and microphthalmia.

H = **H**erpes: look for vesicular skin lesions (with positive Tzanck smears) and history of maternal herpes lesions.

12. What do you need to know about HIV testing and transmission in mother and child?

In untreated HIV-positive patients, HIV is transmitted to the fetus in roughly 25% of cases. Roughly one-third of transmissions occur antenatally, one-third in the peripartum period, and one-third postpartum, most commonly via breastfeeding. Transmission rates are much higher in the setting of acute HIV infection, in which a woman seroconverts during pregnancy.

When multidrug antiretroviral therapy is given to the mother prenatally and zidovudine is given to the infant for 6 weeks after birth, HIV transmission is reduced to less than 2%. A noninfected infant may still have a positive HIV antibody test at birth because maternal antibodies can cross the placenta. Within 6 to 18 months, however, the test reverts to negative. This is why infants of HIV-positive mothers are tested using a direct HIV DNA polymerase chain reaction (PCR) test at birth, at 4 to 6 weeks of age, and 4 months of age. Babies who have these three negative tests should have an HIV antibody test at 12 and 18 months of age. Cesarean section is recommended for viremic women with a viral load greater than 1000 copies at the time of delivery to prevent HIV transmission to the child. Mothers with HIV should avoid breastfeeding, since the virus crosses into breast milk (the WHO recommends that in developing countries mothers continue breastfeeding while the mother or infant takes antiretroviral drugs).

13. What should you do if a pregnant woman has genital herpes?

A decision is generally made when the mother goes into labor, not beforehand. If, at the time of true labor, the mother has active, visible genital herpes lesions, do a cesarean section to prevent transmission to the fetus. If, at the time of true labor, the mother has no visible genital herpes lesions, the child may be delivered vaginally. Women with a history of genital herpes should be offered suppressive therapy with acyclovir to maximize their chance at a vaginal delivery.

14. What should you do for the child if the mother has chronic hepatitis B or chickenpox?

If the mother has chronic hepatitis B confirmed by HBsAg measurement, give the infant the first hepatitis B vaccine shot plus hepatitis B immunoglobulin at birth and a bath as soon as possible. If the mother contracts chickenpox in the last 5 days of pregnancy or the first 2 days after delivery, give the infant varicella-zoster immunoglobulin.

15. What subtype of maternal antibody can cross the placenta?

IgG is the only type of maternal antibody that crosses the placenta. This may be an important diagnostic point: An elevated neonatal IgM concentration is never normal, whereas an elevated neonatal IgG often represents maternal antibodies.

CHAPTER 13

DISORDERS OF BLOOD

SPLENIC DISORDERS

1. What do you need to know about splenic rupture?
   The spleen is the most commonly injured organ in blunt trauma. Patients with splenic rupture, the most severe form of injury, have a history of blunt abdominal trauma, hypotension, tachycardia, shock, and/or **Kehr sign** (referred pain in the left shoulder). Patients with Epstein-Barr virus infection or infectious mononucleosis and splenomegaly should avoid contact sports to prevent rupture. Make sure patients with a history of functional or surgical asplenia have received the pneumococcal, meningococcal, and *Haemophilus influenzae* (i.e., encapsulated bugs) vaccines.

ANEMIAS AND CYTOPENIAS

1. Define anemia.
   Hemoglobin less than 12 mg/dL in women or less than 14 mg/dL in men.

2. What are the signs and symptoms of anemia?
   Signs: tachycardia, pallor (especially of the sclera and mucous membranes), systolic ejection murmurs (from heightened flow), and signs of the underlying cause (e.g., jaundice and/or pigment **gallstones** in hemolytic anemia, positive stool guaiac with a gastrointestinal [GI] bleed).
   Symptoms: fatigue, dyspnea on exertion, lightheadedness, dizziness, syncope, palpitations, angina, and claudication.

3. What are the important elements of the history when anemia is present?
   Important points include medications, blood loss (e.g., trauma, surgery, melena, hematemesis, menorrhagia), chronic diseases (anemia of chronic disease), family history (e.g., hemophilia, thalassemia, sickle cell disease, glucose-6-phosphatase deficiency [G6PD]), and alcoholism (which may lead to iron, folate, and B_{12} deficiencies as well as GI bleeds).

4. What findings help you in the setting of acute blood loss as a cause of anemia?
   The important point is that immediately after blood loss the hemoglobin may be normal; it takes at least 3 to 4 hours, often more, for reequilibration. Look for obvious bleeding, pale and cold skin, tachycardia (often the first sign of acute anemia), and hypotension (a late sign of hypovolemic shock, especially in younger patients with better hemodynamic reserve). Transfuse if indicated, even with a normal hemoglobin in the acute setting. Consider internal hemorrhage in the setting of trauma and abdominal aortic aneurysm in patients with a pulsatile abdominal mass. Consider evaluation with an ultrasonographic FAST (focused assessment with sonography in trauma) exam.

5. What medications can cause anemia? How?
   Many medications can cause anemia through various mechanisms. Methyldopa, penicillins, and sulfa drugs can cause red blood cell (RBC) antibodies with subsequent hemolysis; chloroquine and sulfa drugs cause hemolysis in patients with G6PD; phenytoin causes megaloblastic anemia through interference with folate metabolism; and chloramphenicol, cancer drugs, and zidovudine cause aplastic anemia and bone marrow suppression. Other drugs are also implicated, but this list should get you through the USMLE exam.

6. What test should be ordered first to help determine the cause of anemia?
   The complete blood count (CBC) with RBC indices. The hemoglobin must be below normal to diagnose anemia. The mean corpuscular volume (MCV) tells you whether the anemia is microcytic (MCV <80), normocytic (MCV = 80–100), or macrocytic (MCV >100).

7. What test should be ordered next?
   A peripheral blood smear. Many classic findings can help in making diagnoses:
   - Sickled cells (sickle cell disease; Fig. 13.1)
   - Hypersegmented neutrophils (folate/B12 deficiency; Fig. 13.2)
   - Hypochromic and microcytic RBCs (iron deficiency; Fig. 13.3)
   - Basophilic stippling (lead poisoning; Fig. 13.4)

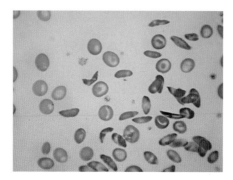

Fig. 13.1 Sickle cells show a sickle or crescent shape resulting from polymerization of hemoglobin S. This smear also shows target cells and boat-shaped cells with a lesser degree of polymerization of hemoglobin S than in a classic sickle cell. (From Goldman L, Schafer Al. *Goldman's Cecil Medicine.* 24th ed. Philadelphia: Saunders; 2011 [fig. 160-7].)

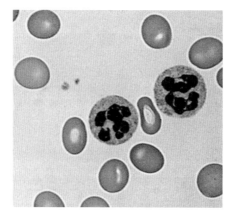

Fig. 13.2 Megaloblastic changes of macrocytosis and a hypersegmented neutrophil. (From Goldman L, Schafer Al. *Goldman's Cecil Medicine.* 24th ed. Philadelphia: Saunders; 2011 [fig. 170-6].)

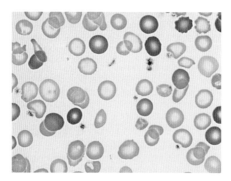

Fig. 13.3 Iron-deficiency anemia. Pale red blood cells with an enlarged central area of pallor. (From McPherson R, Pincus M. *Henry's Clinical Diagnosis and Management by Laboratory Methods.* 21st ed. Philadelphia: Saunders; 2006 [fig. 31-2].)

- Bite cells (classically, G6PD deficiency; other hemolytic anemias; Fig. 13.5)
- Heinz bodies (G6PD deficiency; see Fig. 13.5)
- Howell-Jolly bodies (asplenia; Fig. 13.6)
- Teardrop-shaped RBCs (dacrocytes seen in myelofibrosis; Fig. 13.7)
- Schistocytes, helmet cells, and fragmented RBCs (intravascular hemolysis; Fig. 13.8)

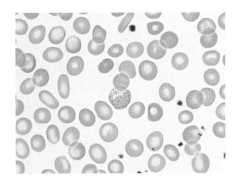

Fig. 13.4 Basophilic stippling. Irregular basophilic granules in red blood cells; often associated with lead poisoning and thalassemia. (From McPherson R, Pincus M. *Henry's Clinical Diagnosis and Management by Laboratory Methods.* 21st ed. Philadelphia: Saunders; 2006 [fig. 29-23].)

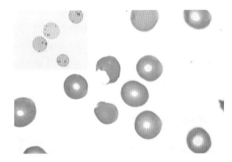

Fig. 13.5 Bite cells with Heinz bodies. (Courtesy Dr. Robert W. McKenna, Department of Pathology, University of Texas Southwestern Medical School, Dallas, TX.)

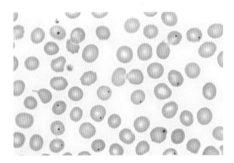

Fig. 13.6 Howell-Jolly bodies in peripheral blood erythrocytes. These nuclear remnants indicate a lack of splenic filtrative function. (From Orkin SH, et al. *Nathan and Oski's Hematology of Infancy and Childhood.* 7th ed. Philadelphia: Saunders; 2009 [fig. 14-4].)

- Spherocytes and elliptocytes (hereditary spherocytosis and elliptocytosis; Fig. 13.9)
- Acanthocytes and spur cells (abetalipoproteinemia; Fig. 13.10)
- Target cells (thalassemia, liver disease; Fig. 13.11)
- Echinocytes, including burr cells and acanthocytes (uremia, liver disease; Fig. 13.12)
- Polychromasia (from reticulocytosis; should alert you to the possibility of hemolysis; Fig. 13.13)
- Rouleaux formation (multiple myeloma; Fig. 13.14)
- Parasites inside RBCs (malaria [Fig. 13.15], babesiosis)
- Iron inclusions (ringed sideroblasts) in RBCs of the bone marrow (sideroblastic anemia; Fig. 13.16)

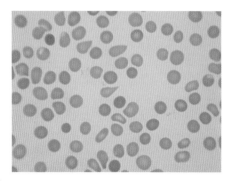

Fig. 13.7 Teardrop red blood cells, usually seen in myelofibrosis. (From Goldman L, Ausiello D. *Cecil Medicine*. 23rd ed. Philadelphia: Saunders; 2008 [fig. 161-13].)

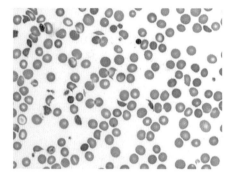

Fig. 13.8 Schistocytes and helmet cells. Red blood cell fragments seen in microangiopathic hemolytic anemia and disseminated intravascular coagulation. (From McPherson R, Pincus M. *Henry's Clinical Diagnosis and Management by Laboratory Methods*. 21st ed. Philadelphia: Saunders; 2006 [fig. 29-19].)

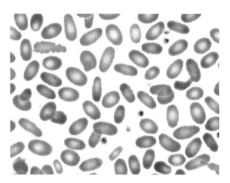

Fig. 13.9 Hereditary elliptocytosis. A blood film reveals characteristic elliptical red blood cells. (From McPherson R, Pincus M. McPherson R, Pincus M. *Henry's Clinical Diagnosis and Management by Laboratory Methods*. 21st ed. Philadelphia: Saunders; 2006 [fig. 30-16].)

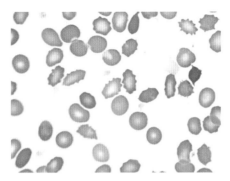

Fig. 13.10 Acanthocytes. Irregularly spiculated red blood cells, frequently seen in abetalipoproteinemia or liver disease. (From McPherson R, Pincus M. *Henry's Clinical Diagnosis and Management by Laboratory Methods*. 21st ed. Philadelphia: Saunders; 2006 [fig. 29-20].)

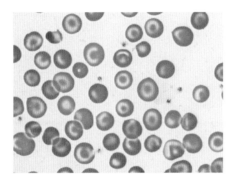

Fig. 13.11 Target cells are frequently seen in hemoglobin C disease and liver disease. (From McPherson R, Pincus M. McPherson R, Pincus M. *Henry's Clinical Diagnosis and Management by Laboratory Methods*. 21st ed. Philadelphia: Saunders; 2006 [fig. 29-18].)

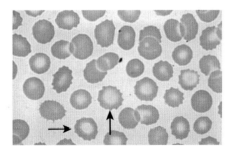

Fig. 13.12 Echinocytes, or burr cells *(arrows)*, are the hallmark of uremia. (From Hoffman R, et al. *Hematology: Basic Principles and Practice*. 5th ed. Philadelphia: Churchill Livingstone; 2008 [fig. 156-1].)

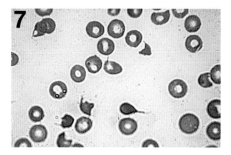

Fig. 13.13 Microangiopathic hemolytic anemia demonstrating red blood cell fragments, anisocytosis, polychromasia, and decreased platelets. (From Tschudy MM, Arcara KM. *The Harriet Lane Handbook*. 19th ed. Philadelphia: Mosby; 2011 [plate 7].)

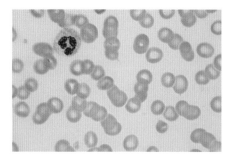

Fig. 13.14 Rouleaux formation of stacked red blood cells seen in multiple myeloma. (From Goldman L, Ausiello D. *Cecil Medicine*. 23rd ed. Philadelphia: Saunders; 2008 [fig. 161-19].)

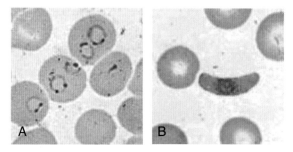

Fig. 13.15 Malaria. Peripheral blood film examples of various stages of *Plasmodium falciparum*. (A) Small ring forms. (B) A crescentic gametocyte with centrally placed chromatin. (From Hoffman R, et al. *Hematology: Basic Principles and Practice*. 5th ed. Philadelphia: Churchill Livingstone; 2008 [fig. 159-5].)

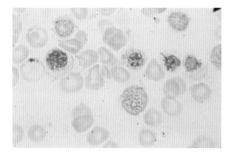

Fig. 13.16 Ringed sideroblasts seen in sideroblastic anemia. (From Goldman L, Ausiello D. *Cecil Medicine*. 23rd ed. Philadelphia: Saunders; 2008 [fig. 163-5].)

8. What are reticulocytes? Why is a reticulocyte count routinely ordered in an anemia workup?

Reticulocytes are immature RBCs. If their count is abnormally decreased in the setting of anemia, the marrow is not responding properly and is thus the site of the problem. A high reticulocyte count should make you think of hemolysis or blood loss as the cause (the marrow is responding properly and is not the problem).

9. Which test comes next?

At this point, it depends. If you have a complete history and results of the other three tests (CBC with RBC indices, peripheral smear, and reticulocyte count), most possibilities will be eliminated, and you can order a confirmatory test. If the answer is still not clear, consider a bone marrow biopsy. For the Step 3 exam, biopsy is unlikely to be necessary unless malignancy is the cause of the anemia.

10. What are the classic causes of microcytic, normocytic, and anemia? Which of these tends to have an inappropriately low reticulocyte count?

Microcytic	*Normocytic*
With Normal or Elevated Reticulocyte Count	**With Normal or Elevated Reticulocyte Count**
Thalassemia/hemoglobinopathy (e.g., sickle cell disease)	Acute blood loss
	Hemolysis (multiple causes)
	Medications (antibody causing)
With Low Reticulocyte Count	**With Low Reticulocyte Count**
Lead poisoning	Cancer/dysplasia (e.g., myelophthisic anemia, acute leukemia)
Sideroblastic anemia	Anemia of chronic disease (some cases)
Anemia of chronic disease (some cases)	Aplastic anemia/medications causing bone marrow suppression
Iron deficiency	Endocrine failure (thyroid, pituitary)
	Renal failure

Macrocytic (All Types Have Low Reticulocyte Count)
Folate deficiency
Vitamin B_{12} deficiency
Medications (methotrexate, phenytoin)
Alcohol abuse (interferes with folate metabolism)
Cirrhosis, liver disease

11. What clues point to hemolysis as the cause for anemia?

- Elevated lactate dehydrogenase (LDH)
- Elevated bilirubin (unconjugated as well as conjugated if the liver is functioning)
- Jaundice
- Low or absent haptoglobin (intravascular hemolysis only)
- Urobilinogen, bilirubin, and hemoglobin in urine (only conjugated bilirubin shows up in the urine; and hemoglobin shows up in the urine only when haptoglobin has been saturated, as in brisk intravascular hemolysis)
- Pigmented gallstones or history of cholecystectomy (usually at a young age)

12. What is the most common cause of anemia in the United States?

Iron-deficiency anemia.

13. Why do people get iron deficiency?

Iron deficiency is common in women of reproductive age because of menstrual blood loss. In all patients over age 40 (men and especially postmenopausal women), it is important to rule out colon cancer as a cause of chronic, asymptomatic blood loss. Increased requirements may also lead to iron deficiency in children and pregnant or breastfeeding women. Give iron-containing formula or iron supplements to all infants except full-term infants who are exclusively breastfed. Start iron supplementation (iron-fortified cereal or daily iron supplement) at 4 to 6 months for full-term infants and at 2 months for preterm infants. Giving cow's milk before 1 year of age may lead to anemia by causing GI bleeding, so avoidance of cow's milk in the first year is essential. Iron supplements also are commonly given during pregnancy and lactation (because of the increased demand).

14. What are the classic laboratory abnormalities in iron-deficiency anemia? What weird cravings may occur with iron deficiency?

Look for low iron and low ferritin levels, elevated total iron-binding capacity (TIBC; also known as transferrin), and low TIBC saturation. Rare patients may develop a craving for ice (pagophagia) or dirt/clay (**pica**).

15. How is iron deficiency treated?

First you must determine the cause. In a menstruating woman, a presumptive diagnosis of menstrual blood loss is often made. In patients over 40 years, be sure to test the stool for occult blood and strongly consider colonoscopy to detect colon cancer. Postmenopausal vaginal bleeding may also cause anemia and warrants screening for gyne-cologic cancer. Treat with iron supplements for 3 to 6 months in uncomplicated cases to replete body iron stores.

16. **How do you recognize anemia of chronic disease?**
First, look for the presence of a disease that causes chronic inflammation (e.g., rheumatoid arthritis, systemic lu-pus erythematosus, cancer, tuberculosis). The anemia is either normocytic or microcytic. Serum iron is low, but so is total iron-binding capacity. Thus the percent saturation may be near normal. Serum ferritin is elevated (because ferritin is an acute-phase reactant, the level should be increased). Treat the underlying disorder to correct the anemia. Do not give iron.

17. **How is thalassemia differentiated from iron deficiency?**
Both cause microcytic, hypochromic anemia, but thalassemia must be differentiated from iron deficiency because iron levels are normal in thalassemia. Iron supplementation is contraindicated in patients with thalassemia because it may cause iron overload. Look for elevations in hemoglobin A2 or hemoglobin F (beta thalassemia only); target cells, nucleated RBCs, and diffuse basophilia on peripheral smears; skull radiograph with "crew-cut" appearance; extramedullary hematopoiesis; splenomegaly; and positive family history. Thalassemia is more common in Blacks, Mediterraneans, and Asians.

18. **What diagnostic test confirms a diagnosis of thalassemia? How is it treated?**
Diagnosis is made by hemoglobin electrophoresis. There are four gene loci for the alpha chain of hemoglobin but only two for the beta chain. Patients with four affected loci produce no alpha globulin (hemoglobin Barts) and die in utero (hydrops fetalis), while patients with three affected loci (hemoglobin H) are symptomatic at birth or early childhood. Patients with beta thalassemia are not symptomatic until 6 months of age.
   No treatment is required for minor thalassemia. Patients are often asymptomatic because they are used to living with a lower level of hemoglobin. Thalassemia major is more symptomatic and severe. Treat with transfu-sions as needed and iron chelation therapy to prevent secondary hemochromatosis.

19. **What two clues on the Step 3 exam often point to a diagnosis of sickle cell disease?**
A peripheral blood smear and race. Eight percent of Blacks are heterozygous for the sickle cell trait. Know what sickled RBCs look like. Patients usually have a high percentage of reticulocytes (8%–20%).

20. **What are the clinical manifestations and complications of sickle cell disease?**
   - Aplastic crises (due to parvovirus B19 infection)
   - Bone pain (due to infarcts; the classic example is avascular necrosis of the femoral head)
   - Dactylitis (also known as hand-foot syndrome, seen in children)
   - Renal papillary necrosis
   - Splenic sequestration crisis
   - Autosplenectomy (increased infections with encapsulated bugs such as *Pneumococcus, Haemophilus,* and *Neisseria* spp.)
   - Acute chest syndrome (mimics pneumonia)
   - Pigment cholelithiasis
   - Priapism
   - Stroke

21. **How is sickle cell disease diagnosed and treated?**
Diagnosis is made by hemoglobin electrophoresis. Screening is done at birth, but symptoms usually do not appear until around 6 months of age because of the lack of adult hemoglobin production. Treat with prophylactic penicillin until at least 5 years of age and perhaps longer, beginning as soon as the diagnosis is made. Proper vaccination includes the pneumococcal, meningococcal, and *H. influenzae* type B vaccines (given to all children anyway), as well as yearly influenza vaccination. Other strategies include folate supplementation, early treatment of infections, and adequate hydration.
   A sickle cell crisis involves severe pain in various sites due to RBC sickling. Treat with oxygen, lots of intravenous fluids, and analgesics (do not be afraid to use narcotics). Consider transfusions if symptoms and/or findings are severe.

22. **What are the commonly tested causes of autoimmune hemolytic anemia?**
   - Systemic lupus erythematosus (or medications that cause lupuslike syndromes, such as procainamide, hydral-azine, and isoniazid) and other autoimmune disorders
   - Drugs (the classic example is methyldopa, but penicillins, cephalosporins, sulfa drugs, and quinidine also have been implicated)
   - Leukemia or lymphoma
   - Infection (the classic examples are mycoplasmosis, Epstein-Barr virus, and syphilis)

23. **What lab test is often positive in patients with autoimmune anemia?**
The **Coombs test** is positive in most autoimmune anemias. You may also see spherocytes on peripheral smear because of incomplete macrophage destruction (extravascular hemolysis) of RBCs.

24. What clues point to lead poisoning as a cause of anemia?

Lead poisoning causes a hypochromic, microcytic anemia, almost always in a child. With acute lead poisoning, look for vomiting, ataxia, colicky abdominal pain, irritability (aggressive behavior, behavioral regression), and encephalopathy, cerebral edema, or seizures. Usually, however, poisoning is chronic and low level with minimal nonspecific symptoms. Watch for basophilic stippling on peripheral smear, elevated free erythrocyte protoporphyrin or lead level, and consider risk factors for lead exposure (a child who eats paint chips or lives in an old, run-down building).

25. True or False: Children with risk factors should be screened for lead poisoning.

True. Screening all asymptomatic children with a serum lead level at 1 and 2 years old regardless of risk is becoming controversial. However, in children with risk factors, screening is very important because chronic low-level exposure may lead to permanent neurologic sequelae. Screening should start at 6 months in children with risk factors, such as pica (especially paint chips and dust in old buildings that may have lead paint), residence in an old or neglected building, and/or residence near or with family members who work at a lead-smelting or battery-recycling plant. Screen and measure symptomatic exposure with serum lead levels (normal value: <10 µg/dL).

26. How is lead poisoning treated?

Treat initially with decreased exposure (best strategy) as well as lead chelation therapy, if needed. Use succimer in children and dimercaprol in adults; in severe cases, use dimercaprol plus ethylenediamine tetraacetic acid (EDTA) for children or adults.

27. How can sideroblastic anemia be recognized on the Step 3 exam? Should the presence of sideroblastic anemia raise concern about other conditions?

The typical description is a microcytic hypochromic anemia with increased or normal iron, ferritin, and TIBC (transferrin). This description should immediately steer you away from iron deficiency. Look for polychromatophilic stippling and the classic ringed sideroblasts in bone marrow (know what it looks like). Sideroblastic anemia may be related to myelodysplasia or future blood dyscrasia. Although you will probably not be asked about management, treatment is supportive. In rare cases, the anemia responds to **pyridoxine.** Do not give iron.

28. Describe the hallmarks of spherocytosis.

This normochromic, normocytic anemia is associated with spherocytes on peripheral smear, positive family history (autosomal dominant), splenomegaly, positive osmotic fragility test, and an increased **mean corpuscular hemoglobin concentration** (the only occasion on which this RBC index is useful for the Step 3 exam). Treatment often involves splenectomy. Spherocytes may also be seen in extravascular hemolysis, but the osmotic fragility test is normal.

29. Why do chronic renal disease patients develop anemia? How do you treat it?

All patients with chronic renal failure develop a normocytic, normochromic anemia with decreased reticulocyte count due to decreased erythropoietin production. If necessary, give erythropoietin to correct the anemia.

30. What clues point to a diagnosis of aplastic anemia?

Although aplastic anemia may be idiopathic, on the Step 3 exam watch for chemotherapy, radiation, malignancy affecting the bone marrow (especially leukemias), benzene, and implicated medications (e.g., chloramphenicol, carbamazepine, sulfa drugs, zidovudine, gold). Decreased white blood cells (WBCs) and platelets accompany the anemia. Treat first by stopping any possible causative medication; then try antithymocyte globulin, colony-stimulating factors (such as erythropoietin, sargramostim, filgrastim, pegfilgrastim), or bone marrow transplant.

31. Define myelophthisic anemia. What clues on the peripheral smear suggest its presence?

Myelophthisic anemia is due to a space-occupying lesion in the bone marrow. The common causes are malignant invasion that destroys bone marrow (most common) and myelodysplasia or myelofibrosis. On the peripheral smear, look for marked anisocytosis (different size), poikilocytosis (different shape), nucleated RBCs, giant and/or bizarre-looking platelets, and **teardrop-shaped** RBCs (dactocytes). A bone marrow biopsy may reveal no cells ("dry tap" if the marrow is fibrotic) or malignant-looking cells.

32. How do you recognize glucose-6-phosphate dehydrogenase deficiency on the USMLE?

This genetic disorder is X-linked recessive, affecting males. It is most common in Blacks and Mediterraneans. Look for sudden hemolysis or anemia after exposure to fava beans or certain drugs (antimalarials, salicylates, sulfa drugs) or after infection. You may see **Heinz bodies** and "bite cells" on peripheral smear. The diagnosis is made with a RBC enzyme assay, which should not be done immediately after hemolysis because of the potential for a false-negative result (all of the older RBCs already have been destroyed, and the younger RBCs are not affected in most patients). Treat with avoidance of precipitating foods and medications; discontinue the triggering medication first.

33. Name some other causes of anemia.

- Endocrine failure (especially pituitary and thyroid; look for endocrine symptoms)
- Mechanical heart valves (hemolyzed RBCs)
- Disseminated intravascular coagulation (DIC), thrombotic thrombocytopenic purpura (TTP), and hemolytic uremic syndrome (look for schistocytes and RBC fragments on smear and other appropriate findings)

- Other hemoglobinopathies (the hemoglobin C and E varieties are fairly common)
- Paroxysmal nocturnal or cold hemoglobinuria
- *Clostridium perfringens* infection, malaria, and babesiosis (causes intravascular hemolysis and fever)
- Hypersplenism (associated with splenomegaly and often with low platelets and WBCs)

34. When is transfusion indicated for anemia (at what hemoglobin level)?

Always transfuse on clinical grounds; observe the symptoms. In other words, treat the patient, not the lab value. There is no such thing as a "trigger value" for transfusion. Having said this, hemoglobin levels less than 7 g/dL are typically an indication for transfusion.

35. What are the common causes of thrombocytopenia? What kinds of bleeding problems are caused by low platelet counts?

Common causes of thrombocytopenia include purpura (idiopathic or thrombotic), hemolytic uremic syndrome, DIC, human immunodeficiency virus (HIV), splenic sequestration, heparin (including heparin-induced thrombocytopenia; treat by first stopping heparin), other medications (especially quinidine and sulfa drugs), autoimmune disease, and alcohol. Bleeding from thrombocytopenia is in the form of petechiae, nosebleeds, and easy bruising.

36. Specify the main differences between thrombotic thrombocytopenic purpura and idiopathic thrombocytopenic purpura (ITP), including presentation and treatment.

	TTP	ITP
Most common age	Young adults	Children or adults
Previous infection	None	Viral (especially in children)
Red blood cell count	Low	Normal
Platelet count	Low	Low
Peripheral blood smear	Hemolysis	Normal
Kidney effects	ARF, proteinuria	None
Treatment	Plasmapheresis, NSAIDs; no platelets[†]	Steroids[*] splenectomy if drugs fail
Key differential points	CNS changes, age	Antiplatelet antibodies

ARF, Acute renal failure; *CNS*, central nervous system; *ITP*, idiopathic thrombocytopenic purpura; *NSAIDs*, nonsteroidal antiinflammatory drugs; *TTP*, thrombotic thrombocytopenic purpura.
*Give steroids only if the patient is bleeding or when platelet counts are very low ($<$20,000 cells/μL).
[†]Do not give platelet transfusions to patients with TTP; clots may form.

BLEEDING DISORDERS

1. How do specific diseases affect clotting tests? What are the main differential points?

Disease	PT	PTT	BT	Platelet Count	RBC Count	Other
von Willebrand disease	Normal	High	High	Normal	Normal	Autosomal dominant (look for family history)
Hemophilia A/B	Normal	High	Normal	Normal	Normal	X-linked recessive, A = low factor VII, B = low factor IX
Hemophilia C	Normal	High	Normal	Normal	Normal	Autosomal recessive, low factor XI
DIC	High	High	High	Low	Normal/low	Appropriate history, low level of factor VIII
Liver failure	High	High	Normal	Normal/low	Normal/low	Jaundice, normal factor 8 level; do not give vitamin K (ineffective); use FFP
Heparin	Normal	High	Normal	Normal/low	Normal	Watch for thrombocytopenia and thrombosis
Warfarin	High	Normal	Normal	Normal	Normal	Vitamin K antagonist (factors II, VII, IX, and X)
ITP	Normal	Normal	High	Low	Normal	Watch for preceding URI
TTP	Normal	Normal	High	Low	Low	Hemolysis (smear), CNS symptoms (hallucinations, altered mental status, headache, stroke); treat with plasmapheresis; do not give platelets!
Scurvy	Normal	Normal	Normal	Normal	Normal	Fingernail and gum hemorrhages, bone hemorrhages; caused by vitamin C deficiency

BT, Bleeding time; *CNS,* central nervous system; *DIC,* disseminated intravascular coagulation; *FFP,* fresh frozen plasma; *ITP,* idiopathic thrombocytopenic purpura; *PT,* prothrombin time; *PTT,* partial thromboplastin time; *RBC,* red blood cell; *TTP,* thrombotic thrombocytopenic purpura; *URI,* upper respiratory infection.

2. What are the most common causes of disseminated intravascular coagulation?
   The most common cause is pregnancy and obstetric complications (roughly 50% of cases), followed by malignancy (33%), sepsis, and trauma (especially head trauma, prostate surgery, and snake bites).

3. How do you recognize and treat disseminated intravascular coagulation in a classic at-risk patient?
   DIC usually manifests with bleeding diathesis but may have thrombotic tendencies. Look for the classic oozing or bleeding from puncture and intravenous sites; prolonged prothrombin time (PT), partial thromboplastin time (PTT), and bleeding time (BT). DIC is the only disorder on the Step 3 exam that prolongs all three tests. Other clues include positive D-dimer, increased fibrin degradation products, thrombocytopenia, decreased fibrin, and decreased clotting factors (including factor VIII).
   Treat the underlying cause (e.g., evacuate the uterus, give antibiotics). You may need to give transfusions with fresh frozen plasma or, in rare cases, heparin (only if thrombosis occurs).

4. Which clotting tests measure which portions of the coagulation cascade? Which medications affect these tests?
   Prothrombin time measures the function of the extrinsic clotting pathway (prolonged by warfarin), activated partial thromboplastin time measures the function of the intrinsic clotting pathway (prolonged by heparin), and bleeding time measures platelet function (prolonged by aspirin).

5. What causes petechiae or "platelet-type" bleeding in the setting of normal platelets?
   Vitamin C deficiency (scurvy) causes bleeding similar to that seen with low platelets (splinter and gum hemorrhages, petechiae); perifollicular and subperiosteal hemorrhages are unique to scurvy. Patients have a poor dietary history (the classic example is hot dogs and soda or tea and toast), myalgias and arthralgias, and capillary fragility (bleeding is due to collagen problems in the vessels). Treat with oral vitamin C.
   Other causes include uremia (results in platelet dysfunction), inherited connective tissue disorders (Ehlers-Danlos syndrome, Marfan syndrome), and chronic corticosteroid use (causes capillary fragility).

6. Which clotting factors are affected by vitamin K? What is the interaction of vitamin K and the liver?
   Vitamin K is needed for hepatic synthesis of factors II, VII, IX, and X as well as proteins C and S. Chronic liver disease (cirrhosis) can cause prolongation of PT and the international normalized ratio (INR) because the liver is unable to synthesize clotting factors even in the presence of adequate vitamin K levels. In the setting of active bleeding, this problem should be corrected with fresh frozen plasma, although the effects will only be temporary. Vitamin K is ineffective in the setting of severe liver disease.

REACTIONS TO BLOOD COMPONENTS

1. What are the indications for the use of various blood products?
   Whole blood: used only for rapid, massive blood loss or exchange transfusions (poisoning, TTP).
   Packed RBCs: used for routine transfusions.
   Washed RBCs: free of traces of plasma, white cells, and platelets; good for immunoglobulin A (IgA) deficiency as well as allergic or previously sensitized patients.
   Platelets: given for symptomatic thrombocytopenia (usually $<10,000/\mu L$).
   Granulocytes: used on rare occasions for neutropenia.
   Fresh frozen plasma: contains all clotting factors; used for bleeding diathesis when you cannot wait for vitamin K to take effect (e.g., DIC, severe warfarin poisoning) or when vitamin K will not work (liver failure).

2. What blood type can be given in an emergency to avoid a transfusion reaction?
   Type O negative blood can be used to avoid a reaction when you cannot wait for blood typing or when the blood bank does not have the patient's blood type.

3. Describe the signs and symptoms of a blood transfusion reaction.
   Look for **febrile reaction** (e.g., chills, fever, headache, back pain) from antibodies to WBCs; **hemolytic reaction** (e.g., anxiety or discomfort, dyspnea, chest pain, shock, jaundice) from antibodies to RBCs; or **allergic reaction** (e.g., urticaria, edema, dizziness, dyspnea, wheezing, and anaphylaxis) to an unknown component in donor serum. Oliguria may be an associated finding.

4. What should you do if you suspect a transfusion reaction?
   The first step is to *stop the transfusion.* If oliguria is present, treat with intravenous fluids and diuresis (mannitol or furosemide).

5. What are the other risks of transfusion?
   There is a small but real risk of infection (usually viral infections such as hepatitis B and C, HIV, and cytomegalovirus), development of noncardiogenic pulmonary edema (transfusion-associated circulatory overload or transfusion-related acute lung injury), and hyperkalemia (from hemolysis). With large transfusions (>5 units packed

RBCs), bleeding diathesis may result from dilutional thrombocytopenia and citrate (a blood preservative and calcium chelator that prevents clotting). Look for oozing from puncture or intravenous sites. With massive transfusion there is a possibility of developing hypocalcemia due to citrate preservative binding to calcium.

MALIGNANT NEOPLASIAS

1. With what conditions is basophilia associated?
   Allergies or neoplasm/blood dyscrasia.

2. What are the key differential points for the commonly tested blood dyscrasias?

Type	Age	What to Look for in Case Description, Trigger Words
ALL	Children (peak age 3–5 yr)	Pancytopenia (bleeding, fever, anemia), history of radiation therapy, Down syndrome
AML	>30 yr	Pancytopenia (bleeding, fever, anemia), Auer rods, DIC
CML	30–50 yr	WBC count >50,000, Philadelphia chromosome (t[9;22]), blast crisis, splenomegaly
CLL	>50 yr	Male gender, lymphadenopathy, lymphocytosis, infections, smudge cells, splenomegaly
Hairy cell leukemia	Adults	Blood smear (hairlike projections), splenomegaly, TRAP staining
Mycosis fungoides/Sézary syndrome	>50 yr	Plaquelike, itchy skin rash that does not improve with treatment, a blood smear shows cerebriform nuclei known as butt cells, Pautrier abscesses in epidermis
Burkitt lymphoma	Children	Associated with Epstein-Barr virus (in Africa), (t[8;14]), "starry sky" on histology
CNS B-cell lymphoma	Adults	Seen in patients with HIV infection, AIDS
T-cell leukemia	Adults	Caused by HTLV-1 virus
Hodgkin disease	15–34 yr	Reed-Sternberg cell, painless cervical lymphadenopathy, night sweats, lymph nodes become painful with alcohol consumption
Non-Hodgkin lymphoma	Any age	Small follicular type has the best prognosis; diffuse large type has the worst prognosis; primary tumor may be located in the gastrointestinal tract
Myelodysplasia/myelofibrosis	>50 yr	Anemia, teardrop cells, dry tap on bone marrow biopsy, high MCV and RDW; associated with CML
Multiple myeloma	>40 yr	Bence Jones protein (IgG 50%, IgA 25%), osteolytic lesions, high serum calcium, anemia, renal impairment
Waldenström macroglobulinemia	>40 yr	Hyperviscosity syndrome, IgM spike, cold agglutinins (Raynaud phenomenon with cold sensitivity)
Polycythemia vera	>40 yr	High hematocrit/hemoglobin, aquagenic pruritus; use phlebotomy
Primary thrombocythemia	>50 yr	Platelet count usually >1,000,000 cells/mL; may have bleeding or thrombosis

AIDS, Acquired immunodeficiency syndrome; *ALL,* acute lymphoblastic leukemia; *AML,* acute myelogenous leukemia; *CLL,* chronic lymphocytic leukemia; *CML,* chronic myelogenous leukemia; *CNS,* central nervous system; *DIC,* disseminated intravascular coagulation; *HIV,* human immunodeficiency virus; *HTLV-1,* human lymphotropic virus 1; *Ig,* immunoglobulin; *MCV,* mean corpuscular volume; *RDW,* red cell distribution width; *TRAP,* tartrate-resistant acid phosphatase; *WBC,* white blood cell.

3. What is the difference between acute leukemia and chronic leukemia?
   For acute leukemia, look for proliferation of minimally differentiated cells such as lymphoblasts and myeloblasts. There should be more than 20% blasts in the bone marrow. Chronic leukemia is marked by proliferation of more differentiated cells such as lymphocytes and myelocytes.

4. Who tends to get acute lymphocytic leukemia (ALL)? What are the presenting symptoms?
   ALL is most common in children and has a higher incidence in those with Down syndrome. Look for nonspecific symptoms such as fever, lethargy, and a sore throat; start thinking ALL if there is persistence of the fever, bone pain, and/or easy bruising.

5. How is acute lymphocytic leukemia diagnosed? How is it treated? What is the prognosis?
   Look for an elevated or depressed WBC count, a markedly decreased platelet count, and elevated LDH and uric acid. Lymphoblasts will be seen on a peripheral blood smear. Confirm the diagnosis with a bone marrow biopsy.

Order a chest x-ray, a computed tomography (CT) scan, and a lumbar puncture to evaluate for extramedullary involvement/metastases. Treat with chemotherapy. Prognosis is determined by the age of onset and the results of cytogenetic studies. Five-year survival rates are now greater than 85% in children but are lower in adults (30%–40% overall cure rate).

6. **Who gets acute myelogenous leukemia (AML)? What are the presenting symptoms?**
Most cases of AML occur in adults. Look for symptoms similar to those for ALL, such as easy bruising, fatigue, fever, anemia, and frequent infections. Patients may also have central nervous system involvement, DIC, or gingival hyperplasia.

7. **How is acute myelogenous leukemia diagnosed?**
Look for an increase in myeloid cell lines, as well as decreased leukocyte alkaline phosphatase (LAP) and elevated uric acid levels. A peripheral blood smear will show a predominance of myeloblasts. Look for Auer rods. Confirm the diagnosis with a bone marrow biopsy.

8. **How is acute myelogenous leukemia treated?**
AML is classified into subtypes; treatment depends on the subtype, but chemotherapy (and sometimes bone marrow transplantation) is the key to treatment.

9. **What is chronic lymphocytic leukemia (CLL)? What are the presenting symptoms?**
CLL is a malignancy of mature lymphocytes that is usually seen in patients older than 65 years. CLL is an indolent disease characterized by fatigue, lymphadenopathy, and hepatosplenomegaly. It is sometimes diagnosed incidentally when a CBC reveals lymphocytosis.

10. **How is chronic lymphocytic leukemia diagnosed? How is it treated?**
Look for lymphocytosis alone on a CBC with normal hemoglobin, hematocrit, and platelet counts. A peripheral blood smear will show many small lymphocytes. Confirm with a bone marrow biopsy; look for smudge cells and CD5$^+$ expression.
Asymptomatic patients do not require treatment. If the patient is symptomatic or has advanced-stage CLL, the treatment is radiation therapy (for localized CLL) or chemotherapy (for advanced CLL).

11. **What is chronic myelogenous leukemia (CML)? Who gets it? What are the presenting symptoms?**
CML is a malignancy of myeloid cells that typically occurs in middle-aged adults. It typically remains in a chronic phase for several years and then transforms into an acute leukemia as a blast crisis, which often results in death within a few months.
CML may be found incidentally on a CBC that reveals leukocytosis. In a symptomatic patient, look for nonspecific symptoms such as fatigue, malaise, fever, weight loss, and night sweats. The symptoms of an acute blast crisis include fever, weight loss, bone pain, and splenomegaly.

12. **How is chronic myelogenous leukemia diagnosed?**
Look for a markedly elevated WBC count (often of the order of 150,000 cells/μL) with leukocytosis, prominence of myeloid cells with basophilia on a peripheral blood smear, decreased LAP, and an elevated vitamin B$_{12}$ level. Confirm the diagnosis with demonstration of the Philadelphia chromosome or the BCR-ABL complex via cytogenetic analysis, fluorescence in situ hybridization (FISH) analysis, or reverse transcription polymerase chain reaction (RT-PCR) for blood or bone marrow samples.

13. **How is chronic myelogenous leukemia treated?**
Tyrosine kinase inhibitors (e.g., imatinib, dasatinib, or nilotinib) are the initial treatment of choice for most patients with CML. Bone marrow transplantation is an option for some patients in the blast phase.

14. **What is Hodgkin lymphoma? What are the presenting symptoms?**
Hodgkin lymphoma is a malignancy of Reed-Sternberg cells (B-cell origin) for which the typical presentation is cervical lymphadenopathy, as well as the so-called B symptoms: fever (>100.4°F [38°C]), night sweats, and weight loss (>10% over ≤6 months).

15. **How is Hodgkin lymphoma diagnosed? What is the treatment?**
Biopsy an enlarged lymph node to make the diagnosis and look for the presence of Reed-Sternberg cells. Staging is based on the Ann Arbor system and includes a number (I–IV according to the anatomic location of the tumor) and either A or B symptoms, where A indicates the absence of symptoms and B symptoms are as described in the previous question. Treatment is with combination chemotherapy.

16. **What is non-Hodgkin lymphoma? What are the presenting symptoms? How is non-Hodgkin lymphoma diagnosed? What is the treatment?**
Non-Hodgkin lymphoma is a diverse group of malignant neoplasms derived from B-cell progenitors, T-cell progenitors, mature T cells, and sometimes natural killer cells. The symptoms and diagnosis are similar to those for Hodgkin lymphoma. Treatment is with combination chemotherapy.

17. **What are the presenting symptoms for multiple myeloma?**
Multiple myeloma is a malignancy of plasma cells that is typically seen in older adults. Look for back pain, pathologic fractures, fatigue, frequent infections, and signs/symptoms of hypercalcemia. Multiple myeloma needs to be included in the differential diagnosis for a patient with hypercalcemia, anemia, renal failure, or bone pain.

18. **How is multiple myeloma diagnosed?**
Order serum protein electrophoresis (SPEP) to look for monoclonal immunoglobulin. Other important tests include a CBC, a chemistry screen (including calcium, albumin, creatinine, LDH, and beta$_2$-microglobulin), and serum free monoclonal light-chain analysis. Perform a bone marrow biopsy to confirm the diagnosis (>10% plasma cells) and a full-body skeletal survey to look for osteolytic lesions of the skull and long bones.

19. **How is multiple myeloma treated?**
There are several chemotherapy regimens for the treatment of multiple myeloma that are beyond the scope of the Step 3 exam. However, remember that you will also need to treat the signs, symptoms, and complications of multiple myeloma:
- Hypercalcemia: hydration, steroids, bisphosphonates such as zoledronic acid and pamidronate
- Renal insufficiency: avoid nephrotoxins, maintain hydration, and perform plasmapheresis or hemodialysis as needed
- Bone pain from skeletal lesions: local radiation, bisphosphonates
- Infections: pneumococcal vaccine, yearly influenza vaccine; prophylactic antibiotic administration is controversial
- Anemia: erythropoietin; RBC transfusions as needed
- Hyperviscosity syndrome: plasmapheresis
- Thrombosis: no specific treatment, but be aware that patients with multiple myeloma are at higher risk of both venous thromboembolism and arterial thromboembolism (stroke, transient ischemic attacks, myocardial infarction, peripheral arterial disease)

20. **What are the most common types of cancer in children and young adults (age <30 years)?**
Leukemia and lymphoma.

INFECTIONS

1. **With what conditions is eosinophilia associated?**
- Allergic or atopic diseases (allergic rhinitis, asthma, allergic bronchopulmonary aspergillosis, eczema, urticaria, atopic dermatitis, milk-protein allergy, drug reactions)
- Parasitic infections
- Fungal infections
- HIV infection
- Malignancies (lymphoma, leukemia, lung cancer, gastric cancer, pancreatic cancer, colon cancer, ovarian cancer)
- Connective tissue/autoimmune diseases (Churg-Strauss vasculitis, rheumatoid arthritis, lupus, scleroderma, eosinophilic fasciitis, Dressler syndrome, inflammatory bowel disease)
- Granulomatous disorders (sarcoidosis)
- Skin disorders (psoriasis, pemphigus)
- Immune disorders (Wiskott-Aldrich syndrome, hyper-IgE syndrome, IgA deficiency, thymoma)
- Adrenal insufficiency
- Pulmonary eosinophilia (Löffler syndrome)
- Cirrhosis
- Atheroembolic disease
- Familial eosinophilia
- Eosinophilia-myalgia syndrome (from using l-tryptophan)

2. **What are the systemic inflammatory response syndrome (SIRS) criteria?**
1. Temperature less than 96.8°F (<36°C) or greater than 100.4°F (>38°C)
2. Heart rate greater than 90 beats/min
3. Respiratory rate greater than 24 breaths/min or PCO$_2$ of less than 32 mm Hg
4. Leukocyte count greater than 12,000 cells/mL or less than 4000 cells/mL, or greater than 10% bands on a peripheral blood smear

3. **How do you define systemic inflammatory response syndrome, sepsis, severe sepsis, and septic shock?**
- SIRS is a serious condition related to systemic inflammation, organ dysfunction, and organ failure, and it can be a sign of sepsis. SIRS can be diagnosed when two of the SIRS criteria are met.
- Sepsis requires at least two of the SIRS criteria with evidence of an infectious process.
- Severe sepsis involves the sepsis criteria plus evidence of organ dysfunction or tissue hypoperfusion (manifesting as hypotension, elevated lactate level, acute kidney injury, or decreased urine output).
- Septic shock is severe sepsis plus persistently low blood pressure that does not respond to fluid resuscitation.

4. What are the principles for the management of sepsis?

Early goal-directed therapy involves adjustments of cardiac preload, afterload, and contractility to balance oxygen delivery with oxygen demand. The main principles for management of sepsis are early initiation of supportive care to correct physiologic abnormalities (e.g., hypotension and hypoxemia) and distinguishing sepsis from SIRS. The standard workup typically includes CBC, lactate, electrolytes, blood urea nitrogen, creatinine, glucose, aspartate aminotransferase, alanine aminotransferase, PT, and PTT tests. Measure arterial blood gas if respiratory failure is a concern. If an infection is present or suspected, identify it and treat it as soon as possible. Studies such as a chest x-ray, urinalysis, urine culture, and blood cultures are usually indicated. Sputum samples, cerebrospinal fluid analysis, and additional imaging such as CT scanning may be required.

- Stabilize respiration: give oxygen and monitor pulse oximetry. Intubate and provide mechanical ventilation if needed for respiratory failure or a depressed level of consciousness.
- Assess perfusion: systolic blood pressure of less than 90 mm Hg or mean arterial pressure (MAP) of less than 70 mm Hg indicates hypotension and inadequate perfusion. Also look for cool vasoconstricted skin, tachycardia, obtundation, or oliguria/anuria. Insert an arterial catheter as needed. An elevated serum lactate level (>1 mmol/L) can indicate organ hypoperfusion, and a level of 4 mmol/L or greater is an independent predictor of septic shock.
- Establish central venous access: patients with septic shock generally require a central venous catheter to infuse vasopressor agents and for hemodynamic monitoring. Patients with severe sepsis generally do not require a catheter because they are fluid responsive and therefore do not need vasopressor agents or invasive hemodynamic monitoring.
- Initial resuscitation: give fluids aggressively (large-volume infusions) in the first 6 hours to increase the central venous pressure (CVP) to 8 to 12 mm Hg, the central venous oxygen saturation to 70%, the MAP to 65 mm Hg or greater, and urine output to 0.5 mL/kg/hour or greater. The newest sepsis guidelines recommend intravenous fluids at 30 mL/kg in patients for whom there is no contraindication to this strategy.
- Vasopressors: use in patients who remain hypotensive despite adequate fluid resuscitation (e.g., when the CVP is 8–12 mm Hg and the MAP remains <65 mm Hg).
- Central venous oxygen: once the CVP and MAP goals are met, if the central venous oxygen saturation is less than 70%, the patient needs an increase in either (1) cardiac output (via dobutamine administration) or (2) oxygen-carrying capacity (via RBC transfusion). If the hemoglobin level is less than 10 g/dL, transfuse; if not, use dobutamine to increase the central venous oxygen saturation to greater than 70%.
- Antibiotics: start intravenous antibiotic therapy immediately after obtaining the appropriate cultures. When choosing the antibiotic, consider the patient's history, Gram stain data, and local resistance patterns. Initial empiric therapy should involve a broad-spectrum antibiotic against gram-positive and gram-negative bacteria. Vancomycin plus either ceftriaxone, piperacillin-tazobactam, or imipenem is a good starting point. If *Pseudomonas* infection is possible, use a regimen such as vancomycin plus ceftazidime plus imipenem.

TOXIC EFFECTS

1. What is the most important side effect of heparin?

Heparin can cause two types of thrombocytopenia. The first is a nonimmune form that is of no clinical consequence and is characterized by a slight fall in platelet count during the first 2 days. The platelet count generally returns to normal with continued heparin administration. The second form is less common but more serious and is called type II heparin-induced thrombocytopenia (HIT). In this immune-mediated disorder, antibodies are formed against the heparin-platelet factor IV complex. In immune-mediated HIT, the platelet count falls by more than 50%, typically 5 to 10 days after heparin therapy is initiated. Immune-mediated HIT can lead to both arterial and venous thrombosis. The diagnosis of HIT is made on clinical grounds but can be confirmed with a functional assay. If HIT is suspected, heparin (and low-molecular-weight heparin) should be discontinued immediately.

Measure CBCs to monitor platelet counts in patients being treated with heparin.

2. How are the effects of aspirin, heparin, and warfarin monitored?

Heparin is monitored in terms of **PTT,** a measure of the internal coagulation pathway. Warfarin is monitored using **PT,** a measure of the external coagulation pathway. Aspirin prolongs **BT,** a measure of platelet function. Clinically, the effect of aspirin is not monitored via laboratory testing but be aware that it prolongs the BT test.

3. How are the effects of low-molecular-weight heparin monitored?

Low-molecular-weight heparin does not affect any of the coagulation parameters mentioned in the previous question, and its effect is not clinically monitored. In rare cases, a special type of factor X assay (anti-Xa) is used to measure its effect.

4. In an emergency, how can you reverse the effects of heparin, warfarin, and aspirin?

Heparin and low-molecular-weight heparin can be reversed with **protamine,** warfarin with fresh frozen plasma (contains clotting factors; immediate effect) and/or vitamin K (takes a few days to work), and aspirin with platelet transfusions and DDAVP.

CHAPTER 14

DISORDERS OF THE MALE REPRODUCTIVE SYSTEM

MALE REPRODUCTIVE SYSTEM

1. List the relevant characteristics of normal semen analysis.
   Ejaculate volume greater than 1.5 mL
   Sperm concentration greater than 15 million/mL
   Initial forward motility greater than 32% of sperm
   Normal morphology greater than 60% of sperm

2. What do you need to know about breast cancer in men?
   Breast cancer is about 100 times more common in women than in men and tends to occur at an older age in men than in women. Rates of breast cancer are higher in Blacks, who also have a poorer prognosis. Risk factors include family history, obesity, sedentary lifestyle, Jewish ancestry, and prior chest-wall irradiation. Invasive ductal breast cancers account for more than 90% of male breast cancers. The typical presenting sign is a painless, firm, subareolar mass.

3. How is male breast cancer diagnosed and treated?
   Mammography is typically performed, but a biopsy is required to confirm the diagnosis and check hormone receptors and HER2 (also known as ERBB2) expression. Simple mastectomy with lymph node evaluation is typically performed. Additional therapies may include chest-wall radiation, tamoxifen, and chemotherapy, depending on the risk of relapse, lymph node involvement, hormone receptor status, and tumor size. Genetic counseling and *BRCA1* and *BRCA2* gene mutation testing should be strongly considered.

4. What are the three main risk factors for prostate cancer?
   Age: prostate cancer is rare in men younger than 40 years old. The incidence increases with age, and about 60% of men older than 80 years have at least microscopic prostate cancer.
   Race: Black greater than White greater than Asian.
   Family history: men who have a family history of prostate cancer are more likely to develop the disease at a younger age and to die from it than men who do not have a family history of prostate cancer.

5. How do you recognize prostate cancer on the Step 3 exam?
   Look for patients older than 50 years. Patients often present late because early prostate cancer is asymptomatic. Look for symptoms typical of benign prostatic hyperplasia (BPH; urinary hesitancy, dysuria, frequency) with hematuria and/or elevated prostate-specific antigen (PSA). Look for prostate irregularities (nodules) on a rectal examination. Patients may also have back pain from vertebral metastases, which are osteoblastic.

6. How is prostate cancer treated?
   Local prostate cancer is treated with surgery (prostatectomy) or local radiation. For metastatic disease, treatment is androgen deprivation therapy (ADT) with surgical or medical orchiectomy to suppress serum testosterone levels. Options include orchiectomy or medical treatment with a GnRH agonist (leuprolide, goserelin, buserelin, triptorelin) combined with an antiandrogen such as an androgen-receptor antagonist (flutamide) or a GnRH antagonist (degarelix). Radiation therapy is used for local disease or pain from bony metastases. Chemotherapy can be combined with ADT for patients with extensive metastatic disease.

7. Define cryptorchidism. When does it occur?
   Cryptorchidism is arrested descent of the testicle(s) between the renal area and the scrotum. The more premature the infant, the greater the likelihood of cryptorchidism. Many arrested testes eventually descend on their own within the first year. Intramuscular human chorionic gonadotropin (hCG) may be used to induce testicular descent. After 1 year, surgical intervention (orchiopexy) is warranted in an attempt to preserve fertility as well as to facilitate future testicular exams. Affected testes have an increased risk for testicular cancer.

8. True or False: It is important to place abdominal testes in the scrotum surgically to decrease the risk of cancer.
   False. Cryptorchidism is a major risk factor for testicular cancer (40 times increased risk), but bringing the testis into the scrotum probably does not alter the increased risk. It does make cancer easier to detect via testicular exam. The higher the testicle is found (the further away from the scrotum), the higher the risk of developing testicular cancer and the lower the likelihood of retaining fertility.

9. **What should you know about testicular cancer?**
It is the most common solid malignancy in adult men younger than 30 years of age. The main risk factor is **cryptorchidism.** Transillumination and ultrasound help to distinguish a hydrocele (which is filled with fluid and transilluminates) from cancer (solid and does not transilluminate). The most common histologic type is seminoma, which is radiosensitive and highly curable. Use ultrasound to make the diagnosis.

10. **How does testicular cancer usually present? Describe the major risk factors, histology, and treatment.**
Testicular cancer usually presents as a painless testicular mass or enlargement of the testes in a young man (15–35 years old). The main risk factor is cryptorchidism. Roughly 90% are germ cell tumors; the most common type is **seminoma.** The non–seminoma germ cell tumors include yolk sac tumors, choriocarcinomas, embryonal carcinomas, and teratomas. Stromal tumors (non–germ cell) include Leydig cell and Sertoli cell tumors. Testicular cancer is generally treated with orchiectomy and radiation; if disease is widespread, use chemotherapy. Alpha-fetoprotein is a marker for yolk sac tumors; human chorionic gonadotropin is a marker for choriocarcinoma. Leydig cell tumors may secrete androgens and cause precocious puberty.

11. **Cover the right-hand columns and specify the classic differences between testicular torsion and epididymitis. What imaging test can diagnose and distinguish these two conditions?**

	Testicular Torsion	*Epididymitis*
Age	<20 yr (usually prepubertal)	>20 yr
Appearance	Testis may be elevated into the inguinal canal; swelling	Swollen testis, overlying erythema, urethral discharge/urethritis, prostatitis
Prehn sign	Pain stays the same or worsens	Pain decreases with testicular elevation
Cremasteric reflex	Abnormal	Normal, present
Treatment	Attempt to reduce, but ultimately most go to immediate surgery to salvage testis; surgical orchiopexy for both testes	Antibiotics*

*In men age <50 years, epididymitis is commonly due to sexually transmitted disease (e.g., chlamydial infection and gonorrhea). Treat with ceftriaxone and doxycycline. In men age >50 years, epididymitis is commonly due to urinary tract infection (e.g., *Escherichia coli*). Treat with trimethoprim-sulfamethoxazole or ciprofloxacin.

Ultrasound is the diagnostic test of choice in the setting of testicular/scrotal pain. It can easily differentiate between these two conditions as well as visualize testicular tumors (which sometimes present with pain, although they are classically painless).

12. **What are the symptoms and sequelae of benign prostatic hyperplasia?**
BPH can cause urinary hesitancy, intermittency, terminal dribbling, decreased size and force of the urinary stream, sensation of incomplete emptying, nocturia, urgency, dysuria, and frequency. It may result in acute urinary retention, urinary tract infections, hydronephrosis, and even kidney damage or failure in severe cases.

13. **How is BPH treated?**
Medical therapy, which is started when the patient becomes symptomatic, includes long-acting alpha$_1$-blockers (e.g., terazosin, doxazosin, tamsulosin, alfuzosin, and silodosin) and 5-alpha-reductase inhibitors (finasteride, dutasteride). Transurethral resection of the prostate (TURP) is used for more advanced cases, especially with repeated urinary tract infections, urosepsis, urinary retention, and/or hydronephrosis or kidney damage due to reflux. Surgical prostatectomy is used in some patients but is associated with a higher complication rate.

14. **How do you recognize and manage acute urinary retention?**
Acute urinary retention generally presents with abdominal pain; palpation of a full, distended bladder on abdominal exam; enlarged prostate on exam and/or a history of BPH in men; and a lack of urination in the past 24 hours or longer. A volume less than 50 mL is a normal postvoid residual volume on bladder scan in patients under 65 years old, and a volume less than 100 mL is normal in patients over 65 years old. The first step is to empty the bladder. If you cannot pass a regular Foley catheter, consider the use of a larger catheter with a firm coudé tip, or alternatively do a suprapubic tap to drain the bladder. Then address the underlying cause—usually BPH, which in this setting is generally treated with TURP.

15. **What are the common causes of erectile dysfunction?**
Erectile dysfunction is caused most commonly by vascular problems and atherosclerosis. Medications are also a common culprit (especially antihypertensive and antidepressant agents). Diabetes can cause impotence through vascular (increased atherosclerosis) or neurogenic (diabetic autonomic neuropathy) compromise. Hypogonadism can also cause impotence (look for small testes and loss of secondary sexual characteristics). Patients undergoing dialysis are often impotent. Remember "**p**oint and **s**hoot": **p**arasympathetics mediate erection; **s**ympathetics mediate ejaculation.

The history often gives you a clue if the cause of impotence is psychogenic. Look for a normal pattern of nocturnal erections, selective dysfunction (the patient has normal erections when masturbating but not with his partner), and a history of stress, anxiety, or fear.

16. **Distinguish between hydrocele and varicocele.**
A **hydrocele** represents a remnant of the processus vaginalis (remember embryology?) and transilluminates. It generally causes no symptoms and needs no treatment. A **varicocele** is a dilatation of the pampiniform venous plexus ("bag of worms," usually on the left). It does not transilluminate, disappears in the supine position, and becomes prominent with standing or the Valsalva maneuver. Varicoceles may cause infertility or pain and can be treated surgically.

17. **Define epispadias and hypospadias. How are they treated?**
Both are congenital penile anomalies. In **hypospadias,** the urethra opens on the ventral (under) side of the penis. In **epispadias,** the urethra opens on the dorsal (top) side of the penis. Epispadias is associated with exstrophy of the bladder. Both are treated with surgical correction.

INFECTIONS

1. **What are the presenting symptoms for prostatitis?**
For acute prostatitis, look for a spiking fever, chills, dysuria, malaise, irritative urinary symptoms (e.g., urgency, frequency, urge incontinence), cloudy urine, and pelvic, perineal, or testicular pain. Pain at the tip of the penis is common. Swelling of the prostate can result in voiding symptoms (e.g., hesitancy and dribbling or even acute urinary retention).

2. **What are the examination findings for prostatitis? What tests should be performed if prostatitis is suspected?**
Look for a tender, firm, edematous prostate gland on digital rectal examination. A urine Gram stain and culture should be performed.

3. **What organisms cause prostatitis? What is the treatment for prostatitis?**
E. coli is responsible for most cases of prostatitis, but *Proteus, Klebsiella, Enterobacter, Serratia,* and *Pseudomonas* spp. also cause prostatitis. Staphylococci, streptococci, and enterococci have been implicated but are much less common. Treat empirically with trimethoprim-sulfamethoxazole or a fluoroquinolone for about 2 weeks (although some physicians treat for up to 6 weeks). Urine culture results can further guide the choice of therapy.

4. **What is the classic cause of orchitis? How is it treated? Does it usually cause infertility?**
Mumps can cause orchitis, which classically presents with a painful, swollen testis in a postpubertal male. The best treatment is prevention (immunization against the mumps virus). Mumps orchitis rarely causes sterility because it is usually unilateral. Bacterial orchitis is typically due to spread from adjacent bacterial epididymitis and is termed epididymo-orchitis.

5. **What do you need to know about syphilis, human immunodeficiency virus (HIV), hepatitis B virus (HBV), and hepatitis C virus (HCV)?**
Syphilis and HIV are discussed in detail in Chapter 15. HBV and HCV are discussed in detail in Chapter 5.

6. **What are the presenting symptoms for genital herpes in men? What causes it?**
Look for painful vesicles in the anogenital region as a result of infection with human herpes simplex virus (HSV), typically type 2. Other signs and symptoms may include tingling in the genital area, fever, headache, myalgias, and tender inguinal lymphadenopathy.

7. **How do you diagnose genital herpes? What is the treatment?**
Genital herpes is often a clinical diagnosis, but it can be confirmed by viral polymerase chain reaction (PCR) after unroofing a vesicle. Primary episodes of genital herpes can be treated with acyclovir, famciclovir, or valacyclovir. Treatment of recurrences depends on the frequency of episodes and severity of symptoms. For frequent episodes or severe symptoms, suppressive therapy with any of the abovementioned medications may be considered.

8. **What causes infectious urethritis in men? What are the presenting symptoms?**
Chlamydia and gonorrhea cause most cases of infectious urethritis in sexually active men, but *Mycoplasma genitalium,* HSV, and *Treponema pallidum* (syphilis) must also be considered. Dysuria is the most common complaint, but other signs and symptoms include itching, burning, and a urethral discharge. Urethral discharges can range from watery to purulent.

9. **How is urethritis diagnosed?**
Diagnosis can be made on the basis of symptoms but can also be supported by the presence of a urethral discharge, polymorphonuclear neutrophils on a Gram stain of a urethral swab, positive leukocyte esterase on a urine dipstick, or 10 or more white blood cells per high-power field on urinalysis. Urine PCR for *Chlamydia* and gonorrhea should be performed in all cases of suspected urethritis.

10. How is urethritis treated?

   Empiric treatment for suspected gonococcal urethritis is 250 mg of ceftriaxone intramuscularly and a single oral dose of 1 g of azithromycin, which treats *Chlamydia trachomatis* (treatment for *Chlamydia* is included because it can be asymptomatic). For patients with confirmed nongonococcal urethritis, treat with 1 g of azithromycin orally or 100 mg of doxycycline twice daily for 7 days.

11. What diseases does human papillomavirus (HPV) infection cause in males? Which HPV subtypes are responsible?

   Most men who get HPV never develop any signs or symptoms. HPV types 6 and 11 cause 90% of genital warts. Anal cancer is rare, but the incidence is rising; HPV types 16 and 18 cause 70% of anal cancers and precancerous anal lesions. HPV is also implicated in the rising incidence of squamous cell carcinoma of the head and neck.

12. What is the current recommendation regarding vaccination against HPV in males?

   The US Advisory Committee on Immunization Practices (ACIP) recommends vaccination against HPV in all boys and girls at ages 11 to 12 years; vaccination can be given starting at age 9 years. Catchup HPV vaccination is recommended for all persons through age 26 years.

TRAUMA AND TOXIC EFFECTS

1. What are the signs of urethral injury?

   Usually urethral injury occurs in the context of pelvic trauma. The four classic findings are an absent or abnormally positioned prostate on exam (i.e., "high-riding prostate"), difficulty or inability to urinate, blood at the urethral meatus, and scrotal/perineal ecchymosis.

2. True or False: Urethral injury is a contraindication to insertion of a Foley catheter.

   True. Always look for the four warning signs of urethral injury. If even one of these signs is present, do not attempt to insert a Foley catheter. Order a retrograde urethrogram to rule out urethral injury in this setting.

CHAPTER 15

DISORDERS OF THE IMMUNE SYSTEM

IMMUNODEFICIENCY DISORDERS

1. What is the most common primary immunodeficiency? How do you recognize it?
Immunoglobulin A (IgA) deficiency, which causes recurrent respiratory and gastrointestinal (GI) infections. IgA levels are always low, and levels of IgG subclass 2 may be low. Do not give immunoglobulins, which may cause anaphylaxis due to development of anti-IgA antibodies. Alternatively, if any patient develops anaphylaxis after immunoglobulin exposure or blood transfusion, you should think of IgA deficiency.

2. How do you recognize Bruton agammaglobulinemia?
Bruton agammaglobulinemia (X-linked agammaglobulinemia) is an X-linked recessive disorder with low or absent B cells due to no B-cell maturation. It is caused by a defect in the *BTK* gene. Infections begin after 6 months when maternal antibodies disappear. Look for recurrent lung or sinus infections with *Streptococcus* and *Haemophilus* spp. and absent/scanty lymph nodes and tonsils. Therapy includes immunoglobin replacement therapy and prophylactic antibiotics in certain situations.

3. What is the classic cause of severe combined immunodeficiency (SCID)? How does it present?
SCID may be autosomal recessive or X-linked. The classic cause is **adenosine deaminase deficiency** (autosomal recessive), though X-linked is the most common cause of SCID (i.e., a defect in the interleukin-2 [IL2] receptor gamma chain). Patients have B- and T-cell defects and severe infections in the first few months of life. Other symptoms include failure to thrive, cutaneous anergy, chronic diarrhea, and absent or dysplastic thymus and lymph nodes. Treatment is stem cell transplant.

4. Describe the pathophysiology of chronic granulomatous disease (CGD).
CGD is usually an X-linked recessive disorder that affects males. Because of a defect in the activity of the enzyme nicotinamide adenine dinucleotide phosphate (NADPH) oxidase, patients have recurrent infections with catalase-positive organisms (e.g., *Staphylococcus aureus*, *Pseudomonas* sp., *Aspergillus*, *Candida*). Diagnosis is clinched if the question mentions deficient nitroblue tetrazolium (NBT) dye reduction by granulocytes. This test measures the respiratory burst, which patients with CGD lack. The patient will have a yellow/colorless NBT test (a positive test is blue and means that the respiratory burst is intact). On the USMLE, if you see "CGD," then look for "NBT" in the answer choices. Another test that might be mentioned is the dihydrorhodamine test, which is essentially flow cytometry.

5. Complement deficiencies of C5 through C9 cause recurrent infections with which genus of bacteria?
Neisseria species.

6. Define chronic mucocutaneous candidiasis.
Chronic mucocutaneous candidiasis is a cellular immunodeficiency specific for candida infection. Patients have thrush and candidal infections of the scalp, skin, and nails as well as anergy to *Candida* sp. with skin testing. It is often associated with hypothyroidism. The rest of the immune function is intact; no other types of infections are present.

7. Give the classic description of hyper-IgE syndrome (Job-Buckley syndrome).
Patients with hyper-IgE syndrome have recurrent staphylococcal infections (especially of the skin) and extremely high IgE levels. They also commonly have fair skin, coarse facial features, eczema, retained primary teeth, and recurrent fractures.

8. Discuss the mechanism of action of the commonly used immunosuppressant drugs in transplant medicine.
- Steroids inhibit the production of IL1, IL2, and IL6 as well as tumor necrosis factor (TNF)–alpha and interferon (IFN)–gamma. Prednisone is most commonly used.
- Methotrexate is a folic acid antagonist, but the precise mechanism in immunosuppression is unclear.
- Cyclosporine is a calcineurin inhibitor that inhibits IL2 production.
- Tacrolimus is another calcineurin inhibitor that inhibits signaling through the T-cell receptor and production of IL2.

- Mycophenolate prevents T-cell activation.
- Azathioprine is an antineoplastic that is cleaved into mercaptopurine and inhibits DNA/RNA synthesis (which causes decreased production of B and T cells).
- Antithymocyte globulin is an antibody against T cells.
- OKT3 is an antibody to the CD3 receptor on T cells.
- Hydroxychloroquine interferes with antigen presentation.
- Basiliximab is a monoclonal antibody against the IL2 receptor.
- Daclizumab is a monoclonal antibody against the IL2 receptor.

9. **What risks are associated with immunosuppression?**
Immunosuppression carries the risk of infection (with common as well as rare bugs that infect patients with acquired immunodeficiency syndrome [AIDS]) and an increased risk of cancer (especially lymphomas and epithelial cell cancers).

HUMAN IMMUNODEFICIENCY VIRUS (HIV)

1. **What sexually transmitted infectious infection should be considered when a patient presents with a sore throat and mononucleosis-like syndrome?**
Acute HIV infection because initial seroconversion usually presents as a mononucleosis-like syndrome (e.g., fever, malaise, pharyngitis, rash, lymphadenopathy). Also consider gonococcal pharyngitis in sexually active young persons with severe pharyngitis and nontender cervical lymphadenopathy.

2. **How is HIV diagnosed? How long after exposure does the HIV test become positive?**
Most organizations now recommend that screening be performed with a fourth-generation combination immunoassay for the p24 antigen and HIV-1/2 antibodies with confirmatory testing via a HIV-1/2 antibody differentiation immunoassay. It takes 3 weeks for antibodies to develop in the majority of patients. Antibodies are present by 6 months in 95% of patients. Therefore if a patient requests testing because of recent high-risk sexual behavior or if a known exposure has occurred, Centers for Disease Control and Prevention (CDC) guidelines call for testing at 4 weeks, 12 weeks, and 24 weeks if third-generation (enzyme-linked immunosorbent assay [ELISA]) testing is used, or at 16 weeks if fourth-generation testing is used. If the exposure occurred within the last 72 hours, postexposure prophylaxis (PEP) should be offered. PEP consists of taking a fully active three-drug regimen (tenofovir/emtricitabine plus raltegravir) for 28 days.

　　Rapid tests, which usually result within a few minutes to hours, are available, but as the positive predictive value varies with the prevalence of HIV infection in the population, preliminary positive tests require confirmatory testing with ELISA and Western blot. Negative test results are reliable unless the patient is in the window period, which is generally considered to be 3 weeks with the third-generation tests and about 16 days with fourth-generation tests incorporating p24 antigen. If acute HIV infection is suspected, it is necessary to send HIV viral load in addition to HIV antibody.

3. **Are control tests needed when a purified protein derivative (PPD) test is done in HIV-positive patients?**
Most authorities no longer recommend control (also known as anergy) testing when a PPD test is done in HIV-positive patients; however, serum testing with IFN-gamma release assays (IGRAs; e.g., QuantiFERON Gold) is becoming increasingly popular for the diagnosis of latent tuberculosis infection both in HIV-positive patients and in the general population.

4. **Cover the right-hand column, then answer the questions about HIV management on the left.**

Question	Answer
After human immunodeficiency virus (HIV) diagnosis, how often do you check the CD4 count?	Every 3–4 mo initially, then every 6–12 mo for patients who are adherent to therapy with sustained viral suppression and stable clinical status for more than 2–3 yr
When do you start antiretroviral therapy?	Since 2011, the Centers for Disease Control and Prevention has recommended HIV treatment with highly active antiretroviral therapy (HAART) regardless of CD4 count. However, HAART is contraindicated in the setting of a preexisting opportunistic infection due to potential for immune reconstitution inflammatory syndrome.

Continued on following page

Question	Answer
What are the acquired immunodeficiency syndrome (AIDS)–defining illnesses?	*Pneumocystis jirovecii* pneumonia (PCP) Esophageal or other invasive candidiasis Wasting syndrome Kaposi sarcoma Disseminated *Mycobacterium avium* infection Tuberculosis Cytomegalovirus disease Disseminated histoplasmosis Progressive multifocal leukoencephalopathy HIV-associated dementia or encephalopathy Recurrent bacterial pneumonia Toxoplasmosis Immunoblastic lymphoma Chronic or extrapulmonary cryptosporidiosis Burkitt lymphoma Invasive cervical cancer Chronic herpes simplex Chronic intestinal isosporiasis Recurrent *Salmonella* infection
When do you start PCP prophylaxis?	When the CD4 count is $<200/mm^3$
What is the drug of choice for PCP prophylaxis?	Trimethoprim-sulfamethoxazole (Bactrim)
What other agents are used in patients with allergy or intolerance to Bactrim?	Dapsone, aerosolized pentamidine, and atovaquone
When should you start *Mycobacterium avium* complex (MAC) prophylaxis?	MAC prophylaxis with a macrolide had been common practice with a CD4 count $<50/mm^3$, but this is no longer routine in the era of effective antiretroviral therapy.
True or False: Once the CD4 is $<200/mm^3$, the patient is automatically considered to have AIDS (even without opportunistic infections).	True
True or False: Give the measles-mumps-rubella vaccine.	True (CD4 count must be $>200/mm^3$)
True or False: Give the varicella vaccine.	True, if patient does not have evidence of immunity to varicella (CD4 count must be $>200/mm^3$)
True or False: Do not give annual influenza vaccines.	False (give every year to all HIV-infected patients)
True or False: Pneumococcal vaccine should be given.	True. It should be given to all HIV-infected patients, and revaccination every 5 yr should be considered.
True or False: Give hepatitis A vaccine.	True, if the patient has chronic liver disease or is at increased risk for hepatitis A infection
True or False: Give hepatitis B vaccine.	True
True or False: Purified protein derivative testing should be done annually.	True, if the initial test is negative and the patient is high risk
True or False: Oral polio vaccine should be given to patients who are at risk of exposure through travel or work.	False (use inactive polio vaccine injection)
The risk of which cancer is increased on the skin and in the mouth?	Kaposi sarcoma
The risk of which type of blood cell cancer is increased?	Non-Hodgkin lymphoma (usually primary B-cell lymphomas of central nervous system [CNS])
What do positive India ink preparations of the cerebrospinal fluid indicate?	*Cryptococcus neoformans* meningitis
What do ring-enhancing lesions in the brain on computed tomography or magnetic resonance imaging scans usually indicate?	Toxoplasmosis, cysticercosis/*Taenia solium*, or primary CNS lymphoma

Question	Answer
True or False: HIV may cause thrombocytopenia.	True
True or False: HIV can cause dementia.	True
True or False: HIV protects against peripheral neuropathies.	False. HIV can cause them.
True or False: HIV-positive mothers may breastfeed their infants.	False. HIV can be transmitted through breast milk.
First-choice agent for cytomegalovirus retinitis	Valganciclovir
Second-choice agents for cytomegalovirus retinitis	Ganciclovir, foscarnet, or cidofovir
True or False: Pregnant patients should receive antiretroviral therapy.	True. Three-drug therapy is currently recommended (no different for the pregnant female; earlier administration is best).
True or False: Low-risk infants born to HIV-positive mothers should take zidovudine.	True (for at least 6 wk after delivery). There are separate guidelines for high-risk infants, who take a three-drug regimen akin to postexposure prophylaxis.
True or False: Cesarean section increases maternal HIV transmission.	False. Cesarean section is the recommended mode of delivery for HIV+ women with viral load >1000 copies to prevent perinatal transmission. Women with viral load <1000 copies may be offered vaginal delivery if appropriate.
Most likely cause of pneumonia in HIV-positive patient	*Streptococcus pneumoniae*
Most likely cause of opportunistic pneumonia in HIV-positive patient	*P. jirovecii*
Stain used on sputum to detect PCP	Silver (Wright-Giemsa or Giemsa)
Two pathogens that cause chronic diarrhea only in AIDS	*Cryptosporidium* and *Isospora* spp.
True or False: Herpes-zoster infection in young adults = possible HIV infection.	True (suggests immunodeficiency)
True or False: Thrush in young adults may mean HIV infection.	True (also associated with diabetes, leukemia, and steroids)
True or False: A positive HIV antibody test in a newborn is unreliable.	True. Maternal antibodies in the neonate can give a false-positive result for the first 4–6 mo and is considered unreliable in neonates; definitive testing is done with HIV DNA polymerase chain reaction.

VASCULAR AND ARTERIAL DISORDERS

1. What is Henoch-Schönlein purpura?

   Henoch-Schönlein purpura (IgA vasculitis) is a vasculitis that may present with GI bleeding and abdominal pain. Look for a history of upper respiratory infection, characteristic rash (palpable purpura) on the lower extremities and buttocks, swelling in hands and feet, arthritis, and/or hematuria and proteinuria. It is associated with ileoileal intussusception. Treat supportively with hydration, rest, and pain relief. Severe cases may require steroids.

2. Describe the usual presentation of Kawasaki disease. How is it treated?

   Kawasaki disease usually affects children younger than 5 years; it is more common in Japanese and female children. Patients have a truncal rash, high fever (which lasts >5 days), conjunctival injection, cervical lymphadenopathy, strawberry tongue, late skin desquamation of the palms and soles, and/or arthritis. Patients may develop coronary vessel vasculitis and subsequent aneurysms, which may thrombose and cause a myocardial infarction. Kawasaki disease should be suspected in any child who has a heart attack. Treat during the acute stage with aspirin and intravenous immunoglobulins to reduce the risk of coronary aneurysm. Kawasaki disease can be remembered by the mnemonic **CRASH and burn:** **c**onjunctivitis, **r**ash, **a**denopathy, **s**trawberry tongue, and **h**ands/feet desquamation (CRASH; burn is for the 5 days of fever). For complete Kawasaki disease, the patient must have at least four of these five signs in addition to the 5 days of fever. Incomplete (previously called atypical) Kawasaki disease can be diagnosed if the patient has two or three of these signs and laboratory abnormalities that are consistent with Kawasaki disease (e.g., elevated C-reactive protein or erythrocyte sedimentation rate, hypoalbuminemia, anemia). Patients should be screened for coronary aneurysms and other cardiac complications via echocardiography and electrocardiography.

3. How does Takayasu arteritis present?

Takayasu arteritis tends to affect Asian women between the ages of 15 and 30 years. It is called the "pulseless disease" because you may not be able to feel the pulse or measure blood pressure on the affected side. The vasculitis affects large vessels, typically the aortic arch and its branches. Carotid involvement may cause neurologic signs or stroke, and congestive heart failure is not uncommon. Angiogram shows the characteristic lesions. Treat with steroids.

4. What autoimmune disorders affect the lungs and kidneys?

Granulomatosis with polyangiitis and Goodpasture syndrome. These are discussed in more detail in Chapter 10.

MUSCULOSKELETAL/CONNECTIVE TISSUE DISORDERS

1. What disease classically causes a false-positive result for the rapid plasma reagin (RPR) or Venereal Disease Research Laboratory (VDRL) syphilis test?

Systemic lupus erythematosus (SLE). A false-positive result on the RPR or VDRL test is actually one of the diagnostic criteria for SLE.

2. What conditions are associated with an increased risk of malignancy?

Diseases with an increased incidence of cancer include dermatomyositis, polymyositis, immunodeficiency syndromes, Bloom syndrome, and Fanconi anemia. Breast, ovarian, and colon cancer have well-known familial tendencies (as well as some other types of cancer), but rarely can a Mendelian inheritance pattern be demonstrated (e.g., *BRCA1* and *BRCA2* genes account for about 5% of breast cancers).

3. What are the signs and symptoms of dermatomyositis?

Dermatomyositis is essentially polymyositis (see the next question) plus skin involvement (a **heliotrope rash around the eyes** with associated periorbital edema is classic). Additional skin findings include a shawl sign (a V-shaped rash around the neck), Gottron papules (scaly eruptions over the metacarpophalangeal and interphalangeal joints of the hands), and mechanic hands (rough, cracked skin on the hands). Patients usually have trouble rising from a chair or climbing steps because of the effects on proximal muscles. Muscle enzymes are elevated, and electromyography is irregular. Muscle biopsy establishes the diagnosis. The incidence of malignancy is higher in affected patients. See Chapter 7 for a complete discussion of dermatomyositis and polymyositis.

4. How do you distinguish among fibromyalgia, polymyositis, and polymyalgia rheumatica?

	Fibromyalgia	*Polymyositis*	*Polymyalgia Rheumatica*
Classic age/sex	Young adult women	Female aged 40–60 yr	Female >age 50 yr
Location	Various	Proximal muscles	Pectoral and pelvic girdles, neck
ESR	Normal	Elevated	Markedly elevated (often >100)
EMG/biopsy	Normal	Abnormal	Normal
Classic findings	Anxiety, stress, insomnia, point tenderness over affected muscles	Elevated CPK, abnormal EMG/biopsy, higher risk of cancer	Temporal arteritis, great response to steroids, very high ESR, elderly patients
Treatment	Antidepressants, NSAIDs, trigger point injections, pregabalin, physical activity	Steroids	Steroids

CPK, Creatine phosphokinase; *EMG,* electromyography; *ESR,* erythrocyte sedimentation rate; *NSAIDs,* nonsteroidal antiinflammatory drugs.

5. Describe the hallmarks of systemic lupus erythematosus.

SLE can cause malar rash, discoid rash, photosensitivity, renal insufficiency, arthritis, pericarditis and pleuritis, positive **antinuclear antibody (ANA),** positive anti-Smith antibody, positive syphilis results (on the VDRL and RPR screening tests, with negative *Treponema pallidum* particle agglutination (TP-PA) assay and direct syphilitic testing), positive lupus anticoagulant, blood disorders (thrombocytopenia, leukopenia, anemia, or pancytopenia), neurologic disturbances (depression, psychosis, seizures), and oral ulcers. Any of these may be presenting symptoms. Use the ANA titer as an initial diagnostic test (high sensitivity, low specificity) and confirm with the **anti-Smith antibody** test (higher specificity). Treat with nonsteroidal antiinflammatory drugs, hydroxychloroquine, corticosteroids, or immunosuppressive/immunomodulating agents (methotrexate, cyclophosphamide, cyclosporine, azathioprine, mycophenolate, tacrolimus, leflunomide, or belimumab).

6. Describe the hallmarks of scleroderma.

Scleroderma (also known as progressive systemic sclerosis) classically presents with **CREST** symptoms (**c**alcinosis, **R**aynaud phenomenon, **e**sophageal dysmotility with dysphagia, **s**clerodactyly, and **t**elangiectasia), heartburn, and masklike, leathery facies. Use the ANA test for the initial diagnostic test; confirm the diagnosis with the **anticentromere antibody** test (for CREST symptoms only) and the **antitopoisomerase antibody** (for full-blown scleroderma). Treatment depends on the symptoms. Sclerotic skin lesions can be treated with topical glucocorticoids, calcipotriol, or methotrexate. Systemic therapy depends upon the organs affected.

7. What are the hallmarks of Sjögren syndrome?

Sjögren syndrome causes dry eyes (keratoconjunctivitis sicca) and dry mouth (xerostomia) and is often associated with other autoimmune diseases. Patients tend to have SS-A (Ro) and SS-B (La) antibodies. Treat with eye drops and good oral hygiene. A classic question on the obstetrics-gynecology and pediatrics sections is that SS-A/SS-B antibody positivity in pregnant mothers is associated with congenital heart block.

8. With what is polyarteritis nodosa associated? How is it diagnosed?

Polyarteritis nodosa is a type of vasculitis classically associated with hepatitis B infection and cryoglobulinemia. Patients present with fever, abdominal pain, weight loss, renal disturbances, and/or peripheral neuropathies. Lab abnormalities include elevations in erythrocyte sedimentation rate and C-reactive protein, leukocytosis, anemia, and hematuria or proteinuria. Patients often have a positive **antineutrophil cytoplasmic antibody** titer. The vasculitis involves medium-sized vessels. Biopsy of an affected organ is the gold standard for diagnosis.

9. How do you recognize Behçet syndrome on the Step 3 exam?

Behçet syndrome classically occurs in young men in their 20s and involves painful oral and genital ulcers. Patients may also have uveitis, arthritis, and other skin lesions (especially erythema nodosum). Steroids are the mainstay of therapy.

VACCINATIONS AND CHEMOTHERAPY

1. What do you need to know about vaccinations?

Vaccinations are reviewed in detail in Chapter 1.

ANAPHYLAXIS/IMMUNOLOGIC REACTIONS

1. List the four classic types of hypersensitivity reactions.
   - Anaphylactic (type I)
   - Cytotoxic (type II)
   - Immune complex mediated (type III)
   - Cell mediated/delayed (type IV)

2. What causes type I hypersensitivity? Give the classic clinical examples.

Type I (immediate) hypersensitivity is due to preformed IgE antibodies that cause release of vasoactive amines (e.g., histamine, leukotrienes) from mast cells and basophils. Examples are anaphylaxis, angioedema, atopy, allergic rhinitis, urticaria, and some forms of asthma. Anaphylaxis may be due to bee stings, food allergy (especially peanuts and shellfish), medications (especially penicillins and sulfa drugs), or latex allergy.

3. Describe the clinical findings with chronic type I hypersensitivity.

Look for eosinophilia, elevated IgE levels, positive family history, and seasonal exacerbations. Patients may also have allergic "shiners" (bilateral infraorbital edema) and a transverse nasal crease ("allergic salute sign") due to frequent nose rubbing. Pale, bluish, edematous nasal turbinates with many eosinophils in clear, watery nasal secretions are also classic.

4. What causes type II hypersensitivity? List some classic clinical examples.

Type II (cytotoxic) hypersensitivity is due to preformed IgG and IgM antibodies that react with the antigen and cause secondary inflammation. Examples include the following:
   - Autoimmune hemolytic anemia (classically caused by methyldopa, penicillins, or sulfa drugs) or other cytopenias caused by antibodies (e.g., idiopathic thrombocytopenic purpura)
   - Transfusion reactions
   - Erythroblastosis fetalis (Rh incompatibility)
   - Goodpasture syndrome (identified by linear immunofluorescence on kidney biopsy)
   - Myasthenia gravis
   - Graves disease
   - Pernicious anemia
   - Pemphigus vulgaris
   - Hyperacute transplant rejection (as soon as the anastomosis is made at transplant surgery, the transplanted organ deteriorates in front of the surgeon's eyes)

5. **What lab test is usually positive with a type II hypersensitivity that causes anemia?**
Coombs test (usually the direct Coombs test).

6. **What causes type III hypersensitivity? List some classic clinical examples.**
Type III (immune complex-mediated) hypersensitivity is due to antigen-antibody complexes that deposit in vessels and cause an inflammatory response. Examples include serum sickness, SLE, rheumatoid arthritis, polyarteritis nodosa, cryoglobulinemia, and certain types of glomerulonephritis (e.g., from chronic hepatitis).

7. **What causes type IV hypersensitivity? How is it related to tuberculosis testing?**
Type IV (cell-mediated/delayed) hypersensitivity is due to sensitized T lymphocytes that release inflammatory mediators. The tuberculosis skin test (i.e., PPD) exploits this immune system reaction. Other examples include contact dermatitis (especially poison ivy, nickel earrings, cosmetics, and medications), chronic transplant rejection, diabetes mellitus type 1, and granulomas (e.g., sarcoidosis).

8. **How do you recognize and treat true anaphylaxis?**
Look for the classic triggers mentioned earlier just before the patient becomes tachycardic, hypotensive, and flushed and develops itching or hives (urticaria), facial swelling (angioedema), and difficulty breathing. Symptoms tend to develop rapidly and dramatically. Nausea, vomiting, and abdominal pain are also concerning for anaphylaxis, since similar receptors are present in the gut wall.
　　Treat immediately by securing the airway (laryngeal edema may prevent intubation, in which case do a cricothyroidotomy, if needed). Give intramuscular epinephrine, histamine-1 (H1) and H2 receptor blockers, and corticosteroids. If symptoms continue or hypotension develops, consider pressor support and intravenous epinephrine.

9. **What usually causes hereditary angioedema?**
A deficiency of **C1 esterase inhibitor** (complement) is the usual cause of hereditary angioedema. Patients have diffuse swelling of the lips, eyelids, and possibly the airway, unrelated to allergen exposure. The disease is autosomal dominant; look for a positive family history. C4 complement levels are low. Some benefit has been shown with administration of fresh frozen plasma to replace C1 esterase. Androgens are used for long-term treatment because they increase liver production of C1 esterase inhibitor.

10. **What type of testing can identify an allergen if it is not obvious?**
Skin or patch testing.

INFECTIONS

1. **What triad indicates the diagnosis of Wiskott-Aldrich syndrome?**
Wiskott-Aldrich deficiency is an X-linked recessive disorder. The classic triad consists of eczema, thrombocytopenia (look for bleeding), and recurrent infections (usually respiratory). A mnemonic to remember this disease is WATER: **W**iskott-**A**ldrich, **t**hrombocytopenia, **e**czema, and **r**ecurrent pyogenic infections.

2. **How do you recognize Chediak-Higashi syndrome?**
Chediak-Higashi syndrome is an autosomal recessive disorder characterized by giant granules in neutrophils, pyogenic infections, and often oculocutaneous albinism. The underlying defect is abnormal organellar protein trafficking due to a mutation in the *CHS1/LYST* gene, resulting in impaired phagocytosis.

3. **Cover the right-hand column, then specify what each Gram stain result most likely represents?**

Gram Stain Result	Meaning
Blue/purple color	Gram-positive organism
Red color	Gram-negative organism
Gram-positive cocci in chains	Streptococci
Gram-positive cocci in clusters	Staphylococci
Gram-positive cocci in pairs (diplococci)	*Streptococcus pneumoniae*
Gram-negative coccobacilli (small rods)	*Haemophilus* sp.
Gram-negative diplococci	*Neisseria* sp. (sexually transmitted disease, septic arthritis, meningitis) or *Moraxella* sp. (lungs, sinusitis)
Plump gram-negative rod with thick capsule (mucoid appearance)	*Klebsiella* sp.
Gram-positive rods that form spores	*Clostridium* sp., *Bacillus* sp.
Pseudohyphae	*Candida* sp.
Acid-fast organisms	*Mycobacterium* (usually *M. tuberculosis*), *Nocardia* sp.

Gram Stain Result	Meaning
Gram-positive with sulfur granules	*Actinomyces* sp. (pelvic inflammatory disease in intrauterine device users; rare cause of neck mass/cervical adenitis)
Silver staining	*Pneumocystis jirovecii,* Cryptococcus, Candida, Legionella, *H. pylori,* Treponema, and *Bartonella henselae* (cat-scratch disease)
Positive India ink preparation (thick capsule)	*Cryptococcus neoformans*
Spirochete	*Treponema* sp., *Leptospira* sp. (both seen only on dark-field microscopy), *Borrelia* sp. (seen on regular light microscope)

4. Cover the middle and right-hand columns, then specify which bugs are associated with each type of infection and what type of empiric antibiotic should be used while waiting for culture results.

Condition	Main Organism(s)	Empiric Antibiotics
Urinary tract infection	*Escherichia coli*	Nitrofurantoin (avoid in the elderly and those with decreased renal function), TMP/SMX, fosfomycin, amoxicillin-clavulanate, cephalosporins, quinolones
Bronchitis	Viruses, *Haemophilus influenzae, Mycoplasma, Chlamydia pneumonia, Moraxella* spp.	Usually no benefit from antibiotics. May consider macrolides or doxycycline (in cases such as a purulent cough >1 wk in duration)
Pneumonia (classic)	*Streptococcus pneumoniae, H. influenzae*	Azithromycin, third-generation cephalosporin, levofloxacin
Pneumonia (atypical)	*Mycoplasma, Chlamydia* spp., *Legionella*	Macrolide antibiotic, doxycycline
Osteomyelitis	*Staphylococcus aureus, Salmonella* spp., *Pseudomonas aeruginosa*	Vancomycin, ceftazidime, piperacillin/tazobactam; oxacillin, nafcillin, and cefazolin for methicillin-susceptible *S. aureus*
Cellulitis	Staphylococci, Streptococci	Cephalexin, dicloxacillin, trimethoprim-sulfamethoxazole, doxycycline, or clindamycin are often used as first-line agents due to the emergence of methicillin-resistant *S. aureus*
Erysipelas	Staphylococci, Streptococci	Penicillin, amoxicillin for uncomplicated cases, otherwise treat like cellulitis
Meningitis (neonate)	Streptococci B, *E. coli,* Listeria spp.	Ampicillin + aminoglycoside (usually gentamicin). An expanded spectrum third-generation cephalosporin (cefotaxime) should be added if a gram-negative organism is suspected
Meningitis (child/adult)	*S. pneumoniae, Neisseria meningitidis**	Cefotaxime or ceftriaxone + vancomycin
Endocarditis (native valve)	Staphylococci, streptococci	Vancomycin
Endocarditis (prosthetic valve)	Numerous different organisms	Vancomycin + gentamicin + cefepime or a carbapenem
Sepsis	Gram-negative organisms, streptococci, staphylococci	Third-generation penicillin/cephalosporin + aminoglycoside, or imipenem
Septic arthritis‡	*S. aureus*	Vancomycin
	Gram-negative bacilli	Ceftazidime or ceftriaxone
	Gonococci	Ceftriaxone, ciprofloxacin, or spectinomycin

H. influenzae is no longer as common a cause of meningitis in children because of widespread vaccination. In a child with no history of immunization, *H. influenzae* is the most likely cause of meningitis.
‡Think of staphylococci if the patient is monogamous or not sexually active. Think of gonorrhea for younger adults who are sexually active.

5. Cover the right-hand columns, then specify the empiric antibiotic of choice for each organism.

Organism*	Antibiotic	Other Choices
Streptococcus A or B	Penicillin, cefazolin	Erythromycin
S. pneumoniae	Third-generation cephalosporin (ceftriaxone) + vancomycin	Fluoroquinolone (levofloxacin)
Enterococcus	Penicillin or ampicillin + aminoglycoside (gentamicin)	Vancomycin + aminoglycoside
Staphylococcus aureus	Antistaphylococcus penicillin (e.g., methicillin)	Vancomycin, trimethoprim-sulfamethoxazole, doxycycline, clindamycin, daptomycin, or linezolid for methicillin-resistant *S. aureus*
Gonococcus[†]	Ceftriaxone	Cefixime or high-dose azithromycin followed by test of cure in 1 wk
Meningococcus	Cefotaxime or ceftriaxone	Chloramphenicol or penicillin G if proven to be penicillin susceptible
Haemophilus	Second- or third-generation cephalosporin	Amoxicillin
Pseudomonas	Antipseudomonal penicillin (ticarcillin, piperacillin) +/− beta lactamase inhibitor (clavulanate, tazobactam)	Ceftazidime, cefepime, aztreonam, imipenem, ciprofloxacin
Bacteroides	Metronidazole	Clindamycin
Mycoplasma	Erythromycin, azithromycin	Doxycycline
Treponema pallidum	Penicillin	Doxycycline
Chlamydia	Doxycycline, azithromycin	Erythromycin, ofloxacin
Lyme disease (*Borrelia* spp.)	Cefuroxime, doxycycline, amoxicillin	Erythromycin

*Always use culture sensitivities to guide therapy once available.
[†]With genital infections, always treat for presumed *Chlamydia* coinfection with azithromycin or doxycycline.

6. Cover the two right-hand columns, then specify the organism after looking at its associated scenario.

Scenario	Organism(s)	Comments
Stuck with thorn or gardening	*Sporothrix schenckii*	Treat with itraconazole
Aplastic crisis in sickle cell disease	Parvovirus B19	
Sepsis after splenectomy	*S. pneumoniae, H. influenzae, N. meningitis* (encapsulated bugs)	Encapsulated organisms
Pneumonia in the US Southwest (California, Arizona)	*Coccidioides immitis*	Treat with itraconazole or fluconazole, amphotericin B for severe disease
Pneumonia after cave exploring or exposure to bird droppings in Ohio and Mississippi river valleys	*Histoplasma capsulatum*	Majority are self-limited and do not require treatment
Pneumonia after exposure to a parrot or exotic bird	*Chlamydia psittaci*	Treat with doxycycline or azithromycin
Fungus ball/hemoptysis after tuberculosis or cavitary lung disease	*Aspergillus* sp.	Treat with voriconazole
Pneumonia in a patient with silicosis	*Mycobacterium tuberculosis*	
Diarrhea after hiking/drinking from a stream	*Giardia lamblia*	Stool cysts; treat with metronidazole

Scenario	Organism(s)	Comments
Pregnant woman with cats	*Toxoplasma gondii*	Treat infected pregnant women with pyrimethamine and sulfadiazine
B$_{12}$ deficiency and abdominal symptoms	*Diphyllobothrium latum* (intestinal tapeworm)	
Seizures with ring-enhancing brain lesion on computed tomography	*Taenia solium* (cysticercosis) or toxoplasmosis	Treat neurocysticercosis with albendazole or praziquantel, usually with steroids Consider anticonvulsants
Squamous cell bladder cancer in Middle East or Africa	*Schistosoma haematobium*	
Worm infection in children	*Enterobius* sp.	Positive tape test, perianal itching. Treat with mebendazole or albendazole
Fever, muscle pain, eosinophilia, and periorbital edema after eating raw meat	*Trichinella spiralis* (trichinosis)	
Gastroenteritis in young children	Rotavirus, Norwalk virus	
Food poisoning after eating reheated rice	*Bacillus cereus*	Infection is usually self-limited
Food poisoning after eating raw seafood	*Vibrio parahaemolyticus*	
Diarrhea after travel to Mexico	*E. coli* (Montezuma revenge)	ETEC. Treat with ciprofloxacin.
Diarrhea after antibiotics	*Clostridioides difficile*	Use oral vancomycin or fidaxomicin. Oral metronidazole may be used in settings where access to vancomycin or fidaxomicin is limited for an initial episode of nonsevere *C. difficile* infection
Baby paralyzed after eating honey	*Clostridioides botulinum*	Toxin blocks acetylcholine release
Genital lesions in children in the absence of sexual abuse or activity	Molluscum contagiosum	
Cellulitis after cat/dog bites	*Pasteurella multocida*	Treat animal bite wounds with prophylactic amoxicillin-clavulanate
Slaughterhouse worker with fever	*Brucella* spp. (brucellosis)	
Pneumonia after being in hotel or near air conditioner or water tower	*Legionella pneumophila*	May have diarrhea and hyponatremia Treat with azithromycin or levofloxacin
Burn wound infection with blue/green color	*Pseudomonas* sp.	*Staphylococcus aureus* is also a common burn infection, but it lacks blue-green color

7. **How is syphilis diagnosed?**
   Screen for syphilis with RPR or VDRL test. Confirm a positive test with a fluorescent treponemal antibody absorbed (FTA-ABS) or microhemagglutination (MHA-TP) test because false positives occur with the RPR and VDRL tests, classically in patients with antiphospholipid syndrome (or SLE with antiphospholipid antibodies). Once syphilis is treated, the RPR and VDRL tests become negative, whereas the FTA-ABS and MHA-TP tests often remain positive for life. You can also scrape the base of a genital chancre or condyloma latum and look for spirochetes on dark-field microscopy.

8. **Describe the three stages of syphilis.**
   Primary stage: look for painless chancre that resolves on its own within 8 weeks.
   Secondary stage: roughly 6 weeks to 18 months after infection; look for condyloma lata, maculopapular rash (classically involves palms and soles of feet) (Fig. 15.1), and lymphadenopathy.

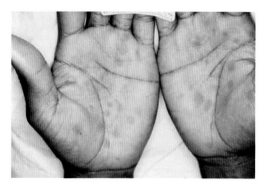

Fig. 15.1 Hyperpigmented macules on the palms due to secondary syphilis. (From Brinster NK, Liu V, Diwan AH, et al. *Dermatopathology: High-Yield Pathology.* Saunders; 2011:228-230 [fig 3 courtesy of J Nunley MD; Virginia Commonwealth University, Richmond].)

Tertiary stage: years after initial infection (between the secondary and tertiary stages is the latent phase, in which the disease is quiet and asymptomatic). Look for gummas (granulomas in many different organs), neurologic symptoms and signs (e.g., neurosyphilis, Argyll-Robertson pupil, dementia, paresis, tabes dorsalis, Charcot joints), and thoracic aortic aneurysms.

9. How is syphilis treated?
   With penicillin. Use doxycycline for penicillin-allergic patients.

10. Describe the classic findings of Epstein-Barr virus (EBV) infection (infectious mononucleosis).
    Fatigue, fever, pharyngitis, and cervical lymphadenopathy in a young adult. The signs and symptoms are similar to those of streptococcal pharyngitis, but malaise tends to be prolonged and pronounced in EBV infection. To differentiate from streptococcal pharyngitis, look for the following:
    • Splenomegaly (patients are at increased risk of splenic rupture and should avoid contact sports and heavy lifting)
    • Hepatomegaly
    • Atypical lymphocytes (bizarre forms that may resemble leukemia) with lymphocytosis, anemia, or thrombocytopenia
    • Positive serology (heterophile antibodies [e.g., Monospot test]) or specific EBV antibodies (viral capsid antigen, Epstein-Barr nuclear antigens)

11. What is an important differential diagnosis of Epstein-Barr virus infection or influenza infection?
    Acute HIV infection, which can cause a mononucleosis-type syndrome.

12. What is the association between Epstein-Barr virus and cancer?
    EBV is associated with nasopharyngeal cancer, African Burkitt lymphoma, and posttransplant lymphoproliferative disorder.

13. Describe the classic clinical vignette for Rocky Mountain spotted fever. What causes it? What is the treatment?
    Look for history of a tick bite (especially in a patient on the East Coast) 1 week before the development of high fever/chills, severe headache, and prostration or severe malaise. A rash appears roughly 4 days later on the palms/wrists and soles/ankles and spreads rapidly to the trunk and face (unique pattern of spread). Patients often look quite ill (e.g., disseminated intravascular coagulation, delirium). The infection is caused by *Rickettsia rickettsii.* Treat with doxycycline; chloramphenicol is a second choice.

14. In what clinical scenario does rabies occur in the United States? Describe the classic physical findings.
    Rabies in the United States is due to bites from bats, skunks, raccoons, or foxes; rabies due to bites from dogs is rare due to vaccination. The incubation period is usually around 1 to 2 months. The classic findings are hydrophobia (fear of water due to painful swallowing) and central nervous system (CNS) signs (e.g., paralysis).

15. What should you do after a patient is bitten by an animal?
    1. Treat the local wound. Cleanse thoroughly with soap. Do *not* cauterize or suture the wound. Amoxicillin-clavulanate is often given for cellulitis prophylaxis.
    2. Observe the animal. If possible, capture and observe the dog or cat to see if it develops rabies. If a wild animal is caught, it should be killed and the brain tissue examined for rabies.

3. If the wild animal escapes or has rabies, give rabies immunoglobulin and vaccinate the patient. In cases of a dog or cat bite, do *not* give prophylaxis or vaccine unless the animal acted strangely or bit the patient without provocation and rabies is prevalent in the area (rare). Do not give prophylaxis or vaccine for rabbit or small rodent bites (e.g., rats, mice, squirrels, chipmunks).

16. What are the two main infections caused by *Streptococcus pyogenes* (group A *Streptococcus*)? What are the common sequelae?
    S. pyogenes causes pharyngitis and skin infections. Sequelae include rheumatic fever, scarlet fever, and poststreptococcal glomerulonephritis.

17. Other than pneumonia, what infections does *Streptococcus pneumoniae* commonly cause?
    Otitis media, meningitis, sinusitis, and spontaneous bacterial peritonitis.

18. What are the main infections caused by *Staphylococcus aureus*?
    The list is long. *S. aureus* is a common cause of the following infections:
    • Skin and soft tissue abscesses (especially in the breast after breastfeeding or in the skin after a furuncle)
    • Endocarditis (especially in drug users)
    • Osteomyelitis (the most common cause, unless sickle cell disease is present)
    • Septic arthritis
    • Food poisoning (via a preformed toxin)
    • Toxic shock syndrome (via a preformed toxin)
    • Scalded skin syndrome (via a preformed toxin; affects younger children who often have impetigo and subsequent desquamation)
    • Impetigo
    • Cellulitis
    • Wound infections
    • Pneumonia (often forms a lung abscess or empyema)
    • Furuncles and carbuncles

19. What is the treatment of choice for staphylococcal infections on the USMLE?
    An antistaphylococcal penicillin (e.g., methicillin, dicloxacillin). Use vancomycin, clindamycin, doxycycline, trimethoprim-sulfamethoxazole, or linezolid if the staphylococcal species is known to be methicillin resistant or if methicillin-resistant *S. aureus* (MRSA) is suspected. MRSA is a rapidly growing problem. Most abscesses (regardless of the causative organism) must be treated first with surgical incision and drainage because antibiotics cannot penetrate through the walls of an abscess cavity.

20. Distinguish between preorbital (preseptal) and orbital cellulitis.
    Both conditions may present with swollen lids; fever; a history of facial laceration, trauma, insect bite, or sinusitis; and chemosis (edema of the conjunctiva). Orbital cellulitis can mimic preorbital cellulitis early in its course. However, if ophthalmoplegia, proptosis, severe eye pain, double vision, decreased eye movements, or decreased visual acuity is present, the patient has orbital cellulitis. Orbital cellulitis is an ophthalmologic emergency because it may extend into the skull, causing meningitis, venous thromboses, and/or blindness. Computed tomography scan of the orbits and sinuses is the imaging modality of choice for evaluation of suspected orbital cellulitis.

21. What are the common bacterial causes of preorbital and orbital cellulitis? How are they treated?
    The most common bugs in both are *Streptococcus pneumoniae, Haemophilus influenzae* type b, and *S. aureus* or streptococcal species (in patients with a history of trauma). Treat orbital cellulitis with blood cultures and administration of broad-spectrum intravenous antibiotics until culture results are known. In preorbital cellulitis, blood cultures are not routinely collected, as they are rarely positive and cultures from the site are difficult to obtain. Empiric oral antibiotics for preorbital cellulitis consist of monotherapy with trimethoprim-sulfamethoxazole or combination therapy with clindamycin plus either amoxicillin or amoxicillin-clavulanic acid or cefpodoxime or cefdinir. A typical regimen for orbital cellulitis is vancomycin plus either ceftriaxone or cefotaxime or ampicillin-sulbactam, or piperacillin-tazobactam. Although preorbital cellulitis may be treated on an outpatient basis with close follow-up, orbital cellulitis requires hospital admission and intravenous antibiotics.

22. What prophylactic medication should be given to contacts of a patient with *Neisseria meningitidis* infection?
    Rifampin, ciprofloxacin, or ceftriaxone.

CHAPTER 16

CLINICAL CASE SCENARIOS

CASE 1

History of present illness (HPI): A 60-year-old man with a history of hypertension has right lower leg redness, swelling, and warmth. He states that about 1 week ago he hit his shin while working on his car, which left a small laceration on his skin. Initially it seemed to heal well, but for the past 3 days the skin around the site has become increasingly red, warm, painful, and swollen and is now "the size of a half-dollar." He says that he felt like he may have had a fever at home but did not take his temperature. He denies any other symptoms.

Vital signs: Temperature 98.2°F (36.8°C), pulse 80 beats/min, blood pressure (BP) 140/78 mm Hg, respiratory rate (RR) 16 breaths/min.

Additional history: The patient takes hydrochlorothiazide for hypertension. He occasionally consumes alcohol; he denies smoking and drug use. His vaccinations are up to date.

1. What is the differential diagnosis?
   Cellulitis, erysipelas, fasciitis, thrombophlebitis, stasis dermatitis.

2. What components of the physical examination do you perform?
   General appearance, cardiovascular, lungs, skin/extremities.
   Physical examination:
   General: Well-developed, overweight man in no apparent distress.
   Cardiovascular: Within normal limits (WNL).
   Lungs: WNL
   Skin/extremities: 4×4-cm^2 region of poorly demarcated erythema on the anterolateral surface of the right midcalf with associated warmth and edema. Small (1-cm) laceration at the middle of the erythema, healed, without purulence or discharge. No crepitus, no tenderness proximally, no other skin changes. Distal pulses 2+. Sensation intact. Strength 5/5 bilateral lower extremities.

3. What are your initial orders?
   Complete blood count (CBC), chemistry 8 panel (chem 8), analgesia (e.g., acetaminophen PO), antibiotics (e.g., trimethoprim/sulfamethoxazole, cephalexin, or doxycycline).
   Advance clock: CBC WNL, no leukocytosis. Chem 8 WNL. Patient feels better after analgesia.

4. What are your follow-up actions?
   Discharge with a prescription for appropriate antibiotics and analgesics, follow up in 2 to 3 days for wound check.
   Advance clock:
   The patient has been taking antibiotics as prescribed. The erythema has significantly decreased.
   Case ends.
   Critical actions: Recognition of cellulitis, understanding of causative organisms (e.g., *Staphylococcus* and *Streptococcus*), administration of appropriate antibiotics, follow-up for wound check, consideration of more serious infections.
   Discussion: This patient has cellulitis, an infection of the dermis and subcutaneous tissue. Infections of skin and soft tissue range from erysipelas involving the superficial layers of the dermis to cellulitis affecting the dermis and subcutaneous tissue to fasciitis affecting the fascia. The erythema in erysipelas, because of its superficial nature, typically has very well-demarcated borders and is raised; this is typically caused by *Streptococcus* species. Cellulitis has less well-defined margins and varying degrees of erythema and is typically caused by either *Streptococcus* or *Staphylococcus aureus*. Fasciitis affects deeper layers and can be life threatening, such as in the case of necrotizing fasciitis, and the presenting symptoms can include even fewer skin signs given its deep nature. Scenarios describing necrotizing fasciitis tend to have findings in the history and physical, including pain out of proportion to exam, tenderness to palpation outside of margins of swelling, bullae formation, crepitus, and skip lesions, which are patchy areas of inflammation and injury appearing to "skip" areas that are unaffected. This infection is usually polymicrobial but can be due to *Streptococcus pyogenes* or *Clostridium* species. Differentiating erysipelas, cellulitis, and fasciitis is important in prognosis and in management.
   Diagnosis of cellulitis is primarily clinical. On examination, the affected areas will be warm, erythematous, and tender. The area should be examined for areas of fluctuance that signify abscess formation. Systemic symptoms may include fever and chills. Risk factors include skin breakdown (trauma, burns, bites, etc.), poor circulation to the affected area (resulting from diabetes, lymphatic stasis, peripheral vascular disease), and poor immune

function (human immunodeficiency virus infection/acquired immunodeficiency syndrome [HIV/AIDS], renal or hepatic failure, steroid use).

Simple cellulitis can be diagnosed clinically and treated on an outpatient basis, but patients with more severe involvement or immunocompromised states should be hospitalized for parenteral antibiotic administration. An outpatient regimen in an immunocompetent host should cover *Staphylococcus* if the patient has cellulitis with purulence or evidence of an abscess (and drain the abscess if indicated) and *Streptococcus* for cellulitis without purulence or abscess. Trimethoprim-sulfamethoxazole would cover *Staphylococcus* (including methicillin-resistant *S. aureus* [MRSA]), and cephalexin would cover *Streptococcus*, and both would be examples of appropriate antibiotics.

Diagnosis: Cellulitis.

CASE 2

HPI: An 11-day-old previously healthy and ex–full-term infant boy is brought to his pediatrician by his concerned parents because his "skin and eyes look yellow." The parents state that they think that he has been yellow now for about 2 days but are unsure. They state that he is interacting with them normally, is wetting a normal number of diapers, has normal bowel movements, is breastfeeding exclusively, and is breastfeeding the appropriate number of times (about 10 times a day, 20 minutes per breast each time). No fever, vomiting, cough, runny nose, or other concerns.

Vital signs: Temperature 98.2°F (36.8°C), pulse 120 beats/min, BP 72/40 mm Hg, RR 35 breaths/min.

Additional history: Unremarkable prenatal course. No birth complications. Mother delivered at 39 weeks via normal spontaneous vaginal delivery; no cephalohematoma or bruising during delivery. According to the pediatrician's records, the patient is growing appropriately and is at the 80th percentile for height and weight.

1. What is the differential diagnosis?
   Neonatal hyperbilirubinemia: breast milk jaundice, breastfeeding jaundice, physiologic jaundice (but too old), breakdown of blood (e.g., from cephalohematoma), infection, hemolysis, genetic defects, biliary atresia.

2. What components of the physical examination do you perform?
   General appearance, skin, cardiovascular, lungs, abdomen, genitalia.
   Physical examination:
     General: Well-developed, well-nourished infant in no distress, latching appropriately onto the mother's breast with good sucking. Cries when examined with good tear production but is easily consoled by parents.
     Skin: Good skin turgor, capillary refill less than 2 seconds. Jaundiced from face to midchest. No signs of skin or soft tissue infection.
     Cardiovascular: WNL
     Lungs: WNL
     Abdomen: WNL
     Genitalia: Normal uncircumcised boy, testes descended bilaterally.

3. What are your initial orders?
   Bilirubin level.
   Advance clock: Bilirubin level: 8 mg/dL.

4. What are your follow-up actions?
   Counseling on disease process, follow-up bilirubin check.
   Advance clock:
     The parents are relieved that you reassured them about the jaundice. They return in 1 week and the bilirubin level is 2 mg/dL.
     Case ends.
   Critical actions: Recognition of neonatal hyperbilirubinemia, consideration of benign and serious causes of hyperbilirubinemia, recognition of treatment levels when bilirubin is significantly abnormal.
   Discussion: This patient has breast milk jaundice, which is caused by an unknown mechanism in breast milk that leads to increased bilirubin levels, usually in the second week of life. Neonatal jaundice (hyperbilirubinemia) is extremely common: over half of full-term neonates (and more than three-quarters of preterm neonates) will have jaundice. Neonatal jaundice is usually benign and does not require treatment. However, jaundice that is present at birth (or within 24 hours), increases rapidly, or occurs in an ill-appearing baby is pathologic and requires a workup to identify the underlying cause (sepsis, hemolysis, congenital infection, etc.). Very high bilirubin levels can be associated with kernicterus, irreversible brain damage caused by deposition of bilirubin. Very high bilirubin levels (see later discussion) require phototherapy or exchange transfusion. Jaundice can be caused by several conditions:
   - **Physiologic jaundice:** Caused by immature hepatic conjugation combined with fetal erythrocyte breakdown.
   - **Breastfeeding jaundice** (should be called *lack of* breastfeeding jaundice): Caused by inadequate intake of calories and resolves when nutritional intake is adequate.

- **Breast *milk* jaundice**: Breast milk itself can cause increased bilirubin levels through a mechanism that is unclear but may include increased enterohepatic recycling of bilirubin and/or substances in breast milk that block conjugation of bilirubin. In this patient, given that feeding and growth are normal and the level of bilirubin is not dangerous, the mother can continue to breastfeed. In instances in which the bilirubin is high enough to warrant treatment, some physicians recommend stopping breastfeeding and switching to formula briefly.
- **Extravascular blood**: Breakdown of blood products leads to increased bilirubin. If an infant suffers from cephalohematoma or bruising during birth, the blood involved will break down and cause increased bilirubin production.

In infants with more severe hyperbilirubinemia or those who appear ill, other causes such as infection, hemolysis (from ABO compatibility or rhesus factor [Rh] alloimmunization), genetic defects (including conjugation diseases such as Crigler-Najjar syndrome, red blood cell [RBC] defects such as spherocytosis, and inborn errors of metabolism), or obstructed bile flow (such as biliary atresia, etc.) should be investigated. Treatment levels for hyperbilirubinemia depend on the patient's risk factors (e.g., premature), age in hours, and level of bilirubin (this can be plotted on a nomogram to determine whether phototherapy is indicated). In general, any level greater than 20 mg/dL at any time is abnormal and warrants treatment. Phototherapy converts unconjugated bilirubin into a water-soluble molecule that the kidneys can excrete. Exchange transfusion replaces newborn blood with donor blood, removing bilirubin in the process, and is indicated only for very high bilirubin levels, neurologic symptoms consistent with kernicterus or encephalopathy, or failure of phototherapy.

Diagnosis: Breast milk jaundice.

CASE 3

HPI: A 36-year-old woman presents to the urgent care center complaining of 1 day of chills, fever, and a cough that produces rust-colored sputum. She states that she has had a runny nose, dry cough, and sore throat for a week but thought she was getting better until today. She denies any hemoptysis, prolonged immobilization, shortness of breath, or other symptoms.

Vital signs: Temperature 100.7°F (38.6°C), pulse 96 beats/min, BP 118/68 mm Hg, RR 18 breaths/min.

Additional history: Previously healthy, no medications except acetaminophen for the fever (last dose 10 hours before arrival). Denies tobacco, drug, or alcohol use. Sexually active with protection with one male partner. Denies travel outside the country, incarceration, recent hospitalization, or close contact with individuals with tuberculosis (TB).

1. What is the differential diagnosis?
   Community-acquired pneumonia, viral upper respiratory tract infection, TB, pulmonary embolism.

2. What components of the physical examination do you perform?
   General appearance; head, eyes, ears, nose, and throat (HEENT); cardiovascular; lungs; abdomen.
   Physical examination:
   General: Well-developed, well-nourished woman in no apparent distress, coughing up rust-colored sputum during examination.
   HEENT: No sinus tenderness, oropharynx WNL.
   Cardiovascular: WNL
   Lungs: Crackles heard in the left lower lobe on auscultation.
   Abdomen: WNL

3. What are your initial orders?
   Chest x-ray (CXR), acetaminophen.
   Advance clock: CXR shows an infiltrate that silhouettes the left diaphragm. Temperature 1 hour after acetaminophen administration is 99.7°F (37.6°C) and the heart rate is now 90 beats/min.

4. What are your follow-up actions?
   Discharge with a prescription for amoxicillin or (if local resistance <25%) a macrolide antibiotic such as azithromycin for 5 days, with a follow-up appointment in 1 week. Counseling on the disease process.
   Advance clock:
   The patient is seen 7 days later for a follow-up appointment: her symptoms have resolved, and she is asymptomatic.
   If the patient is reexamined, there will be no crackles in the left lower lobe of the lung.
   Case ends.
   Critical actions: Recognition of pneumonia, appropriate treatment, recognition that the patient does not need to be treated as an inpatient.
   Discussion: This patient has community-acquired pneumonia, usually caused by "typical" pathogens such as *Streptococcus pneumoniae* and *Haemophilus influenzae* or atypical pathogens such as *Mycoplasma*, Legionella, and *Chlamydophila pneumoniae* (previously referred to as *Chlamydia pneumoniae*). In the time frame of an emergency department (ED) or urgent care visit, the type of bacteria causing the pneumonia will not be identified, therefore antibiotic coverage against the most likely agents is appropriate. This is typically done on an inpatient basis with ceftriaxone (for typical bacteria) and azithromycin (for atypical bacteria because some lack a cell wall,

and therefore beta-lactam antibiotics are ineffective). Outpatient regimens for a young healthy adult are typically amoxicillin monotherapy, macrolide antibiotic monotherapy (such as azithromycin), or doxycycline monotherapy. Patients with comorbidities such as chronic heart, lung, liver, or renal disease or conditions that are otherwise immunosuppressing should instead receive a respiratory fluoroquinolone (e.g., levofloxacin or moxifloxacin) or a macrolide plus amoxicillin/clavulanate. Pneumonia associated with a health care setting or pneumonia in those with an underlying lung disease (such as bronchiectasis) typically requires broader coverage because bacteria such as *S. aureus* and *Pseudomonas aeruginosa* are also possible infectious agents.

Diagnosis of pneumonia is based on history, physical examination, and x-ray imaging. The history typically involves a cough that produces purulent sputum with a fever and possibly shortness of breath. On examination of the lungs, localized crackles in the area of the pneumonia are common. Imaging may show a lobar infiltrate or patchy interstitial infiltrates. The possibility of unusual organisms should be considered by identifying risk factors: (1) Is the patient immunocompromised (e.g., on steroids, risk factors for HIV)? (2) Could the patient have aspirated fluid (risk of *Klebsiella* and polymicrobial anaerobic infections)? (3) Has the patient recently been hospitalized or taken antibiotics (risk of MRSA or *Pseudomonas*)? (4) Could the patient have TB?

The most important decision after diagnosing pneumonia is whether the patient can be treated as an outpatient or needs to be admitted to the hospital. Many prediction rules have been developed to help in this decision. One approach is to apply the CURB-65 criteria, whereby you assign 1 point each for confusion, urea (blood urea nitrogen [BUN] >19 mg/dL), RR greater than 30 breaths/min, BP less than 90 mm Hg systolic or 60 mm Hg diastolic, and age older than 65 years. Patients with a score of 0 or 1 can be treated as outpatients, those with a score of 4 or 5 should be admitted, and the decision for those with an intermediate score (2 or 3) should be on a case-by-case basis. The more complicated PORT score is another decision tool. In this case, the patient appears well, is young, has no other comorbidities, and can be safely treated as an outpatient without the need to draw blood tests. Some guidelines recommend that patients with risk factors for malignancy (e.g., smoking history) should have a follow-up CXR 6 weeks later to confirm resolution of the infiltrate. Failure of the infiltrate to resolve requires additional evaluation such as a computed tomography (CT) scan to assess the possibility of an underlying malignancy.

Diagnosis: Pneumonia.

CASE 4

HPI: A 26-year-old woman presents to her primary care doctor with right arm weakness and numbness that started gradually 2 days ago while she was working outside. She states that she could still move the arm, but that it felt much weaker than usual and as if "pins and needles" were sticking into her. She denies any numbness or weakness elsewhere or trauma to her arm. She states that her symptoms have already significantly improved, but she is scared that the condition could be permanent.

Vital signs: Temperature 98.2°F (36.8°C), pulse 76 beats/min, BP 155/78 mm Hg, RR 16 breaths/min.

Additional history: The patient was diagnosed with optic neuritis 6 months ago, but this has since resolved and she essentially has normal vision. There is no other medical history. No medications, allergies, or use of alcohol, drugs, or tobacco.

1. What is the differential diagnosis?

   Transient ischemic attack (TIA), stroke, cervical radiculopathy, peripheral neuropathy, multiple sclerosis (MS), acute disseminated encephalomyelitis, subacute combined degeneration of the spinal cord, HIV-associated neuropathies (e.g., progressive multifocal leukoencephalopathy), vasculitis (e.g., polyarteritis nodosa), neuromyelitis optica.

2. What components of the physical examination do you perform?

   General appearance, HEENT/neck, lungs, cardiovascular, neuro/psych.

   Physical examination:

   General: Well-developed, well-nourished woman in no distress.

   HEENT/neck: On flexion of the neck, the patient says she feels as if "shocks of electricity" are going down her spine.

   Cardiovascular: WNL

   Lungs: WNL

   Neuro/psych: Alert and oriented to name, time, place, situation. Cranial nerves II to XII intact. Strength of right arm 4+/5, rest of body 5/5. Minimally diminished sensation to a light touch and pinprick over the right arm.

3. What are your initial orders?

   CBC, chem 8, antinuclear antibody (ANA), erythrocyte sedimentation rate (ESR), vitamin B_{12} level, HIV screening, brain CT, magnetic resonance imaging (MRI) scan of the brain/spine.

   Advance clock:

   CBC, chem 8, ANA, ESR, B_{12}, HIV all negative/WNL.

   Brain CT negative.

   MRI of the brain/spine shows multiple demyelinating plaques in various stages throughout the central nervous system (CNS).

4. What are your follow-up actions?

Counseling on the disease process. Consult with neurology to start disease-modifying therapy (e.g., interferon-beta or natalizumab).

Advance clock: Case ends.

Critical actions: Recognition of MS as a likely cause of the patient's symptoms, investigation of disease with MRI brain, consultation with neurology, and/or initiation of disease-modifying therapy.

Discussion: This patient has MS, an autoimmune disorder in which CNS neurons become demyelinated. Depending on where the demyelination occurs, patients can have a variety of symptoms; the most common include optic neuritis, sensory or motor changes in the extremities, and ataxia. The demyelination does not occur all at once but rather over time, so MS is described as involving lesions separated in space (multiple locations within the CNS) and time (multiple episodes). MS can follow one of four general courses: relapsing remitting (most common, characterized by exacerbations and remissions); primary progressive (slowly worsening symptoms without marked exacerbations or remissions); secondary progressive (after an initial relapsing remitting course); and progressive relapsing (least common; progressive but with exacerbations on top of the progression). The cause of MS is unknown, but as for many autoimmune diseases, it is more common in women than in men. It is also more common in younger individuals (age 20–40 years).

Diagnosis of MS is on the basis of a history and physical examination leading to clinical suspicion of the disease and confirmation on MRI brain/spine revealing demyelination in multiple areas. In equivocal cases cerebrospinal fluid (CSF) analysis showing oligoclonal bands, or visual/auditory evoked potentials showing subclinical demyelinating disease, can support the diagnosis. Other causes of demyelination should be investigated and ruled out (e.g., HIV, vitamin B_{12} deficiency, other autoimmune conditions). There is no cure for MS. The mainstay of treatment for exacerbations is steroids, which decrease duration and severity of symptoms during an exacerbation but do not alter the long-term course for MS. For maintenance, medications such as natalizumab or interferon-beta are prescribed in conjunction with a neurologist. Additional immunocompromising medications may be considered. Prior to initiation of immunomodulators, patients should be evaluated for viral hepatitis infections and for latent TB infection.

Diagnosis: MS.

CASE 5

HPI: A 40-year-old woman presents to her primary care doctor and reports 8 months of progressive weakness, dizziness, and fatigue. She states that whenever she stands up, she feels like she is "going to pass out" and finds it hard to even get out of bed in the morning. She states that despite not going outside much because of her weakness, her skin has been getting darker. She has lost 20 lb over the 8-month period and states she does not have much of an appetite, but her husband remarks on how much salt she uses at the dinner table. She affirms that she is too thin and wants to gain her weight and strength back. She denies any syncopal episodes.

Vital signs: Temperature 98.2°F (36.8°C), pulse 60 beats/min, BP 108/60 mm Hg, RR 16 breaths/min.

Additional history: No suicidal ideation, homicidal ideation, or auditory or visual hallucinations. No medical or psychiatric history. Denies use of alcohol, tobacco, or drugs.

1. What is the differential diagnosis?

Chronic adrenal insufficiency (Addison disease), anorexia nervosa, occult malignancy, hemochromatosis, hypothyroidism.

2. What components of the physical examination do you perform?

General appearance, HEENT, cardiovascular, lungs, neuro/psych.

Physical examination:

General: Thin woman in no apparent distress with generalized hyperpigmentation.

HEENT: No goiter or palpable thyroid nodules. Buccal mucosal hyperpigmentation. Dry mucous membranes.

Cardiovascular: WNL

Lungs: WNL

Neuro/psych: WNL

3. What are your initial orders?

Orthostatic vital signs, electrocardiography (ECG), CBC, chem 8, thyroid-stimulating hormone (TSH).

Advance clock: Orthostatic vital signs are positive; BP on standing 80/50 mm Hg and pulse 108 beats/min. ECG shows normal sinus rhythm. CBC and TSH WNL, chem 8 remarkable for a potassium level of 5.5 mEq/dL, sodium of 134 mEq/dL, and bicarbonate of 20 mmol/L.

4. What are your follow-up actions?

Early-morning cortisol level. Fluid replacement.

Advance clock: Early-morning cortisol is undetectable.

5. What are your follow-up actions?

Consult endocrinology and/or start hydrocortisone and fludrocortisone replacement.

Advance clock:
  The patient feels much better.
  Case ends.
Critical actions: Recognition of chronic primary adrenal insufficiency, appropriate workup (e.g., chem panel and cortisol level) and treatment (e.g., steroid replacement).
Discussion: This patient has chronic primary adrenal insufficiency, also known as Addison disease. The adrenal cortex has three layers: the zona glomerulosa (which makes aldosterone, a mineralocorticoid), the zona fascicu-lata (which makes cortisol, a glucocorticoid), and the zona reticularis (which makes dehydroepiandrosterone sulfate [DHEAS], an androgen). Aldosterone acts to reclaim sodium and excrete potassium and acid in the distal nephron, so loss of this hormone leads to hypotension and hyperkalemic metabolic acidosis. Cortisol also has a role in catecholamine sensitization, and loss of this hormone can lead to resistant hypotension. Loss of the androgenic hormones is less noticeable.

Addison disease is most commonly of autoimmune origin in developed countries, but TB is the most com-mon cause worldwide. Loss of cortisol production causes increased adrenocorticotropic hormone (ACTH) levels; one breakdown product of this is alpha-melanocyte–stimulating hormone (alpha-MSH), which leads to character-istic hyperpigmentation, especially in the buccal mucosa, genital area, and areola. Symptoms include fatigue, salt craving, memory impairment, depression, and vague nonspecific symptoms.

Acute adrenal insufficiency can be seen with sepsis, especially infections with *Neisseria meningitidis* causing Waterhouse-Friderichsen syndrome. Iatrogenic causes such as acute cessation of chronic steroid therapy or ad-ministration of medications that inhibit cortisol production (e.g., etomidate, ketoconazole) are also precipitating factors.

Screening can be performed via measurement of the early-morning cortisol level; a level greater than 20 μg/dL excludes adrenal insufficiency, very low levels (<3 μg/dL) are diagnostic, and intermediate levels require further investigation. An ACTH (cosyntropin) stimulation test can be performed in which baseline cortisol is measured, ACTH is administered, and 30- and 60-minute cortisol levels are measured. Low initial and 30- and 60-minute levels confirm the diagnosis of primary adrenal insufficiency. A low initial level and normal 30- and 60-minute levels indicate pituitary dysfunction because the pituitary gland is functional (normal ACTH response) but is not secreting enough ACTH, or the hypothalamus is not sending enough corticotropin-releasing hormone (CRH) to the pituitary.

Management involves administration of hydrocortisone and fludrocortisone, with increases in the hydrocorti-sone dose during illness or before a stressful medical procedure to mimic the body's endogenous cortisol spikes during these times.
Diagnosis: Adrenal insufficiency.

CASE 6

HPI: A 12-year-old boy presents to the ED complaining of a sore throat and fever for the past 2 days. He denies a
  cough, runny nose, or sick contacts. He states that he has significant pain on swallowing that is limiting his ability
  to eat. He can drink fluids without difficulty.
Vital signs: Temperature 101.8°F (38.8°C), pulse 94 beats/min, BP 116/70 mm Hg, RR 18 breaths/min.
Additional history: Denies sexual activity. No known drug allergies. Vaccinations up to date.

1. What is the differential diagnosis?
   Viral pharyngitis, streptococcal pharyngitis, infectious mononucleosis, peritonsillar abscess, retropharyngeal abscess, diphtheria, Lemierre syndrome, gonococcal pharyngitis.

2. What components of the physical examination do you perform?
   General appearance, HEENT, cardiovascular, lungs, skin.
   Physical examination:
   General: Mild distress due to throat pain, speaks with a normal voice in full sentences.
   Cardiovascular: WNL
   Lungs: WNL
   HEENT: Tonsillar exudates bilaterally; tender, diffuse, anterior cervical lymphadenopathy; erythematous and in-
      flamed posterior oropharynx; mild petechiae on the palate; uvula midline; no meningismus; and full range of
      motion of the neck.
   Skin: WNL

3. What are your initial orders?
   Acetaminophen or ibuprofen. Group A Strep rapid antigen detection test (RADT). PO challenge.
   Advance clock:
     + Group A Strep RADT.
   Patient feels much better, his symptoms have improved.

4. What are your follow-up actions?
One dose of intramuscular (IM) benzathine penicillin or a 10-day course of PO penicillin or amoxicillin.
Follow-up in 1 week.
Advance clock: Case ends.
Critical actions: HEENT examination to rule out peritonsillar abscess or more serious cause of the sore throat; analgesics; diagnosis of group A Strep and initiation of antibiotics.
Discussion: Streptococcal pharyngitis accounts for approximately 30% of acute pharyngitis in children and is caused by group A beta-hemolytic streptococci (*S. pyogenes*). Once the diagnosis of acute pharyngitis is established clinically, the Centor criteria can be applied to direct who to test, whereby 1 point is given for each of the following: (1) tonsillar exudates, (2) tender anterior cervical lymphadenopathy, (3) fever, and (4) absence of cough. For the modified Centor criteria, add 1 point for age younger than 15 years and subtract 1 point for age older than 44 years. However, strep throat in children younger than 3 years is very rare.
  A score of 0 or 1 has a positive predictive value (PPV) of 1% to 5% for strep throat, which means that testing should not be undertaken because the likelihood of disease is so low that positive tests are likely to be false positives. A score of 4 points has a high PPV for disease; however, confirmatory testing is still generally recommended prior to initiation of antibiotics. Testing can be performed using the RADT or a throat culture.
  Complications of strep throat include suppurative complications such as peritonsillar abscesses, otitis media, retropharyngeal abscess, Lemierre syndrome, and mastoiditis. Nonsuppurative complications can also occur such as acute rheumatic fever (can be prevented with antibiotics) and poststreptococcal glomerulonephritis (PSGN; cannot be prevented with antibiotics).
  Diagnosis: Streptococcal pharyngitis.

CASE 7

HPI: A 22-year-old woman was brought in by her boyfriend 4 hours after she ingested an unknown number of pills from her medicine cabinet. Emergency medical service personnel stated that there were no prescription medications in the cabinet—just aspirin and acetaminophen. The patient states that she feels fine and wants to go home. She denies any nausea, vomiting, abdominal pain, or current suicidal ideation.
Vital signs: Temperature 98.2°F (36.8°C), pulse 80 beats/min, BP 112/64 mm Hg, RR 16 breaths/min.
Additional history: None

1. What is the differential diagnosis?
Overdose of acetaminophen, salicylates, ferrous sulfate, and other medications.

2. What components of the physical examination do you perform?
General appearance, cardiovascular, lungs, abdomen, neuro/psych.
Physical examination:
General: No acute distress, no scleral icterus. Pupils equal and round, reactive to light and accommodation (PERRLA). No diaphoresis.
Cardiovascular: WNL
Lungs: WNL
Abdomen: WNL
Neuro/psych: WNL

3. What are your initial orders?
Chem 8, CBC, coagulation studies, liver function tests (LFTs), acetaminophen level, salicylate level, ethanol (EtOH) level, urinary toxicology screen, urinary pregnancy test, ECG.
Advance clock: CBC, chemistry panel, coagulation studies, LFTs, salicylate level, EtOH level, pregnancy test, and ECG are all WNL/negative. Acetaminophen level is 200 µg/L (high). Urine toxicology screen is positive for cannabinoids.

4. What are your follow-up actions?
Administration of *N*-acetylcysteine (NAC) IV or PO, consultation with poison control, psychiatry consultation for involuntary hold and further psychiatric evaluation, admission to a monitored bed for continued NAC therapy and monitoring of LFTs.
Advance clock: Case ends.
Critical actions: Recognition of acetaminophen toxicity, appropriate treatment even in the absence of symptoms (because early symptoms are rare), admission for continued therapy.
Discussion: This patient presented to the hospital without symptoms after a suicide attempt involving ingestion of pills. The lack of symptoms does not rule out such ingestion because many cases are initially asymptomatic. This patient had a negative laboratory workup except for an elevated acetaminophen level. At 4 hours, the treatment threshold for acetaminophen ingestion is 150 µg/L according to the Rumack-Matthew nomogram, which was

surpassed in this patient. In addition, if the amount of acetaminophen ingested is known, acute ingestion of more than 150 mg/kg acetaminophen is also an indication for treatment.

The initial treatment is 150 mg/kg NAC, which helps to inactivate the hepatotoxic metabolic product *N*-acetyl-*p*-benzoquinone imine and prevents the complications of acetaminophen overdose. Therapy is then typically continued for 72 hours on an inpatient basis (although shorter regimens are becoming more popular). The patient should also have a comprehensive psychiatric evaluation. Because the ingestion occurred more than 1 to 2 hours prior to presentation, activated charcoal would not be beneficial. For acute ingestion or ingestion of time-release medications for which the ingested substance can bind to charcoal, administration of activated charcoal can be beneficial. Without treatment, acetaminophen overdose can cause drug-induced liver injury with fulminant hepatitis.

It is important to rule out coingestion of other medications/substances. The patient had a normal ECG and no access to prescription medications, making tricyclic antidepressant (TCA) overdose less likely (the classic three *C*s for TCA overdose are *c*ardiotoxicity, *c*onvulsions, and *c*oma). The patient's salicylate level was negligible, and salicylate toxicity would be expected to produce a mixed acid-base disorder of respiratory alkalosis (tachypnea from direct stimulation of medullary respiratory centers) and metabolic acidosis (uncoupling of oxidative phosphorylation). A significant dose of opioids should cause symptoms and signs such as respiratory depression and miosis. There is no evidence of a sympathomimetic agent (e.g., cocaine, amphetamine) or cholinergic toxidrome. The lack of metabolic acidosis (normal bicarbonate) makes ingestion of a substance such as methanol or ethylene glycol much less likely.

Diagnosis: Acetaminophen toxicity.

CASE 8

HPI: A 40-year-old woman who was previously healthy presents to the ED after having had two car accidents in which she had hit parked cars. She states that she did not see them in her peripheral vision and is usually a good driver. She is also concerned because although she typically has regular menstrual cycles, she has not had menses in 3 months. She notes that she has had some bilateral nipple discharge.

Vital signs: Temperature 98.2°F (36.8°C), pulse 76 beats/min, BP 114/64 mm Hg, RR 16 breaths/min.

Additional history: No other medical history. The patient has not been sexually active for more than 2 years.

1. What is the differential diagnosis?
   Prolactinoma, pregnancy, hypothyroidism, primary brain malignancy.

2. What components of the physical examination do you perform?
   General appearance, HEENT, breast, neuro/psych.
   Physical examination:
   General: WNL
   HEENT: WNL
   Breast: A small amount of milky discharge can be expressed from each nipple. No masses are palpable.
   Neuro/psych: Bitemporal hemianopsia, otherwise WNL.

3. What are your initial orders?
   CBC, chem 8, prolactin level, TSH, brain MRI, urinary pregnancy test.
   Advance clock: Prolactin level 200 ng/mL (elevated). TSH is WNL. Pregnancy test negative. Brain MRI reveals a 12-mm mass in the anterior pituitary gland, with a mass effect on the optic chiasm.

4. What are your follow-up actions?
   Consult endocrinology and begin dopamine agonist therapy (e.g., bromocriptine, cabergoline).
   Consult neurosurgery; no surgical intervention recommended at this time.
   Counsel the patient regarding her disease.
   Advance clock:
   The patient's visual complaints have resolved. (If follow-up MRI ordered, the mass has shrunk on treatment to 5 mm.)
   Case ends

Critical actions: Recognition of prolactinoma, ordering of a pregnancy test for a woman of reproductive age with amenorrhea (regardless of reported sexual activity), endocrinology consultation or initiation of appropriate therapy for prolactinoma (dopamine agonist therapy).

Discussion: This patient has a prolactinoma, a benign tumor of the lactotroph cells in the anterior pituitary gland. This is the most common tumor of the pituitary. Prolactin secretion by a prolactinoma causes downregulation of the release of sex hormones and therefore amenorrhea, infertility, and/or loss of libido can occur. Prolactin stimulates milk production, so affected females often have bilateral nipple discharge.

As the size of the tumor increases (>10 mm is classified as a macroadenoma vs a smaller microadenoma), there can be mass effect on the optic chiasm, which compresses the crossing fibers from the nasal retina, causing bitemporal hemianopsia. In this patient, loss of these visual fields caused her to accidentally hit the parked cars that were outside her visual field.

The cornerstone of therapy is dopamine agonists such as bromocriptine or cabergoline. Dopamine exerts negative feedback on the anterior pituitary gland, decreasing prolactin release. This causes the tumor to produce less prolactin and decrease in size, therefore the patient had an improvement in visual symptoms after treatment. The differential diagnosis for hyperprolactinemia includes medication use (e.g., dopamine antagonists), renal failure (from decreased clearance and disordered hypothalamic regulation), and hypothyroidism (because thyrotropin-releasing hormone [TRH] stimulates prolactin release). Surgical therapy is an option, but dopamine agonist therapy is the first-line treatment for most patients.

Diagnosis: Prolactinoma.

CASE 9

HPI: You are called to the inpatient unit because a 10-year-old boy started shaking and became unresponsive; the episode was witnessed by his parents and the nursing staff. The boy was visiting his mother, who is ill. He started shaking 3 minutes ago. He has never had this problem before. The parents deny any trauma or ingestions. The patient was apparently sitting and talking with his mother when he suddenly became unresponsive, his entire body started convulsing, and he exhibited urinary incontinence. He is currently still shaking and is unresponsive.

Vital signs: Temperature 98.2°F (36.8°C), pulse 110 beats/min, BP 110/60 mm Hg, RR 22 breaths/min.

Additional history: No medical history, vaccines up to date, no allergies.

1. What is the differential diagnosis?
   Seizure secondary to epilepsy, hypoglycemia, hypoxemia, toxin ingestion, infection (meningitis, encephalitis), trauma, mass lesion, bleeding, electrolyte disturbances (e.g., hyponatremia), or conversion disorder.

2. What components of the physical examination do you perform?
   Defer examination because the patient requires immediate intervention.

3. What are your initial orders?
   Cardiac monitoring, pulse oximetry, oxygen, fingerstick blood glucose, lorazepam.
   Advance clock: Oxygen saturation 100%, fingerstick glucose 108 mg/dL. After administration of one dose of lorazepam, the seizure stops.

4. What are your follow-up actions?
   Transfer to the ED; perform CBC, chem 8, noncontrast head CT scan, physical examination.

5. What components of the physical examination do you perform?
   General appearance, HEENT/neck, lungs, cardiovascular, abdomen, neuro/psych.
   Physical examination:
   General: Slowly responds to questions, no shaking activity, breathing on his own.
   HEENT/neck: No meningismus, small superficial laceration to the lateral tongue.
   Cardiovascular: WNL
   Lungs: Tachypnea.
   Abdomen: WNL
   Neuro/psych: Moving all his extremities, alert and oriented to name only, no focal neurologic deficits.
   Advance clock:
   CBC, chem 8, noncontrast head CT scan all WNL.
   Patient returns to baseline, no neurologic deficits, alert and oriented to name, time, place, situation, and conversing normally.

6. What are your follow-up actions?
   Counseling on the disease process, neurology consult, electroencephalography (EEG) as an outpatient, MRI scan of the brain as an outpatient, discharge with follow-up appointment.
   Advance clock: Case ends.
   Critical actions: Recognition of active seizure, immediate supportive care and treatment with benzodiazepine, appropriate workup for seizure.
   Discussion: This patient had a generalized tonic-clonic seizure. Seizures are due to uncontrolled firing of neurons in the brain resulting from any number of possible inducing agents (e.g., infections, toxins, trauma). Seizure types include generalized tonic-clonic seizures, partial (focal) seizures with or without impairment of awareness (previously complex vs simple), or secondarily generalized seizures (start as partial, then become generalized). Absence seizures are characterized by numerous episodes of short seizures with abrupt impairment of consciousness and a blank stare lasting for seconds each time. This patient cannot have had a febrile seizure because he does not have a fever and is also outside the typical age range for febrile seizures (6 months–6 years). The current definition of status epilepticus (SE) is a seizure lasting more than 5 minutes or two seizures without a return to baseline between seizures (i.e., the patient is still postictal when the second seizure occurs). SE is a life-threatening condition.
   Treatment for active seizures includes standard supportive care (oxygen, monitoring, airway management if required), followed by benzodiazepines (e.g., lorazepam) as first-line agents. Repeated doses of benzodiazepines should be given if needed. Phenytoin (or the more soluble fosphenytoin), levetiracetam, or phenobarbital are

second-line therapies if the patient does not respond. The blood sugar level should be checked for all patients who have a seizure or are actively seizing because glucose administration can stop seizures in hypoglycemic patients. A woman of child-bearing age should have a pregnancy test. After the seizure terminates, basic laboratory tests are helpful in excluding electrolyte abnormalities (e.g., hyponatremia). A head CT or MRI should be obtained for all patients with first-time seizures (except simple febrile seizures; see Case 44 for details). Outpatient EEG and MRI scanning are indicated for most patients. Counsel patients that 40% of cases will have another seizure.

Diagnosis: Seizure.

CASE 10

HPI: A 60-year-old woman presents to the ED with chronic constipation, fatigue, memory deficits, and nausea for months. She was referred to the ED by her primary care physician when lab tests for these symptoms showed that her calcium level was elevated. She denies any weight loss, night sweats, or other symptoms.
Vital signs: Temperature 98.6°F (37°C), pulse 96 beats/min, BP 140/90 mm Hg, RR 16 breaths/min.
Additional history: Kidney stones, spine compression fracture, hip fracture with prosthetic hip replacement.

1. What is the differential diagnosis?
   Hypercalcemia due to primary hyperparathyroidism (PHPT) or malignancy. Less likely causes include medications, milk alkali syndrome, hyperthyroidism, immobilization.

2. What components of the physical examination do you perform?
   General appearance, cardiovascular, lungs, abdomen.
   Physical examination:
   General: Comfortable woman with appearance in agreement with stated age, dry mucous membranes.
   Cardiovascular: WNL
   Lungs: WNL
   Abdomen: Mild diffuse tenderness on palpation of the abdomen, no rebound or guarding.

3. What are your initial orders?
   Chem 14, CBC (because the calcium level is known to be elevated already, parathyroid hormone [PTH] measurement can be ordered at this point or later), ECG, and albumin (for correct determination of the calcium level) or ionized calcium (not impacted by the albumin level).
   Advance clock: Chem 14 remarkable for a calcium level of 13.6 mg/dL (albumin level normal). CBC unremarkable. If an ECG is ordered it shows a normal sinus rhythm with a short QT interval.

4. What are your follow-up actions?
   IV fluid administration, calcitonin, bisphosphonate, PTH level.
   Advance clock:
   PTH result 55 pg/mL (normal 10–60 pg/mL).
   Patient feels much better after IV fluid administration.
   If imaging of the parathyroid glands (e.g., sestamibi scan, ultrasound) is ordered, scans will show a solitary parathyroid adenoma.
   Surgery consultation.
   If any other imaging is ordered (e.g., CXR, CT scan), the results will be negative.
   If the PTH-related protein (PTHrP) level is measured, it will be undetectable.
   Case ends.
   Critical actions: Recognition of hypercalcemia, treatment with at least IV fluids, recognition that high normal PTH in the setting of high calcium levels is abnormal and confirms the diagnosis of PHPT. Referral for definitive surgical treatment. Initiation of bisphosphonate therapy to reduce the risk of worsening osteoporosis in a patient who already has multiple fractures, presumably because of her underlying condition.
   Discussion: This patient has hypercalcemia, a calcium level greater than 10.5 mg/dL. Although the differential diagnosis for hypercalcemia is broad, over 90% of cases result from one of two conditions: (1) PHPT or (2) malignancy. Abnormal PTH production in PHPT is typically due to a solitary parathyroid adenoma that overproduces PTH (80%), diffuse parathyroid hyperplasia (15%), or, in rare cases, parathyroid carcinoma (5%).
   Malignancy can cause hypercalcemia either directly because of bone degradation or via PTHrP. In this case, the PTH level was high for the level of calcium (in the presence of hypercalcemia the PTH level should be less than the lower normal limit because of negative feedback). This confirms the diagnosis of PHPT.
   Treatment of hypercalcemia is threefold: (1) IV fluids to reduce calcium levels and improve symptoms, (2) calcitonin to temporarily decrease calcium levels (not a long-term solution because of tachyphylaxis), and (3) bisphosphonate therapy to prevent further bone loss. Further treatment depends on the cause of the patient's hypercalcemia. In PHPT, surgical treatment is first-line therapy. Loop diuretics such as furosemide were previously used as first-line therapy but are now reserved for when urine output is inadequate despite aggressive fluid resuscitation. Sestamibi scans or ultrasound can show whether the parathyroid glands have an adenoma or diffuse hyperplasia. In cases of malignancy, the underlying cancer must be treated.
   Diagnosis: Hypercalcemia due to PHPT.

CASE 11

HPI: A 72-year-old man presents to his primary care physician complaining of red urine for the past 3 months. Initially his urine was just slightly off-colored and brown, and the patient thought he was dehydrated, but it has since progressed to a deep red color every time he urinates. The patient denies dysuria, hesitancy, or nocturia. He denies any fevers or chills or weight loss.

Vital signs: Temperature 98.2°F (36.8°C), pulse 76 beats/min, BP 135/78 mm Hg, RR 16 breaths/min.

Additional history: Takes hydrochlorothiazide for hypertension. No other medications and no allergies. Previously smoked for 40 years, 2 packs/day, but quit 3 years ago. Occasional alcohol consumption, no drug use.

1. What is the differential diagnosis?
   Hematuria due to bladder cancer, renal cancer, urinary tract infection (UTI), interstitial cystitis, nephrolithiasis, or prostate cancer; nephritic syndrome if urinalysis (UA) for hematuria reveals RBC casts.

2. What components of the physical examination do you perform?
   General appearance, cardiovascular, lungs, abdomen.
   Physical examination:
   General: Well-developed, well-nourished man in no apparent distress.
   Cardiovascular: WNL
   Lungs: WNL
   Abdomen: Firm mass in the pelvis, otherwise WNL.

3. What are your initial orders?
   CBC, chem 8, coagulation profile, UA, urine culture, urine cytology.
   Advance clock: CBC normal except hemoglobin (Hb) 11 mg/dL and a mean corpuscular volume (MCV) of 70 fL. Chem 8 and coagulation profile WNL. UA reveals a high level of blood with too many RBCs to count, no RBC casts, otherwise WNL. Urine culture and cytology pending.

4. What are your follow-up actions?
   CT urogram, urology consult for cystoscopy and biopsy.
   Advance clock:
   CT urogram demonstrates a 5-cm bladder mass without evidence of hydronephrosis or metastatic disease. Cystoscopy is performed and demonstrates a bladder mass; biopsy and urine cytology both consistent with transitional cell carcinoma of the bladder. Urine culture negative.
   Case ends.
   Critical actions: Recognition that painless hematuria in an older patient has a high likelihood of malignancy, ordering of appropriate workup including UA and imaging such as CT urogram. Urology referral for cystoscopy and biopsy.
   Discussion: This patient has bladder cancer. Painless gross hematuria is the most common presentation, and almost 100% of patients with bladder cancer will have some amount of microscopic hematuria on UA. Hematuria is often the only symptom, but patients can also have dysuria or frequent urination. A patient may experience urinary retention if the lesion is obstructive. Bladder cancer is more common in men than in women (3:1), older patients (median age is >70 years), and those with a history of smoking. Patients may have multiple tumors in the bladder at the same time because of the field effect, whereby the entire bladder is exposed to urinary carcinogens (e.g., from smoking), so multiple malignant foci can be present simultaneously.
   Diagnosis is on the basis of a history of painless hematuria in an appropriately aged patient, followed by UA, urine culture, and urine cytology. A CT urogram can define the anatomy and assess for obstruction and metastatic disease and is recommended for all patients thought to have a malignancy of the urinary system. Although the CT urogram is excellent at detecting renal malignancies, the sensitivity is lower for bladder malignancies. Therefore, for completion of workup and definitive diagnosis of a bladder malignancy, cystoscopy with biopsy is necessary. Transitional cell carcinoma (urothelial carcinoma) is the most common type of bladder cancer in the United States (almost all cases), followed by the much rarer squamous cell carcinoma and adenocarcinoma. All patients should be assessed for obstruction or severe anemia.
   Treatment depends on the depth of invasion and the presence or absence of metastatic disease. Low-grade lesions can be completely resected via transurethral resection of bladder tumor (TURBT) and intravesical bacillus Calmette-Guérin (BCG) treatment, but more advanced disease can require radical cystectomy with or without chemotherapy and possibly radiation if isolated metastases exist. The 5-year survival for localized lesions is good (>75%), but for metastatic disease the prognosis is poor.
   Diagnosis: Hematuria due to bladder cancer.

CASE 12

HPI: A 50-year-old woman presents to the ED complaining of a headache. She says that she was watching television, and at 5:13 pm (approximately 8 hours ago) she instantly developed a severe headache over her entire head that caused her to vomit twice. She states that lights now bother her, and her neck feels stiff, as if she "slept on it wrong." She denies any history of headaches, except for 1 week ago when she had a similar episode lasting for hours, but that episode was less severe and she did not seek medical evaluation.

Vital signs: Temperature 98.2°F (36.8°C), pulse 98 beats/min, BP 120/78 mm Hg, RR 18 breaths/min.

Additional history: Occasional alcohol use, no use of drugs or tobacco. No medical or surgical history.

1. What is the differential diagnosis?

   Subarachnoid hemorrhage (SAH), migraine, meningitis, hemorrhagic stroke, intracranial hemorrhage, mass lesion, obstructive hydrocephalus.

2. What components of the physical examination do you perform?

   General appearance, HEENT/neck, cardiovascular, lungs, neuro/psych.

   Physical examination:

   General: Well-developed, well-nourished woman in moderate distress due to pain.

   HEENT/neck: Meningismus, PERRLA.

   Cardiovascular: WNL

   Lungs: WNL

   Neuro/psych: Normal strength, sensation, reflexes, and tone. Cranial nerves intact.

3. What are your initial orders?

   Stat noncontrast head CT scan. CBC, chem 8, coagulation profile, analgesics (e.g., acetaminophen).

   Advance clock:

   Noncontrast head CT scan: negative for bleeding or a mass effect.

   CBC, chem 8, coagulation profile: WNL

   Patient feels slightly better after analgesia.

4. What are your follow-up actions?

   Lumbar puncture with a cell count and differential, protein, glucose, Gram stain, culture.

   Advance clock: Lumbar puncture shows more than 100,000 RBCs in all tubes, + xanthochromia, otherwise normal.

5. What are your follow-up actions?

   CT angiogram head/neck, nimodipine PO, neurosurgery consult, blood pressure control if hypertensive (e.g., IV nicardipine), admit to the intensive care unit (ICU).

   Advance clock: Case ends.

   Critical actions: Recognition of the possibility of SAH, appropriate diagnostic testing (CT scan and, if negative, a lumbar puncture), admission to the ICU for close monitoring.

   Discussion: This patient has a SAH, which is blood inside the subarachnoid space (where the CSF resides), a life-threatening condition. This is usually due to rupture of a preexisting saccular aneurysm in the circle of Willis but can also be traumatic in origin. The classic presentation is a sudden-onset "thunderclap" headache, which is the worst of the patient's life, with or without loss of consciousness. The blood irritates the meninges, so patients can exhibit neck stiffness, nausea, vomiting, seizures, and an altered level of consciousness. Some patients with SAH have a sentinel bleed days to weeks previously, which this patient exhibited.

       Diagnosis can initially be made based on a noncontrast CT scan of the head that demonstrates blood inside the subarachnoid space. If positive, the diagnosis is clear and treatment can proceed. If the CT scan is negative, this does not necessarily rule out SAH (CT is not sensitive enough if performed >6 hours after presentation) and therefore the patient requires a lumbar puncture for detection of blood in the CSF (or xanthochromia from blood breakdown if the bleed is slightly older). After diagnosis, treatment includes BP management (avoiding hypertension and hypotension), volume management (avoiding hypovolemia), preventing vasospasm with nimodipine (a calcium channel blocker), and preventing seizures with anticonvulsants (typically levetiracetam, but anticonvulsants are controversial for SAH). These patients should be admitted to the ICU for close observation for complications such as continued bleeding, vasospasm, hyponatremia, and obstructive hydrocephalus. In cases of aneurysmal SAH, the aneurysm can be coiled or clipped to prevent future episodes of bleeding.

   Diagnosis: SAH.

CASE 13

HPI: A 22-year-old woman presents to the clinic at her university for a rash on her lip. She says that she has had fatigue and a mild fever (maximum temperature recorded 100.4°F [38.0°C]). Today she developed a painful rash on her left lower lip. She denies any history of similar symptoms. She admits that she had protected sex with a man she met at a party last week but says he did not have any rashes that she noticed.

Vital signs: Temperature 99.7°F (37.6°C), pulse 58 beats/min, BP 118/58 mm Hg, RR 16 breaths/min.

Additional history: Twenty lifetime sexual partners, all male, occasional protection. Last menses 3 weeks ago. Moderate alcohol use. No cigarette use, smokes marijuana weekly. No medical problems, medications, allergies, or surgeries.

1. What is the differential diagnosis?

   Primary herpes simplex virus (HSV) infection, impetigo, herpangina, aphthous stomatitis, herpes zoster, primary syphilis, chancroid, perioral dermatitis.

2. **What components of the physical examination do you perform?**
General appearance, HEENT, cardiovascular, lungs.
Physical examination:
General: Well-developed, well-nourished woman in no apparent distress.
HEENT: Groups of vesicles on an erythematous base at the vermillion border of the left lower lip measuring 8 mm
in total. No intraoral lesions. Submandibular and cervical lymphadenopathy. No meningismus.
Cardiovascular: WNL
Lungs: WNL

3. **What are your initial orders?**
Urinary pregnancy test; *Chlamydia,* gonorrhea, rapid plasma reagin (RPR), HIV screening. Counsel the patient on
safe sex techniques, birth control. Optional: HSV polymerase chain reaction (PCR) of lesion.
Advance clock: Urinary pregnancy test, *Chlamydia,* gonorrhea, RPR, HIV negative. HSV PCR of lesion, if ordered,
will be positive.

4. **What are your follow-up actions?**
Acyclovir or valacyclovir treatment. Counseling on disease.
Advance clock: Case ends.
Critical actions: Recognition of the signs and symptoms of primary HSV infection. Appropriate screening for sexually
active young adults, counseling. Treatment of HSV.
Discussion: This patient has a primary infection with HSV. HSV-1 classically causes oral herpes, whereas HSV-2
classically causes genital herpes, but either one can cause an infection in either location. Outbreaks can be classified as primary or secondary and have different signs and symptoms. The first outbreak (primary) of oral herpes is
usually much more severe than subsequent outbreaks and is characterized by mononucleosis-like symptoms
such as fever, fatigue, and headache often associated with lymphadenopathy. The rash is vesicular, and a small
group of vesicles will manifest itself, usually on the outer edge of the vermillion border. Recurrent outbreaks occur
on reactivation of the herpes virus (which is latent in the nerve), are less severe, and often have a prodrome of
neuropathic pain and burning before the vesicular lesion "cold sore or fever blister" appears. HSV can also infect
the genital region, cause encephalitis (HSV-1 is the most common cause of viral encephalitis), infect the skin via
direct contact (herpes gladiatorum), infect skin that is susceptible because of eczema (eczema herpeticum), infect
the fingers (herpetic whitlow), or infect the cornea (herpetic keratitis).
    The diagnosis is made on a clinical basis because many individuals have asymptomatic infections, and anti-
body tests are of limited use. A viral culture or PCR can be used if the clinical diagnosis is not straightforward. For
cases of suspected encephalitis, a lumbar puncture should be performed and sent for HSV PCR; imaging if obtained will typically show involvement of the medial temporal lobes, and patients should receive IV acyclovir. For
herpetic keratitis, a fluorescein dye used on the eye will demonstrate dendritic lesions. Herpetic keratitis is treated
with oral or topical acyclovir. Steroid eye drops should be avoided because they will greatly exacerbate the infection.
    Treatment is with acyclovir or valacyclovir for primary infection and to prevent or treat recurrences. Those
with a primary HSV infection may never have another outbreak. Patients should be counseled on transmission of
HSV and asymptomatic shedding, whereby the virus can still be transmitted even if no lesions are visible. As an
aside, the Centers for Disease Control and Prevention recommends annual screening for *Chlamydia* for all sexually
active women younger than 25 years; screening for gonorrhea is indicated for those at risk of infection, and HIV
screening should be discussed.
    Diagnosis: HSV-1 primary infection.

CASE 14

HPI: A 56-year-old man with a medical history of alcoholic cirrhosis is brought to the ED by his wife. He complains of
1 day of gradually worsening, dull abdominal pain. The pain is now moderate and associated with subjective fever.
He denies coffee-ground emesis or blood in his stool.
Vital signs: Temperature 100.8°F (38.2°C), pulse 105 beats/min, BP 110/78 mm Hg, RR 12 breaths/min.
Additional history: Diagnosed with alcoholic cirrhosis 2 years previously. No longer drinks alcohol.

1. **What is the differential diagnosis?**
Spontaneous bacterial peritonitis (SBP), secondary bacterial peritonitis, appendicitis, diverticulitis, cholecystitis,
pancreatitis, perforated viscus.

2. **What components of the physical examination do you perform?**
General appearance, HEENT, cardiovascular, lungs, abdomen, extremities.
Physical examination:
General: No acute distress.
HEENT: Dry cracked lips, scleral icterus.
Cardiovascular: Tachycardia, otherwise WNL.
Lungs: WNL

Abdomen: Distended with a fluid wave and shifting dullness; soft, moderate tenderness that is diffuse; no rebound or guarding.
Extremities: Pitting edema (score 2+) to the knees.

3. What are your initial orders?
Pulse oximetry, BP/cardiac monitor, CBC, chem 8, LFTs, prothrombin time (PT)/partial thromboplastin time (PTT), lipase/amylase, blood cultures, UA, urine culture, paracentesis (cell count, protein, albumin, glucose, lactate dehydrogenase [LDH], Gram stain, culture).
Advance clock:
Elevated white blood cell (WBC) count, mild anemia and thrombocytopenia, elevated PT/PTT, low albumin.
Ascitic fluid: More than 250 polymorphonuclear neutrophil (PMN) cells/mL, total protein less than 1 g/dL, glucose greater than 50 g/dL, LDH greater than 225 U/L, Gram stain reveals gram-negative rods.
Other studies: WNL

4. What are your follow-up actions?
Ceftriaxone IV, albumin IV, admit to inpatient unit. Vital signs observed every 4 hours, CBC and chem 8 next day. Counseling before discharge.
Advance clock:
Culture is positive for *Escherichia coli* on hospital day 2. Sensitive to ceftriaxone.
WBC count normalizes, vital signs normalize, and the patient's symptoms are greatly improved.
Case ends.
Critical actions: Abdominal examination, paracentesis with ascitic fluid studies, IV antibiotics, admit to inpatient unit.
Discussion: SBP is a serious medical condition that typically occurs in cirrhotic patients with existing large-volume ascites. The classic presenting symptoms are fever, diffuse abdominal pain/tenderness, and altered mental status. All three of these features may be subtle, however, because cirrhotic patients tend to be hypothermic at baseline and the presence of ascites obscures the physical examination finding of an acute rigid abdomen. Altered mental status may take the form of full delirium or a subtle behavioral change (and can be obscured by baseline hepatic encephalopathy). The most common organisms responsible for SBP are *E. coli*, *Streptococcus*, and *Klebsiella*.

SBP is diagnosed on the basis of an ascites PMN count of greater than 250 cells/mL. Gram stain is often negative as the total bacterial counts in SBP are generally low. A diagnosis of SBP can only be established, however, in the absence of a secondary cause of peritonitis. To assess for secondary bacterial peritonitis, other ascites studies include ascitic protein, albumin, glucose, LDH, and amylase. Ascites findings that indicate secondary peritonitis include protein greater than 1 g/dL, glucose less than 50 mg/dL, and LDH greater than 225 U/L. Elevated amylase or bilirubin in ascitic fluid may indicate pancreatic or biliary causes of peritonitis. If secondary bacterial peritonitis cannot be ruled out, a search for a secondary source must begin. CT imaging can help in evaluating for most pancreatic, biliary, and bowel pathologies. Once a diagnosis of SBP is established, the patient should be treated with a third-generation cephalosporin (ceftriaxone) with adjustment of treatment following identification of sensitivities and susceptibilities of culprit pathogens. Albumin IV is administered to patients who have a creatinine above 1 mg/dL, BUN greater than 30 mg/dL, OR if the total bilirubin is greater than 4 mg/dL as it has been shown to prevent hepatorenal syndrome and decreases mortality. Patients at high risk of recurrence may be discharged on a prophylactic antibiotic regimen such as trimethoprim/sulfamethoxazole.
Diagnosis: SBP.

CASE 15

HPI: A 36-year-old woman presents to the ED after noticing swelling and pain in her left leg. She does not recall any trauma to the leg. She noticed that the leg was painful and tender this morning when she tried to walk. She has had no fevers, chills, chest pain, cough, or shortness of breath. She was recently on a flight from Australia to New York.
Vital signs: Temperature 98.6°F (37.0°C), pulse 78 beats/min, BP 110/78 mm Hg, RR 15 breaths/min.
Additional history: The patient takes an oral contraceptive. No other medical history or medications. No use of drugs, tobacco, or alcohol.

1. What is the differential diagnosis?
Deep venous thrombosis (DVT), superficial thrombophlebitis, cellulitis, muscle strain, fracture, venous insufficiency.

2. What components of the physical examination do you perform?
General appearance, HEENT, cardiovascular, lungs, abdomen, extremities.
Physical examination:
General: No acute distress.
HEENT: WNL
Cardiovascular: WNL
Lungs: WNL
Abdomen: WNL
Extremities: Swelling and erythema of left calf compared to right. Tenderness along the posterior calf with a deep palpable cord. Peripheral pulses 2+.

3. What are your initial orders?
Pulse oximetry, ultrasound of the leg, CBC, chem 8, PT/PTT, urine pregnancy test.
Advance clock: Ultrasound reveals a noncompressible popliteal vein consistent with venous thrombosis. All other studies WNL.

4. What are your follow-up actions?
Apixaban or rivaroxaban without a low molecular weight heparin (LMWH) bridge, versus LMWH bridge with edoxaban, dabigatran, or warfarin. If using warfarin, follow up in 3 days to check PT/international normalized ratio (INR), discontinue oral contraceptive pill (OCP), counseling.
Advance clock: Case ends.
Critical actions: Examination of the extremities, ultrasound of the leg, discontinuation of OCP, anticoagulation therapy (e.g., LMWH and warfarin).
Discussion: This patient has unilateral swelling of the leg with risk factors for DVT (OCP use and recent travel). The physical examination in this case is suggestive of DVT, and further diagnostic testing is warranted. In patients with low risk of DVT, a single negative d-dimer result may be sufficient to rule out thrombosis. In this intermediate-risk patient (based on history and physical findings), the workup should proceed directly to ultrasound because a negative d-dimer result is insufficient to rule out DVT. Most cases of DVT can be treated on an outpatient basis with anticoagulation therapy. Depending on medication accessibility, this can be performed with (1) a direct oral anticoagulant (DOAC) such as rivaroxaban, apixaban, edoxaban, or dabigatran, or (2) warfarin. Dabigatran, edoxaban, and warfarin require LMWH bridging, whereas rivaroxaban and apixaban do not. The initial laboratory screening tests can identify those at risk of anticoagulation complications. If warfarin is used, patients should be scheduled for follow-up in 2 to 3 days to check the PT/INR and adjust warfarin dosage. When applicable, OCPs should be discontinued, and patients should be counseled about alternative contraceptive methods. In first-time provoked (known risk factors such as OCP use) cases of DVT, anticoagulation therapy is continued for 3 to 6 months and screening for hypercoagulability is generally not warranted. In patients with unprovoked or recurrent DVT, a hypercoagulable workup is performed that includes testing for protein C, protein S, antithrombin III, factor V Leiden, antiphospholipid antibodies, and prothrombin G20210A gene mutation. These tests are usually ordered at follow-up because some are influenced by oral anticoagulation use and the clotting event itself. The evaluation and treatment of DVT are primarily to prevent the complications of venous thromboembolism, including pulmonary embolism (discussed separately). Any patient with DVT should be evaluated for signs and symptoms related to pulmonary embolism (chest pain, shortness of breath, hypoxia).
Diagnosis: DVT.

CASE 16

HPI: A 4-year-old boy is brought to the ED by his parents, who are concerned about their child's fever. They state that they have taken his temperature for the past 6 days and it was always greater than 100.4°F (38°C) and did not seem to resolve on acetaminophen or ibuprofen administration. The patient denies a cough, runny nose, urinary problems, or sore throat. The parents state that he has had red eyes for the past 2 days but that they do not hurt, and on the first day of illness he had a rash on his chest that felt rough but has since resolved.
Vital signs: Temperature 101.5°F (38.6°C), pulse 120 beats/min, BP 110/80 mm Hg, RR 20 breaths/min.
Additional history: No medical history, no hospitalizations, all vaccines up to date.

1. What is the differential diagnosis?
Kawasaki disease, viral exanthem, conjunctivitis (e.g., adenovirus), infectious mononucleosis.

2. What components of the physical examination do you perform?
General appearance, HEENT, skin, cardiovascular, lungs, abdomen.
Physical examination:
General: Well-developed, well-nourished boy in no acute distress.
HEENT: Bilateral conjunctivitis with perilimbal sparing, no exudates. Tongue has diffuse inflamed red papillae. Anterior cervical adenopathy bilaterally, largest 2 cm.
Skin: No rashes.
Cardiovascular: WNL
Lungs: WNL
Abdomen: WNL

3. What are your initial orders?
Admit to the inpatient unit, aspirin, IV immunoglobulin (IVIG), transthoracic echocardiogram (TTE).
Advance clock: The patient's fever resolves with treatment. TTE shows no evidence of coronary artery aneurysm.

4. What are your follow-up actions?
Discharge with follow-up for serial TTE and recheck.
Advance clock: Case ends.
Critical actions: Recognition of Kawasaki disease as a clinical diagnosis; initiation of treatment.

Discussion: This patient has Kawasaki disease, an acute vasculitis of childhood primarily involving the coronary arteries. The diagnosis is on a clinical basis, but for incomplete Kawasaki disease (previously called atypical), laboratory findings support the diagnosis (see later). Untreated patients are at much higher risk (20%–25%) of coronary artery aneurysms than treated patients (4%), so prompt recognition is essential.

The clinical diagnosis of Kawasaki disease can be remembered by the "CRASH and burn" mnemonic. The burn refers to the 5 days of fever, and CRASH is a mnemonic for conjunctivitis (nonexudative bilateral, perilimbil sparing), rash (anything but petechiae), adenopathy (cervical), strawberry tongue or other oral mucous membrane changes, and hands and feet (erythema, edema, desquamation). At least four of the CRASH mnemonic findings must be present, as well as fever for 5 days. If two or three CRASH findings are present, then there are laboratory criteria to support the diagnosis of incomplete Kawasaki disease (hypoalbuminemia, anemia, alanine aminotransferase [ALT] elevation, thrombocytosis, leukocytosis, urinary WBCs).

Treatment is with IVIG and acute high-dose aspirin administration, followed by low-dose aspirin for a longer period of time (6–8 weeks). TTE should be performed on initial diagnosis and at 2 weeks and 2 months to rule out interval development of coronary artery aneurysms.

Diagnosis: Kawasaki disease.

CASE 17

HPI: A 35-year-old woman presents to the ED with intense, intermittent right flank pain for the past 2 days. During this time, she has also noticed that her urine has taken on a darker appearance. She states that when she has the pain, she cannot seem to get comfortable; the pain is alleviated somewhat by ibuprofen. She denies any history of similar symptoms. No fevers, cough, dysuria, nausea, vomiting, or trauma.
Vital signs: Temperature 98.2°F (36.8°C), pulse 64 beats/min, BP 115/68 mm Hg, RR 16 breaths/min.
Additional history: No use of drugs, alcohol, or tobacco. No medical history.

1. What is the differential diagnosis?
   Nephrolithiasis, pyelonephritis, right lower lobe pneumonia, musculoskeletal pain, abdominal aortic aneurysm (AAA), cholecystitis.

2. What components of the physical examination do you perform?
   General, cardiovascular, lungs, abdominal, back.
   Physical examination:
   General: Well-developed and well-nourished woman in moderate distress due to pain, writhing uncomfortably on the gurney.
   Cardiovascular: WNL
   Lungs: WNL
   Abdomen: WNL
   Back: Moderate right-sided flank tenderness. No overlying skin changes or evidence of trauma.

3. What are your initial orders?
   CDC, chem 0, UA, urinary pregnancy test, (after pregnancy test results negative) nonsteroidal antiinflammatory drug (NSAID; e.g., ketorolac, ibuprofen).
   Advance clock: CBC and chem 8 WNL. UA blood 3+ with more than 182 RBCs per high-power field (hpf), otherwise WNL. Urinary pregnancy test negative. Patient feels much better after pain medication.

4. What are your follow-up actions?
   Noncontrast CT scan of the abdomen/pelvis.
   Advance clock: CT scan shows 6-mm kidney stone at the right ureterovesical junction (UVJ) with mild hydronephrosis.

5. What are your follow-up actions?
   Prescription for ibuprofen, +- an opioid, and tamsulosin. Follow-up after 1 week. Counsel the patient on the disease process and advise her to strain her urine.
   Advance clock:
   Patient returns stating she passed the stone, and her pain has resolved; she was unable to catch the stone.
   Case ends.
   Critical actions: Recognition of nephrolithiasis, appropriate treatment, and follow-up.
   Discussion: This patient has urolithiasis (a kidney stone) in the urogenital tract. Kidney stones typically cause severe intermittent (colicky) pain due to intermittent spasm of an irritated ureter. The three most common locations of stones are the ureteropelvic junction (where the renal pelvis joins the ureter), the pelvic brim (where the stone can get caught as the ureter passes over the iliac arteries), and the UVJ (where the ureters enter the bladder). The likelihood of stone passage is related to the size and location of the stone. Stones smaller than 5 mm usually pass, whereas stones larger than 10 mm almost never pass spontaneously. The most common stone is a calcium oxalate stone, but other stones can also occur. Struvite stones can occur when patients have infections from urea-splitting organisms such as *Proteus* because the free ammonia from the split urea makes up part of the struvite stone; these stones can completely fill the renal pelvis and are referred to as staghorn calculi.

Diagnosis is by history and physical examination. For patients who have a kidney stone without a prior history of stones, a CT scan is typically performed to evaluate the size and location of the stone, and rule out alternative diagnoses. If patients have typical symptoms and a history of kidney stones, a renal ultrasound is preferred. The ultrasound rarely visualizes a ureteral stone, but it can assess for complications. Complications include obstructing stones (which block urinary flow from the kidney and are associated with hydronephrosis), infected stones (which can prevent infected urine from passing), and renal failure if obstruction persists for too long. Management is with a combination of NSAIDs, acetaminophen, + opioids (the NSAIDs help prevent prostaglandin-mediated ureter pain). Tamsulosin is an alpha-antagonist that helps dilate the smooth muscle in the urogenital tract to facilitate stone passage. Tamsulosin's evidence to facilitate stone passage is strongest for stones between 5 and 10 mm in size. Patients with uncomplicated nephrolithiasis can be managed as outpatients with urologic follow-up if the stone is unlikely to be passed on its own. Urgent urologic consultation and/or admission are indicated for concurrent infection and hydronephrosis, renal failure, uncontrollable pain, or inability to tolerate oral intake. In older patients, even with symptoms classic for nephrolithiasis, other emergent conditions such as AAA must always be considered.

Diagnosis: Nephrolithiasis

CASE 18

HPI: A 26-year-old man is brought to the ED by his friends because he "wasn't making sense" when he talked and was becoming less responsive. The friends say that he takes insulin but ran out a little less than 1 week ago and has not been able to get a refill. They deny any ingestion or any other complaints from the patient.

Vital signs: Temperature 98.2°F (36.8°C), pulse 120 beats/min, BP 100/70 mm Hg, RR 28 breaths/min.

Additional history: Unknown.

1. **What is the differential diagnosis?**
   Altered mental status: **AEIOU TIPS** mnemonic: **a**cidosis; **e**lectrolytes, **e**ncephalopathy, **e**ndocrine (e.g., diabetic ketoacidosis [DKA]); **i**nsulin causing hypoglycemia; **o**piates or **o**verdose; **u**remia; **t**rauma, **t**emperature, **t**oxemia; **i**nfections; **p**ulmonary embolism or **p**sychogenic; **s**pace-occupying lesions, **s**trokes, **s**hock, **s**eizure.

2. **What components of the physical examination do you perform?**
   General appearance, cardiovascular, lungs, neuro/psych.
   Physical examination:
   General: Obtunded but able to be aroused, breathing rapidly and deeply.
   Cardiovascular: Tachycardic but no murmurs, rubs, or gallops.
   Lungs: WNL
   Neuro/psych: Able to say name on stimulation, knows year. No obvious focal neurologic deficits but limited examination secondary to obtundation.

3. **What are your initial orders?**
   Fingerstick blood glucose, CBC, chem 8, serum ketones, UA, ECG, venous blood gas, portable CXR, IV fluids.
   Advance clock: CBC shows leukocytosis of 16 × 103 cells/mL with a left shift but no bandemia; otherwise normal. Chem 8 remarkable for sodium 130 mEq/L, potassium 4.8 mEq/L, bicarbonate 10 mEq/L (anion gap 26 mEq/L), normal creatinine, and glucose 500 mg/dL; otherwise normal. Serum ketones elevated. UA reveals a high ketone level, high specific gravity, and a high glucose level; otherwise negative. ECG sinus tachycardia at 125 beats/min. Venous blood gas pH 7.05. Portable CXR negative. After IV fluids, the heart rate decreases to 110 beats/min.

4. **What are your follow-up actions?**
   Begin regular insulin IV drip, continue high rate of IV fluid administration with potassium supplementation, admit to the ICU.
   Advance clock: Case ends.
   Critical actions: Check point-of-care glucose in patient with altered mental status, recognition of DKA as the cause of the patient's altered mental status; fluid resuscitation, waiting for potassium value before starting insulin.
   Discussion: This patient has DKA secondary to running out of insulin. Lack of insulin causes increased gluconeogenesis and lipolysis, leading to ketosis and acidosis. These factors, paired with an inability to import glucose into cells, lead to significant hyperglycemia. After diagnosis, fluid resuscitation should be initiated because osmotic diuresis arising from hyperglycemia typically causes profound hypovolemia. In children, however, there is controversy about whether aggressive fluid resuscitation causes cerebral edema so intravenous fluids should be given with caution. Insulin therapy should not be initiated until a potassium level is obtained. Patients experience whole-body potassium depletion but often have normal or high serum potassium values because of acidosis. If potassium is low (<3.3 mEq/L), insulin should not be administered until potassium is replete because insulin will drive potassium intracellularly and further lower serum potassium. If the potassium is normal, potassium can be added to IV fluids; if high (>5.5 mEq/L), no potassium should be added. The dose of insulin is 0.1 U/kg/hr via a regular insulin IV drip; an initial bolus of 0.1 U/kg is controversial and probably unnecessary. Sodium is often classically low because hyperglycemia causes water to shift into the intravascular space, where it dilutes sodium. The correction is 1.6 mEq/L (some use 2 mEq/L) added for every 100 mg/dL by which glucose exceeds 100 mg/dL.

Although missing insulin doses are a common precipitant for DKA, there should be a high index of suspicion for alternative causes. Infection is a common inducing factor, as are myocardial infarction (MI) and substance ingestion. Alcoholic ketoacidosis should also be included in the differential diagnosis. Close monitoring of electrolytes and glucose is required, and once glucose falls below 250 mg/dL, glucose should be added to the IV fluids. The insulin drip can be stopped once the acidosis and ketosis resolve while overlapping with subcutaneous insulin. Admission to a monitored bed or ICU is usually warranted for initial management.

Diagnosis: DKA.

CASE 19

HPI: An 84-year-old man is brought to his primary care physician by his family because of concerns about increased forgetfulness. The family states that for the past 5 to 6 years he has progressively worsened in his ability to remember things. Initially, he needed help with his finances and taxes but otherwise was able to live independently and carry out his daily activities. However, over the past year or so he has been getting lost when he goes out driving or walking and has been forgetting to do things like turn off the stove and forgetting the names of family members. The patient denies being forgetful and says that he never gets lost. The family and the patient deny any abrupt decline in function, changes in medication, or new exposures. The patient does not have any difficulty in walking, sleeping, or eating, and has no weakness.

Vital signs: Temperature 98.2°F (36.8°C), pulse 66 beats/min, BP 135/78 mm Hg, RR 16 breaths/min.

Additional history: History only significant for hyperlipidemia, for which he takes atorvastatin. No other medical problems or allergies. No use of drugs, alcohol, or tobacco.

1. What is the differential diagnosis?

   Dementia: Alzheimer (most likely), vascular, frontotemporal, Lewy body. Other causes: hypothyroidism, vitamin B_{12} deficiency, HIV infection, neurosyphilis, calcium derangement, depression, medication effects.

2. What components of the physical examination do you perform?

   General appearance, lungs, cardiovascular, neuro/psych.

   Physical examination:

   General: Well-developed, well-nourished man in no apparent distress.

   Cardiovascular: WNL

   Lungs: WNL

   Neuro/psych: Cranial nerves II through XII intact. Strength, sensation, reflexes, and gait all WNL. Alert and oriented to name only. Remembers 0/3 objects at 5 minutes. Cannot subtract serial 7s from 100, and cannot spell *WORLD* backwards. Can name a pen, but not a watch. Can follow one-step commands, but not more complicated commands.

3. What are your initial orders?

   CBC, chem 8, ESR, vitamin B_{12}, thyroid function tests, HIV, RPR, noncontrast MRI brain.

   Advance clock: All the studies ordered are WNL.

4. What are your follow-up actions?

   Counseling on the disease process and the need to stop driving, social work consult, consider starting medication such as donepezil.

   Advance clock: Case ends.

   Critical actions: Recognition of dementia, basic evaluation to rule out reversible causes, counseling on disease process and prognosis.

   Discussion: This patient has dementia, a chronic and often irreversible global decline in cognitive function. Dementia has many subtypes, including Alzheimer disease (most common), vascular dementia, frontotemporal dementia, and Lewy body dementia, among others. It is important to rule out a reversible cause of dementia and its mimics (e.g., hypothyroidism, pseudodementia caused by depression, HIV infection, neurosyphilis, medication effects in older individuals leading to cognitive impairment), as well as delirium (change in level of consciousness with acute or subacute onset, often caused by a medical problem and usually reversible if identified).

   Diagnosis is on the basis of history and physical examination and a ruling out of reversible causes. A mental status examination should be performed in all patients to evaluate their cognitive function. Basic laboratory tests such as CBC, serum chemistry (to rule out electrolyte/metabolic disturbances and uremia), vitamin B_{12} level (evaluate for subacute combined degeneration of the spinal cord), thyroid tests (evaluate for hypothyroidism), fourth-generation HIV antigen/antibody testing to evaluate for HIV-related dementia, and RPR to evaluate for neurosyphilis should be performed, and a CT or MRI of the brain is often ordered to rule out hydrocephalus and other lesions. Depending on the history, additional tests may be required (e.g., autoimmune disease, carotid ultrasound if vascular dementia is being considered, LFTs if hepatic encephalopathy is considered, ESR if screening for occult inflammatory states or malignancy). Treatment is mainly supportive because current medications (e.g., donepezil, memantine) have limited efficacy. Ensuring a safe home environment, counseling patients and their caregivers/family on the disease course, and appropriate follow-up to track disease progression are required.

   Diagnosis: Dementia.

CASE 20

HPI: An 18-month-old boy is brought to the ED with abdominal pain for the past 24 hours. The mother states that he appears well and is acting normally but then periodically starts to cry and brings his legs to his chest and vomits. During these episodes he says "Ow" and points to his abdomen. He has also been eating less and making fewer wet diapers during this time. The mother denies any changes in bowel movements.

Vital signs: Temperature 99.7°F (37.6°C), pulse 110 beats/min, BP 100/70 mm Hg, RR 30 breaths/min.

Additional history: All vaccinations up to date. Delivered at full term. No previous surgeries.

1. What is the differential diagnosis?

   Intussusception, incarcerated hernia, adhesions (if patient had history of surgery), constipation (if change in bowel movements), volvulus, testicular torsion.

2. What components of the physical examination do you perform?

   General appearance, cardiovascular, lungs, abdomen, genitalia.

   Physical examination:

   General: Well-appearing infant who occasionally has fits of crying and appears to be in moderate distress due to pain.

   Cardiovascular: WNL

   Lungs: WNL

   Abdomen: Soft, nondistended, tender to palpation during episodes of pain, sausage-like mass in the right abdomen.

   Genitalia: Testes descended bilaterally and nontender.

3. What are your initial orders?

   Ultrasound of abdomen; optional kidney, ureter, bladder (KUB) X-ray; UA.

   Advance clock: Ultrasound demonstrates the target sign, suggestive of intussusception.

4. What are your follow-up actions?

   Air/barium enema, surgical consult, admission to inpatient unit, counseling.

   Advance clock: Case ends.

   Critical actions: Recognition of intussusception as the cause of the abdominal pain, ordering appropriate workup, appropriate disposition. Checking the testes in male patients with abdominal pain because testicular torsion can cause referred pain to the abdomen.

   Discussion: This patient has ileocolic intussusception, whereby one part of the bowel (the intussusceptum) invaginates into a distal adjoining part of the bowel (the intussuscipiens). This typically occurs in patients between 3 months and 2 years of age but can also occur in older individuals with a lead point that drags the proximal bowel into the distal bowel. Examples are polyps, lymphoid hyperplasia from infections or lymphoma, a Meckel diverticulum, and submucosal hematomas seen in Henoch-Schönlein purpura.

   The classic presentation of intussusception involves the triad of intermittent colicky abdominal pain, vomiting, and a stool resembling red currant jelly, which is a late finding due to intestinal necrosis. The patient may draw the legs up during episodes of pain, and the vomiting due to the intestinal obstruction may be bilious. Infants may also present with lethargy with or without abdominal symptoms. On examination there may be a sausage-like mass that can be palpated. Diagnosis is made on the basis of ultrasound showing a target sign, but plain x-rays can also be beneficial.

   An air (or barium) enema is both diagnostic and therapeutic because the intussusception is often reduced by the enema (90% of cases). Management also includes fluid resuscitation if needed, antibiotics if there is evidence of peritonitis due to perforation, and a surgical consult. Admission to the hospital is usually warranted because recurrence risk is highest within the first 24 hours.

   Diagnosis: Intussusception.

CASE 21

HPI: A 66-year old man presents to the clinic complaining of several weeks of decreased energy. He feels so fatigued that he can barely get out of bed. When he does move he feels short of breath. He has found several large bruises over his body as a result of minor trauma. He cut himself while preparing dinner last week, and the bleeding did not stop for an abnormally long time.

Vital signs: Temperature 99.3°F (37.4°C), pulse 92 beats/min, BP 110/76 mm Hg, RR 18 breaths/min.

Additional history: No medical history. No use of drugs, tobacco, or alcohol.

1. What is the differential diagnosis?

   Anemia, thrombocytopenia, leukemia, congestive heart failure (CHF), pneumonia, viral infection, depression.

2. What components of the physical examination do you perform?

   General appearance, skin, lymph nodes, HEENT, cardiovascular, lungs, abdomen, extremities, neuro/psych.

Physical examination:
General: No acute distress.
Skin/lymph nodes: Two 5×5-cm^2 ecchymoses over lateral thigh and arm.
HEENT: Conjunctival pallor.
Cardiovascular: WNL
Lungs: WNL
Abdomen: WNL
Extremities: WNL
Neuro/psych: WNL

3. What are your initial orders?
Pulse oximetry, CBC with differential, peripheral smear, chem 8, PT/PTT, CXR.
Advance clock: CBC reveals 72,000 WBCs/mL with a high percentage of blasts, Hb 9.1 mg/dL, MCV 92 fL, platelets 82,000 cells/µL. Peripheral smear notable for presence of Auer rods. Other studies WNL.

4. What are your follow-up actions?
Uric acid, LDH, LFTs, oncology consult, bone marrow biopsy.
Advance clock: Case ends.
Critical actions: CBC, hematology-oncology consult.
Discussion: This patient has vague symptoms of fatigue and shortness of breath. Although this indicates a broad differential, the signs and symptoms of easy bruising indicate the possibility of a hematologic issue. CBC is an excellent screening test for hematologic issues, and the peripheral smear can offer more specific information. A thorough physical examination and CXR can exclude some other causes in the differential. The presence of hyperleukocytosis ($>$50,000 WBCs/mL), anemia, and thrombocytopenia points to a hematologic malignancy. The presence of blasts is suggestive of leukemia, and the presence of Auer rods is highly suggestive of acute myelogenous leukemia (AML). Once leukemia is suspected, a hematologist-oncologist should be consulted. The hematologist-oncologist will perform a bone marrow biopsy to confirm the diagnosis.
Urgent considerations in management include the exclusion of complications such as tumor lysis syndrome, leukostasis, and infection. Tumor lysis syndrome is evidenced by very high levels of uric acid, LDH, potassium, and phosphorus. It causes renal, cardiac, and neurologic complications. Treatment involves IV hydration, correction of electrolyte abnormalities, and administration of uric-acid–lowering agents such as rasburicase. Leukostasis may occur because of the high viscosity of the blood, particularly when the WBC count exceeds 100,000 cells/mL. This may cause renal, neurologic (e.g., headache and confusion), and pulmonary symptoms (dyspnea and hypoxia). Treatment for leukostasis is aggressive hydration and a hematology consult for induction therapy and possible leukapheresis. Patients with leukemia may be febrile secondary to the disease process or to bacterial infection. It is often difficult to distinguish the cause so cultures should be sent and empiric antibiotic therapy should be initiated in patients with leukemia and fever.
Diagnosis: AML.

CASE 22

HPI: A 53-year-old woman presents to the ED complaining of 2 days of fatigue and 1 day of mild confusion. Her daughter says she is normally in excellent health but has had difficulty getting out of bed over the past several days. She has felt feverish, but no temperature was recorded at home. Her daughter also noted a few small purple specks on her mother's skin. Today her mother seemed very confused so her daughter brought her to the ED.
Vital signs: Temperature 100.6°F (38.1°C), pulse 92 beats/min, BP 120/76 mm Hg, RR 18 breaths/min.
Additional history: No medical history. No use of drugs, tobacco, or alcohol.

1. What is the differential diagnosis?
Anemia, thrombocytopenia, leukemia, immune thrombocytopenic purpura (ITP), stroke, thrombotic thrombocytopenic purpura (TTP), vasculitis, infection (including pneumonia, UTI, meningitis, influenza), disseminated intravascular coagulation (DIC).

2. What components of the physical examination do you perform?
General appearance, skin, lymph nodes, HEENT, cardiovascular, lungs, abdomen, extremities, neuro/psych.
Physical examination:
General: No acute distress.
Skin: Few scattered petechiae.
Lymph nodes: WNL
HEENT: Conjunctival pallor.
Cardiovascular: WNL
Lungs: WNL
Abdomen: WNL
Extremities: WNL
Neuro/psych: Alert and oriented to person and place but not time, no focal neurologic deficits, neck supple.

3. What are your initial orders?

Pulse oximetry, CBC with differential, peripheral smear, chem 14, PT/PTT, CXR, UA.

Advance clock: CBC reveals platelets 25,000 cells/μL, Hb 7 mg/dL. Peripheral smear notable for presence of schistocytes. Mildly elevated BUN, creatinine, and bilirubin. UA blood 2+. Other studies WNL.

4. What are your follow-up actions?

Reticulocyte count, haptoglobin, LDH, hematology consult for plasma exchange, corticosteroids (e.g., prednisone), fresh frozen plasma (FFP) transfusion, admit to ICU.

Advance clock: Case ends.

Critical actions: CBC, hematology-oncology consult, admission, avoid transfusion of platelets.

Discussion: TTP is recognized clinically by a pentad described by the mnemonic FAT RN: *f*ever, *a*nemia (microangiopathic hemolytic anemia [MAHA]), *t*hrombocytopenia, *r*enal failure, and *n*eurologic deficits. The condition is caused by a deficiency of the protease ADAMTS13, usually due to autoantibodies. Under normal conditions, ADAMTS13 cleaves von Willebrand factor (vWF) multimers into smaller parts. ADAMTS13 deficiency causes vWF to agglutinate platelets in small vessels. As platelets clump in the small vessels, they create a shearing force on passing RBCs that causes MAHA (characterized by anemia, schistocytes, and elevated bilirubin). Occlusion of the microvasculature also causes renal failure and neurologic signs (e.g., coma, confusion, seizures). The complete pentad is present in only 50% of cases, however, so the presence of MAHA and thrombocytopenia should trigger a hematology consult. The diagnosis may not be suspected until routine laboratory tests for evaluation of the presenting complaint have been completed. CBC will reveal thrombocytopenia and anemia. A chemistry panel may reveal renal insufficiency. A peripheral smear will reveal schistocytes. LDH, bilirubin, and reticulocytes will all be elevated. Unlike DIC, the PT/PTT/INR will be normal because these parameters are not affected in TTP.

Treatment of TTP is initiated in consultation with a hematologist. The treatment of choice is plasmapheresis, which removes the patient's autoantibodies and ultralarge vWF. Then dysfunctional ADAMTS13 is replaced with functional ADAMTS13 in FFP. Plasmapheresis is rarely available immediately so temporizing measures should be undertaken. These include corticosteroid administration to address the autoimmune component and FFP transfusion to replace dysfunctional ADAMTS13. Despite often profound thrombocytopenia, platelets should not be transfused. Additional platelets will also become occluded in small vessels, worsening the microangiopathic process.

Although hemolytic uremic syndrome (HUS) and TTP appear similar clinically, they are caused by different mechanisms, and ADAMTS13 is not implicated in HUS. HUS is more likely to occur in children, to be accompanied by diarrhea, and to have more profound kidney injury. Classically, HUS is caused by *E. coli* O157:H7. TTP is more likely to have neurologic sequelae. TTP may also be confused with meningitis since patients may have fever, confusion, and petechiae in both conditions. Thrombocytopenia is a contraindication to lumbar puncture so patients may need to be treated empirically with antibiotics if there is diagnostic uncertainty.

Diagnosis: TTP.

CASE 23

HPI: A 19-year-old man is brought to the ED by ambulance after becoming confused in his dormitory. He was complaining of a headache and fever before he became confused. Two other students in the same dormitory have recently been hospitalized for similar symptoms.

Vital signs: Temperature 102.2°F (39°C), pulse 130 beats/min, BP 90/62 mm Hg, RR 20 breaths/min.

Additional history: No medical history, no use of drugs, alcohol, or tobacco.

1. What is the differential diagnosis?

Meningitis, encephalitis, sepsis, intracranial hemorrhage, brain abscess, hemolytic uremic syndrome, TTP, Rocky Mountain spotted fever, other rickettsial disease.

2. What components of the physical examination do you perform?

General appearance, HEENT, cardiovascular, lungs, abdomen, skin, neuro/psych.

Physical examination:

General: Lethargic, not answering questions appropriately, alert and oriented to name only.

HEENT: Withdraws when light is shined in eyes. Neck stiff to movement, positive Brudzinski sign.

Cardiovascular: Tachycardic.

Lungs: WNL

Abdomen: WNL

Skin: Diffuse, scattered petechiae, nonblanching.

Neuro/psych: Difficult to assess given mental status, but moving all extremities. Positive Kernig and Brudzinski signs.

3. What are your initial orders?

Head CT scan, ceftriaxone 2 g IV, vancomycin 1 g IV, with or without dexamethasone before antibiotics, CBC, chem 8, coagulation studies, IV fluids, antipyretics.

Advance clock: Head CT scan normal. CBC remarkable for WBC count of 26,000 cells/mL with 20% bands. Chem 8 unremarkable. Coagulation studies unremarkable. After IV fluid administration, the patient's BP has improved to 118/70.

4. What are your follow-up actions?

Lumbar puncture with CSF cell count, glucose, protein, Gram stain, culture.

Advance clock: Lumbar puncture demonstrates opening pressure of 35 cm H_2O (elevated), 2400 WBCs/mL (95% neutrophils), protein 500 mg/dL, glucose 20 mg/dL. Gram stain shows numerous gram-negative diplococci.

5. What are your follow-up actions?

Admit to the ICU, antibiotic prophylaxis of close contacts, counseling.

Critical actions: Recognition of meningitis, ordering a CT scan before a lumbar puncture in a patient with altered mental status. Ordering appropriate antibiotics. Ordering a lumbar puncture and CSF studies.

Discussion: This patient has meningococcal meningitis caused by *Neisseria meningitidis*, an encapsulated, aerobic, gram-negative diplococcus that classically occurs in crowded living situations such as military camps and dormitories. *N. meningitidis* causes a spectrum of disease that includes occult bacteremia, meningococcal meningitis, and septicemia with adrenal hemorrhage (called Waterhouse-Friderichsen syndrome). Although meningitis of any cause typically leads to fever, headache, and eventually neck stiffness and confusion, only meningococci cause petechial lesions. Petechiae occur because *N. meningitidis* releases blebs of endotoxin into the bloodstream that lodge in capillaries and cause inflammatory reactions that break down the capillary bed.

The treatment of meningitis in adults involves recognition, early administration of dexamethasone (as discussed later) and appropriate antibiotics. A noncontrast head CT is indicated if the patient has focal neurologic deficits, altered mental status, recent seizure, known CNS lesion, immunocompromised state, age older than 60 years, or papilledema. If the CT scan does not show evidence of increased intracranial pressure, it is safe to perform a lumbar puncture. It has been shown that dexamethasone improves outcomes in pneumococcal meningitis but not necessarily in other forms of meningitis, and it must be given before antibiotics to be effective. A lumbar puncture in a patient with bacterial meningitis classically shows elevated opening pressure, a high WBC count with neutrophil predominance, high protein, and low glucose. In this case the patient demonstrated all of these signs and the Gram stain showed *N. meningitidis*, confirming the diagnosis. Because of his hypotension, admission to the ICU for close monitoring in case of adverse effects such as adrenal hemorrhage is warranted.

The other possible causes of bacterial meningitis in this age group include *Streptococcus pneumoniae* and, albeit much less likely, *Listeria monocytogenes*. Ceftriaxone provides excellent coverage for both *N. meningitidis* and *S. pneumoniae*, and vancomycin can be added to ensure coverage for any resistant *S. pneumoniae* species. Ampicillin can be added for coverage of *L. monocytogenes* in susceptible patients (immunocompromised, pregnant, or patients <1 month or >50 years of age). All close contacts should be given prophylaxis with either rifampin (600 mg PO every 12 hours for 2 days) or ciprofloxacin (500 mg PO, single dose) to prevent the development of meningitis.

Diagnosis: Meningitis.

CASE 24

HPI: A 70-year-old man presents to his primary care physician because yesterday he suddenly felt part of his face and his right arm go numb and limp while eating dinner. His wife states that his face looked asymmetric and he was unable to speak or move his right arm. She thinks those symptoms lasted about 20 minutes but then completely resolved. She wanted to go to the ED last night but he refused because his symptoms had resolved. He denies any history of similar symptoms and currently "feels okay."

Vital signs: Temperature 98.2°F (36.8°C), pulse 80 beats/min, BP 160/98 mm Hg, RR 16 breaths/min.

Additional history: Has a history of type 2 diabetes, hypertension, and dyslipidemia. Takes metformin, glipizide, hydrochlorothiazide, amlodipine, and simvastatin. No allergies. Occasional alcohol use, no tobacco or drugs.

1. What is the differential diagnosis?

TIA, hypoglycemia, complicated migraine, seizure with Todd paralysis, demyelinating diseases.

2. What components of the physical examination do you perform?

General appearance, lungs, cardiovascular, neuro/psych.

Physical examination:

General: Overweight man in no apparent distress.

Cardiovascular: WNL

Lungs: WNL

Neuro/psych: Cranial nerves II through XII intact. Strength 5/5 and symmetric over all extremities. Normal sensation, reflexes 2+ throughout, downgoing Babinski response bilaterally. No ataxia, no dysdiadochokinesia, normal gait.

3. What are your initial orders?

Fingerstick blood glucose, CBC, chem 8, coagulation profile, ECG, CXR, UA, noncontrast head CT scan.

Advance clock:

CBC, chem 8, coagulation profile, fingerstick glucose, ECG, CXR, UA are WNL.

Noncontrast head CT scan unremarkable.

4. What are your follow-up actions?

Admit to inpatient unit, bedside swallow evaluation, aspirin, neurology consult. Order TTE, MRI brain, carotid ultrasound, fasting lipid panel, hemoglobin A1c. Counseling on disease process.

Advance clock:

TTE, MRI, and carotid ultrasound negative. Fasting lipid panel WNL. Hemoglobin A1c 8.2%.

Case ends.

Critical actions: Recognizing TIA in a high-risk patient, performing a neurologic exam, checking blood glucose, obtaining a head CT scan before starting antiplatelet therapy, admission for high-risk TIA and neurologic consult. Inpatient workup of TIA, including TTE, MRI, carotid ultrasound, and fasting lipid panel with hemoglobin A1c for risk stratification.

Discussion: This patient has had a TIA, which is "a transient episode of neurologic dysfunction caused by focal brain, spinal cord, or retinal ischemia, *without* acute infarction" according to the American Stroke Association (previously it was defined as resolving within 24 hours). If acute infarction has occurred, the patient would instead be diagnosed with a stroke. Although this patient's symptoms have completely resolved, the risk of a subsequent stroke is high; the highest risk of a subsequent stroke is in the first week after a TIA, and 17% of patients will have a stroke within the first 3 months after their TIA. Predisposing factors include hypertension, diabetes, dyslipidemia, and atrial fibrillation (AF).

Diagnosis is based on history and physical examination demonstrating a neurologic deficit that follows a vascular distribution, therefore knowledge of the basic vascular distribution of the brain is important. Blood glucose should be checked in all such patients because hypoglycemia can mimic stroke symptoms. An immediate head CT or MRI should be obtained for any patient suspected of having had a stroke or TIA to rule out hemorrhage because antiplatelet and thrombolytic agents are contraindicated in such patients. Treatment of a TIA (if not contraindicated) involves antiplatelet agents, such as aspirin, and control of the patient's risk factors. Additional neurologic evaluation includes MRI (if not obtained initially), TTE, carotid ultrasound (or other carotid imaging), and fasting lipid panel.

Diagnosis: TIA.

CASE 25

HPI: A 42-year-old man presents to his primary care physician because of dizziness. He says that this morning he rolled over in bed and all of a sudden "the whole room was spinning" and he vomited once. The entire episode was severe and lasted about 30 seconds before resolving. Since then, whenever he turns to the right the symptoms are reproduced, and he feels nauseated. Symptoms never last for more than 30 seconds, and when he continues to turn right, the symptoms get less and less severe each time. He denies any trauma, numbness, weakness, changes in hearing, recent or current illness, or other symptoms. As long as he sits still, he says he feels fine.

Vital signs: Temperature 98.2°F (36.8°C), pulse 76 beats/min, BP 126/68 mm Hg, RR 16 breaths/min.

Additional history: No medical history. Has smoked 1 pack of cigarettes per day for 10 years, occasional alcohol consumption, no drug use. No surgeries or allergies.

1. What is the differential diagnosis?
   - Peripheral vertigo: Benign positional paroxysmal vertigo (BPPV), labyrinthitis, vestibular neuronitis, Ménière disease, perilymphatic fistula, herpes zoster oticus, otosclerosis, cholesteatoma.
   - Central vertigo: Cerebellar or brainstem infarction or bleeding, tumors such as acoustic neuroma, demyelinating disease such as MS.

2. What components of the physical examination do you perform?

General appearance, HEENT/neck, lungs, cardiovascular, neuro/psych.

Physical examination:

General: Well-developed, well-appearing male in no distress when sitting still, but severe distress when moving head to the right.

HEENT/neck: Neck with full range of motion, no carotid bruit, bilateral ear canals and tympanic membranes normal.

Cardiovascular: WNL

Lungs: WNL

Neuro/psych: Cranial nerves II through XII intact, strength 5/5 in bilateral upper and lower extremities, reflexes 2+ throughout, normal sensation throughout, PERRLA without nystagmus. When the patient is rapidly laid down with his head tilted 45 degrees to the right, he develops nystagmus and his symptoms are reproduced.

3. What are your initial orders?

Epley maneuver, fingerstick glucose.

Advance clock:

Fingerstick glucose 105 mg/dL.

Epley maneuver performed; patient states he no longer has symptoms.

4. What are your follow-up actions?

Disease counseling, meclizine prescription, follow-up after 1 week.

Table 16.1 Differentiation of Central Vertigo From Peripheral Vertigo

	PERIPHERAL	CENTRAL
Onset	Sudden	Sudden or slow
Severity	Intense	Less intense, ill defined
Pattern	Paroxysmal, intermittent	Persistent
Worse with motion	Yes	Sometimes
Nausea	Often	Rarer
Fatigue of symptoms on movement	Yes	No
Other neurologic findings	No	Often

Advance clock:
Patient states that he had occasional episodes of symptoms soon after the visit, but they have since resolved. Case ends.

Critical actions: Recognition of vertigo, consideration of central versus peripheral causes.

Discussion: This patient has vertigo, a perception of abnormal movement (usually a sensation that the room is spinning). Any patient who complains of dizziness must further describe what they mean because "dizziness" can mean lightheadedness (presyncope), imbalance (ataxia), or vertigo. For a patient with vertiginous symptoms, it should be determined whether the vertigo is likely to be central or peripheral.

Causes of central vertigo include lesions in the brainstem or cerebellum (e.g., infarction, bleeding, tumors, toxins, or demyelination [e.g., MS]) and are typically more serious. Peripheral vertigo can be caused by lesions in the inner ear or vestibular system, including BPPV (caused by otolith displacement from the normal position in the utricle into one of the semicircular canals), labyrinthitis (inflammation of the vestibular organs, usually due to a virus), vestibular neuronitis (inflammation of the vestibular nerve, also usually caused by a virus) or Ménière disease (increased volume of endolymph in semicircular canals, characterized by vertigo, hearing loss, feeling of ear fullness, and tinnitus). There are also rarer causes of peripheral vertigo such as perilymphatic fistulas, herpes zoster oticus (Ramsay Hunt syndrome), otosclerosis, and cholesteatomas, which are not covered here.

The general characteristics that can help in differentiating central from peripheral vertigo are listed in Table 16.1.

In this case, the patient has symptoms and an examination consistent with peripheral vertigo, specifically BPPV, and has a positive Dix-Hallpike test. The otoliths can be repositioned using the Epley maneuver, but medications often have to be prescribed to ameliorate symptoms given that the maneuver can provoke episodes of vertigo until full recovery (1–2 weeks). First-line treatment is with an anticholinergic medication such as meclizine or scopolamine, with possible addition of a benzodiazepine such as diazepam if needed. Antiemetic agents can also be added for symptom control. In general, patients with peripheral vertigo can be discharged home. Patients with central vertigo will need urgent imaging (CT or MRI brain), a neurologic consult, and admission to the hospital.

Diagnosis: Vertigo due to BPPV.

CASE 26

HPI: An 8-year-old boy presents to his pediatrician because his mother thinks his urine "has looked funny" for the past 2 days. The boy says he feels tired all the time since the condition started and thinks his body "seems puffy" as well. He has never had similar symptoms before and otherwise feels okay. His mother accompanies him on the visit and is concerned that this is some type of reaction to the antibiotic he received 2 weeks ago for a sore throat (finished a 10-day course a few days ago). The patient denies any joint pain, rashes, nausea, vomiting, dysuria, or shortness of breath.

Vital signs: Temperature 98.2°F (36.8°C), pulse 80 beats/min, BP 130/90 mm Hg, RR 16 breaths/min.

Additional history: Culture-positive group A streptococcal pharyngitis 2 weeks ago, treated with penicillin twice daily for 10 days. No other medical history. No other medications or allergies.

1. **What is the differential diagnosis?**
   Glomerular disease, probably nephritic syndrome: PSGN, rapidly progressive glomerulonephritis, immunoglobulin A (IgA) nephropathy (Berger disease), HUS, lupus nephritis.
   Nonglomerular hematuria: interstitial cystitis, UTI.

2. **What components of the physical examination do you perform?**
   General appearance, cardiovascular, lungs, abdomen.

Physical examination:
General: Well-developed, well-nourished boy in no apparent distress. Mildly edematous, especially in the periorbital area.
Cardiovascular: WNL
Lungs: WNL
Abdomen: Mild tenderness over bilateral flanks.

3. **What are your initial orders?**
CBC, chem 8, coagulation profile, UA (with microscopy).
Advance clock:
CBC, chem 8, coagulation profile all WNL.
UA demonstrates a high level of blood with numerous RBC casts, moderate protein; otherwise WNL.

4. **What are your follow-up actions?**
Antistreptolysin O (ASO) titer, anti-DNAse B titer, serum C3 and C4 levels, nephrology consult. Follow-up appointment for rechecking of laboratory tests. Counseling.
Advance clock:
ASO and anti-DNAse B titers are strongly positive. Serum C3 and C4 undetectable.
Nephrology has no recommendations at this time; supportive care only.
Patient follow-up in 3 days and repeat laboratory tests are all WNL, hematuria is decreasing, patient states that he feels better.
Case ends.
Critical actions: Check UA and renal function. Recognition of nephritic syndrome, consideration of PSGN as the likely cause, supportive care.
Discussion: This patient has PSGN, an immunologic response after an infection with group A beta-hemolytic streptococcal (GAS) infection. In children and young adults, PSGN can follow either a skin infection (e.g., impetigo) or an infection of the pharynx (e.g., streptococcal pharyngitis, strep throat). Young children (age <7 years) are most commonly affected. Unfortunately, treatment of the initial infection with antibiotics does not prevent this immunologic complication. There are other forms of postinfectious glomerulonephritis; IgA nephropathy (Berger disease) classically occurs after a viral infection of the upper respiratory tract. IgA nephropathy has a faster onset (1–2 days, often called "synpharyngitic" because the nephropathy occurs with the infection) than PSGN (weeks). PSGN is a nephritic syndrome and therefore there will be RBC casts in the urine and some proteinuria.
   Diagnosis of PSGN is on the basis of a history suggestive of recent infection (as well as laboratory testing to confirm recent GAS infection with ASO and anti-DNAse B titers) and evidence of a nephritic syndrome. Urine microscopy will demonstrate RBC casts and moderate proteinuria. If complement levels (e.g., C3, C4) are ordered, they will be low, but these are not specific to PSGN. A renal biopsy is not required in stable patients for whom the diagnosis is clear, but patients who rapidly deteriorate or have an unclear diagnosis may require a biopsy to exclude other treatable causes. Treatment is primarily supportive, guided in conjunction with a nephrologist, and may include antihypertensive medication and/or diuresis. Any underlying infection should be treated (although antibiotics do not seem to prevent PSGN, patients with PSGN and an active GAS infection do better with early antibiotic treatment).
   Diagnosis: PSGN.

CASE 27

HPI: A 21-year-old man with known sickle cell disease presents to the ED with severe aches and pains in his ribs and both legs. The pain started while he was playing soccer outside earlier today with friends. He describes the pain as an ache of 10/10 in intensity consistent with multiple prior exacerbations of his condition. He has these exacerbations approximately twice a year. He usually takes oral hydromorphone at home to help with mild to moderate pain, but he ran out of his home medication. He denies fevers or vomiting.
Vital signs: Temperature 97.7°F (36.5°C), pulse 112 beats/min, BP 122/84 mm Hg, RR 18 breaths/min.
Additional history: Takes hydroxyurea. No other medical history. No use of tobacco, alcohol, or drugs.

1. **What is the differential diagnosis?**
Sickle cell pain crisis, acute chest syndrome, muscle strain.

2. **What components of the physical examination do you perform?**
General appearance, HEENT, cardiovascular, lungs, abdomen, extremities.
Physical examination:
General: Moderate distress secondary to pain.
HEENT: Dry mucous membranes, conjunctival pallor, mild scleral icterus.
Cardiovascular: Tachycardic.
Lungs: WNL
Abdomen: WNL
Extremities: WNL

3. **What are your initial orders?**
   Pulse oximetry, normal saline IV, analgesia (e.g., IV hydromorphone), CBC, CXR, reticulocyte count.
   Advance clock: The patient's pain is well controlled, heart rate normalizes. O_2 saturation 100% on room air. Hb 9 g/dL; other studies WNL.

4. **What are your follow-up actions?**
   Discharge home with hydromorphone PO and follow-up after 1 week. Counseling.
   Advance clock: Case ends.
   Critical actions: Recognition of sickle cell pain crisis, aggressive analgesia, consideration of other complications of sickle cell disease.
   Discussion: Sickle cell anemia is a genetic condition caused by homozygosity for the atypical Hb molecule HbS. This form of Hb is prone to polymerization under conditions of stress and causes erythrocytes to form a sickle shape that can lead to vasoocclusive events. Acute painful episodes are the most common manifestation of vasoocclusive events. They may be triggered by exertion, hypoxia, or dehydration, but often there is no recognizable underlying trigger. The mainstay of management for acute painful episodes is aggressive analgesia, often requiring IV opioids. Correction of reversible causes should be addressed. This patient appears dehydrated after playing soccer and will benefit from hydration. Correction of hypoxia, when present, is also warranted. It is also important to consider other sickle cell crises. Patients with chest pain, cough, or fever should be evaluated for acute chest syndrome using CXR. The presence of acute chest syndrome warrants hospital admission and antibiotics because it cannot be clinically distinguished from pneumonia, with specific coverage for *Streptococcal* species because of high rates of functional asplenia from autoinfarction. Patients with neurologic symptoms should be evaluated for stroke. Sickle cell patients with stroke or hypoxia from acute chest syndrome should be evaluated by a hematologist for possible exchange transfusion. Hb measurement can help in screening for hemolytic and aplastic crises when compared to baseline data. Hydroxyurea increases the presence of HbF in the circulation, which decreases the frequency of vasoocclusive events and the need for transfusions but is not helpful in the acute setting. Hydroxyurea is indicated for patients with more than two vasoocclusive events per year and those with other severe complications (e.g., acute chest syndrome).
   Diagnosis: Sickle cell pain crisis.

CASE 28

HPI: A 40-year-old woman with a history of hypertension complains of chronic fatigue that started months ago and has not abated. She admits not sleeping well and not being able to stay focused on her job because of her fatigue. She also states she has gained 20 lb during this time and complains of dry scaly skin. She feels that she is losing more hair than normal but attributes this to the stress of her inability to sleep.
Vital signs: Temperature 98.2°F (36.8°C), pulse 60 beats/min, BP 110/78 mm Hg, RR 16 breaths/min.
Additional history: Takes amlodipine for hypertension. Denies suicidal ideations, homicidal ideations, or auditory or visual hallucinations.

1. **What is the differential diagnosis?**
   Hypothyroidism (caused by Hashimoto thyroiditis, iodine deficiency, de Quervain thyroiditis, Reidel thyroiditis), chronic fatigue syndrome, depression, anemia.

2. **What components of the physical examination do you perform?**
   General appearance, HEENT, cardiovascular, lungs, abdomen, neuro/psych.
   Physical examination:
   General: Well-developed woman, no pallor, no apparent distress.
   HEENT: Slightly enlarged thyroid, nontender, no nodules.
   Cardiovascular: WNL except for bilateral nonpitting edema of the extremities.
   Lungs: WNL
   Abdomen: WNL
   Neuro/psych: Normal strength and sensation; reflexes abnormal because of prolonged relaxation phase.

3. **What are your initial orders?**
   CBC, chem 8, TSH (free T4, T3, can order once TSH result comes back).
   Advance clock: CBC and chem 8 WNL, no anemia. TSH markedly elevated and free T4 nearly undetectable.

4. **What are your follow-up actions?**
   Levothyroxine PO, follow-up appointment.
   Advance clock:
   Patient's symptoms significantly improved, feels much better.
   Case ends.
   Critical actions: Recognition of hypothyroidism and differential diagnosis that includes depression and anemia. Appropriate workup and treatment.

Discussion: This patient has hypothyroidism, which is underproduction of thyroid hormone. The most common cause is Hashimoto thyroiditis, an autoimmune disease affecting the thyroid gland. Unlike Graves disease, in which autoantibodies stimulate the TSH receptor, in Hashimoto thyroiditis, antibodies block the TSH receptor and thyroid peroxidase (TPO) and elicit T-cell attack of the thyroid gland. Other causes of hypothyroidism include iodine deficiency (incredibly rare in industrialized countries), thyroiditis syndromes, hypothalamic/pituitary causes, and drug-related causes, but all of these are much rarer than Hashimoto thyroiditis.

Symptoms of hypothyroidism are consistent with generalized slowing of the metabolism (because thyroid hormone is the main metabolic regulator). These symptoms include dry, rough skin; brittle nails; myxedema because of decreased turnover of glycosaminoglycans; cold intolerance because of a decrease in body heat production; fatigue; constipation; and weight gain. Patients can also experience myopathy characterized by proximal muscle weakness, myalgias, elevated creatine kinase (CK) levels, and stiffness; a decreased relaxation phase may also be apparent during reflex responses.

Diagnosis is via laboratory testing, which reveals elevated TSH and decreased free T4. Treatment is with levothyroxine (synthetic T4). Myxedema coma is a life-threatening complication of untreated hypothyroidism for which the symptoms are hypothermia, altered mental status, and hypotension; it is treated with high-dose thyroid hormone.

Diagnosis: Hypothyroidism.

CASE 29

HPI: A 40-year-old man presents to his primary care physician complaining of progressive weakness in his legs and arms for the past year. He denies any changes in sensation. His weakness has worsened to the point that he cannot perform his normal daily activities and can no longer work. His symptoms are similar all day and do not seem to get better or worse with continued use of his muscles. He has also noticed that his tongue wiggles continuously.

Vital signs: Temperature 98.6°F (37°C), pulse 80 beats/min, BP 118/60 mm Hg, RR 16 breaths/min.

Additional history: None. Previously healthy, no medications. Works as a day laborer, denies exposure to any chemicals.

1. **What is the differential diagnosis?**
   Amyotrophic lateral sclerosis (ALS; Lou Gehrig disease), tick paralysis, MS, spinal muscular atrophy, myasthenia gravis (MG), Lambert-Eaton myasthenic syndrome.

2. **What components of the physical examination do you perform?**
   General appearance, cardiovascular, lungs, neuro/psych.
   Physical examination:
   General: Comfortable, speaking in full sentences.
   Cardiovascular: WNL
   Lungs: Slightly shallow breaths; no cyanosis, wheezes, crackles, or rhonchi.
   Neuro/psych: Diffuse atrophy of all muscle groups, visible fasciculations of the tongue and the thigh and arm. Normal sensation to light tough, pinprick, and vibration. Hyperreflexia of the upper extremities and hyporeflexia of the lower extremities. Abnormal Babinski sign on the right foot but normal on the left. Cranial nerves intact.

3. **What are your initial orders?**
   Neurology consult, pulmonary function tests, admit to a monitored bed, electromyography (EMG)/nerve condition studies (optional), MRI scan of the brain/spinal cord (optional).
   Advance clock:
   EMG/nerve conduction studies show evidence of both upper and lower motor neuron disease.
   Pulmonary function tests show low risk of respiratory compromise.
   If MRI of the brain and spinal cord is ordered, the results are normal.

4. **What are your follow-up actions?**
   Start riluzole therapy, counsel the patient on the disease, physical therapy.
   Advance clock: Case ends.
   Critical actions: Recognition of both upper and lower motor neuron disease as characteristics of ALS, prompt neurology consult, pulmonary function tests to ensure the patient is not at risk of respiratory compromise.
   Discussion: This patient has ALS, a progressive, incurable, and ultimately fatal disease affecting both upper and lower motor neurons in the brain, brainstem, and spinal cord. Although some cases of ALS are genetic (associated with superoxide dismutase mutations), most are sporadic, and onset typically occurs between the ages of 40 and 70 years. Other motor neuron diseases and autoimmune diseases are initially in the differential diagnosis. Patients with spinal muscular atrophy should have only lower motor neuron signs; patients with MS would not have a normal MRI scan and would be unlikely to have such an abrupt and diffuse onset; those with MG should have symptoms that worsen on repeated muscle use; and those with Lambert-Eaton myasthenic syndrome should have symptoms that improve on repeated muscle use.

Treatment of ALS is mostly supportive, aided by physical, occupational, and speech therapy. There is one medication approved for use, riluzole, which lengthens survival by slowing disease progression, but the survival benefit is measured in months, not years. Patients will eventually need to decide if they want more aggressive measures, such as a feeding tube and ventilator, as their disease progresses further.

Diagnosis: ALS.

CASE 30

HPI: A 28-year-old woman presents to the outpatient clinic complaining of increased fatigue and occasional blurry vision. She states that she works as a receptionist, and for the past 2 months has noticed that by the end of the day she is extremely tired and "can barely keep her eyes open," and the screen becomes blurry. If she takes a break she can go back to work, but the symptoms then start again. She states she is getting enough sleep, does not use caffeine or drink alcohol, and overall feels well other than this complaint. She says her diet is good, but she has moved to eating softer foods recently because she is so tired that even chewing can be difficult. She denies any history of similar symptoms and any numbness or tingling.

Vital signs: Temperature 98.2°F (36.8°C), pulse 76 beats/min, BP 120/70 mm Hg, RR 16 breaths/min.

Additional history: No medical history, no medications, no allergies.

1. **What is the differential diagnosis?**

   MG, botulism, Lambert-Eaton myasthenic syndrome, cholinergic crisis/toxicity, depression.

2. **What components of the physical examination do you perform?**

   General appearance, lungs, cardiovascular, neuro/psych.

   Physical examination:

   General: Well-developed, well-nourished woman in no apparent distress.

   Cardiovascular: WNL

   Lungs: WNL

   Neuro/psych: Strength initially 5/5 but on repetitive testing becomes weaker and weaker to 3/5. Ptosis bilaterally. PERRLA, extraocular movements intact, but during a sustained gaze to one side the patient develops diplopia in about 30 seconds. Sensation intact, reflexes 2+ throughout, cranial nerves II through XII intact but motor cranial nerves fatigue on test repetition.

3. **What are your initial orders?**

   EMG; ice pack test.

   Advance clock:

   EMG demonstrates decreasing amplitude of muscle contraction on repetitive muscle stimulation, relieved by rest.

   Ice pack test performed; when ice pack is placed on the face patient has improvement in ptosis.

4. **What are your follow-up actions?**

   Neurology consult, start acetylcholine esterase inhibitor (e.g., pyridostigmine) treatment, counseling on the disease process. Follow-up appointment.

   Advance clock:

   Patient states she has good symptom control with the new medication.

   Case ends.

   Critical actions: Recognition of the classic presentation of MG, ordering basic diagnostic tests (mostly a clinical diagnosis), neurology consult or starting medication for symptom control.

   Discussion: This patient has MG, an autoimmune disorder in which autoantibodies attack and block acetylcholine receptors at the neuromuscular junction. This leads to generalized muscle weakness, including the eye muscles (diplopia, ptosis), that is worse on repetitive movement. This worsening on repetitive movement is unlike Lambert-Eaton myasthenic syndrome (anti–calcium channel antibodies), which gets *better* on repetitive movement because of an increase in calcium release with each movement. Myasthenic crisis is a potentially life-threatening condition in which there is an acute increase in weakness; if the weakness involves the respiratory muscles, respiratory failure can occur.

   Diagnosis of MG is on the basis of history and physical examination but can be supported by laboratory testing (such as acetylcholine receptor autoantibody screens [AChR-Ab] and antibodies against muscle-specific receptor tyrosine kinase [anti-MuSK]), EMG showing decreased amplitude of contraction with repetitive stimulation, and the ice pack test. The edrophonium test is no longer used. All patients with MG should be investigated for the presence of a thymoma; thymomas are common in MG, and improvements in symptoms can occur if the thymoma is removed.

   Treatment involves three different approaches: (1) symptom control, (2) immunosuppression, and (3) surgical removal of any thymoma. Symptom control with pyridostigmine is common; by increasing the amount of acetylcholine in the neuromuscular junction, patients will have increased strength. Immunosuppression with prednisone or other immunosuppressants helps to decrease autoantibody production. Lastly, thymectomy should be considered.

A myasthenic crisis can be treated with plasmapheresis to remove autoantibodies from the blood or with IVIG. In myasthenic crisis, the patient's respiratory status must be closely monitored (e.g., forced vital capacity and/or negative inspiratory force) to watch for any deterioration.

Diagnosis: MG.

CASE 31

HPI: An 18-month-old boy is brought to the ED because of "high-pitched sounds" on breathing in for the past 2 hours. His parents state that the patient has had a fever, runny nose, and cough for 2 days. The parents deny any possibility of foreign body ingestion.

Vital signs: Temperature 101.5°F (38.6°C), pulse 130 beats/min, BP 96/60 mm Hg, RR 40 breaths/min.

Additional history: Ex-full term, no complications, no hospitalizations, no medical history, medications, or allergies. Vaccinations are up to date.

1. **What is the differential diagnosis?**
   Stridor due to laryngotracheobronchitis (croup), foreign body, epiglottitis, bacterial tracheitis, laryngomalacia, subglottic stenosis, or retropharyngeal abscess.

2. **What components of the physical examination do you perform?**
   General appearance, HEENT, cardiovascular, lungs.
   Physical examination:
   General: Well-developed, well-nourished infant in moderate respiratory distress. A barking cough is present.
   HEENT: No foreign body visualized on inspection of the oropharynx. Clear rhinorrhea. Moist mucous membranes.
   Cardiovascular: Tachycardic, regular.
   Lungs: Tachypneic. Diffuse symmetric inspiratory stridor at rest with some expiratory wheezes. Using subcostal and intercostal accessory muscles.

3. **What are your initial orders?**
   Racemic epinephrine via nebulizer, dexamethasone. Antipyretics. CXR optional. Cool mist optional.
   Advance clock: After administration of racemic epinephrine and dexamethasone, the patient no longer exhibits stridor and is breathing comfortably without accessory muscle use. If a CXR is ordered, it will show a steeple sign in the upper airway.

4. **What are your follow-up actions?**
   Observe for 4 hours; if stridor returns before then, admit to the hospital; if not, discharge with return precautions.
   Advance clock: Case ends.
   Critical actions: Recognition of croup as a common cause of stridor, administration of racemic epinephrine and dexamethasone, observation for an appropriate amount of time before disposition.
   Discussion: This patient has laryngotracheobronchitis (croup) caused by parainfluenza virus or other viruses. Croup typically occurs between 6 months and 3 years of age and causes (as the name implies) predominantly upper airway obstruction that leads to stridor. The classic cough associated with croup resembles a seal barking. Croup lasts for 3 to 5 days, but the second or third night is when the most intense symptoms typically occur, as in this case. There is another condition called spasmodic croup that is noninfectious and affects those with a history of upper airway disease and/or reactive airway disease.

   Diagnosis of croup is primarily clinical. Foreign body aspiration must be ruled out because a foreign body in the upper airway can cause stridor. In this case, the viral symptoms, barking cough, and lack of aspiration history make this situation less likely. Epiglottitis is a particularly dangerous cause of stridor, as is bacterial tracheitis; patients with these conditions typically appear much more ill. Clinical scenarios involving epiglottitis will typically describe a child that is drooling/unable to manage secretions and may indicate the patient has not completed vaccination series for *Haemophilus influenzae*. Findings on x-ray in epiglottitis typically include the thumbprint sign, whereby the enlarged epiglottis looks like a thumb-sized mark on the lateral view.

   Management of croup of any severity includes dexamethasone administration to decrease airway inflammation. Severe croup, in which patients have stridor at rest, should be treated with racemic epinephrine via a nebulizer, which decreases swelling and inflammation with effects lasting approximately 2 hours. This is why patients must be observed for 4 hours, even if they appear well immediately after treatment, to watch for the return of symptoms after the epinephrine wears off (dexamethasone takes hours to have an effect but is long lasting). Cool mist has been used in croup for decades, but there is no evidence that it provides benefit; however, there is little harm in cool mist administration, so this strategy is optional.

   Diagnosis: Croup.

CASE 32

HPI: A 60-year-old man with a history of small cell lung cancer complains of headache, nausea, weakness, generalized fatigue, and muscle cramps for the past 3 days. He states that the symptoms all occurred progressively and there was no inducing event. He denies any vomiting, fever, chills, visual changes, or significant changes in weight.
Vital signs: Temperature 98.2°F (36.8°C), pulse 92 beats/min, BP 150/80 mm Hg, RR 16 breaths/min.
Additional history: Localized small cell lung cancer diagnosed 1 year ago without evidence of metastatic disease; 50 pack-year smoking history (quit after diagnosis). The patient denies alcohol or drug use. No recent chemotherapy or radiotherapy.

1. **What is the differential diagnosis?**
   Metastases to brain, paraneoplastic syndrome such as syndrome of inappropriate antidiuretic hormone (SIADH) causing hyponatremia, malnutrition from cachexia, other electrolyte imbalances, hyperglycemia or hypoglycemia, chemotherapy side effects, tumor lysis syndrome.

2. **What components of the physical examination do you perform?**
   General appearance, cardiovascular, lungs, neuro/psych.
   Physical examination:
   General: Mildly cachectic male, sleeping but can be aroused and converses appropriately.
   Cardiovascular: WNL, no jugular venous distention (JVD), no pitting edema.
   Lungs: Dullness on percussion and decreased breath sounds in the right upper lobe.
   Neuro/psych: Strength 4/5 diffusely, sensation intact, gait normal, cranial nerves II through XII intact, no papilledema, visual fields full, PERRLA, reflexes normal.

3. **What are your initial orders?**
   Noncontrast head CT scan, fingerstick blood glucose, oxygen saturation, CBC, chem 8.
   Advance clock: Head CT scan shows no evidence of bleeding, metastatic disease, or midline shift. Fingerstick blood glucose 115 mg/dL. Oxygen saturation 97% on room air. CBC is WNL. Chem 8 significant for sodium 120 mEq/L, all other electrolytes WNL. If a uric acid level is ordered to evaluate for tumor lysis syndrome, it is normal.

4. **What are your follow-up actions?**
   Serum osmolality (will be low), urine osmolality (will be inappropriately high), urine electrolytes (urine sodium will be high), admit to a ward bed, fluid restriction, start IV saline with correction no faster than 0.5 mEq/L, serial sodium checks.
   Advance clock: Case ends.
   Critical actions: Checking glucose and oxygen saturation for altered patient, head CT or MRI in a patient with headache and malignancy, recognition of SIADH as a common paraneoplastic syndrome for small cell lung cancer, admission and appropriate treatment of hyponatremia.
   Discussion: This patient has hyponatremia, which is a sodium level of less than 135 mEq/L. However, the sodium value should first be corrected for hyperglycemia, if present. There are many causes of hyponatremia; the condition is usually classified as hypovolemic, euvolemic, or hypervolemic hyponatremia, each with different causes. Hypovolemic hyponatremia is usually due to extrarenal fluid losses via diarrhea, third spacing of fluids, poor intake, and increased insensible losses. Hypovolemic hyponatremia can also be due to renal losses caused by diuretic usage, cerebral salt wasting, and mineralocorticoid deficiency. Euvolemic hyponatremia (what this patient has) is typically due to SIADH but in rare cases can be due to primary polydipsia, in which the patient drinks gallons of water a day, or tea and toast syndrome. Hypervolemic hyponatremia can be caused by hypervolemic states such as CHF, cirrhosis, nephrotic syndrome, and renal failure.
   The first step in the workup is measurement of plasma and urine osmolality and assessment of volume status during a physical examination. This patient is euvolemic and has low plasma osmolality but high urine osmolality. The body should completely shut off ADH production to dilute the urine as much as possible to correct low plasma osmolality. In this case, the kidneys are inappropriately concentrating the urine, exacerbating the problem. This is known as SIADH. This patient has a history of small cell lung cancer, which can secrete ADH. Pulmonary disease broadly can cause SIADH as well, with this occurring in patients who have developed pneumonia or patients who have chronic obstructive pulmonary disease (COPD) or interstitial lung disease. Treatment involves fluid restriction and slow correction of the sodium level to normal using saline, salt tablets, or a vasopressin antagonist (e.g., vaptan drugs such as conivaptan and tolvaptan). Rapid correction can lead to osmotic demyelination syndrome, an irreversible and potentially fatal condition. Various guidelines suggest different correction rates; generally, correction is safe at 6 to 8 mEq/day.
   Diagnosis: Hyponatremia.

CASE 33

HPI: A 23-year-old woman presents to your clinic because of jitteriness and weight loss. She states that she feels her heart racing intermittently and she sweats easily; she wears much less clothing than her friends for this reason.

She has also lost 10 lb unintentionally in the past 3 months, and states that her appetite has decreased. She denies any caffeine or stimulant use, any history of similar symptoms, and any significant life stressors.

Vital signs: Temperature 98.2°F (36.8°C), pulse 90 beats/min, BP 120/70 mm Hg, RR 16 breaths/min.

Additional history: Works as a cashier. No medical history and no medications. No recent infections.

1. **What is the differential diagnosis?**

   Hyperthyroidism (Graves disease, toxic multinodular goiter [TMG], toxic adenoma, de Quervain thyroiditis, hashi-toxicosis, exogenous thyroid hormone use), anxiety disorder, panic disorder, pheochromocytoma, stimulant abuse.

2. **What components of the physical examination do you perform?**

   General appearance, HEENT, cardiovascular, lungs.

   Physical examination:

   General: Well-developed woman in no apparent distress.

   HEENT: Mild goiter noted, palpation of the thyroid gland reveals no tenderness and no discrete nodules. Lid lag is noted.

   Cardiovascular: Rate 96 beats/min and regular, holosystolic murmur throughout the precordium.

   Lungs: WNL

3. **What are your initial orders?**

   ECG, urine human chorionic gonadotropin (hCG), TSH (optional free T4 and T3, but should be ordered if TSH is abnormal if not ordered now).

   Advance clock: ECG shows normal sinus rhythm, rate 96 beats/min. TSH undetectable, free T4 and T3 elevated. (If TSH were normal, consider urine metanephrines for pheochromocytoma and a urine toxicology screen for evidence of stimulant abuse.)

4. **What are your follow-up actions?**

   Counsel the patient on disease, endocrinology consult, propranolol for symptomatic relief, methimazole or propyl-thiouracil to decrease thyroid hormone production, appointment to reassess symptoms. Consider measurement of anti-TPO antibodies, ordering a thyroid uptake scan, or endocrinology referral for radioactive iodine ablation.

   Advance clock: Case ends.

   Critical actions: Recognition of the symptoms of hyperthyroidism, appropriate diagnostic testing (e.g., at least TSH), consult endocrinology or initiate treatment (symptom control with propranolol, blockade of thyroid hormone production with methimazole or propylthiouracil).

   Discussion: This patient has hyperthyroidism, characterized by increased thyroid hormone levels in the setting of decreased TSH levels. Graves disease is the most common cause of hyperthyroidism in children and young adults; it is an autoimmune disease characterized by stimulatory antibodies that bind to TSH receptors, causing increased thyroid hormone production. TMG is the most common cause of hyperthyroidism in older individuals. Graves disease stimulates fibroblasts and causes lymphocytic infiltration in the periorbital space so patients can have exophthalmos, a finding specific to this disease. The most common cause of hypothyroidism is Hashimoto thyroiditis (also an autoimmune disease), and early in its course inflammation in the thyroid can cause thyroid hormone to leak out, leading to transient hyperthyroidism (hashitoxicosis). Painful (and rarer) causes of hyperthyroidism include de Quervain thyroiditis (a postviral thyroiditis) and postpartum thyroiditis.

   Diagnosis of hyperthyroidism is on the basis of increased T3 or free T4 levels (not total T4) and decreased TSH. If the cause of the hyperthyroidism is in question, a radioiodine uptake scan can be performed. In Graves disease, diffuse overproduction of thyroid hormone leads to diffuse radioiodine uptake. In TMG there are multiple nodules of uptake. In exogenous thyroid ingestion and thyroiditis, there is little uptake because the thyroid gland is not stimulated to produce thyroid hormone. Treatment is aimed at reducing symptoms from high sympathetic tone (e.g., a nonselective beta-blocker such as propranolol), reducing TPO enzyme activity to decrease hormone production (with methimazole or propylthiouracil) and possibly administering radioactive iodine to ablate the thyroid gland and destroy it permanently.

   Diagnosis: Hyperthyroidism.

CASE 34

HPI: A 5-year-old girl is brought to the pediatrician by her father. Her parents have noticed that her gums have been bleeding a small amount when they brush her teeth. They have also noticed that small purple dots have appeared on her ankles. She has been acting normally and does not appear to be bothered by the skin changes. She has always been a healthy child although she occasionally suffers from viral respiratory infections. She had symptoms of an upper respiratory tract infection approximately 2 weeks ago.

Vital signs: Temperature 98.2°F (36.8°C), pulse 80 beats/min, BP 100/70 mm Hg, RR 20 breaths/min.

Additional history: No other medical history. Vaccinations up to date.

1. **What is the differential diagnosis?**

   Immune/idiopathic thrombocytopenic purpura (ITP), HUS, TTP, drug-induced thrombocytopenia, leukemia.

2. **What components of the physical examination do you perform?**
General appearance, HEENT, skin/lymph nodes, cardiovascular, lungs, abdomen, neuro/psych.
Physical examination:
General: No acute distress.
HEENT: WNL
Skin/lymph nodes: Scattered bilateral petechiae over the lower extremities, no lymphadenopathy.
Cardiovascular: WNL
Lungs: WNL
Abdomen: WNL, no splenomegaly.
Neuro/psych: WNL

3. **What are your initial orders?**
CBC, peripheral smear, chem 14, PT/PTT.
Advance clock: Platelets 28,000 cells/mL, other studies WNL.

4. **What are your follow-up orders?**
Prednisolone PO, repeat CBC in 5 days, follow-up in 5 days and 2 weeks.
Advance clock: After 2 weeks the patient's platelet count has normalized and her symptoms have resolved.
Critical actions: Skin examination, lymph node examination, abdominal examination, CBC, peripheral smear, consideration of steroid therapy.
Discussion: ITP is a condition characterized by platelet counts of less than 100,000 cells/mL and symptoms of thrombocytopenia (petechiae, bruising, bleeding). The condition can range from mild asymptomatic thrombocytopenia to severe life-threatening hemorrhage, including intracranial hemorrhage. In children, ITP is most common between the ages of 2 and 5 years. It tends to be acute in onset and resolves spontaneously or with steroid administration. ITP is often preceded by a viral infection during the previous month. In adults, ITP tends to be more indolent. It occurs over a long period of time and is more refractory to treatment. A careful history and physical examination can reveal suspicion of thrombocytopenia, and a CBC can quickly provide a platelet count. Once a diagnosis of thrombocytopenia is established, other causes should be evaluated. A normal peripheral smear helps to rule out TTP. In patients at risk, infectious causes should be evaluated, including HIV and *Helicobacter pylori*. The size of the spleen should be evaluated using at least a physical examination, and any suspicion of splenomegaly warrants advanced imaging. Any precipitating agents should be stopped if possible; common offenders are antihistamines, proton pump inhibitors (PPIs), and sulfa drugs. Children with mild manifestations can usually be monitored as outpatients and do not need treatment. Moderate cases can be treated with steroids alone. Severe cases require steroids, IVIG, platelet transfusion, and a hematology consult. Refractory cases may benefit from splenectomy. A bone marrow biopsy is indicated in patients who are refractory to treatment and those in whom malignancy is a possibility (e.g., lymphadenopathy, weight loss, atypical cells on smear).
Diagnosis: ITP.

CASE 35

HPI: A 9-year-old girl is brought to an urgent care clinic because of redness and swelling around her right eye for the past day that is worsening. There is no discharge from the eye according to her mother, and she states that the child is using her eye normally otherwise. The patient states that she has 6/10 pain over the skin around the eye but no pain in the eye itself. She recently had sinusitis, which has since resolved. The patient denies neck stiffness, pain on eye movements, and visual changes.
Vital signs: Temperature 98.2°F (36.8°C), pulse 80 beats/min, BP 110/60 mm Hg, RR 16 breaths/min.
Additional history: Immunizations up to date.

1. **What is the differential diagnosis?**
Periorbital (preseptal) cellulitis, orbital cellulitis, conjunctivitis, dacryoadenitis, dacryocystitis, hordeolum, chalazion.

2. **What components of the physical examination do you perform?**
General appearance, HEENT.
Physical examination:
General: Well-developed, well-nourished girl in no apparent distress.
HEENT: Right eye has significant periorbital swelling, warmth, and erythema encircling the skin around the entire eye and upper and lower eyelids. No conjunctival injection. No proptosis. PERRLA. Extraocular movements intact. Visual acuity 20/20 in both eyes.

3. **What are your initial orders?**
Antibiotics (e.g., oral amoxicillin-clavulanate for 10 days), analgesia. Discharge home with follow-up appointment in 24 to 48 hours for recheck. Counseling on periorbital cellulitis.
Advance clock: The patient has been taking antibiotics as prescribed, and the erythema has significantly receded.

4. **What are your follow-up actions?**
Follow-up appointment in 7 to 10 days to ensure complete resolution.
Advance clock: Case ends.
Critical actions: Recognition of periorbital cellulitis, consideration of other causes of redness around the eye, ruling out orbital cellulitis according to the history and physical examination.
Discussion: This patient has periorbital (also known as preseptal) cellulitis, which is a bacterial cellulitis involving the area of the orbits and limited to tissues anterior to the orbital septum. Periorbital cellulitis is typically caused by spread from the paranasal sinuses, and therefore infection is most commonly due to organisms involved in sinusitis (*Streptococcus* species, *H. influenzae*, anaerobes, and *S. aureus*). The infection causes warmth, swelling, and erythema of the eyelid and skin around the orbit. Periorbital cellulitis must be distinguished from the emergent condition orbital cellulitis. Orbital cellulitis has more severe symptoms and may involve proptosis, decreased or painful extraocular motility, ocular pain, and visual changes. Whereas periorbital cellulitis can often be treated with antibiotics (such as amoxicillin-clavulanate) on an outpatient basis with close follow-up, orbital cellulitis is an emergency and requires admission to the hospital for parenteral antibiotics, ophthalmology evaluation, and a CT scan of the orbits to rule out retroorbital air or abscess formation.

There should always be close follow-up of patients with periorbital cellulitis because complications can occur. Periorbital cellulitis can progress to orbital cellulitis. The veins that drain the periorbital area lead into the cavernous sinus; the infection can predispose patients to cavernous sinus thrombosis. The close proximity of the paranasal sinuses to the CSF also means that meningitis is a possible complication.
Diagnosis: Periorbital cellulitis.

CASE 36

HPI: A 38-year-old woman with recent diagnoses of hypertension and diabetes presents to her primary care doctor for follow-up. She says that she had numerous symptoms in the time around her diagnoses, including fatigue, insomnia, and inability to concentrate. She also says she is embarrassed to say that she is gaining weight around her abdomen and is developing stretch marks and that she has recently had to shave her facial hair, although she has never had this problem before. She is concerned about these changes in her body because she was previously healthy, exercised frequently, and never had any complaints.
Vital signs: Temperature 98.2°F (36.8°C), pulse 90 beats/min, BP 160/90 mm Hg, RR 16 breaths/min.
Additional history: Diagnosed with hypertension and diabetes 2 months ago. Takes hydrochlorothiazide, amlodipine, metformin, and glipizide. No allergies. No surgeries. No use of alcohol, tobacco, or drugs. Not sexually active, menses previously regular every 4 weeks but currently irregular for the past 4 or 5 months.

1. **What is the differential diagnosis?**
Hypercortisolism: excess exogenous glucocorticoid, ACTH-dependent endogenous glucocorticoid production (e.g., pituitary adenoma, ectopic ACTH production), ACTH-independent endogenous glucocorticoid production (e.g., adrenal tumor). Depression, polycystic ovarian syndrome, metabolic syndrome.

2. **What components of the physical examination do you perform?**
General appearance, HEENT, cardiovascular, lungs, abdomen, extremities, neuro/psych.
Physical examination:
General: Overweight woman in no apparent distress.
HEENT: Presence of a dorsocervical fat pad, moon facies, acne, mild hirsutism.
Cardiovascular: WNL
Lungs: WNL
Abdomen: Centripetal obesity with purple-red striae.
Extremities: Decreased muscle mass over extremities, peripheral edema 1+.
Neuro/psych: 4/5 strength in proximal muscle groups diffusely, otherwise 5/5 strength. Exam otherwise WNL.

3. **What are your initial orders?**
CBC, chem 8, CK, UA, urinary pregnancy test, hypercortisolism screening (24-hour urinary free cortisol or salivary cortisol or dexamethasone suppression test).
Advance clock: CBC is WNL. Chem 8 demonstrates blood glucose 240 mg/dL and potassium 3 mEq/L but otherwise WNL. CK is WNL. UA is WNL and urinary pregnancy test negative. Marked elevation of 24-hour urinary free cortisol. Salivary cortisol markedly elevated. Dexamethasone suppression test shows no suppression at a low dose but suppression at a high dose.

4. **What are your follow-up actions?**
ACTH level.
Advance clock: ACTH level markedly elevated.

5. **What are your follow-up actions?**
Brain CT/MRI.
Advance clock: CT or MRI scan of the brain shows a pituitary mass.

6. **What are your follow-up actions?**
Neurosurgery consult, transsphenoidal surgery to remove the mass.
Advance clock:
The pituitary mass is removed. The patient sees you in 6 months and now has no symptoms.
Case ends.
Critical actions: Recognition of hypercortisolism as a likely cause of the patient's symptoms, testing for hypercortisolism, determination of the cause of the hypercortisolism, and initiation of appropriate treatment.
Discussion: This patient has hypercortisolism (Cushing syndrome) caused by an ACTH-secreting pituitary adenoma (Cushing disease). Hypercortisolism can be caused by a number of factors, ranging from exogenous intake of glucocorticoids (e.g., prolonged steroid use), excess stimulation of glucocorticoid release (e.g., pituitary tumor secreting ACTH, ectopic ACTH-secreting tumor, or CRH-producing tumor), or a tumor of the zona fasciculata of the adrenal glands that directly produces glucocorticoids. Knowledge of the physiology of glucocorticoid release will help in understanding the diagnosis and treatment. In brief, the hypothalamus secretes CRH, leading to ACTH release by the anterior pituitary gland. This ACTH then acts on the zona fasciculata of the adrenal gland to promote secretion of glucocorticoids, which then exert negative feedback on the hypothalamus and pituitary gland to decrease CRH and ACTH production, respectively. This ensures tight control of glucocorticoid production.

Diagnosis is on the basis of history and a physical examination showing classic central obesity, dorsocervical fat pad ("buffalo hump"), moon facies (rounded face), acne, hirsutism, and hemorrhagic purple-red striae. Basic laboratory tests may reveal hyperglycemia arising from the diabetogenic effect of glucocorticoids in increasing insulin resistance, and vital signs may demonstrate hypertension because glucocorticoids in high doses have mineralocorticoid-like effects (act like aldosterone). Diagnosis of hypercortisolism involves first determining that hypercortisolism exists, usually by measurement of urinary free cortisol or late-night salivary cortisol. A dexamethasone suppression test can be performed to assess if the hypercortisolism decreases when dexamethasone (a steroid) is administered; this should cause ACTH suppression via negative feedback. In the case of an ACTH-secreting pituitary tumor, high-dose dexamethasone will suppress production. However, if the ACTH is being secreted by another ectopic source (e.g., small cell carcinoma of the lung) or the tumor was not ACTH-dependent to begin with (e.g., tumor in the adrenal gland that directly secretes cortisol), no negative feedback will occur. An ACTH level can also help in differentiating between an adrenal tumor (low ACTH because of negative feedback) and an ACTH-dependent tumor. Treatment depends on the cause: If exogenous steroid use is the cause, tapering of the steroid regimen is warranted; if the cause is endogenous (e.g., a tumor), surgery is the therapy of choice.

Diagnosis: Hypercortisolism from Cushing disease.

CASE 37

HPI: A 50-year-old woman presents to clinic because of heavy vaginal bleeding and fatigue. Until 1 year ago she had regular menses every month that lasted for 5 days with a normal flow. She now has irregular menses that last as long as 14 days and has bleeding between cycles. She has a very heavy flow and occasional passage of clots. Recently she has also been feeling fatigued. She has never lost consciousness, although at times she does have a vague lightheaded sensation. She has no personal or family history of bleeding disorders.
Vital signs: Temperature 99.1°F (37.3°C), pulse 88 beats/min, BP 112/77 mm Hg, RR 18 breaths/min.
Additional history: No medical history. No use of drugs, tobacco, or alcohol.

1. **What is the differential diagnosis?**
Vaginal bleeding due to abnormal uterine bleeding (AUB), fibroids, endometrial carcinoma, endometrial polyp, cervical lesion, bleeding disorder.

2. **What components of the physical examination do you perform?**
General appearance, lymph nodes, HEENT, cardiovascular, lungs, abdomen, extremities, genitalia.
Physical examination:
General: No acute distress.
Lymph nodes: WNL
HEENT: Conjunctival pallor.
Cardiovascular: WNL
Lungs: WNL
Abdomen: WNL
Extremities: WNL
Genitalia: Scant blood visualized in the vaginal vault. No cervical lesions.

3. **What are your initial orders?**
CBC with differential, PT/PTT, TSH, pelvic ultrasound, Papanicolaou (Pap) smear, urinary pregnancy test, endometrial biopsy.
Advance clock: CBC reveals Hb 10.1 mg/dL, MCV 69 fL. Other studies WNL.

4. **What are your follow-up actions?**
Ferrous sulfate PO, medroxyprogesterone IM (Depo-Provera), follow up in 2 months.
Advance clock: Case ends.
Critical actions: Genitalia examination, CBC, endometrial biopsy, hormonal treatment of AUB.
Discussion: This patient has heavy menstrual bleeding (previously termed *menorrhagia*) and intermenstrual bleeding (previously termed *metrorrhagia*). She is in the perimenopausal period, and in this setting AUB due to anovulatory cycles is the most common cause. Anovulatory AUB arises from the unopposed effect of estrogen on the endometrium. Without ovulation, the corpus luteum is not able to secrete progesterone to stabilize the endometrial lining. The lining thus builds up and sheds in an irregular pattern with a heavy flow. Although AUB is the most common cause of perimenopausal bleeding, AUB is a diagnosis of exclusion, and other causes of vaginal bleeding should be investigated. A Pap smear can evaluate the cervical pathology, and pelvic ultrasound can assess for structural problems such as uterine fibroids and endometrial polyps. Endometrial biopsy is indicated in women older than 35 years with abnormal vaginal bleeding to assess for endometrial carcinoma. For any patient with concerning bleeding, a CBC should be performed to assess Hb and platelet levels. Transfusion may be indicated in some patients with symptomatic anemia, but ferrous sulfate is often sufficient to replenish iron stores. Although many hormonal methods can be used to treat AUB, in the perimenopausal period, medroxyprogesterone IM (Depo-Provera) is often used to address the underlying hormonal imbalance. Nonpharmacologic therapies are also available for patients with contraindications to hormonal treatment or refractory symptoms despite hormonal treatment. Endometrial ablation and hysterectomy provide definitive management of AUB.
Diagnosis: AUB.

CASE 38

HPI: An 85-year-old woman with a history of hypertension is brought to the ED by ambulance after she fell at her assisted living facility. Caregivers saw the patient slip and fall while getting out of the bath this morning. Initially she complained of a mild headache but did not lose consciousness. According to the caregivers she has become progressively more confused over the past 6 hours. They deny any possibility of syncope or seizure as a cause of the fall. The caregivers say she normally knows her name and the date and can carry on a conversation, but now does not make sense when she talks.
Vital signs: Temperature 98.2°F (36.8°C), pulse 80 beats/min, BP 145/80 mm Hg, RR 16 breaths/min.
Additional history: No use of alcohol, tobacco, or drugs. Medical history only significant for hypertension controlled with hydrochlorothiazide. No history of dementia.

1. **What is the differential diagnosis?**
Blunt head trauma causing epidural hematoma, subdural hematoma, SAH, intraparenchymal hemorrhage, traumatic brain injury, diffuse axonal injury.
    Altered mental status arising from another cause: infection/sepsis, stroke/TIA, opioid overdose, alcohol overdose, acute renal failure, electrolyte derangement, calcium derangement, hypoglycemia, MI.

2. **What components of the physical examination do you perform?**
General appearance, skin, HEENT/neck, lungs, cardiovascular, abdomen, extremities, neuro/psych.
Physical examination:
General: Confused and disoriented.
HEENT/neck: 5-cm hematoma over the right frontal bone, no evidence of a depressed skull fracture. No posterior auricular hematoma, no hemotympanum. Pupils are 6 mm and reactive bilaterally.
Lungs: WNL
Cardiovascular: WNL
Abdomen: WNL
Extremities: WNL
Neuro/psych: Alert and oriented to name only. Opens eyes spontaneously, localizes pain but does not obey simple commands. Speaks in sentences, but the sentences do not make sense (Glasgow Coma Scale 4-5-4).

3. **What are your initial orders?**
IV fluids, pulse oximetry, cardiac monitor. Fingerstick blood glucose. CBC, chem 8, coagulation profile. Immediate noncontrast head CT scan. ECG. Consider troponin, CXR, UA/culture.
Advance clock:
Pulse oximetry 100% O_2 saturation. Fingerstick blood glucose 160 mg/dL. Other laboratory tests WNL.
Noncontrast head CT scan reveals a right-sided concave density consistent with subdural hematoma. No evidence of midline shift.

4. **What are your follow-up actions?**
Neurosurgery consult. IV levetiracetam. Admit to ICU.
Advance clock: Case ends.
Critical actions: Recognition and evaluation of altered mental status, stabilization of the patient, evaluation of intracranial pathology in a patient with head trauma, neurosurgery consult.

Discussion: This patient has an acute subdural hematoma, a life-threatening neurosurgical emergency. It most commonly occurs as a result of injury to the bridging veins in the skull that penetrate the dura, leading to bleeding in the potential space between the dura and the arachnoid (because the bleeding is under the dura, it is a *sub*dural hematoma). In patients with atrophic brains (e.g., older individuals, alcoholic patients), the causative trauma can be minor. As the bleed expands, the patient is at risk of herniation and death.

Diagnosis is on the basis of a noncontrast CT scan of the brain showing a sickle-shaped (concave) bleed that can cross suture lines (unlike epidural hematomas). Management is first supportive (airway, breathing, circulation) with reversal of anticoagulation if the patient is taking an anticoagulant. Seizure prophylaxis is typically given as well with levetiracetam. Treatment includes admission to an ICU and possible neurosurgical intervention, depending on the extent of the bleeding and the patient's symptoms.

Diagnosis: Subdural hematoma.

CASE 39

HPI: A 62-year-old man presents to the ED complaining of weakness for the past few days. He has a history of diabetes and oliguric end-stage renal disease on hemodialysis, but he admits that he has missed the past two dialysis sessions because of his hectic work schedule. When asked to elaborate on his weakness, he states, "I don't know, I just can't walk as far as normal, and I feel like my whole body isn't as strong as it usually is."

Vital signs: Temperature 98.2°F (36.8°C), pulse 54 beats/min, BP 166/94 mm Hg, RR 16 breaths/min.

Additional history: Occasional alcohol use.

1. What is the differential diagnosis?
   Hyperkalemia, fluid overload, hyperglycemia, other electrolyte derangements (e.g., hypercalcemia), CHF, uremia, anemia.

2. What components of the physical examination do you perform?
   General appearance, cardiovascular, lungs, abdomen, neuro/psych.
   Physical examination:
   General: Comfortable.
   Cardiovascular: WNL
   Lungs: WNL
   Abdomen: WNL
   Neuro/psych: 4+/5 strength in all extremities, symmetric.

3. What are your initial orders?
   ECG, chem 14, CBC, CXR, brain natriuretic peptide (BNP), troponin, LFTs.
   Advance clock:
   ECG shows sinus bradycardia with diffuse peaked T waves, a PR interval of 0.24 sec, and a QRS duration of 0.16 sec.
   Chem 14 remarkable for potassium 7.4 mEq/L, BUN 80 mg/dL, creatinine 12 mg/dL.
   CBC remarkable for Hb 11.2 mg/dL.
   CXR shows mild cephalization of the pulmonary vasculature, no pulmonary edema or effusions, no cardiomegaly.

4. What are your follow-up actions?
   Calcium gluconate, insulin and glucose, albuterol, furosemide, sodium zirconium cyclosilicate (Lokelma), urgent nephrology consult for hemodialysis, admit to inpatient unit.
   Advance clock: Case ends.
   Critical actions: Recognition of hyperkalemia, rapid intervention with potassium shifting/lowering medications, nephrology consult, and/or definitive treatment with dialysis.
   Discussion: This patient has potentially life-threatening hyperkalemia as a result of missing dialysis sessions. Normally, individuals take in more potassium than they need, and the excess is excreted by the kidneys. However, patients with renal failure are prone to accumulation of excess potassium and the development of hyperkalemia. The presenting symptoms for hyperkalemia can be generalized weakness/malaise, palpitations because of cardiac arrhythmia, or cardiac arrest. A potassium level greater than 5 mEq/L is generally considered hyperkalemia. The differential diagnosis for generalized weakness in a renal failure patient should also include fluid overload from a decreased glomerular filtration rate, as well as anemia due to decreased erythropoietin production.

   Causes of hyperkalemia fall into three categories: (1) decreased elimination of potassium (renal insufficiency, medications such as angiotensin-converting enzyme [ACE] inhibitors, conditions with decreased aldosterone such as adrenal insufficiency), (2) increased potassium release from cells (rhabdomyolysis, hemolysis, acidosis), and (3) excessive potassium intake (rare; common dietary sources include bananas, prunes, chocolate). These must be distinguished clinically from a laboratory error caused by RBC hemolysis during blood draw from the patient, leading to spuriously elevated potassium levels.

   Treatment of hyperkalemia involves three targets: (1) temporary stabilization of the myocardium to prevent arrhythmias using calcium chloride or calcium gluconate; (2) a temporary shift in intracellular potassium using agents such as insulin (IV, not SC, and with glucose administration to prevent hypoglycemia), and albuterol; and (3) elimination of potassium from the body, which can be accomplished via the urine with loop diuretics (furosemide), via the stool with ion exchange resins sodium zirconium cyclosilicate (Lokelma), and via the blood with dialysis. It should be emphasized that (1) and (2) are merely temporizing measures: The myocardial stabilizing activity of calcium lasts for just 30 minutes, and the activity of agents that shift potassium intracellularly typically last for a few hours. In all cases of hyperkalemia, the underlying cause should be determined and corrected if possible.

   Diagnosis: Hyperkalemia.

CASE 40

HPI: A 10-day-old infant boy is brought to the ED because of poor feeding, vomiting, fever, and abdominal distention for 1 day. The parents state that he was born at 35 weeks of gestation, and the mother had preeclampsia, but the hospital stay was uncomplicated, and they were released from the hospital just 3 days previously, after the infant's feeding was monitored.

Vital signs: Temperature 102.2°F (39°C), pulse 160 beats/min, BP 64/40 mm Hg, RR 60 breaths/min.

Additional history: None. Received birth vaccinations. Breastfed only.

1. **What is the differential diagnosis?**
   Necrotizing enterocolitis (NEC), malrotation/midgut volvulus, strangulated hernia, neonatal sepsis.

2. **What components of the physical examination do you perform?**
   General appearance, cardiovascular, lungs, abdomen.
   Physical examination:
   General: Lethargic, ill-appearing neonate, unresponsive but breathing.
   Cardiovascular: Tachycardic, weak and thready pulses, no murmur.
   Lungs: Tachypneic, but lungs clear on auscultation; using accessory muscles.
   Abdomen: Distended, diffusely tender to palpation, absent bowel sounds.

3. **What are your initial orders?**
   IV fluid bolus of normal saline, nothing by mouth (NPO), nasogastric/orogastric tube, blood cultures, CBC, chem 14, UA, urine culture, broad-spectrum antibiotics (e.g., ampicillin, gentamicin, metronidazole), fingerstick blood glucose, abdominal x-ray.
   Advance clock:
   After fluid resuscitation the patient's BP is 90/60 mm Hg and the heart rate is 140 beats/min.
   An abdominal x-ray shows pneumatosis intestinalis and dilated loops of bowel.
   Blood glucose is normal.
   CBC demonstrates leukocytosis with a left shift.

4. **What are your follow-up actions?**
   Surgery consult. Admit to ICU.
   Advance clock: Case ends.
   Critical actions: Recognition of vital sign abnormalities in the neonate, resuscitation. Recognition of NEC as a possible cause of the abdominal pain, ordering an appropriate workup, including abdominal imaging, surgical consult, hospital admission.
   Discussion: NEC is the most common neonatal GI emergency, with high morbidity and mortality. NEC is caused by bowel ischemia, which causes translocation of bacteria through the bowel wall. Risk factors are prematurity and any cause of a low-flow state to the bowel, including congenital heart disease, maternal cocaine use, maternal preeclampsia, and hypotension. NEC presentation to the ED is uncommon because it classically occurs in more premature or otherwise ill neonates who would have reasons to remain in hospital. In term babies, NEC typically occurs within the first week of life, and within weeks 2 to 3 of life in premature babies.
       The presenting symptoms for NEC are abdominal distention, fever, irritability, and possibly peritoneal signs, with progression to shock. Plain abdominal x-rays are often sufficient to make the diagnosis and classically show (1) pneumatosis intestinalis, (2) free portal vein air, and/or (3) dilated loops of bowel.
       Management includes NPO, nasogastric or orogastric tube placement, fluid resuscitation, blood cultures, broad-spectrum antibiotics, glucose testing, abdominal x-ray, and ICU admission. In this case the neonate was hypotensive and needed fluid resuscitation. Normal systolic BP in a child can be calculated as: minimum systolic BP = 70 + [2 × age in years] up to age 10 years and 90 mm Hg thereafter. Poor glycogen stores in neonates necessitate blood sugar checks for all ill-appearing patients.
   Diagnosis: NEC.

CASE 41

HPI: A 27-year-old man attends the clinic complaining of 1 week of fever and malaise. He states that he has been feeling "hot" all week and has had frequent shaking chills. He has also noticed some pink patches on his skin that are painful to touch. He has never had any similar symptoms. He denies a cough, shortness of breath, other skin changes, sick contacts, or recent travel history.

Vital signs: Temperature 100.8°F (38.2°C), pulse 90 beats/min, BP 125/78 mm Hg, RR 16 breaths/min.
Additional history: No medical history. Uses IV heroin two or three times per week, smokes marijuana, drinks occasional alcohol, and smokes one pack of cigarettes daily. Not currently sexually active.

1. What is the differential diagnosis?
   Bacteremia, endocarditis, autoimmune disease, malignancy.

2. What components of the physical examination do you perform?
   General appearance, HEENT, cardiovascular, lungs, extremities.
   Physical examination:
   General: Mildly disheveled male in no apparent distress.
   HEENT: Fundoscopy shows small retinal hemorrhages with pale white centers, no papilledema, otherwise WNL.
   Cardiovascular: IV/VI holosystolic murmur at the left lower sternal border, otherwise WNL.
   Lungs: Occasional crackles throughout the lung fields bilaterally.
   Extremities: Multiple tender erythematous nodules on the hands and feet. Splinter hemorrhages seen on the nail beds of the hands and feet bilaterally.

3. What are your initial orders?
   CBC, chem 8, blood cultures, lactate, rapid HIV test, CXR, antipyretics (e.g., acetaminophen).
   Advance clock: CBC remarkable for leukocytosis of 17,000 cells/mL with neutrophil predominance. Chem 8 WNL. Blood cultures pending. Rapid HIV test negative. CXR shows evidence of septic pulmonary emboli in both lung fields.

4. What are your follow-up actions?
   Admit to monitored bed. Initiation vancomycin and ceftriaxone IV. Echocardiogram. Infectious disease consult.
   Advance clock: Echocardiogram shows vegetation on the tricuspid valve. Blood cultures grow methicillin-sensitive *S. aureus*.

5. What are your follow-up actions?
   Narrow antibiotics to oxacillin administration via a peripherally inserted central catheter line for 4 to 6 weeks.
   Advance clock: Case ends.
   Critical actions: Recognition of infective endocarditis (IE), admission, ordering of appropriate workup, including blood cultures, initiation of appropriate treatment.
   Discussion: This patient has IE, an infection of the endocardium of the heart, typically on the valvular surfaces. The most common causes are *S. aureus* (especially for acute presentations) and Viridans group *Streptococcus* species (for subacute presentations). In this individual with a history of IV drug use, *S. aureus* is the most likely agent. IE should be suspected in patients with fever and a heart murmur. Classic examination findings in IE include Roth spots (retinal emboli causing hemorrhages, often with white or pale centers); splinter hemorrhages in the nailbed; Janeway lesions, which are nontender purple macular lesions; and Osler nodes, which are similar to Janeway lesions but are raised and painful (remember Osler—Ow!).
   The diagnosis of IE is made according to the Duke criteria whereby (1) two major criteria or (2) one major and three minor criteria or (3) five minor criteria are met. The two major criteria are:
   1. Positive blood cultures for organisms causing endocarditis (e.g., Viridans group streptococci, *S. aureus*, and HACEK species).
   2. Evidence of endocardial involvement (e.g., a positive echocardiogram showing a vegetation or new valvular regurgitation).
   The minor criteria are conditions that are also common to many other diseases and therefore are not as specific for endocarditis. They are:
   1. Fever.
   2. Predisposition (e.g., IV drug use, damaged heart valve).
   3. Vascular phenomena (e.g., emboli, Janeway lesions).
   4. Immunologic phenomena (e.g., Osler nodes, Roth spots).
   5. Positive blood cultures that do not meet major criteria. Typically, multiple sets of blood cultures will need to be obtained before antimicrobial treatment is started to ensure adequate isolation of the causative organism.
   Treatment is with long-term parenteral antibiotics (4–6 weeks). An infectious disease consult should be sought to ensure appropriate antimicrobial coverage and follow-up of blood cultures as an outpatient to ensure clearance. Abscess formation, heart block, hemodynamic instability, persistent blood culture positivity, significant embolic burden to the brain, and other forms of decompensation are all indications for surgical management. Fungal endocarditis also generally requires cardiothoracic surgery evaluation. The most common two complications are CHF from valvular dysfunction and embolization (through the pulmonary circulation [lungs] for tricuspid vegetations or the systemic circulation [e.g., brain, kidneys] for mitral and aortic vegetations). The disposition for all patients with suspected or confirmed endocarditis is admission.
   Diagnosis: IE.

CASE 42

HPI: A 36-year-old woman presents to her regular doctor 48 hours after receiving a tuberculin skin test (TST) as a condition of her new employment as a nurse at a nursing home. Since the skin test was placed on her right forearm she has noticed the development of a large bump in the area. She has worked at other nursing homes in the past and her TST was always negative. She denies any cough, fevers, chills, night sweats, weight loss, or other symptoms.

Vital signs: Temperature 98.2°F (36.8°C), pulse 76 beats/min, BP 115/68 mm Hg, RR 16 breaths/min.

Additional history: No medical history. Occasional alcohol use, denies smoking or use of other drugs. Sexually active with one male partner. Born in Mexico and has received the BCG vaccine.

1. **What is the differential diagnosis?**
   TB: latent versus active.

2. **What components of the physical examination do you perform?**
   General appearance, cardiovascular, lungs, extremities.
   Physical examination:
   General: Well-developed, well-nourished woman in no apparent distress.
   Cardiovascular: WNL
   Lungs: WNL
   Extremities: 11-mm induration over the volar aspect of the right forearm.

3. **What are your initial orders?**
   CXR, CBC, chem 7, LFTs.
   Advance clock: CXR negative. CBC, chem 7, and LFTs all WNL.

4. **What are your follow-up actions?**
   Begin isoniazid and pyridoxine treatment for 9 months. Counsel patient on disease. Consider periodic LFTs to monitor for isoniazid-induced hepatitis.
   Advance clock: Case ends.
   Critical actions: Recognition of what classifies a positive TST in each risk group, understanding the difference between latent and active TB, appropriate treatment.
   Discussion: This patient has latent TB, a contagious bacterial infection due to *Mycobacterium tuberculosis.* TB has a wide spectrum of disease, ranging from latent (asymptomatic) TB to primary or reactivated pulmonary TB to disseminated TB. An asymptomatic individual with a newly positive TST and no evidence of active disease has latent TB; treatment for these patients involves 9 months of isoniazid therapy. Active TB is characterized by clinical symptoms such as chronic cough, hemoptysis, fever, night sweats, and weight loss. TST and QuantiFERON-Gold test negativity are not sufficient to rule out active TB in patients with high suspicion, and further evaluation with induced sputum for acid-fast bacilli smears and *Mycobacterium tuberculosis* PCR is usually required in the instance of pulmonary TB. TB may also affect other organ systems (e.g., TB pericarditis, TB pleuritis) and will require appropriate tissue sampling for evaluation. Patients with active TB are often treated with four drugs (isoniazid, rifampin, pyrazinamide, and ethambutol) for 2 months and then two drugs (isoniazid and rifampin) for a further 4 months over a total treatment time of 6 months. This can be remembered by the "4-for-2 and 2-for-4" mnemonic (4 drugs for 2 months, 2 drugs for 4 months). Extrapulmonary TB is typically treated in the same way as active TB, except a longer course is used for spinal involvement (Pott disease) and TB meningitis. Consider adding pyridoxine (vitamin B_6) to patients on isoniazid, because isoniazid can cause pyridoxine deficiency and subsequently lead to neuropathy and seizures.

   Multidrug-resistant (MDR) TB is becoming more common and is resistant to isoniazid and rifampin, requiring other agents such as fluoroquinolones. However, an even more resistant strain called extensively drug-resistant (XDR) TB is emerging and is resistant to many of these second-line drugs as well. Patients with HIV have a 10% per year risk of reactivation of latent TB; this is in contrast to immunocompetent individuals, who have a 10% lifetime risk of reactivation.

   A positive TST is defined differently for different risk groups, but the measurement (in millimeters) is always based on induration (not erythema). Whether or not the patient has received the BCG vaccine should not impact management:

   - 5 mm or greater for high-risk patients, including HIV-positive individuals, immunosuppressed individuals, patients with a CXR consistent with TB, and individuals who have had recent contact with someone known to have active TB.
   - 10 mm or greater for intermediate-risk patients, including immigrants from a high-prevalence country, IV drug users, residents or employees of a high-risk setting (e.g., jail, homeless shelter, nursing home, hospital), and individuals with a high-risk comorbid condition (e.g., diabetes, chronic kidney disease).
   - 15 mm or greater for low-risk patients who have no risk factors for TB.

   The patient in this case falls into the category for which the TST is positive at 10 mm because she is a health care worker in a high-risk environment. Therefore she should be treated. She did not have evidence of active TB and therefore has latent TB.
   Diagnosis: Latent TB.

CASE 43

HPI: A 6-week-old infant boy is brought to the ED because he is "throwing up everything he eats" according to his parents. For the past few days, his condition has worsened to the point that he was vomiting 100% of his meals. Initially the patient would want to feed immediately afterward, but recently has been less interactive with his mother. The mother describes the vomitus as "the same color as the formula" with no blood.

Vital signs: Temperature 98.2°F (36.8°C), pulse 170 beats/min, BP 60/40 mm Hg, RR 50 breaths/min.

Additional history: Ex-full term, no complications.

1. **What is the differential diagnosis?**
   Pyloric stenosis, malrotation with midgut volvulus, duodenal atresia, gastroesophageal reflux disease (GERD), antral web or atresia, adrenal insufficiency, inborn error of metabolism, improper feeding practices.

2. **What components of the physical examination do you perform?**
   General appearance, cardiovascular, lungs, abdomen, skin, extremities.
   Physical examination:
   General: Lethargic infant, responding poorly to stimuli but breathing on his own.
   Cardiovascular: Tachycardic for age, holosystolic murmur throughout the precordium.
   Lungs: Tachypneic but lungs clear on auscultation.
   Abdomen: Soft, nontender, nondistended, small olivelike structure palpated superiorly and to the right of the umbilicus.
   Skin: No rash.
   Extremities: Delayed capillary refill.

3. **What are your initial orders?**
   Blood glucose test, CBC, chem 8, IV fluid bolus, abdominal ultrasound when stable.
   Advance clock: After a bolus of normal saline, the patient's heart rate is 140 beats/min and BP is 80/55 mm Hg. He is now interacting with his mother. Blood glucose 30 mg/dL. CBC remarkable for hemoconcentration. Chem 8 remarkable for potassium 3 mEq/L, bicarbonate 30 mEq/L, chloride 80 mEq/L, normal renal function. Abdominal ultrasound shows a hypertrophied pylorus.

4. **What are your follow-up actions?**
   IV 10% dextrose, maintenance fluids 5% dextrose in quarter-strength normal saline with KCl 20 mEq/L, NPO, surgery consult, admit.
   Advance clock: Case ends.
   Critical actions: Checking blood glucose in ill-appearing neonate, abdominal ultrasound for diagnosis of pyloric stenosis, consideration of other life-threatening causes, correction of metabolic abnormalities, patient stabilization, admission and surgical consult.
   Discussion: This patient has pyloric stenosis caused by hypertrophy of the gastric pylorus leading to obstruction. This classically occurs early in life, between the ages of 2 and 8 weeks. The vomiting is always nonbilious because bile is introduced in the duodenum, and the blockage is proximal. As the hypertrophy progresses, the patient vomits more frequently and forcefully (projectile vomiting), which often leads to dehydration and lethargy.
       Findings are typically hypochloremic and hypokalemic metabolic acidosis arising from both vomiting of HCl and K^+ from the stomach and upregulation of the renin-angiotensin-aldosterone system. An olive-type mass can sometimes be palpated over the area of the pylorus, as in this case. Definitive diagnosis is via ultrasound, which will demonstrate a thick wall (>3 mm) and a long length (>16 mm) for the pylorus.
       Management is with fluid resuscitation, if required, and correction of metabolic abnormalities (electrolyte derangements, hypoglycemia because of poor glycemic stores). Surgical pyloromyotomy is definitive but not emergent because the patient will stabilize once resuscitated.
   Diagnosis: Pyloric stenosis.

CASE 44

HPI: A 4-year-old, previously healthy boy is brought to the ED by his parents after he had a single 30-second episode of "shaking of his whole body." He was unresponsive during this episode and was briefly confused afterward but has since returned to normal.

Vital signs: Temperature 102.2°F (39°C), pulse 120 beats/min, BP 100/64 mm Hg, RR 24 breaths/min.

Additional history: Patient has had a runny nose, cough, and fever for the past 3 days. No history of ingestions, headache, or vision changes.

1. **What is the differential diagnosis?**
   Seizure secondary to febrile illness, meningitis, intracranial hemorrhage, toxic ingestion, intracranial mass.

2. **What components of the physical examination do you perform?**
   General appearance, HEENT, cardiovascular, lungs, neuro/psych.

Physical examination:
General: Well-developed, well-nourished boy in no distress, nontoxic, smiling.
HEENT: No evidence of trauma, neck supple without meningeal signs. Mild posterior oropharynx erythema and cobblestoning. Small lateral tongue abrasion. Rhinorrhea. Tympanic membranes normal.
Cardiovascular: WNL
Lungs: WNL
Neuro/psych: Appropriate for developmental age. Normal strength, sensation, and reflexes. Cranial nerves II through XII intact. No focal neurologic deficits.

3. **What are your initial orders?**
Fingerstick glucose test, acetaminophen PO.
Advance clock: Glucose 110 mg/dL, repeat temperature check 99.7°F (37.6°C).

4. **What are your follow-up actions?**
Counsel the parents on simple febrile seizures.
Follow up with primary doctor.
Advance clock: Case ends.
Critical actions: Recognition of simple febrile seizure, ruling out of more serious etiologies (e.g., meningitis) according to the history and physical examination, not pursuing an aggressive workup (such as CT or lumbar puncture) for simple febrile seizure.
Discussion: This patient had a simple febrile seizure. A simple febrile seizure occurs in patients aged 3 months to 6 years with a temperature of 100.4°F (38°C) or greater and must meet all of the following criteria: (1) generalized tonic-clonic seizure, (2) less than 15 minutes in duration, (3) only occurs once in a 24-hour period, and (4) no focal features. Any exceptions to these four criteria will classify the condition as a complex febrile seizure, which may require a more thorough workup.
   The differential diagnosis for a patient who otherwise meets all the criteria for a simple febrile seizure includes any febrile illness (usually viral) but can also include more serious causes such as meningitis, intracranial hemorrhage, toxic ingestion, and intracranial mass. These other causes should be ruled out on the basis of the history and physical examination alone. In this case, the child currently appears well and nontoxic, does not have meningeal signs, has no abnormalities on neurologic examination, and has an examination consistent with an alternative diagnosis (viral upper respiratory tract infection). Therefore the patient and his parents can be reassured that this condition is common (up to 5% of the population), is not harmful, and does not require antiepileptic medications.
   Diagnosis: Simple febrile seizure.

CASE 45

HPI: A 70-year-old woman attends your clinic for follow-up of thoracic back pain that has persisted for the past 3 weeks. She denies any similar history of pain. She denies any antecedent trauma or numbness or weakness in her body. She states that her back pain still occurs with activity and describes it as knifelike and nonradiating. She has also noticed that her posture has changed; she stoops forward from her upper back since the pain began.
Vital signs: Temperature 98.2°F (36.8°C), pulse 76 beats/min, BP 130/68 mm Hg, RR 16 breaths/min.
Additional history: 20–pack-year smoking history, quit 30 years ago. Hypertension controlled with amlodipine.

1. **What is the differential diagnosis?**
Vertebral compression fracture secondary to osteoporosis, malignancy (pathologic fracture, especially lung cancer in this former smoker), hyperparathyroidism, Cushing syndrome or steroid use, Paget disease of bone.

2. **What components of the physical examination do you perform?**
General appearance, back, neuro/psych.
Physical examination:
General: Well-developed female in no apparent distress.
Back: Significant kyphosis with a dowager hump, mild tenderness to palpation over the midthoracic vertebrae, no paraspinal tenderness.
Neuro/psych: Normal strength, sensation, and reflexes in all extremities. Cranial nerves II through XII intact.

3. **What are your initial orders?**
CBC, chem 8, thoracic spine x-ray, acetaminophen or other analgesia.
Advance clock: CBC and chem 8 normal, no evidence of hypercalcemia. Thoracic spine x-ray shows wedge fractures of T6 and T7 vertebrae and generalized decreased bone density with degenerative joint disease.

4. **What are your follow-up actions?**
Dual-energy x-ray absorptiometry (DXA) scan, counseling on osteoporosis.
Advance clock: DXA scan shows osteoporosis with a T score of −3.0. The patient's pain has improved with acetaminophen.

5. **What are your follow-up actions?**

Vitamin D (can order a vitamin D level before supplementation), calcium, bisphosphonate (e.g., alendronate).

Advance clock: Case ends.

Critical actions: Recognition of osteoporosis, appropriate workup, and treatment.

Discussion: This patient has osteoporosis, which is decreased bone density characterized by a DXA T value of -2.5 or lower (-1 to -2.5 is osteopenia). This value is the number of standard deviations by which the patient's density differs from a normal peak bone density. A DXA scan should be performed for women older than 65 years, men older than 70 years, and individuals older than 50 years with a fracture. Those with risk factors for osteoporosis (e.g., chronic glucocorticoid use) should be screened at an earlier age.

Treatment of osteoporosis includes lifestyle modifications (e.g., smoking cessation, increased weight-bearing exercise), nutrition (e.g., vitamin D and calcium supplementation), and pharmacologic therapy (e.g., bisphosphonates, PTH analogues such as teriparatide).

In a patient without prior trauma, underlying malignancy must remain in the differential diagnosis, particularly for older patients and for this patient, who is a former smoker. Remember the mnemonic "BLT with a kosher pickle" for malignancies that commonly metastasize to bone: breast, lung, thyroid, kidney, and prostate. Also remember multiple myeloma as a possible cause of bone pain that is commonly missed in the initial evaluation of a patient. Further clues to multiple myeloma include anemia and renal impairment.

Diagnosis: Osteoporosis.

CASE 46

HPI: A 28-year-old man presents to the ED complaining of bilateral lower extremity weakness for 4 days. He states that his symptoms began gradually, with his feet tripping as he walked up stairs, but they have now progressed, and he finds it difficult to walk on flat ground. He denies any trauma or travel history.

Vital signs: Temperature 98.2°F (36.8°C), pulse 76 beats/min, BP 155/78 mm Hg, RR 16 breaths/min.

Additional history: Occasional marijuana use. Had diarrhea that was occasionally bloody 2 weeks ago, but this has since completely resolved.

1. **What is the differential diagnosis?**

Guillain-Barré syndrome (GBS), transverse myelitis, spinal cord compression, tick paralysis, vitamin B_{12} deficiency resulting in subacute combined degeneration of the spinal cord (Lichtheim disease).

2. **What components of the physical examination do you perform?**

General appearance, cardiovascular, lungs, neuro/psych.

Physical examination:

General: Comfortable, no distress, speaking in full sentences.

Cardiovascular: WNL

Lungs: Unlabored breathing.

Neuro/psych: Strength in bilateral upper extremities 5/5, strength in hips 4/5, strength in knees 3/5, strength in ankles 3/5. No patellar or Achilles reflexes. Mild decreased sensation to pinprick in bilateral lower extremities. Cranial nerves intact.

3. **What are your initial orders?**

Chem 14, CBC, bedside pulmonary function tests, lumbar puncture (CSF cell count with differential, protein, glucose, Gram stain and culture), vitamin B_{12} level.

Advance clock: Chem 14 and CBC unremarkable. Bedside pulmonary function tests WNL. Lumbar puncture shows high protein but normal cell count and no organisms on Gram stain. Vitamin B_{12} level normal.

4. **What are your follow-up actions?**

Neurology consultation, plasmapheresis or IVIG, admit to inpatient unit.

Advance clock: Case ends.

Critical actions: Recognition of GBS, appropriate diagnostic testing, including lumbar puncture, assessment of pulmonary function to predict early respiratory compromise, admission to a monitored bed.

Discussion: This patient has GBS, an autoimmune disease affecting the Schwann cells of the peripheral nervous system and characterized by ascending paralysis with areflexia and sensory changes. GBS classically follows an infection, especially with *Campylobacter jejuni*, as in this patient, but it can also occur without a known prior infection. GBS is also rarely (1 in 1 million) associated with influenza vaccination.

There are different GBS subtypes. The most important variant is Miller Fisher syndrome, which has *descending* paralysis, affects the cranial nerves, and is associated with positive anti-GQ1b antibodies. Although at times severe enough to require intubation, GBS commonly resolves completely in most patients. The hallmark diagnostic finding in GBS is albuminocytologic dissociation in the CSF, meaning that there is a high protein level without a corresponding increase in cell count.

The treatment for GBS is plasmapheresis to remove autoantibodies or IVIG to neutralize them. Supportive care with pulmonary function tests and close monitoring is also a cornerstone of therapy to ensure that the patient does not develop respiratory compromise.

Diagnosis: GBS.

CASE 47

HPI: A 26-year-old, previously healthy woman presents to the ED complaining of fever and right-sided back pain for the past 3 days. She states that the pain started approximately 1 week ago with a burning sensation during urination but has now progressed to significant pain in her back. She denies any history of similar symptoms. She states that she has had mild nausea but no vomiting.

Vital signs: Temperature 101.1°F (38.4°C), pulse 120 beats/min, BP 110/68 mm Hg, RR 18 breaths/min.

Additional history: 1-week history of dysuria and urinary urgency and frequency. Denies hematuria. Denies IV drug use. Denies sexual activity.

1. What is the differential diagnosis?

   Pyelonephritis (with or without perinephric abscess), lower UTI (e.g., cystitis), urethritis (e.g., gonococcal or nongonococcal), pelvic inflammatory disease (PID), nephrolithiasis, pregnancy (including ectopic pregnancy).

2. What components of the physical examination do you perform?

   General appearance, cardiovascular, abdomen, back, genitalia.

   Physical examination:

   General: Uncomfortable female sitting up in bed, mild distress.

   Cardiovascular: WNL

   Abdomen: Tenderness to palpation in the suprapubic area without rebound or guarding.

   Back: Costovertebral angle tenderness on the right side. No midline tenderness.

   Genitalia: No urethral prolapse, no vaginal discharge. No vaginal, cervical, or vulvar lesions. No cervical motion tenderness.

3. What are your initial orders?

   UA with microscopy, urine culture, CBC, chem 8, urinary pregnancy test, analgesia/antipyretics/antiemetics (e.g., acetaminophen and ondansetron), IV fluids. (Consider gonococcal and *Chlamydia* testing.)

   Advance clock:

   UA with microscopy significant for positive leukocyte esterase and nitrites, 50 WBCs/hpf, 5 RBCs/hpf, no squamous epithelial cells. Urinary pregnancy test negative.

   CBC significant for leukocytosis of 16,000 cells/mL with 95% neutrophils. Other studies WNL.

   Patient feels much better after analgesics, antipyretics, and antiemetics.

   After IV fluids, her heart rate is 80 beats/min.

   If gonococcal/*Chlamydia* testing is ordered, it will be negative.

4. What are your follow-up actions?

   Appropriate antibiotics for pyelonephritis (e.g., fluoroquinolone such as ciprofloxacin for 10–14 days). Appropriate analgesics and antiemetics (e.g., hydrocodone/acetaminophen, ondansetron). Assess for PO tolerance. Counseling. Discharge with close follow-up.

   Advance clock: Case ends.

   Critical actions: Diagnosis of acute pyelonephritis, assessment of pregnancy status, appropriate analgesia and supportive care, antibiotics appropriate for treatment of acute pyelonephritis.

   Discussion: This patient has a UTI that initially started as cystitis then ascended further to the kidneys, causing pyelonephritis. By far the most common cause of UTIs is *E. coli*, followed by *Staphylococcus saprophyticus*. Whereas cystitis typically does not cause fever, pyelonephritis often leads to fever because bacteria can now reach the bloodstream. UTIs can be divided into complicated and uncomplicated. Uncomplicated UTIs only occur in otherwise healthy women with a normal urinary tract who are not pregnant. Therefore any patient who does not meet these criteria has, by definition, a complicated UTI (e.g., all males, all pregnant women, any patient with a Foley catheter).

   Diagnosis of a UTI is based on history, physical examination, and results of UA with microscopy. A positive nitrite test on UA is the most specific indicator of a UTI (e.g., a positive result in the right clinical context virtually guarantees a UTI) but is not sensitive because only some bacteria (including *E. coli*) have the ability to reduce nitrate to nitrite, and the reaction is slow. Leukocyte esterase is a more sensitive (e.g., more likely to be positive in the presence of a UTI) but less specific indicator. In sexually active patients with symptoms of urethritis (e.g., dysuria, frequency), *Chlamydia* or gonorrhea should be considered.

   If a patient with uncomplicated pyelonephritis can take PO medication, has adequate pain control, and has appropriate follow-up, she can be treated as an outpatient with a 10- to 14-day course of a fluoroquinolone such as ciprofloxacin or levofloxacin; folate inhibitors such as trimethoprim/sulfamethoxazole are second-line agents because of resistance patterns. In general, a patient with pyelonephritis should receive one dose of an IV cephalosporin or aminoglycoside prior to discharge (can be omitted if local resistance to PO antibiotics prescribed is very low). Patients with PO intolerance will require admission for intravenous antibiotics.

Diagnosis: Pyelonephritis.

CASE 48

HPI: A 12-year-old girl presents to the ED complaining of a severe, nonproductive cough for the past 5 days. She says that the cough comes in forceful spurts, and she needs to catch her breath afterward. She has vomited twice today because of the coughing. She says that a week or two ago her condition started with mild fever, a runny nose, and a normal cough, but her parents did not take her to see the doctor because they thought it was a common cold.

Vital signs: Temperature 98.2°F (36.8°C), pulse 76 beats/min, BP 115/68 mm Hg, RR 16 breaths/min.

Additional history: No medical history; unknown vaccination history.

1. **What is the differential diagnosis?**
   Pertussis, cough-variant asthma, viral upper respiratory tract infection, viral bronchitis, viral laryngotracheitis (croup), group A streptococcal tonsillopharyngitis, pneumonia, mononucleosis, TB, foreign body aspiration.
   For older patients, consider other causes of chronic cough: GERD, postnasal drip, ACE-associated cough, COPD exacerbation.

2. **What components of the physical examination do you perform?**
   General appearance, HEENT, cardiovascular, lungs, abdomen.
   Physical examination:
   General: Well-developed, well-nourished girl, occasionally coughing in forceful paroxysms and inhaling forcefully afterward.
   HEENT: WNL
   Cardiovascular: WNL
   Lungs: WNL
   Abdomen: WNL

3. **What are your initial orders?**
   Pulse oximetry. CXR optional. Pertussis PCR. Azithromycin for patient and close contacts.
   Advance clock:
   Pertussis PCR positive for *Bordetella pertussis*.
   Pulse oximetry: 97% on room air.

4. **What are your follow-up actions?**
   Counseling on disease process and mandatory vaccinations if not performed already (Tdap).
   Advance clock: Case ends.
   Critical actions: Recognition of pertussis, azithromycin to reduce the infectivity of patient and close contacts. Counseling on childhood vaccination schedule.
   Discussion: Pertussis (whooping cough) is a bacterial infection with droplet transmission caused by *B. pertussis*, a gram-negative rod bacterium. There are classically three stages of pertussis: (1) the catarrhal stage, characterized by typical upper respiratory tract symptoms such as rhinorrhea and cough; followed by (2) the paroxysmal stage, with the classic cough in paroxysms followed by an inspiratory whoop and posttussive emesis; and finally (3) the convalescent stage, during which a chronic cough develops that lasts for weeks. Unfortunately, very young individuals do not have the classic symptoms and can have apnea as the presenting symptom.
   Diagnosis is mostly on a clinical basis, but the recommended diagnostic test is a pertussis PCR of a nasopharyngeal swab. Culture on Bordet-Gengou medium can also be performed. If a CBC is ordered, it may show severe leukocytosis with marked lymphocytosis because of a stimulating factor made by the bacteria (called a leukemoid reaction because the high WBC count is similar to that seen in acute leukemia). Treatment is with azithromycin (or erythromycin) for 5 days, which reduces infectivity but does not significantly impact symptom duration or severity unless started very early in the course of the illness. Other alternatives are clarithromycin twice a day (BID) for 7 days or Bactrim DS daily for 14 days. Close contacts should be treated as well, regardless of immunization status.
   Diagnosis: Pertussis.

CASE 49

HPI: A 65-year-old man presents to the ED complaining of right knee pain and swelling for the past day that prevent him from being able to walk without extreme pain. The symptoms are associated with fever and malaise. He denies any trauma or a history of similar symptoms.

Vital signs: Temperature 101.8°F (38.8°C), pulse 100 beats/min, BP 155/78 mm Hg, RR 16 breaths/min.

Additional history: History of hypertension and diabetes, moderately controlled. One sexual partner, monogamous. Occasional alcohol consumption, no use of tobacco or drugs.

1. **What is the differential diagnosis?**
   Monoarticular arthritis: septic arthritis, gout, pseudogout, trauma, osteoarthritis (OA), psoriatic arthritis. (If patient were a child, transient synovitis would be included in the differential.)
   Oligoarticular arthritis: Gonococcal arthritis.

2. **What components of the physical examination do you perform?**
   General appearance, cardiovascular, lungs, musculoskeletal/extremities, genitourinary, skin.
   Physical examination:
   General: Well-developed, well-nourished man in mild distress due to pain.
   Cardiovascular: WNL
   Lungs: WNL
   Extremities: Right knee joint swollen with evidence of large effusion. Markedly diminished range of motion because of pain. Distal sensation, motion, and pulses intact. Further examination of the knee limited because of pain. Skin intact, no evidence of skin infection or breakdown.
   Skin: No rashes, lesions, lacerations, abrasions.
   Genitourinary: Nonedematous, nonerythematous, nontender; without purulence, lesions, vesicles; without masses or deformities

3. **What are your initial orders?**
   CBC, chem 8, x-ray series of the right knee, ESR, C-reactive protein (CRP), arthrocentesis of right knee (with Gram stain, culture, cell count with differential, crystal analysis), analgesics and antipyretics (e.g., acetaminophen).
   Advance clock: CBC remarkable for leukocytosis of 17,000 cells/mL with neutrophil predominance. Chem 8 unremarkable. ESR 80 mm/hr and CRP 10 mg/dL (both elevated). X-ray series of the right knee remarkable for joint effusion; otherwise no evidence of fracture, dislocation, or osteomyelitis. Arthrocentesis of the right knee produces purulent liquid for which a Gram stain shows gram-positive cocci in clusters and a cell count of 120,000 WBCs/μL with a neutrophil predominance, culture pending.

4. **What are your follow-up actions?**
   IV vancomycin, admit for antibiotic therapy, serial aspiration. Orthopedic surgery consult for arthrotomy or serial arthrocentesis.
   Advance clock: Case ends.
   Critical actions: Recognition of septic arthritis, arthrocentesis to confirm diagnosis, IV antibiotics, and admission.
   Discussion: This patient has septic arthritis, which is infection of a joint space. Most often, septic arthritis is monoarticular, involves a painful and swollen joint, and may have systemic symptoms such as fever. The cause is usually *S. aureus* (such as in this case); in patients with gonococcal arthritis (which can be monoarticular or oligoarticular), the causative agent is *Neisseria gonorrhoeae*. Septic arthritis should be considered in any patient with acute monoarticular arthritis, although the differential includes gout, pseudogout, trauma, OA, psoriatic arthritis, and transient synovitis (in children; previously called toxic synovitis). Transient synovitis is a common condition in children aged 3 to 10 years (peak incidence 5–6 years) and differs from septic arthritis in that there will typically be no fever, the child will be able to bear weight, and the ESR and WBC count will not be as elevated as in septic arthritis (and if joint aspiration is performed there will be no evidence of infection). Transient synovitis is self-limiting and will resolve with supportive measures (decreased activity, NSAIDs).
       Definitive diagnosis of septic arthritis is on the basis of joint aspiration. The most important test is a bacterial culture, but if enough fluid is aspirated, a Gram stain, cell count with differential, and crystal analysis should be performed. A cell count greater than 50,000 cells/μL, a positive Gram stain, or a positive culture requires immediate treatment. The initial antibiotic choice depends on what the likely organism is and the patient's age, but definitive management is via serial needle aspiration with antibiotic therapy and/or surgical drainage of the joint. Studies have shown that for most joints (not the hip and not for joints with prostheses in them), serial needle aspiration is as effective as surgical drainage of the joint. All patients with septic arthritis should be admitted for parenteral antibiotic therapy and definitive management. Evaluation for further extent of infection (osteomyelitis, endocarditis) may also be warranted if physical exam findings are suggestive.
       Diagnosis: Septic arthritis.

CASE 50

HPI: An 80-year-old man presents to the ED because of sudden-onset weakness and numbness of the left arm and left lower face that started 90 minutes ago. He was watching television when the symptoms suddenly started, and they have not improved at all since onset. He says that it feels like the left side of his mouth is not moving when he speaks and that he cannot move his left arm at all but can still walk. He denies any history of similar symptoms and at baseline takes care of himself and lives with his wife. He denies any recent falls or trauma.

Vital signs: Temperature 98.2°F (36.8°C), pulse 76 beats/min, BP 160/90 mm Hg, RR 16 breaths/min.

Additional history: Has hypertension controlled with amlodipine. No other medical problems, medications, or allergies. No alcohol, tobacco, or drug use.

1. What is the differential diagnosis?

Acute stroke (ischemic vs hemorrhagic), TIA, recrudescence of old stroke, hypoglycemia, seizure with Todd paralysis, cerebral aneurysm rupture, SAH.

2. What components of the physical examination do you perform?

General appearance, lungs, cardiovascular, neuro/psych.

Physical examination:

General: Well-developed, well-nourished man in no apparent distress.

Cardiovascular: WNL; no evidence of carotid bruits auscultated.

Lungs: WNL

Neuro/psych: Cranial nerves II through XII intact except the left lower face has 1/5 strength; left upper face normal. Strength 5/5 and symmetric over all extremities except for the left arm, which has 1/5 strength. Decreased sensation to light touch and pinprick over the left arm. No ataxia, no dysdiadochokinesia, normal gait.

3. What are your initial orders?

Fingerstick blood glucose, CBC, chem 8, coagulation profile, troponin, UA, CXR, immediate noncontrast head CT scan, activate Code Stroke/consult neurology.

Advance clock:

CBC, chem 8, coagulation profile, fingerstick blood glucose WNL.

Noncontrast head CT scan unremarkable, no evidence of intracranial hemorrhage.

4. What are your follow-up actions?

Neurology consult. NPO. Head of bed at least 30 degrees. Thrombolytic agents (e.g., tissue plasminogen activator [tPA]). MRI/MRA stroke protocol. Admit to ICU for close monitoring after thrombolytic administration. Counseling on disease process.

Advance clock:

Patient admitted to ICU after thrombolytic administration.

Patient's weakness resolves and he returns to baseline.

Case ends.

Critical actions: Recognition of acute stroke; ruling out hypoglycemia and hemorrhagic stroke by fingerstick glucose and head CT scan, respectively; and thrombolytic administration for patients who are within the time window and do not have contraindications. Code Stroke activation with neurology consult.

Discussion: This patient had an ischemic stroke, an infarction of an area of brain due to interruption of arterial blood flow. Strokes can be either ischemic (85%) or hemorrhagic (15%). It is important to determine which type of stroke has occurred (with a head CT scan) because their management differs greatly. Strokes are sudden-onset neurologic deficits that follow a vascular distribution, so it is important to understand the vascular distribution of the brain. Strokes are the third leading cause of death in adults in the United States and often occur in older individuals with risk factors for atherosclerosis (hypertension, diabetes, dyslipidemia, tobacco use) and/or emboli (AF).

Diagnosis is on the basis of history and physical examination. Blood glucose should be measured in all patients suspected of having a stroke because hypoglycemia can mimic stroke symptoms. An immediate noncontrast head CT scan should be performed. Early in the course of an *ischemic* stroke, a head CT scan will often be normal or show subtle changes. However, the CT scan is important to exclude a hemorrhagic stroke. Of note, some stroke centers have moved to MRI as first protocol in acute stroke; however, the CT first protocol is most testable. If a diagnosis of stroke is made, the next step is to find out for exactly how long the symptoms have been present. Thrombolytic agents are recommended for patients who do not have contraindications and arrive at the hospital within 3 hours of symptom onset (and some patients within 4.5 hours, but this is less likely to be tested). Some patients between 6 and 24 hours benefit from thrombectomy if they meet certain criteria such as a large-vessel occlusion (since then the clot can be accessed by the thrombectomy catheter) and perfusion imaging (MRI or CT perfusion) showing that most of the territory is ischemic penumbra rather than infarcted (there is brain tissue to salvage). Patients receiving tPA may require IV medications (e.g., nicardipine) to keep BP below 185/110. For those not receiving tPA, treatment of ischemic stroke includes permissive hypertension, whereby BP of up to 220/120 mm Hg should be allowed initially because acute BP lowering can increase the infarct size and extent. All patients should have an emergent neurology consult, especially if thrombolytic agents are considered. All patients should be admitted to a monitored bed for cardiac monitoring in case the stroke was caused by an arrhythmia; if thrombolytic agents are administered, ICU admission should be strongly considered because these patients have a 6% risk of intracranial hemorrhage.

Diagnosis: Ischemic stroke.

CASE 51

HPI: A 45-year-old man presents to his primary care physician because he was at a health fair last week and was told his blood sugar was 300 mg/dL. He was not sure if the result was accurate because he says that he does not have any problems. He denies any polyuria or polydipsia, changes in vision, weight changes, or other symptoms. He read online that you should not eat before you get your blood sugar checked so he has not eaten today.

Vital signs: Temperature 98.2°F (36.8°C), pulse 76 beats/min, BP 120/70 mm Hg, RR 16 breaths/min.

Additional history: Body mass index 30 (obese). Patient works as a receptionist and does not exercise. No medical history, no medications, no allergies. Occasional alcohol consumption, no use of tobacco or drugs.

1. **What is the differential diagnosis?**
   Hyperglycemia due to diabetes, medication effect (but patient not on medications), other endocrine disorders (e.g., hypercortisolism, hypothyroidism), infections (UTI, pneumonia) leading to hyperosmolar hyperglycemic syndrome.

2. **What components of the physical examination do you perform?**
   General appearance, HEENT, cardiovascular, lungs, neuro/psych, skin.
   Physical examination:
   General: Obese male in no apparent distress.
   HEENT: Fundoscopic examination shows mild nonproliferative diabetic retinopathy. Moist mucous membranes.
   Cardiovascular: WNL
   Lungs: WNL. No increased work of breathing (WOB).
   Neuro/psych: AAOx4. Sensation intact to pinprick, light touch, and two-point discrimination in all extremities. Proprioception in distal extremities intact. Rest of neurologic examination WNL.
   Skin: Normal skin turgor

3. **What are your initial orders?**
   Fingerstick blood glucose, HbA$_{1c}$, CBC, chem 8, Mg, Phos, ABG if serum bicarb significantly reduced or patient shows increased WOB, UA, serum beta-hydroxybutyric acid if UA positive for ketones, fasting lipid panel, ECG (to evaluate for electrolyte changes and cardiac conduction).
   Advance clock:
   Fingerstick blood glucose (fasting): 200 mg/dL.
   HbA$_{1c}$: 7.9%.
   CBC WNL; chem 8 glucose 200 mg/dL, otherwise WNL; low-density lipoprotein (LDL) 65 mg/dL.
   UA: Moderate glucose, trace protein, otherwise WNL.

4. **What are your follow-up actions?**
   Counsel patient on disease process, lifestyle modification, diet, weight loss, and exercise. Initiate metformin therapy. Measure urinary microalbumin. Refer for retinal photography. Follow-up appointment in 2 to 3 months.
   Advance clock: Patient returns for visit. States that he has not had medication side effects and has lost 20 lb since changing his diet and starting to exercise. Fingerstick glucose (fasting) 120 mg/dL. Urinary microalbumin negative. Retinal photography shows mild nonproliferative diabetic retinopathy.
   Case ends.
   Critical actions: Recognition of hyperglycemia, knowing diagnostic criteria, initiation of treatment for (likely) type 2 diabetes mellitus (T2DM). Ordering chem 8 to calculate anion gap.
   Discussion: This patient has T2DM, a chronic disorder characterized by insulin resistance and dysfunction of the insulin-producing beta cells in the islets of Langerhans in the endocrine pancreas. Individuals most at risk include those with a positive family history, obesity, a sedentary lifestyle, and increasing age. Hyperosmolar hyperglycemic state (HHS) is an acute complication of T2DM in which severe hyperglycemia occurs without significant ketosis because there is enough insulin to prevent fatty acid breakdown and ketone production. Another acute complication is DKA, which can occur in T2DM when beta cells have failed over time, leading to a marked insulin deficiency and thus hyperglycemia and ketosis. Chronic complications include retinopathy, nephropathy, neuropathy, and accelerated atherosclerosis (leading to increased rates of stroke and MIs, as well as peripheral vascular disease and impotence).
       Diagnosis is on the basis of any two of the following criteria: HbA$_{1c}$ of 6.5% or greater, fasting glucose of 126 mg/dL or greater, and/or random plasma glucose of 200 mg/dL or greater *with symptoms of hyperglycemia*. A 2-hour glucose tolerance test (75 g) with a result of 200 mg/dL or greater can also be applied as a criterion, but this is rarely used outside of pregnancy. Results should be confirmed by a second test unless the results are unequivocal (e.g., fasting glucose of 250 mg/dL certainly represents diabetes). After diagnosis, patient testing should include HbA$_{1c}$, basic laboratory tests, urinary albumin to assess for nephropathy, a fasting lipid profile to assess for concomitant dyslipidemia, referral for retinal photography to assess for retinopathy, counseling on the disease process, and instructions to check the feet daily for foot ulcers (because sensation is diminished with diabetic neuropathy). Treatment always includes lifestyle modifications (patient education, dietary modification, and exercise) with an HbA$_{1c}$ goal of less than 7% in most patients. The first-line medication is metformin to increase insulin sensitivity and decrease hepatic gluconeogenesis, as long as there are no contraindications (e.g., renal failure). Second-line agents include oral drugs such as a sulfonylurea (e.g., glipizide), a glucagon-like peptide-1 (GLP-1) receptor agonist, a SGLT-2 inhibitor (e.g., empagliflozin) or insulin. Insulin is now being recommended earlier in the management of diabetes, especially for patients with marked hyperglycemia. Management of comorbidities is also important. Patients with dyslipidemia should be started on a statin and BP should be controlled with a systolic goal of less than 140/80 mm Hg. An ACE inhibitor or angiotensin receptor blocker (ARB) is the first-line therapy for patients with diabetes and either hypertension or albuminuria. Aspirin therapy is a more evolving recommendation with a recent study in 2018 showing that aspirin for primary prevention in patients with diabetes did decrease serious vascular events but also increased the risk of major bleeding.
       Diagnosis: Uncontrolled T2DM.

CASE 52

HPI: A 29-year-old man presents to the ED with altered mental status. He was brought in by his friend, who says that he was walking home with the patient when they were both assaulted about 1 hour ago. The patient was hit on the right side of his head with a baseball bat and was unconscious for 1 minute, but then felt normal. He did not want to go to the hospital and wanted to "sleep it off." However, before they got home the patient became less responsive and could no longer walk, so his friend called 911. The friend does not think the patient has any other medical problems or injuries.

Vital signs: Temperature 98.2°F (36.8°C), pulse 50 beats/min, BP 175/98 mm Hg, RR 14 breaths/min.

Additional history: Unknown. Patient's friend denies any alcohol or drug use before the assault.

1. **What is the differential diagnosis?**
   Blunt head trauma and concussion causing: epidural hematoma, subdural hematoma, SAH, intraparenchymal hemorrhage, traumatic brain injury (including coup contrecoup)/diffuse axonal injury.
   Altered mental status from another cause: opioid overdose, alcohol overdose.

2. **What components of the physical examination do you perform?**
   General appearance, skin, HEENT/neck, lungs, cardiovascular, abdomen, extremities, neuro/psych.
   Physical examination:
   General: Lethargic, responds to painful stimuli but not voice. Obvious trauma to the right temporal area of his head. Breathing irregularly.
   HEENT/neck: Depression of the skull over the right temporal bone without any laceration. No posterior auricular hematoma, no hemotympanum. Pupils are 6 mm and reactive bilaterally.
   Lungs: Irregular respirations but lungs clear bilaterally on auscultation.
   Cardiovascular: Bradycardic, otherwise WNL.
   Abdomen: WNL
   Extremities: WNL
   Neuro/psych: Opens eyes to verbal stimuli, localizes pain but does not follow commands, and utters inappropriate words (Glasgow Coma Scale 3-5-3). Moving all extremities equally.

3. **What are your initial orders?**
   IV fluids, pulse oximetry, cardiac monitor. Elevate head of bed. Fingerstick blood glucose. EtOH level. CBC, chem 8, coagulation profile. Immediate noncontrast head CT scan.
   Advance clock:
   Pulse oximetry: 100% O_2 saturation on room air.
   Fingerstick blood glucose: 160 mg/dL.
   CBC, chem 8, coagulation profile WNL.
   Noncontrast head CT scan: Right-sided biconvex density consistent with acute epidural hematoma. Midline shift of 5 mm. Depressed skull fracture of right temporal bone.
   EtOH level: 0 mg/dL.

4. **What are your follow-up actions?**
   Neurosurgery consult, admit to the ICU. Intracranial pressure management including head of bed elevation, hyperosmolar therapy (hypertonic saline or mannitol), tranexamic acid (CRASH-3 trial).
   Advance clock: Case ends.
   Critical actions: This patient has an epidural hematoma, a life-threatening neurosurgical emergency. The condition most commonly occurs as a result of injury to the middle meningeal artery during trauma, leading to bleeding in the potential space between the dura and the skull (above the dura, and hence *epi*dural, vs a venous *sub*dural hematoma with bleeding below the dura). The classic presentation is a patient who has suffered significant head trauma (often with loss of consciousness) followed by an asymptomatic lucid period during which the patient is bleeding but has not developed symptoms. As the bleed progresses, the patient will exhibit a rapid deterioration in consciousness and potentially brain herniation and death. This patient has Cushing triad, a combination of bradycardia, hypertension, and irregular breathing, which indicates increased intracranial pressure and should raise the level of suspicion for an intracranial bleed.
   Discussion: Diagnosis is on the basis of a noncontrast CT scan of the brain showing a lens-shaped bleed that does not cross suture lines (because the dura adheres to the skull at the suture lines, the blood cannot cross). Treatment includes stabilizing the patient (airway, breathing, circulation), correcting any underlying coagulopathy, reducing intracranial pressure if signs of herniation are present, and an emergent neurosurgical consult for craniotomy and hematoma evacuation. Seizure prophylaxis (e.g., levetiracetam) is also commonly given to such patients. The CRASH-3 trial showed a benefit of tranexamic acid, an antifibrinolytic agent, in most patients with traumatic brain injury and should be considered. Note the trial did not find a benefit in severe injury but it is possible that this is because there may be a true benefit but the effect size is lower and could not be detected with their trial size (e.g., a patient with a GCS of 3 is likely to do poorly regardless of intervention, even if a moderately effective intervention exists).
   Diagnosis: Epidural hematoma.

CASE 53

HPI: A 30-year-old man presents to the ED with a headache and lightheadedness that began after he woke up this morning. The headache is described as affecting "the whole head" and is a dull pain that is nonradiating. No visual changes, fever or chills, weakness or numbness. The lightheadedness has been occurring all day, is not positional, and is not associated with vertigo or unsteadiness. The patient reports that he lives with his girlfriend and his brother, both of whom are in the ED with the same symptoms.

Vital signs: Temperature 98.2° F (36.8° C), pulse 80 beats/min, BP 125/78 mm Hg, RR 16 breaths/min.

Additional history: No medical history. Denies use of alcohol, tobacco, or drugs.

1. **What is the differential diagnosis?**
   Carbon monoxide (CO) poisoning, cyanide poisoning, headache (migraine, tension, etc.), sedative overdose, toxin withdrawal (alcohol, caffeine), hypoxemia, meningitis, encephalitis, viral syndrome, intracranial mass, SAH (less likely), cerebral vasculitis (less likely).

2. **What components of the physical examination do you perform?**
   General appearance, HEENT, cardiovascular, lungs, neuro/psych.
   Physical examination:
   General: No apparent distress.
   HEENT: WNL; sclera white, conjunctiva pink, red reflex present, PERRL
   Cardiovascular: No cyanosis, WNL.
   Lungs: WNL
   Neuro/psych: AAOx4. Cranial nerves II through XII intact; motion, sensation, and reflexes normal. No focal neurologic deficits.

3. **What are your initial orders?**
   Pulse oximetry, arterial or venous blood gas with co-oximetry, CBC, chem 8, ECG, EtOH level, Utox.
   Advance clock: Pulse oximetry reveals 100% O_2 saturation on room air, blood gas normal except for a CO level of 20%. CBC, chem 8, ECG, EtOH level, Utox all WNL.

4. **What are your follow-up actions?**
   Oxygen via nonrebreather mask (100%), admit for observation.
   Advance clock: Case ends.
   Critical actions: Recognition of CO toxicity as a cause of headache and dizziness, especially in multiple patients in the same building. Treatment with 100% oxygen.
   Discussion: This patient has CO poisoning. CO is produced when there is incomplete combustion of fuel, such as by gas-powered heaters, barbecues, or any fire. CO binds avidly to Hb and therefore prevents oxygen from binding. Although the oxygen-carrying capacity is diminished, the oxygen saturation as measured by normal pulse oximetry will be normal because pulse oximetry cannot distinguish between the waveforms of CO bound to Hb and oxygen bound to Hb. Symptoms are classically flulike symptoms, headaches, and dizziness. Diagnosis of CO poisoning is on the basis of blood gas analysis demonstrating elevated levels of CO in the blood.
   Treatment is via high-flow oxygen (e.g., a nonrebreather mask) because the half-life of CO is about 4 to 6 hours on room air but decreases to 1 hour on 100% oxygen (and even lower with hyperbaric oxygen therapy). Indications for hyperbaric treatment are controversial but include altered mental status, syncope, pregnancy, CO level greater than 25, and cardiovascular compromise.
   Diagnosis: CO poisoning.

CASE 54

HPI: A 67-year-old woman presents to the ED with shortness of breath. The patient has noticed 1 week of gradually worsening dyspnea. She is now unable to walk at all without becoming short of breath. She has never smoked cigarettes and has no history of asthma.

Vital signs: Temperature 98.8°F (37.1°C), pulse 115 beats/min, BP 90/70 mm Hg, RR 30 breaths/min.

Additional history: Metastatic breast cancer.

1. **What is the differential diagnosis?**
   Pulmonary embolism, CHF, pericardial effusion, cardiac tamponade, pneumothorax, pulmonary metastatic disease, malignant pleural effusion.

2. **What components of the physical examination do you perform?**
   General appearance, HEENT, cardiovascular, lungs, abdomen, extremities (looking for Homan/dorsiflexion sign).
   Physical examination:
   General: Tachypneic.
   HEENT: WNL
   Cardiovascular: Elevated jugular venous pressure (JVP), tachycardia, muffled heart sounds. No friction rub appreciated.

Lungs: Tachypnea but otherwise WNL.
Abdomen: WNL
Extremities: WNL

3. **What are your initial orders?**
Pulse oximetry, BP/cardiac monitoring, CBC, chem 8, coagulation panel, blood typing and screening, troponin, arterial blood gas, ECG, CXR, TTE, IV fluids.
Advance clock:
ECG: Low voltage throughout, alternation of QRS amplitude between beats.
CXR: Enlarged cardiac silhouette.
Transesophageal echocardiography (TEE): Pericardial effusion with tamponade physiology.
CT Chest: No PE.
All other studies WNL
Patient update: The patient's dyspnea worsens and she becomes hypotensive.

4. **What are your follow-up actions?**
Pericardiocentesis (the patient's symptoms improve and vital signs normalize). Cardiothoracic surgery consult. Admit to the ICU; morning ECG, CXR, CBC, chem 8. Counseling.
Advance clock: Case ends.
Critical actions: Cardiac and pulmonary examination, ECG, echocardiogram, pericardiocentesis.
Discussion: This patient has a pericardial effusion with tamponade physiology, probably secondary to her metastatic breast cancer. Other causes of pericardial effusion include aortic dissection, radiation, trauma, and uremic/infectious/autoimmune pericarditis. The patient's chief complaint of shortness of breath has a broad differential, but the physical examination strongly suggests pericardial effusion. Furthermore, the triad of JVD, muffled heart sounds, and hypotension is consistent with tamponade. You may also observe pulsus paradoxus, which is an abnormally large decrease in systolic BP greater than 10 mm Hg, as well as stroke volume pulse wave amplitude, with inspiration. As soon as tamponade is suspected, the patient should be given a large bolus of IV fluids as a temporizing measure. IV fluids can increase the preload and cardiac output, which are compromised because the effusion prevents adequate right atrium filling and subsequent left ventricle contraction. CXR may reveal an enlarged cardiac silhouette, and ECG may reveal electrical alternans. TTE may show diastolic collapse of the RA and/or right ventricle as well as right ventricular dilation with bowing into the left ventricle (25% patients with hemodynamic compromise and very specific to cardiac tamponade). The diagnosis of pericardial effusion should be confirmed with an echocardiogram, and an unstable patient should be treated promptly with pericardiocentesis. A cardiothoracic surgery consult should be requested to consider definitive management with a pericardial window. This intervention is probably necessary in this patient because malignant effusions tend to recur.
    Diagnosis: Cardiac tamponade.

CASE 55

HPI: A 50-year-old woman presents to the clinic complaining of burning epigastric abdominal pain that radiates to the throat. It is worse when she lies flat and improves when she is upright for a prolonged period. It has been occurring daily for several months and is worse after large meals. She reports occasional difficulty in swallowing foods such as steak and bread. She says that these foods sometimes feel stuck in her throat. She denies weight loss, odynophagia, and early satiety. She has never noticed blood in her stool.
Vital signs: Temperature 98.8°F (37.1°C), pulse 72 beats/min, BP 115/75 mm Hg, RR: 16 breaths/min.
Additional history: No medical history. No use of tobacco, alcohol, or drugs.

1. **What is the differential diagnosis?**
GERD, esophageal malignancy, achalasia, peptic ulcer disease, coronary artery disease (CAD).

2. **What components of the physical examination do you perform?**
General appearance, skin, lymph nodes, HEENT, cardiovascular, lungs, abdomen, extremities, neuro/psych.
Physical examination:
General: No acute distress.
Skin/lymph nodes/HEENT: WNL
Cardiovascular: WNL
Lungs: WNL
Abdomen: WNL
Extremities: WNL
Neuro/psych: WNL

3. **What are your initial orders?**
CBC to evaluate for anemia, counseling (including diet and lifestyle modifications), omeprazole PO, referral to GI clinic for upper GI tract endoscopy, consider H. pylori testing, follow-up in primary care clinic in 1 month.

Advance clock:
Endoscopy: WNL. No signs of Barrett esophagus or peptic ulcer disease.
Patient returns to clinic and symptoms have greatly improved.
Case ends.
Critical actions: Abdominal examination, upper GI tract endoscopy, PPI or H_2 blocker.
Discussion: This patient has classic GERD symptoms and a physical examination that is nonconcerning. Red flag GERD symptoms that should be evaluated early in the encounter include new onset of dyspepsia in patient older than 60 years, dysphagia, odynophagia, weight loss, early satiety, iron-deficiency anemia, anorexia, persistent vomiting, and GI cancer in a first-degree relative. It is also imperative to evaluate for other etiologies such as CAD, particularly in female patients, so an ECG and troponin may be considered in patients who also endorse chest pain (this patient appears to have low risk for CAD, but you would not lose points if you ordered one in this case).

Initially, CBC should be evaluated to assess for iron-deficiency anemia due to chronic GI bleeding. All patients with GERD should receive dietary counseling and advice on elevating the head of the bed. Calcium carbonate can be used as needed for occasional symptom relief, but the fact that this patient has daily symptoms indicates the need for an H_2 blocker or a PPI. Either would be a reasonable starting agent in this case. However, if the H_2 blocker does not relieve her symptoms, a change to a PPI would be indicated. This patient's mild dysphagia is reason enough to perform upper GI tract endoscopy to assess for Barrett esophagus and dysplasia. If Barrett esophagus with low-grade dysplasia is present, surveillance endoscopy should initially be performed every 6 months. High-grade dysplasia is treated with esophagectomy or endoscopic ablative therapies. The selection of the modality is beyond the scope of Step 3.
Diagnosis: GERD.

CASE 56

HPI: A 28-year-old woman presents to the ED with acute-onset shortness of breath and a sharp chest pain that is worse when she takes a deep breath. She has had no fever, but does report a mild, nonproductive cough. She takes no medications except for an OCP.
Vital signs: Temperature 99.9°F (37.7°C), pulse 103 beats/min, BP 130/80 mm Hg, RR 31 breaths/min.
Additional history: No tobacco, alcohol, or drug use. Car accident 2 months previously that resulted in a fractured tibia.

1. **What is the differential diagnosis?**
   Pneumonia, pneumothorax, pulmonary embolism, asthma, costochondritis, pericarditis.

2. **What components of the physical examination do you perform?**
   General appearance, HEENT, cardiovascular, lungs, abdomen, extremities.
   Physical examination:
   General: Increased WOB.
   HEENT: WNL
   Cardiovascular: Tachycardic.
   Lungs: Tachypneic, breath sounds normal.
   Abdomen: WNL
   Extremities: WNL

3. **What are your initial orders?**
   Pulse oximetry/oxygen, BP/cardiac monitor, CXR, CBC, chem 8, PT/PTT, arterial blood gas, troponin, ECG, urinary pregnancy test, supplemental O_2, start peripheral IVs.
   Advance clock:
   O_2 saturation: 94% on room air, arterial blood gas shows hypoxia.
   Laboratory and radiologic studies: WNL
   ECG: Sinus tachycardia

4. **What are your follow-up actions?**
   Chest CT-angiogram, lower extremity ultrasound.
   Advance clock:
   Chest CT-angiogram chest: Pulmonary embolism on the left.
   Lower extremity ultrasound: Common femoral vein DVT.
   Troponin undetectable

5. **What are your follow-up actions?**
   Stop the OCP (okay to start nonhormonal birth control); start anticoagulation (e.g., LMWH, unfractionated heparin [UFH] drip, or rivaroxaban). Admit to ward. Can discharge home on oral agent when the patient has stable vital signs on room air, and pain is controlled. Follow-up after 1 week. Counseling.
   Case ends.

Critical actions: Pulmonary examination, extremity examination, pulse oximetry and/or oxygen, CT-angiogram, anticoagulation such as LMWH, UFH, a DOAC such as rivaroxaban, or warfarin (with LMWH or UFH as a bridging agent).

Discussion: This patient's history alone raises concerns for pulmonary embolism. She should be evaluated using a reliable imaging method. CT-angiography has largely taken the place of ventilation-perfusion scans. A d-dimer test alone would be insufficient to confirm or rule out pulmonary embolism in this high-probability pretest setting. Pulmonary embolisms are subclassed into three categories: (1) low risk (hemodynamically stable, no end-organ damage), (2) intermediate risk or "submassive" (hemodynamically stable but evidence of right heart strain on cardiac echo or positive cardiac biomarkers such as troponin or B-type natriuretic peptide), and (3) high risk or "massive" (hemodynamically unstable defined as SBP <90 mm Hg for >15 minutes, hypotension requiring vasopressors, or clear evidence of shock). This patient is hemodynamically stable and has a low-risk pulmonary embolism.

For hemodynamically stable patients, treatment includes O_2 supplementation and initiation of anticoagulation. Massive pulmonary embolism may require fluid resuscitation, O_2 supplementation, intubation, and systemic thrombolytic therapy with tPA.

Management of submassive pulmonary embolism is an evolving area of research and unlikely to be tested but may include embolectomy or catheter-directed tPA. A hypercoagulability workup is unlikely to award any extra points in the setting of acute/provoked DVT, but it is not likely that points would be deducted. This patient's therapy should be continued for a minimum of 3 months because she has had a provoked first episode. If you select warfarin as an anticoagulant, INR should be monitored in the outpatient setting. Patients with recurrent pulmonary embolism or persistent risk factors may require lifelong anticoagulation therapy.

Diagnosis: Pulmonary embolism.

CASE 57

HPI: A 51-year-old man arrives by ambulance complaining of three episodes of passage of bright red blood from the rectum. He has no abdominal pain and denies nausea and vomiting. He has previously had a few episodes of a maroon-colored stool but has never passed frank blood. He denies recent weight loss.

Vital signs: Temperature 98.2°F (36.8°C), pulse 92 beats/min, BP 120/75 mm Hg, RR 15 breaths/min.

Additional history: No medical or surgical history.

1. What is the differential diagnosis?
   Lower GI tract bleed: Arteriovenous (AV) malformation, bleeding rectal hemorrhoids, bleeding diverticulosis, colon cancer/polyps, angiodysplasia/AV malformations, anal fissure, colonic ischemia, inflammatory bowel disease (IBD; Crohn disease, ulcerative colitis).
   Brisk upper GI tract bleed: Peptic ulcer disease, varices.

2. What components of the physical examination do you perform?
   General appearance, HEENT, cardiovascular, lungs, abdomen, rectal.
   Physical examination:
   General: Mild pallor.
   HEENT: WNL
   Cardiovascular: WNL
   Lungs: WNL
   Abdomen: WNL
   Rectal: Bright red blood in the rectal vault.

3. What are your initial orders?
   Pulse oximetry, cardiac/BP monitor, CBC, chem 8, LFTs, PT/PTT, blood type and crossmatch, IV normal saline, NPO, GI consult, colonoscopy, admit to inpatient unit.
   Advance clock:
   Hb 8.9 g/dL.
   Colonoscopy reveals bleeding diverticulosis. Hemostasis is achieved with intervention.
   All other studies WNL.

4. What are your follow-up actions?
   CBC every 4 hours (can decrease frequency if stable). Counseling before discharge (including dietary counseling), follow-up in 1 week.
   Advance clock: Case ends.
   Critical actions: CBC. Transfuse pRBCs if Hb is below 7 g/dL. Abdominal examination, rectal examination, GI consult, colonoscopy.
   Discussion: This patient has hematochezia, defined as the passage of fresh (commonly red) blood through the anus. This is typically suggestive of a lower GI tract bleed, anatomically defined as bleeding distal to the ligament of Treitz, or a brisk upper GI tract bleed. The vast majority of lower GI tract bleeds localize to the colon, and the small intestine is a rare source of bleeding.

Presenting symptoms for slow lower GI tract bleeds may be microcytic anemia with occult blood. Bright red blood passed through the rectum corresponds to a high degree of suspicion for a lower GI tract source; however, brisk upper GI tract bleeds may also cause frankly bloody stools. In the United States, diverticular bleeding is the most common cause of lower GI tract bleeding. Diverticula tend to occur around the vasa recta, where the penetrating blood vessels create local areas of weakness. The associated vasa recta are then protected only by the overlying mucosa and are at risk of bleeding.

The first step in assessing an acute GI bleed is to stabilize the patient. This patient's stable vital signs indicate that he does not need aggressive resuscitation or transfusion, but he should be monitored closely. If he is tachycardic or hypotensive, you should have more concern that he has lost significant blood and may be bleeding rapidly. Transfusion strategies vary widely but almost always include transfusion for Hb of less than 7 g/dL or hemodynamic instability. Although most lower GI tract bleeds resolve spontaneously, they should be evaluated with colonoscopy for diagnostic and therapeutic purposes. Treatment strategies for actively bleeding sites include mechanical clips, injection of epinephrine, and bipolar coagulation. Upper GI tract endoscopy would be indicated if colonoscopy were negative to evaluate for a brisk upper GI tract bleed.

Almost all upper GI bleeds are managed as an inpatient (except Mallory-Weiss tears). Many lower GI bleeds, however, can be managed as an outpatient. Patients with stable vital signs, mild bleeding, no significant anemia, no significant comorbidities, and no anticoagulation can be discharged home with plans for outpatient colonoscopy. This patient has significant anemia so requires admission. Once bleeding is controlled, the patient can be monitored and eventually discharged home with counseling and close follow-up with his primary care physician as well as GI referral.

Diagnosis: Bleeding diverticulosis.

CASE 58

HPI: A 42-year-old man is brought by ambulance to the ED. He was observed sitting at a bus stop when he suddenly slumped over, fell to the ground, and had total body convulsions. These convulsions stopped spontaneously, and he was brought directly to the ED.

Vital signs: Temperature 98.6°F (37.0°C), pulse 110 beats/min, BP 145/90 mm Hg, RR 19 breaths/min.

Additional history: Patient is unable to provide additional history.

1. **What is the differential diagnosis?**
   Seizure from: Hypoglycemia, underlying primary generalized epilepsy, alcohol withdrawal, hyponatremia, encephalitis/meningitis, brain lesions (rare), head trauma, eclampsia (in pregnant/postpartum females).
   Seizure mimic: convulsive syncope, psychogenic nonepileptic seizure.

2. **What components of the physical examination do you perform?**
   General appearance, HEENT, cardiovascular, lungs. abdomen, neuro/psych.
   Physical examination:
   General: Disheveled appearance, smells of alcohol.
   HEENT: Soft tissue swelling of the scalp over the parietal region.
   Cardiovascular: Tachycardic.
   Lungs: WNL
   Abdomen: WNL
   Neuro/psych: Postictal, alert and oriented to person and place but not time, follows commands, eyes open, tremor of hands and tongue, no focal neurologic deficits.

3. **What are your initial orders?**
   Fingerstick blood glucose, pulse oximetry, IV normal saline, BP/cardiac monitor, IV diazepam (or alternative benzodiazepine), CBC, chem 8, LFTs, serum EtOH level, lipase, urine toxicology, noncontrast head CT scan.
   Advance clock:
   Hb 10.2 g/dL, MCV 107 fL, other studies WNL.
   Tremor improves, heart rate 90 beats/min.
   CT head: No brain lesions, epidural/subdural/parenchymal hemorrhages

4. **What are your follow-up actions?**
   Multivitamin, thiamine, folate, IV/PO benzodiazepine PRN, admit to inpatient unit, vital signs every 4 hours, continuous pulse oximetry, CBC and chem 8 in the morning, social work consult, addiction unit consult, counseling (including alcohol cessation).
   Advance clock: Case ends.
   Critical actions: Glucose level, benzodiazepine (e.g., diazepam, chlordiazepoxide), counseling, thiamine.
   Discussion: An undifferentiated patient with new onset seizures should trigger a broad initial workup, especially because the medical history is often limited. Rapid assessment for hypoglycemia, hyponatremia, pregnancy, and mass/traumatic brain injury (with CT head) can help narrow the differential and guide management. This patient has symptoms suggestive of alcohol withdrawal given his odor of alcohol and macrocytic anemia.

Presenting symptoms for alcohol withdrawal can include agitation, visual hallucinations, delirium tremens (delirium with unstable vital signs), and seizures. The mainstay of alcohol withdrawal treatment is benzodiaze-pines. Mild withdrawal can be treated on an outpatient basis; however, patients with first-time seizures, delirium tremens, or symptoms requiring large doses of benzodiazepines should be admitted to the hospital. It is prudent to give thiamine before administering any glucose because of the theoretic concern of precipitating thiamine de-pletion and Wernicke encephalopathy. Many clinicians also provide folic acid and a multivitamin containing thia-mine since nutritional deficiencies are common in patients with chronic and severe alcohol abuse. Counseling on alcohol cessation should be given to all patients.

Diagnosis: Alcohol withdrawal seizure.

CASE 59

HPI: A 36-year-old woman presents to clinic complaining of several months of joint pain. She has noticed pain in her hands, wrists, elbows, and knees bilaterally that seems to move from joint to joint. During this time, she has had an in-creasing feeling of fatigue and finds it difficult to get out of bed some days. She has also noticed a rash that appears over her face when her symptoms are at their worst. Her symptoms seem to worsen when she is exposed to the sun.

Vital signs: Temperature 99.3°F (37.4°C), pulse 85 beats/min, BP 120/74 mm Hg, RR 18 breaths/min.

Additional history: No medical history. No use of tobacco, drugs, or alcohol. No medications.

1. **What is the differential diagnosis?**
   Systemic lupus erythematosus (SLE), rheumatoid arthritis (RA), Lyme disease, fibromyalgia, OA, depression, dermato-myositis, viral arthritis (parvovirus B19, chikungunya), psoriatic arthritis.

2. **What components of the physical examination do you perform?**
   General appearance, skin, lymph nodes, HEENT, cardiovascular, lungs, abdomen, extremities, neuro/psych.
   Physical examination:
   General: No acute distress.
   Skin/lymph nodes/HEENT: Erythematous rash over the cheeks sparing the nasolabial folds. Painless oral ulcerations.
   Cardiovascular: WNL
   Lungs: WNL
   Abdomen: WNL
   Extremities: Tenderness to palpation over the hand, wrist, and elbow joints. Mild effusion in the knees bilaterally.
   Neuro/psych: WNL

3. **What are your initial orders?**
   Pulse oximetry, CBC, chem 14, PT/PTT, ESR, CRP, ANA, complement screen, UA, rheumatoid factor (RF), x-ray of affected joints, ibuprofen PO (or other NSAID), beta-hCG pregnancy test.
   Advance clock: ESR/CRP elevated, ANA positive, C3/C4 low, other studies WNL. Minimal symptom improvement with NSAIDs.

4. **What are your follow-up actions?**
   Anti-dsDNA (positive), rheumatology consult/referral, prednisone PO, hydroxychloroquine PO, counseling, physical therapy, occupational therapy, follow-up in 4 weeks.
   Advance clock: Case ends.
   Critical actions: Extremities examination, analgesia (NSAID), ANA test, rheumatology consult.
   Discussion: This patient has a migratory symmetric polyarthritis with malar rash, photosensitivity, and oral ulcers suggestive of SLE. The diagnosis of SLE is based on at least 4 of 11 criteria remembered by the mnemonic SOAP BRAIN MD: *s*erositis, *o*ral ulcerations, *a*rthritis, *p*hotosensitivity, *b*lood disorders, *r*enal involvement, *A*NA positive, *i*mmunologic abnormalities, *n*eurologic disease, *m*alar rash, *d*iscoid rash.

   ANA is a fairly sensitive test in screening for SLE, and anti-dsDNA is highly specific. ESR, CRP, and comple-ment levels are nonspecific markers for inflammation but may suggest an active flare of an autoimmune process or an active infection. Once the diagnosis of SLE is suspected, consultation with a rheumatologist is warranted. Other tests such as antiphospholipid, anti-SSA/SSB, antihistone, anti-Smith, and antiribonucleoprotein antibodies may be ordered; however, for testing purposes a rheumatology consult will be sufficient. Most patients will benefit from NSAIDs for analgesia (if renal function is normal)

   Hydroxychloroquine is an immunomodulatory agent that is first-line therapy for symptom management and prevention of lupus flares. When symptoms are not controlled with NSAIDs and hydroxychloroquine alone, corticoste-roids can provide a significant improvement. Given their side effect profile, they should be used at the lowest effec-tive dose for the shortest possible duration. Other immunosuppressants (e.g., methotrexate) or immunomodulatory agents (e.g., rituximab) may be indicated in patients with severe or refractory symptoms. Patients should be regularly monitored by a rheumatologist for symptom control, progression of disease, and systemic complications, typically ev-ery 3 to 4 months if well controlled and at least every 6 months. A nephrology consult may be indicated for patients with renal involvement. Patients on long-term corticosteroids should be monitored for associated complications.

   Diagnosis: SLE.

CASE 60

HPI: A 45-year-old woman presents to the ED. She has had 24 hours of gradually worsening abdominal pain in the right upper quadrant. She has had seven episodes of vomiting and feels like she has a fever.
Vital signs: Temperature 100.8°F (38.2°C), pulse 105 beats/min, BP 156/98 mm Hg, RR 14 breaths/min.
Additional history: Hyperlipidemia, on atorvastatin. No other medical history.

1. **What is the differential diagnosis?**
   Acute cholecystitis, cholangitis, pancreatitis, symptomatic cholelithiasis.

2. **What components of the physical examination do you perform?**
   General appearance, HEENT, cardiovascular, lungs, abdomen.
   Physical examination:
   General: Moderate distress secondary to pain.
   HEENT: Dry cracked lips.
   Cardiovascular: Tachycardia, otherwise WNL.
   Lungs: WNL
   Abdomen: Obese abdomen; soft, severe tenderness to right upper quadrant with voluntary guarding; positive Murphy sign, no rebound.

3. **What are your initial orders?**
   Pulse oximetry, BP/cardiac monitor, urinary pregnancy test, UA, urine culture, CBC, chem 8, LFTs, lipase, blood cultures, gallbladder ultrasound, IV fluids, morphine, ondansetron, acetaminophen.
   Advance clock:
   WBC: Elevated with left shift.
   Gallbladder ultrasound: Gallstones, thickened gallbladder wall, pericholecystic fluid, normal common bile duct, positive sonographic Murphy sign. Other studies WNL.
   The patient's symptoms are moderately improved.

4. **What are your follow-up actions?**
   PT/PTT, blood type and screen, NPO, IV antibiotics to cover gram negative bacteria and anaerobic bacteria (e.g., ceftriaxone and metronidazole), surgery consult for laparoscopic cholecystectomy, admit to inpatient unit. Check vital signs every 4 hours, CBC and chem 8 next day. Counseling before discharge.
   Advance clock: Case ends.
   Critical actions: Gallbladder ultrasound, IV fluids, morphine, ondansetron, antibiotics, surgery consult, laparoscopic cholecystectomy.
   Discussion: Acute-onset abdominal pain in the right upper quadrant should warrant evaluation for hepatobiliary pathology, including cholecystitis, cholangitis, and pancreatitis. Acute pancreatitis can be excluded if a lipase test is normal. The classic presentation of cholangitis is the Charcot triad: fever, right upper quadrant abdominal pain, and jaundice. In cholangitis, LFTs will reveal elevated bilirubin and (usually) alkaline phosphatase. Cholecystitis can be diagnosed according to the combination of historical features, physical examination, laboratory values, and ultrasound.
   Acute cholecystitis is an inflammatory process of the gallbladder usually secondary to stasis arising from a stone lodged in the cystic duct. Acalculous cholecystitis may occur in critically ill patients. Acute cholecystitis is further categorized as complicated if there is evidence of gallbladder gangrene/necrosis, perforation, or emphysematous cholecystitis. Once the diagnosis is established, patients should be given IV fluid and made NPO. *E. coli* is the most common bacterial source, but gram-positive, gram-negative, anaerobic, and aerobic organisms are all possible causes. Broad-spectrum antibiotics such as ceftriaxone and metronidazole are therefore indicated. Early cholecystectomy is generally the preferred approach because prompt surgical intervention decreases hospital readmission rates and mortality. Complicated cholecystitis warrants emergent rather than urgent surgical intervention. Ascending cholangitis is treated with IV fluids, hospital admission, metronidazole/cefepime (or other broad-spectrum combination for gram-negative, gram-positive, and anaerobic bacteria), and endoscopic retrograde cholangiopancreatography to remove the offending gallstone. If the patient had symptomatic cholelithiasis without cholecystitis, the treatment would include control of symptoms (analgesia and antiemetics) and elective surgery.
   Diagnosis: Uncomplicated acute cholecystitis.

CASE 61

HPI: An 18-year-old woman presents to the ED. She has had 12 hours of gradually worsening abdominal pain in the right lower quadrant. She has vomited many times and has been unable to eat or drink anything since the pain started. She has never had similar pain before this event.
Vital signs: Temperature 101.3°F (38.5°C), pulse 115 beats/min, BP 118/78 mm Hg, RR 23 breaths/min.
Additional history: Sexually active with one male partner. No other medical history.

1. **What is the differential diagnosis?**
   Acute appendicitis, PID, tuboovarian abscess, ectopic pregnancy, ovarian torsion, ovarian cyst rupture, nephrolithiasis, pyelonephritis.

2. **What components of the physical examination do you perform?**
   General appearance, HEENT, cardiovascular, lungs, abdomen, pelvis/genitalia.
   Physical examination:
   General: Moderate distress secondary to pain.
   HEENT: WNL
   Cardiovascular: Tachycardia, otherwise WNL.
   Lungs: Tachypnea, otherwise WNL.
   Abdomen: Soft, severe tenderness to right lower quadrant with voluntary guarding, no rebound.
   Back: No CVA tenderness to percussion
   Genitourinary: No cervical motion tenderness or discharge. No adnexal tenderness.

3. **What are your initial orders?**
   Pulse oximetry, cardiac/BP monitoring, urinary pregnancy test, UA, urine culture, CBC, chem 8, LFTs, lipase, blood cultures, wet mount, gonorrhea/*Chlamydia*, CT of the abdomen/pelvis or ultrasound of the lower abdomen, IV fluids, morphine, ondansetron, acetaminophen.
   Advance clock:
   WBC count elevated with neutrophilic predominance shift.
   Ultrasound: Noncompressible, dilated appendix. Periappendiceal fluid collection. No pelvic pathology.
   CT: Acute appendicitis with trace periappendiceal fluid but no abscess or free perforation.
   Other studies WNL.
   The patient feels a moderate improvement in her pain and is no longer nauseated.

4. **What are your follow-up actions?**
   Coagulation panel, blood type and screen, NPO, IV antibiotics (e.g., cefoxitin or a combination of ceftriaxone and metronidazole), surgery consult, appendectomy, admit to inpatient unit, monitor vital signs every 4 hours, CBC and chem 8 next day. Counseling before discharge.
   Advance clock: Case ends.
   Critical actions: Abdominal examination, beta-hCG pregnancy test, pelvic ultrasound, pelvic examination, IV fluids, antibiotics, appendectomy.
   Discussion: Appendicitis is caused by appendiceal obstruction and subsequent inflammation. In adults this is usually caused by a fecalith, whereas in children it is usually caused by lymphoid hyperplasia from a preceding viral illness. This patient's history and physical examination are classic for appendicitis; however, in women of reproductive age, pregnancy must be excluded and ovarian/pelvic pathology must be considered. A thorough history and physical examination by an experienced clinician may be adequate to diagnose appendicitis in the context of a classic presentation. Advanced imaging is necessary, however, in equivocal cases. In this patient, ultrasound has the benefit of assessing the pelvic organs and can diagnose appendicitis mimics such as tuboovarian abscesses and ovarian torsion. Although ultrasound is specific for appendicitis, it is insensitive, especially in overweight patients. A CT scan is both sensitive and specific but is not as good at evaluating for pelvic pathology. A CT scan also has the disadvantage of radiation exposure. MRI is both sensitive and specific, but its availability is limited, and it generally takes longer.
   Once a diagnosis of appendicitis is made, the patient should proceed to surgery as soon as possible for an urgent appendectomy (evolving evidence shows antibiotic therapy only may be appropriate but has a high recurrence rate of appendicitis and is unlikely to be tested at this time). IV fluids are indicated for all septic patients. Antibiotics should be given preoperatively to cover aerobic and anaerobic gram-negative organisms. For simple appendicitis, cefoxitin, metronidazole/ceftriaxone, or ampicillin-sulbactam is often used. Symptom control should also be achieved with antipyretics (e.g., acetaminophen), IV analgesia, and antiemetics (e.g., morphine and ondansetron).
   In cases of a contained perforated appendix (in which an abscess forms around the perforated appendix to "wall off" the infection from surrounding bowel), patients are often treated with a period of bowel rest and IV antibiotics (e.g., ceftriaxone and metronidazole). They may require percutaneous drainage of infected material and/or delayed appendectomy. Patients with a noncontained perforation are often quite ill with an acute abdomen on physical examination. They require immediate surgical management.
   Diagnosis: Acute appendicitis.

CASE 62

HPI: A 68-year-old man is brought by ambulance to the ED. Over the past several days he has been gradually getting more short of breath. Previously he could walk a block without feeling winded, but now he feels out of breath while sitting.

Vital signs: Temperature 97.7°F (36.5°C), pulse 110 beats/min, BP 195/98 mm Hg, RR: 35 breaths/min.
Additional history: Hypertension, high cholesterol, previous MI. On hydrochlorothiazide and simvastatin.

1. What is the differential diagnosis?
   CHF exacerbation, COPD exacerbation, pneumonia, pulmonary embolism, pneumothorax, pericardial effusion, anemia.

2. What components of the physical examination do you perform?
   General appearance, HEENT, cardiovascular, lungs, abdomen, extremities.
   Physical examination:
   General: Sitting upright in bed, increased WOB.
   HEENT: WNL
   Cardiovascular: JVP 10 cm, tachycardic with a regular rhythm, loud S3, displaced point of maximal impulse.
   Lungs: Crackles in bilateral lower and middle lung fields.
   Abdomen: WNL
   Extremities: Bilateral pitting edema 2+ to the knees.

3. What are your initial orders?
   Pulse oximetry, BP/cardiac monitor, CBC, chem 8, ECG, troponin, CXR, BNP, furosemide IV, nitroglycerin.
   Advance clock:
   O_2 saturation: 94% on room air.
   ECG: Sinus tachycardia, Q waves in leads II, III, aV$_f$.
   CXR: Cephalization, alveolar edema, perihilar fullness, and septal lines.
   BNP: 2543 pg/mL
   The patient is still mildly short of breath but feels better.

4. What are your follow-up actions?
   Admit to inpatient unit, continuous monitoring, DVT prophylaxis, cardiology consult. Check vital signs every 4 hours, low-sodium diet, troponin every 8 hours. CBC and chem 8 in morning, TTE (reveals left ventricular ejection fraction [EF] of 40%). Aspirin, ACE inhibitor (lisinopril PO), beta-blocker, spironolactone, statin, counseling (including medication compliance, nutrition), cardiac rehabilitation, follow-up in 1 week.
   Advance clock: Case ends.
   Critical actions: Furosemide, TTE (or measure of left ventricular function), ACE inhibitor, beta-blocker, aspirin, counseling on diet and medication.
   Discussion: This patient has newly diagnosed acute decompensated heart failure. The immediate symptoms can be treated by reducing cardiac preload with nitroglycerin and furosemide. Newly diagnosed CHF warrants initiation of aspirin therapy and an ACE inhibitor. EF should be measured, usually via TTE. A beta-blocker, usually carvedilol, should be initiated for EF of 40% or less (but this patient requires a beta-blocker regardless of EF because of his history of MI). Goal-directed therapy also includes initiation of a statin. Cardiology should be consulted to evaluate for the etiology of his CHF. In his case, ischemic coronary disease is probable given the Q waves seen in the inferior leads, and he may need an outpatient cardiac catheterization to evaluate for coronary plaques. Other etiologies include dysrhythmia, new valvular disease, and anemia.
   Counseling should be part of every case but is particularly important in CHF: Patients should be advised to eat a low-sodium diet, weigh themselves daily (and alert their clinician if their weight increases significantly over a short period of time), and maintain adherence to their complex medication regimen. An implantable cardiac defibrillator is indicated for prevention of sudden cardiac death in patients with EF of less than 35% despite optimal medical therapy or history of a serious dysrhythmia (ventricular fibrillation/tachycardia) and/or cardiac arrest.
   The initial treatment strategy for acute decompensated heart failure can be remembered by the mnemonic UNLOAD ME: *u*pright position, *n*itroglycerin, *l*evophed (norepinephrine; if in cardiogenic shock), *o*xygen with noninvasive positive pressure ventilation (NIPPV), *A*CE inhibitors, *d*iuresis (furosemide), *m*echanical ventilation (if NIPPV does not work), and *e*lectricity (cardioversion if dysrhythmia is the cause of the decompensation).
   Diagnosis: Acute decompensated CHF.

CASE 63

HPI: A 42-year-old man presents to the ED with chest pain. The patient has noticed 1 day of gradually worsening retrosternal chest pain. It has been constant, sharp, and worse when breathing deeply or lying flat.
Vital signs: Temperature 100.0°F (37.8°C), pulse 88 beats/min, BP 110/75 mm Hg, RR 14 breaths/min.
Additional history: 10–pack-year smoker. Drinks three beers a week.

1. What is the differential diagnosis?
   Acute coronary syndrome (ACS), pulmonary embolism, pericarditis (with or without myocarditis), pneumothorax, pneumonia, aortic dissection.

2. What components of the physical examination do you perform?
   General appearance, HEENT, cardiovascular, lungs, abdomen, extremities.

Physical examination:
General: Nothing abnormal detected.
HEENT: WNL
Cardiovascular: Regular rate and rhythm. Normal S1, S2. High-pitched rub.
Lungs: WNL
Abdomen: WNL
Extremities: WNL

3. What are your initial orders?
Pulse oximetry, BP/cardiac monitoring, CBC, chem 8, PT/PTT, ECG, troponin every 8 hours, CXR, ESR, CRP.
Advance clock:
ECG: ST-segment elevations diffusely across all leads. PR-segment depression.
ESR and CRP elevated.
Other studies WNL.

4. What are your follow-up actions?
Administer NSAID (e.g., ibuprofen), colchicine, omeprazole (optional, due to prolonged NSAID use), TTE to evaluate for pericardial effusion/tamponade. Counseling (including diet and smoking cessation). Discharge home with outpatient follow-up after negative cardiac biomarkers and TTE without evidence of large pericardial effusion or tamponade.
Advance clock: Case ends.
Critical actions: Cardiac and pulmonary examination, ECG, echocardiogram, initiate NSAID.
Discussion: This patient's history and physical examination are suggestive of pericarditis. ECG with diffuse ST-segment elevations and PR depression confirms this diagnosis. In more equivocal cases elevation in inflammatory markers (ESR, CRP, WBCs) can support the diagnosis.
   The treatment of choice for pericarditis is an NSAID such as ibuprofen. A PPI should also be considered for GI protection given the large dose of NSAIDs necessary. Colchicine has also been shown to improve symptoms and decrease recurrence. An echocardiogram can rule out a large or complex pericardial effusion that may necessitate pericardiocentesis. Anticoagulation therapy should be avoided given the possibility of bleeding into a pericardial effusion. An afebrile immunocompetent patient without a large pericardial effusion can usually be safely discharged home. In the USMLE, however, a more conservative approach is rarely penalized. Thus admission with serial troponin measurements to rule out ACS and perimyocarditis (in which the inflammation extends into the myocardium) is also a reasonable disposition.
   Diagnosis: Pericarditis.

CASE 64

HPI: A 65-year-old woman presents to the ED with shortness of breath and a cough productive of thick sputum. The symptoms were gradual in onset. She has smoked 1 pack of cigarettes daily for 50 years. About twice yearly she has episodes such as this one that require her to go to the ED.
Vital signs: Temperature 100.0°F (37.8°C), pulse 90 beats/min, BP 135/85 mm Hg, RR 29 breaths/min.
Additional history: No other medical history. No alcohol or drug use.

1. What is the differential diagnosis?
COPD exacerbation, asthma exacerbation, pneumonia, bronchitis, bronchiectasis, CHF exacerbation, pulmonary embolism, ACS.

2. What components of the physical examination do you perform?
General appearance, HEENT, cardiovascular, lungs, abdomen, extremities.
Physical examination:
General: Moderately increased WOB.
HEENT: WNL
Cardiovascular: WNL
Lungs: Tachypneic, diffuse wheezing, hyperresonance, coarse crackles.
Abdomen: WNL
Extremities: WNL

3. What are your initial orders?
Pulse oximetry, BP/cardiac monitor, CXR, albuterol, ipratropium.
Advance clock:
O_2 saturation: 94% on room air.
Venous blood gas: 7.33/40/60/22
The patient's symptoms are improved. CXR reveals a flattened diaphragm and hyperlucent lung fields.

4. **What are your follow-up actions?**
Repeat pulmonary examination (decreased wheezing, improved air movement, no increased WOB). Steroids (prednisone), antibiotics (azithromycin), counseling (including smoking cessation), follow-up in 1 week.
Advance clock: Case ends.
Critical actions: Lung examination, albuterol, ipratropium, steroids, smoking cessation counseling.
Discussion: This patient's acute episode of shortness of breath, cough, sputum production, and significant smoking history is consistent with COPD, especially given the history of several prior exacerbations.

COPD is characterized by airway inflammation with partially reversible bronchospasm (chronic bronchitis) and pulmonary parenchymal destruction (emphysema). The GOLD definition of a COPD exacerbation is two of three criteria: (1) increased dyspnea, (2) increased sputum production, and (3) increased sputum purulence. This patient is having an acute COPD exacerbation that is responsive to initial medical management. Treatment for COPD exacerbation includes inhaled albuterol/ipratropium (Duoneb; to address bronchospasm) and a steroid course (typically prednisone or dexamethasone) to address inflammation. Because the patient has dyspnea, increased sputum production, and sputum purulence, she is a good candidate for antibiotic therapy. Azithromycin is a common outpatient choice, although more intensive gram-positive coverage with a second- or third-generation cephalosporin in addition to a macrolide is also appropriate. Because the patient greatly improved on albuterol and ipratropium, she is a good candidate for discharge and close follow-up. If the case continued, you could consider outpatient pulmonary function tests, pneumococcal vaccine, and influenza vaccine. Long-term management of poorly controlled symptoms may also include long-acting bronchodilators (a beta-agonist such as salmeterol [always given with an inhaled corticosteroid] or an anticholinergic agent such as tiotropium), inhaled corticosteroids, supplemental oxygen (if chronic hypoxia is present), and pulmonary rehabilitation.
Diagnosis: COPD exacerbation.

CASE 65

HPI: A 76-year-old man is brought by ambulance to the ED because of chest pain and back pain. Thirty minutes before arrival he was watching television when he experienced 9/10 tearing retrosternal chest pain that radiated to his back. The pain has been constant ever since.
Vital signs: Temperature 98.6°F (37.0°C), pulse 110 beats/min, BP 195/65 mm Hg, RR 20 breaths/min.
Additional history: Hypertension, ran out of medications.

1. **What is the differential diagnosis?**
Aortic dissection, ACS, pulmonary embolism, pneumothorax, pericarditis, esophageal rupture.

2. **What components of the physical examination do you perform?**
General appearance, HEENT, cardiovascular, lungs, extremities.
Physical examination:
General: Visible discomfort from chest pain.
HEENT: WNL
Cardiovascular: Tachycardia.
Lungs: WNL
Extremities: WNL

3. **What are your initial orders?**
Pulse oximetry, BP/cardiac monitoring, CBC, chem 8, coagulation panel, ECG, troponin, blood type and screen, CXR, analgesia (e.g., morphine). When stable, CT aorta angiogram with contrast (TEE can be considered if hemodynamically unstable).
Advance clock:
CXR: Widened mediastinum.
CT scan: Ascending aortic dissection.
Follow-up: The patient's symptoms are improved. BP 135/70 mm Hg.

4. **What are your follow-up actions?**
Esmolol drip IV, surgery consult, surgical repair of aortic dissection, admit to ICU, continuous monitoring, check vital signs every 2 hours, additional BP control if needed (e.g., nicardipine), CBC, chem 8 in the morning, counseling.
Advance clock: Case ends.
Critical actions: Cardiovascular examination, chest CT scan or TEE, IV beta-blocker (esmolol or labetalol), IV analgesia (e.g., morphine), surgical consult.
Discussion: This patient has a history and physical examination suggestive of aortic dissection. Classically, pain from aortic dissection is sharp or tearing in quality, may radiate to the back, and may be associated with unequal pulses (or unequal BPs). A widened mediastinum on CXR may also suggest the diagnosis. To confirm the diagnosis, you should obtain a CT angiogram (if the patient is stable) or TEE if the patient is unstable. The presence of an ascending aortic dissection (type A) is a surgical emergency. You should stabilize the patient with IV beta-blockers

and immediately ask for a thoracic surgery consult. An esmolol drip (or other beta-blocker) is the medication of choice to control BP and heart rate with a systolic BP goal of 100 to 120 mm Hg and a heart rate of 60 beats/min or lower. If the patient requires further antihypertensive therapy after high-dose beta-blockers, nitroprusside or nicardipine administration can be initiated. It is important not to start those medications first, however, because reflex tachycardia from the afterload reduction can increase wall stress and make the dissection worse.

Unlike BP reduction strategies in most situations, systolic BP can and should be reduced to 100 to 120 mm Hg regardless of the initial BP (recall that in most cases of elevated BP, the mean arterial pressure should not be reduced acutely by more than 25% because of the risk of decreased cerebral perfusion). Aortic dissection can be complicated by cardiac tamponade (if the dissection extends into the pericardium), MI (if the dissection extends into the coronary arteries, usually the right coronary artery), aortic regurgitation, stroke (carotid artery extension), or limb ischemia.

Aggressive analgesia (morphine) should be used to control pain itself and prevent the contribution of severe pain to hypertension/tachycardia. Uncomplicated descending dissections are treated similarly, but they are not surgical emergencies. Nonetheless surgical or endovascular repair should be considered in consultation with a cardiothoracic (thoracic aorta) or vascular surgeon (abdominal aorta).

Diagnosis: Aortic dissection.

CASE 66

HPI: A 23-year-old woman presents to the clinic complaining of heavy vaginal bleeding. She has had irregular periods over the past 10 months, many of which were heavier than usual or lasted longer than usual. She occasionally has intermenstrual bleeding. She takes no medications. She is sexually active with one partner and uses condoms. She does not desire immediate fertility.

Vital signs: Temperature 97.2°F (36.2°C), pulse 92 beats/min, BP 135/78 mm Hg, RR 17 breaths/min.

Additional history: No medical history. No use of tobacco, drugs, or alcohol.

1. What is the differential diagnosis?
   AUB, polycystic ovary syndrome (PCOS), endometriosis, uterine fibroid, endometrial polyp, pregnancy (with possible pathology such as threatened abortion), coagulopathy (ITP, von Willebrand disease, hemophilia, etc.).

2. What components of the physical examination do you perform?
   General appearance, skin, lymph nodes, HEENT, cardiovascular, lungs, abdomen, genitalia, MSK/extremities, neuro/psych.
   Physical examination:
   General: No acute distress.
   Skin: Acne.
   HEENT: Mild hirsutism.
   Lymph nodes: WNL
   Cardiovascular: WNL
   Lungs: WNL
   Abdomen: Obese abdomen, soft, nontender.
   Genitalia: WNL
   MSK/Extremities: WNL
   Neuro/psych: WNL

3. What are your initial orders?
   Pulse oximetry, urinary pregnancy test, CBC, chem 8, PT/PTT, serum testosterone, DHEAS, luteinizing hormone (LH), follicle-stimulating hormone (FSH), TSH, 17-hydroxyprogesterone, prolactin, fasting lipid panel, HbA$_{1c}$, pelvic ultrasound.
   Advance clock: Urinary pregnancy test negative, testosterone elevated, elevated LH/FSH ratio, ultrasound reveals polycystic ovaries. Other studies WNL.

4. What are your follow-up actions?
   Counseling (including diet, weight loss, exercise), OCP, follow up in 8 weeks.
   Advance clock: The patient's symptoms are greatly improved.
   Critical actions: Assessment of anemia (CBC), hyperandrogenism (physical examination and/or serum testosterone), OCP (if patient does not desire fertility), counseling (including weight loss).
   Discussion: AUB is menstrual bleeding of abnormal quantity, duration, or schedule. The most common etiologies are structural uterine pathology (e.g., fibroids, endometrial polyps, adenomyosis), but it is also critical to consider ovulatory dysfunction, disorders of hemostasis, and cancers as potential differential diagnoses. This patient is young, making structural and hematologic etiologies more likely than cancer, though this is also possible. After determining the patient's stability, the first consideration is whether the patient is pregnant. Vaginal bleeding in early pregnancy carries a very different differential (e.g., threatened or inevitable abortion, retained products of conception, ectopic pregnancy). In this patient's case, she is not pregnant, and the symptoms of hirsutism and obesity make PCOS a more likely etiology.

PCOS in adults is diagnosed according to the presence of two of the three Rotterdam criteria: (1) oligo/anovulation, (2) hyperandrogenism, and (3) polycystic ovaries. Oligo/anovulation manifests as irregular menses. Hyperandrogenism may manifest as hirsutism, acne, virilization, or deepening of the voice. A serum testosterone level can confirm the presence of hyperandrogenism. Polycystic ovaries are diagnosed using ultrasound.

The patient should be evaluated for other causes of oligomenorrhea such as prolactinoma and hypothyroidism. Recall that elevated prolactin downregulates gonadotropin-releasing hormone, causing amenorrhea. Furthermore, hypothyroidism causes increased TRH, which stimulates prolactin release, in turn causing amenorrhea. Checking TSH and prolactin levels can screen for these conditions. Checking DHEAS assesses whether an androgen-secreting tumor is the cause of hirsutism. You should also consider diagnosing and treating common comorbidities of PCOS by checking a lipid panel and HbA$_{1c}$.

Treatment for all patients with PCOS begins with weight loss to attempt to restore normal ovulation and menstruation. For those who do not desire immediate fertility, OCPs can regulate menstruation and reduce hirsutism. An antiandrogen (spironolactone) can be added for persistent hirsutism. Metformin should be added for patients with T2DM.

In patients with PCOS who desire fertility, consultation with a gynecologist is recommended. Treatment includes weight loss, clomiphene (to induce ovulation), and metformin.

Diagnosis: PCOS.

CASE 67

HPI: A 55-year-old male presents to the ED with rapid-onset severe pain in his right knee that started 4 hours ago. The pain is now so severe that he can barely put weight on the knee. The patient also noted some swelling and stiffness of the joint over the past several days. He denies fever, trauma, or recent infection.

Vital signs: Temperature 99.1°F (37.3°C), pulse 90 beats/min, BP 135/75 mm Hg, RR 14 breaths/min.

Additional history: Takes hydrochlorothiazide for hypertension. No use of tobacco or drugs. Drinks three glasses of wine daily.

1. What is the differential diagnosis?
   Septic arthritis, gout, pseudogout, hemarthrosis, OA, meniscal tear.

2. What components of the physical examination do you perform?
   General appearance, skin, HEENT, cardiovascular, lungs, abdomen, extremities, neuro/psych.
   Physical examination:
   General: No acute distress.
   Skin/HEENT: WNL
   Cardiovascular: WNL
   Lungs: WNL
   Abdomen: WNL
   Extremities: Moderate swelling of the right knee. Decreased range of motion and inability to bear weight secondary to pain.
   Neuro/psych: WNL

3. What are your initial orders?
   Knee x-ray, knee arthrocentesis (with Gram stain, culture, cell count with differential, crystal analysis), CBC, chem 8, PT/PTT.
   Advance clock: Knee arthrocentesis: 23,000 WBCs/mL, needle-shaped negatively birefringent crystals, Gram stain negative. Other studies WNL.

4. What are your follow-up actions?
   Naproxen (the patient's symptoms greatly improve), discontinue hydrochlorothiazide, counseling (including diet and alcohol cessation), follow-up in 2 weeks, uric acid level at follow-up.
   Advance clock: Case ends.
   Critical actions: Extremity examination, arthrocentesis, NSAID, discontinue hydrochlorothiazide.
   Discussion: This patient has acute monoarticular arthritis. Septic arthritis should be assumed until proven otherwise, and arthrocentesis should not be delayed. The presence of needle-shaped negatively birefringent crystals, however, is diagnostic of gout. Synovial WBCs may be elevated to a count that can range from 1000 to 50,000 cells/mL in inflammatory conditions, whereas WBC counts greater than 50,000 cells/mL are suggestive of septic arthritis. The patient's use of hydrochlorothiazide should also make us suspicious of a gout flare because thiazides lead to hyperuricemia by decreasing the clearance of uric acid.

   Gout is caused by an inflammatory response to monosodium urate crystals in the joint space. Ninety percent of cases involve the first metatarsophalangeal joint, but any joint may be affected. Ninety percent of cases are also caused by underexcretion of uric acid (e.g., use of thiazide medications), and 10% are caused by overproduction of uric acid (Lesch-Nyhan syndrome, phosphoribosyl pyrophosphate excess, tumor lysis syndrome, von Gierke disease).

NSAIDs are the first-line treatment modality for acute episodes of gout. Oral colchicine and steroids are second- and third-line agents, respectively, but are often avoided because of their side effect profiles. They can be used in patients who cannot tolerate NSAIDs or who have insufficient relief of symptoms. Thiazide diuretics should be discontinued because they decrease the renal clearance of uric acid. Patients should also be counseled on dietary triggers. A uric acid level can be checked 2 weeks after the episode (because it may be falsely low during the acute event). Patients with elevated uric acid and repeated attacks may take a urate-lowering drug such as allopurinol. Allopurinol therapy is not typically started during an acute flare (although evidence suggests this is probably fine, for test purposes do not start allopurinol immediately).

Diagnosis: Gout.

CASE 68

HPI: A 29-year-old woman presents to clinic complaining of 5 weeks of diarrhea and mild cramping pain in her lower abdomen. She has been passing around four loose stools per day that are streaked with blood and mucus. She has not been out of the country or camping recently and has no sick contacts.

Vital signs: Temperature 98.2°F (36.8°C), pulse 82 beats/min, BP 125/75 mm Hg, RR 17 breaths/min.

Additional history: No medical history. No use of tobacco, alcohol, or drugs.

1. What is the differential diagnosis?

Infectious colitis, ulcerative colitis, Crohn disease, celiac disease, diverticulitis, giardiasis, amoebiasis.

2. What components of the physical examination do you perform?

General appearance, skin, lymph nodes, HEENT, cardiovascular, lungs, abdomen, rectal, extremities, neuro/psych.

Physical examination:

General: No acute distress.

Skin/lymph nodes/HEENT: WNL

Cardiovascular: WNL

Lungs: WNL

Abdomen: Mild tenderness of the left lower quadrant.

Rectal: Blood and stool in the rectal vault.

Extremities: WNL

Neuro/psych: WNL

3. What are your initial orders?

Pulse oximetry, CBC, chem 8, LFTs, lipase, urinary pregnancy test, stool culture, stool ova and parasites, *C. difficile* PCR, fecal calprotectin, ESR, CRP, colonoscopy.

Advance clock:

Hb 10.9 g/dL, mildly elevated ESR, CRP, and fecal calprotectin. All other laboratory tests WNL.

Colonoscopy with rectal biopsy: Continuous inflammation of the rectum with friability. Biopsy consistent with ulcerative colitis.

4. What are your follow-up actions?

Mesalamine suppository, counseling, referral to GI clinic, follow-up in 2 weeks.

Advance clock:

The patient's symptoms are greatly improved.

Case ends.

Critical actions: Abdominal examination, colonoscopy, 5-aminosalicylic acid (5-ASA) agent (mesalamine).

Discussion: This patient has subacute bloody diarrhea and cramping abdominal pain consistent with colitis. Acute diarrhea often points to infectious (*Shigella, Salmonella, Campylobacter,* etc.), ischemic, radiation, medication induced, or malabsorption (lactose intolerance). Chronic diarrhea would be more suggestive of inflammatory (ulcerative colitis, Crohn disease), chronic infection (*Giardia,* Whipple disease), microscopic colitis, or chronic malabsorption. Given the patient's subacute onset, both categories need to be considered.

Radiation colitis can be ruled out by history, but infectious colitis should be worked up with stool studies. ESR and CRP help determine severity of disease, and a pregnancy test is always a good idea in a woman of reproductive age. A colonoscopy is the best way to differentiate between the other causes of colitis. In this case, it is consistent with ulcerative colitis. Initial therapy consists of mesalamine suppositories (or enema if inflammation extends beyond the rectum). Persistent symptoms can be treated with topical steroids (e.g., hydrocortisone) or oral mesalamine. Systemic steroids are indicated if the patient is having a severe flare (more than five stools daily, severe pain, fever, tachycardia, or ESR >30 mm/hour). The evaluation and treatment of mild Crohn disease are very similar, although oral rather than rectal 5-ASA agents are preferred, and the oral corticosteroid budesonide is considered a first-line agent. The patient should also receive referral to GI clinic for close followup and monitoring. A fecal calprotectin can also help aid in diagnosis, as it is elevated in inflammatory bowel disease (also would be elevated in invasive enteritis).

Diagnosis: Ulcerative colitis.

CASE 69

HPI: A 19-year-old woman (gravida 1 para 0) at 38 + 0 weeks of gestation presents to the ED complaining of intermittent blurry vision and a frontal headache that has not responded to acetaminophen. The headache has been present for 4 hours and is gradually worsening. The pregnancy has been uncomplicated to this point, and the patient has had regular prenatal care. She denies abdominal pain, contractions, loss of fluids, or vaginal bleeding. She takes a prenatal vitamin, but otherwise takes no medications.
Vital signs: Temperature 97.9°F (36.6°C), pulse 91 beats/min, BP 165/100 mm Hg, RR 19 breaths/min.
Additional history: No medical history. No use of tobacco, drugs, or alcohol.

1. **What is the differential diagnosis?**
   Pregnancy-induced hypertension (gestational hypertension), chronic essential hypertension, preeclampsia, HELLP syndrome (**h**emolysis, **e**levated **l**iver **e**nzymes, **l**ow **p**latelets, and right upper quadrant or epigastric **p**ain).

2. **What components of the physical examination do you perform?**
   General appearance, skin/HEENT, cardiovascular, lungs, abdomen, genitalia, extremities, neuro/psych.
   Physical examination:
   General: No acute distress.
   Skin/HEENT: WNL
   Cardiovascular: WNL
   Lungs: WNL
   Abdomen: Fundal height 38 cm, nontender.
   Genitalia: Cervix soft and dilated to 4 cm, 60% effaced, fetal station −1. No pooling of fluids. Cephalic presentation.
   Extremities: Edema 1+ in lower extremities.
   Neuro/psych: WNL

3. **What are your initial orders?**
   Pulse oximetry, BP/cardiac monitor, CBC, chem 8, PT/PTT, LFTs, uric acid, LDH, blood type and screen, UA, 24-hour urinary protein, urine output, fetal ultrasound, fetal monitor, magnesium sulfate IV, labetalol IV, obstetrics consult.
   Advance clock:
   O_2 saturation: 100% on room air.
   Repeat vital signs: BP 128/80 mm Hg.
   Blood type O positive, UA protein 2+, laboratory tests otherwise WNL.
   Symptoms are greatly improved.

4. **What are your follow-up actions?**
   Admit to inpatient unit, induction of labor (misoprostol and/or oxytocin), counseling.
   Advance clock: Case ends.
   Critical actions: Genital examination, neurologic exam, UA, urine output monitoring, fetal monitoring, magnesium IV, obstetrics consult.
   Discussion: Any gravid woman with symptoms suggestive of preeclampsia (headache, blurry vision, right upper quadrant pain, oliguria, edema) should be promptly evaluated for hypertension, proteinuria, thrombocytopenia, elevated liver enzymes, and hemolysis (LDH/uric acid). Preeclampsia is defined by BP greater than 140/90 mm Hg with proteinuria, developed after 20 weeks of gestation in a patient with no prior history of hypertension. BP greater than 160/110 mmHg or the presence of symptoms is sufficient for the diagnosis of severe preeclampsia. Treatment includes seizure prophylaxis using IV magnesium and BP control with labetalol or hydralazine. Once the patient is stabilized, the only definitive treatment is delivery. Because this patient is full term and has a favorable cervix, induction of labor is a reasonable approach; however, prolonged inductions should be avoided, and cesarean section is indicated if the baby cannot be delivered within a reasonable period of time. Induction can be achieved with misoprostol (cervical ripening) and oxytocin (stimulates contractions). On an exam, credit will be given if you simply consult obstetrics. Antenatal corticosteroids are indicated for gestational ages less than 34 weeks. Blood type should be determined for all gravid women, and Rho(D) immune globulin (RhoGAM) should be administered within 72 hours of delivery if the mother is rhesus (Rh) negative.
   Diagnosis: Preeclampsia.

CASE 70

HPI: A 72-year-old man presents to clinic with leg pain. He describes an ache in both calves that occurs after walking two city blocks. If he rests the pain goes away, but further activity brings the pain back. His legs become uncomfortable when he props them up and are relieved by dangling them over the edge of the bed. He denies numbness or weakness. He has a 50–pack-year smoking history and continues to smoke. He does not exercise and has a sedentary lifestyle.
Vital signs: Temperature 97.9°F (36.6°C), pulse 72 beats/min, BP 120/78 mm Hg, RR 16 breaths/min.
Additional history: No alcohol or drug use. History of hypertension, well controlled on hydrochlorothiazide.

1. What is the differential diagnosis?

   Peripheral arterial disease (PAD), spinal stenosis, peripheral neuropathy, venous insufficiency, Raynaud phenomenon, DVT, popliteal entrapment syndrome, thromboangiitis obliterans (Buerger disease).

2. What components of the physical examination do you perform?

   General appearance, HEENT, cardiovascular, lungs, abdomen, extremities, neuro/psych.

   Physical examination:

   General: No acute distress.

   HEENT: WNL

   Cardiovascular: WNL

   Lungs: WNL

   Abdomen: WNL

   Extremities: Hair loss and shiny skin over bilateral lower extremities. Thick toenails. Faint dorsalis pedis and posterior tibial pulses. Lower extremity pallor with passive leg raise. Sensation and strength intact. No ulcerations or skin breakdown.

   Neuro/psych: WNL

3. What are your initial orders?

   Pulse oximetry, ankle brachial index (ABI), HbA$_{1c}$, fasting lipid panel, ECG, vascular surgery consult.

   Advance clock: ABI 0.8, elevated LDL, all other studies WNL.

4. What are your follow-up actions?

   Aspirin PO, statin PO, counseling (including smoking cessation and exercise), follow-up in 1 month.

   Advance clock: Case ends.

   Critical actions: Extremity examination, ABI, lipid profile, aspirin, counseling.

   Discussion: This patient has bilateral lower extremity aching provoked by exercise and relieved by rest. This is the classic presentation of claudication, which represents exercise-induced limb ischemia due to atherosclerotic disease. PAD is a manifestation of atherosclerotic disease that is usually present throughout the vascular system. Claudication is the peripheral equivalent of angina from CAD. Risk factors include age, tobacco use, diabetes mellitus (DM), hypertension, and hyperlipidemia.

   Physical examination often reveals shiny, hairless skin over the lower legs with decreased pulses and brittle nails. ABI is the SBP in the leg divided by the SBP in the arm. It provides information on the presence and severity of disease (normal is >0.9). ABI can also be used to track progression of disease. It should be interpreted with care, however, in patients with calcified vessels, as occurs in DM. Calcified vessels are less compressible and may result in falsely high ankle SBP, leading to false negative ABIs. All patients should be assessed for critical limb ischemia, which manifests as the six *P*s (*p*ain at rest, *p*ulselessness, *p*allor, *p*aresthesia, *p*aralysis, and *p*oikilothermia [cold]). A cold, pulseless foot is an emergency that requires initiation of anticoagulation therapy (heparin drip) and an emergent vascular surgery consult.

   Treatment for ABI begins with risk factor modification to prevent progression of disease. Smoking cessation and an exercise regimen can improve symptoms and prevent progression of disease. Assessment for and control of BP, hyperlipidemia, and diabetes are also important in disease management. Aspirin reduces disease progression and the risk of stroke and MI, which often occur together in vasculopathic patients. Clopidogrel (in place of aspirin), and cilostazol, a phosphodiesterase inhibitor that decreases platelet aggregation and directly vasodilates vessels, may also be considered for patients with PAD, but only if they have failed lifestyle modifications. New onset PAD warrants a consultation with a vascular specialist to identify any need for procedural revascularization, including stenting or bypass grafting.

   Diagnosis: PAD.

CASE 71

HPI: A 29-year-old woman, gravida 1 para 0, at 9 weeks of gestation presents to clinic complaining of intractable nausea and vomiting. She has been vomiting four or five times daily for the past 10 days. Today she has been unable to drink or eat anything without immediately vomiting. She has lost 4 kg in weight since her last visit. The pregnancy has been uncomplicated up to this point. She takes no medications other than a prenatal vitamin. She denies fever, chills, constipation, diarrhea, and abdominal pain.

Vital signs: Temperature 98.4°F (36.9°C), pulse 111 beats/min, BP 120/80 mm Hg, RR 17 breaths/min.

Additional history: No medical history. No tobacco, drugs, or alcohol use.

1. What is the differential diagnosis?

   Hyperemesis gravidarum, viral gastroenteritis, pyelonephritis, cholecystitis, appendicitis, hepatitis.

2. What components of the physical examination do you perform?

   General appearance, skin, lymph nodes, HEENT, cardiovascular, lungs, abdomen, genitalia, extremities, neuro/psych.

   Physical examination:

   General: Mild distress due to nausea. Dry mucous membranes.

   Skin/lymph nodes/HEENT: WNL

Cardiovascular: Tachycardic, regular rhythm.
Lungs: WNL
Abdomen: WNL
Genitalia: WNL
Extremities: WNL
Neuro/psych: WNL

3. **What are your initial orders?**
   Pulse oximetry, CBC, chem 8, orthostatic vital signs, fetal ultrasound, UA, IV metoclopramide, IV fluids.
   Advance clock:
   UA ketones 2+, otherwise studies WNL.
   The patient's symptoms have mildly improved, but she is still unable to tolerate fluids without emesis.

4. **What are your follow-up actions?**
   Admit to ward, pyridoxine, doxylamine, metoclopramide, repeat chem 8 and UA, replete electrolytes, counseling.
   Advance clock:
   UA WNL with no ketones.
   The patient's symptoms have greatly improved. She is able to tolerate a full diet.
   Case ends.
   Critical actions: Abdominal examination, IV fluids, antiemetics.
   Discussion: Nausea and vomiting are common symptoms during pregnancy, although other intraabdominal processes should also be considered in the differential diagnosis. When pregnancy-induced vomiting causes dehydration, weight loss, or ketonuria, it is on the severe side and is termed *hyperemesis gravidarum*. Diagnostic criteria for hyperemesis gravidarum include weight loss of greater than 5% of the pre-pregnancy weight and prolonged severe nausea and vomiting, after ruling out other causes. It is thought to be caused by the emetogenic properties of hCG and other hormonal changes in pregnancy. It normally starts at 4 weeks of gestation and resolves by 20 weeks. Evaluation should include orthostatic vital signs, chem 8, and UA to assess ketonuria. Treatment of all nausea and vomiting in pregnancy begins with IV fluids as needed. Mild symptoms can be treated with dietary changes and consideration of ginger supplementation alone. Pyridoxine with doxylamine is considered first-line medication therapy for mild to moderate symptoms. Persistent symptoms are usually treated with metoclopramide. Other agents considered safe in pregnancy include diphenhydramine and prochlorperazine. The use of ondansetron is controversial in pregnancy because of a possible association with fetal abnormalities. Patients are stable for discharge home when any ketonuria resolves, they can tolerate PO, and their symptoms are controlled without IV medications.
   Diagnosis: Hyperemesis gravidarum.

CASE 72

HPI: A 19-year-old woman presents to the ED complaining of 2 days of abdominal pain in the right lower quadrant. The pain was gradual in onset and associated with one episode of vomiting. She has had a moderate amount of green vaginal discharge. The patient came to the ED today because she thought she had a fever.
Vital signs: Temperature 102.6°F (39.2°C), pulse 115 beats/min, BP 122/80 mm Hg, RR 14 breaths/min.
Additional history: Sexually active with one male partner. No tobacco, alcohol, or drug use.

1. **What is the differential diagnosis?**
   Acute appendicitis, ectopic pregnancy, PID, septic abortion, pyelonephritis, ovarian torsion, ruptured ovarian cyst.

2. **What components of the physical examination do you perform?**
   General appearance, skin, lymph nodes, HEENT, cardiovascular, lungs, abdomen, genitalia, extremities, neuro/psych.
   Physical examination:
   General: Moderate distress secondary to pain.
   Skin/lymph nodes/HEENT: WNL
   Cardiovascular: Tachycardia.
   Lungs: WNL
   Abdomen: Soft, moderate tenderness in the right lower quadrant without guarding or rebound.
   Genitalia: Right adnexal tenderness, positive cervical motion tenderness, moderate mucopurulent discharge from the cervical os.

3. **What are your initial orders?**
   Pulse oximetry, cardiac/BP monitor, urinary pregnancy test, UA, urine culture, CBC, chem 8, LFTs, lipase, blood cultures, lactate, wet mount, *Gonococcus, Chlamydia,* abdomen/pelvis ultrasound, IV fluids, cefoxitin IV, doxycycline PO, morphine, ondansetron, acetaminophen.
   Advance clock:
   WBC: $14.0 \times 10^3/\mu L$
   Urinary pregnancy test: Negative.

Gonococcus antigen: Positive.
Ultrasound: Thickening of fallopian tube. No tuboovarian abscess.
The patient feels mild improvement but remains in significant pain. She continues to be nauseated.
Temperature 101.1°F (38.4°C), pulse 101 beats/min, BP 130/82 mm Hg, RR 13 breaths/min.

4. **What are your follow-up actions?**
   Admit to inpatient unit, check vital signs every 4 hours, HIV antibody test, RPR. CBC and chem 8 next day. Counseling (including safe sex and partner treatment). Continue cefoxitin and doxycycline. Discharge home when vital signs are normalized, symptoms have improved, and the patient is tolerating food. Transition to PO doxycycline only and continue a 14-day course.
   Advance clock: Case ends.
   Critical actions: CBC, abdominal examination, pelvic examination, pelvic ultrasound, IV fluids, testing for sexually transmitted illnesses, antibiotics for gonorrhea and *Chlamydia*.
   Discussion: PID is an ascending infection that spreads from the lower genital tract to involve the uterus, fallopian tubes, ovaries, and/or peritoneum. It typically begins with the sexually transmitted organisms *N. gonorrhoeae* and *Chlamydia trachomatis*, although PID is a polymicrobial process and must be treated as such. The differential for lower abdominal pain and pelvic pain is broad in female patients. We can substantially limit our differential immediately by ruling out pregnancy. PID is a clinical diagnosis that is suggested by the physical examination (adnexal tenderness, cervical motion tenderness, mucopurulent cervical discharge). Diagnostic tests can support the diagnosis, especially if they detect gonorrhea or *Chlamydia*. Ultrasound can provide further evidence of PID while assessing for other conditions in the differential diagnosis (appendicitis, ovarian cyst, ovarian torsion). Ultrasound can also evaluate potential complications such as tuboovarian abscess secondary to PID.
   Because the patient is septic with significant symptoms, she meets admission criteria and will need IV antibiotics that cover *N. gonorrhoeae* and *C. trachomatis*. IV cefoxitin with PO doxycycline is the first-line inpatient regimen that provides coverage for gram-negative enteric organisms, streptococci, and anaerobes. Once patients have been stabilized for 24 hours (sustained clinical improvement reflected by resolution of fever, nausea, vomiting, and abdominal pain), they may be transitioned to PO doxycycline for a total course of 14 days. If a pelvic abscess is visualized on ultrasound, metronidazole may be added to the 14-day course for anaerobic coverage. The CDC in 2021 issued a weak recommendation to add empiric metronidazole to all patients with PID based on increased clearance of anaerobes but not on patient-oriented outcomes. Patients who have simple PID without systemic symptoms may be treated with a single dose of IM ceftriaxone and a course of PO doxycycline. Patients should also be tested for other sexually transmitted infections, and their sexual partners should be treated.
   Diagnosis: PID.

CASE 73

HPI: A 47-year-old male presents to clinic complaining of decreased energy. For the past 6 weeks he has felt like he lacks his normal amount of energy. He has been waking early in the morning and having trouble getting back to sleep. He believes that this has affected his concentration and caused him to perform poorly at work, which makes him feel guilty about not meeting his team's expectations. He feels sad most days. He denies hallucinations, delusions, past manic episodes, suicidal ideation, and homicidal ideation. He has not recently experienced the death of a loved one.
Vital signs: Temperature 98.2°F (36.8°C), pulse 65 beats/min, BP 115/75 mm Hg, RR 17 breaths/min.
Additional history: No medical history. No tobacco, alcohol, or drug use.

1. **What is the differential diagnosis?**
   Major depressive disorder, dysthymia, adjustment disorder, bipolar disorder, hypothyroidism, anemia, substance abuse disorder, insomnia, obstructive sleep apnea (OSA)/obesity hypoventilation syndrome (OHS).

2. **What components of the physical examination do you perform?**
   General appearance, skin, lymph nodes, HEENT, cardiovascular, lungs, abdomen, extremities, neuro/psych.
   Physical examination:
   General: No acute distress.
   Skin/lymph nodes/HEENT: WNL
   Cardiovascular: WNL
   Lungs: WNL
   Abdomen: WNL
   Extremities: WNL
   Neuro/psych: Depressed mood/affect. No focal neurologic deficits.

3. **What are your initial orders?**
   CBC, chem 8, TSH, Utox, follow-up in 2 weeks, therapy, counseling.
   Advance clock: Studies WNL.

4. **What are your follow-up actions?**
   Citalopram low dose; advise to follow up with primary care physician to uptitrate and monitor for improvement or side effects. Psychotherapy referral.

Advance clock:
The patient's symptoms are improved.
Case ends.

Critical actions: Neuro/psych examination, CBC, TSH, antidepressant (selective serotonin reuptake inhibitor [SSRI] or serotonin-norepinephrine reuptake inhibitor [SNRI]), follow-up.

Discussion: This patient has depressed mood/affect, guilt, sleep disturbance, low energy, and poor concentration. These symptoms have caused functional impairment and lasted for longer than 2 weeks. The *Diagnostic and Statistical Manual of Mental Disorders,* Fifth Edition (DSM-V) diagnosis of depression is depressed mood for more than 2 weeks that is a change in baseline and causes impaired function and specific symptoms. The specific symptoms are at least five of the following eight, which can be remembered by the mnemonic SIG E CAPS: (1) sleep changes, (2) interest loss (anhedonia), (3) guilt, (4) energy decrease, (5) cognition/concentration reduction, (6) appetite decrease, (7) psychomotor changes (agitation or lethargy), and (8) suicide/death preoccupation, usually for at least 6 months. All medical etiologies must be first ruled out. Thyroid disturbances can lead to a depressive-like presentation, as well as substance use (substance-induced mood disorder), and OSA/OHS. This patient fits the diagnostic criteria for depression. If he has a triggering incident such as the death of a loved one, and he is within 6 months of that event, we may also consider grief. Treatment can begin with psychotherapy, counseling, and an SSRI or SNRI. Symptoms may not improve for 4 to 6 weeks despite appropriate therapy. It is important to schedule regular follow-up to reassess for suicidal thinking.

Diagnosis: Depression.

CASE 74

HPI: A 45-year-old woman presents to clinic complaining of several months of gradually worsening joint pain and stiffness. The pain mostly affects the small joints of her hands and has recently included her wrists as well. Both the right and left sides are affected equally. The patient finds the pain and stiffness worse in the morning. Her symptoms are somewhat improved by activity. She notes occasional swelling of the affected joints. She has not had any rash or fever.

Vital signs: Temperature 99.0°F (37.2°C), pulse 79 beats/min, BP 115/75 mm Hg, RR 16 breaths/min.

Additional history: No medical history. No tobacco, alcohol, or drug use.

1. **What is the differential diagnosis?**
   RA, OA, psoriatic arthritis, SLE, fibromyalgia, gout, Lyme disease.

2. **What components of the physical examination do you perform?**
   General appearance, skin, lymph nodes, HEENT, cardiovascular, lungs, abdomen, extremities, neuro/psych.
   Physical examination:
   General: No acute distress.
   Skin/lymph nodes/HEENT: WNL
   Cardiovascular: WNL
   Lungs: WNL
   Abdomen: WNL
   Extremities: Tenderness to palpation over interphalangeal (IP), metacarpophalangeal (MCP), and wrist joints, with moderate swelling and effusion present. Subcutaneous nodules over MCP joints. No visible bony deformities. Decreased range of motion in wrists bilaterally.
   Neuro/psych: WNL

3. **What are your initial orders?**
   Pulse oximetry, CBC, chem 14, ESR, CRP, RF, ANA, dsDNA, cyclic citrullinated peptide antibody (anti-CCP), x-ray of affected joints, ibuprofen (or other NSAID), synovial fluid analysis (cell count, crystals, bacterial culture).
   Advance clock:
   CBC mild anemia, ESR and CRP elevated. RF strongly positive, anti-CCP positive.
   Other studies WNL.

4. **What are your follow-up actions?**
   Rheumatology consult, counseling, methotrexate or other disease-modifying antirheumatic drug (DMARD), physical therapy, occupational therapy, exercise, follow-up in 4 weeks.
   Advance clock:
   The patient's symptoms have improved.
   Case ends.
   Critical actions: Extremities examination, analgesia (NSAIDs or acetaminophen), methotrexate (or other DMARD).
   Discussion: This patient has gradual onset of symmetric joint pain, morning stiffness, and inflammation suggestive of RA. RA usually involves smaller joints, especially of the hands (proximal IPs) and feet. Wrists, elbows, shoulders, knees, and hips may also be affected. Involvement of the distal IP joints, obesity, or history of

excessive weight-bearing activity is more suggestive of OA. The presence of effusions and rheumatoid nodules in this patient are highly suggestive of RA and should trigger a laboratory assessment for this condition. There is no test that is both sensitive and specific for RA, but several laboratory tests can suggest the disease. Anti-CCP is the most specific test at greater than 90%, but it is not sensitive. RF is 70% sensitive and 85% specific. Other nonspecific findings include increased ESR and CRP and the presence of microcytic anemia. Her constellation of symptoms may also represent lupus, so ANA and dsDNA would be reasonable to send as well. Arthrocentesis with synovial fluid analysis may be helpful if there is ongoing diagnostic uncertainty, and a joint effusion is present. Synovial fluid may reveal mild inflammation and can be useful in distinguishing from septic arthritis and gout when these are in the differential diagnosis. X-rays may reveal osteopenia, joint space narrowing, and deformities consistent with RA.

Barring contraindications, most patients with undifferentiated arthritis will benefit from therapy with NSAIDs. Once a diagnosis of RA has been established, initiation of DMARD therapy will not only improve symptoms but also prevent progression of disease. Methotrexate is the most frequently used DMARD, but leflunomide, sulfasalazine, and hydroxychloroquine also have efficacy. In acute flares, a brief course of corticosteroids may be indicated. Patients with severe or refractory disease should be evaluated for treatment with a biologic agent such as etanercept (TNF-alpha antagonist), with testing of TB prior to initiation. Patients on biologic agents are at higher risk of infectious complications. Counseling, physical therapy, and occupational therapy all play a role in disease management as well.

Diagnosis: RA.

CASE 75

HPI: A 23-year-old woman (gravida 1 para 0) at 36 weeks of gestation presents to the ED complaining of vaginal bleeding. The bleeding started approximately 6 hours ago and has included passage of clots. She does not think that her water has broken, but she has been experiencing frequent contractions. She admits using cocaine several times during the pregnancy, including earlier today. She takes no medications other than a prenatal vitamin.

Vital signs: Temperature 98.8°F (37.1°C), pulse 90 beats/min, BP 118/74 mm Hg, RR 19 breaths/min.

Additional history: No medical history. Smokes two packs of cigarettes per week. Uses cocaine twice per month. No alcohol.

1. What is the differential diagnosis?
   Placental abruption, placenta previa, preterm labor, uterine rupture, vasa previa, subchorionic hematoma.

2. What components of the physical examination do you perform?
   General appearance, skin, lymph nodes, HEENT, cardiovascular, lungs, abdomen, genitalia, extremities, neuro/psych.
   Physical examination:
   General: No acute distress.
   Skin/lymph nodes/HEENT: WNL
   Cardiovascular: WNL
   Lungs: WNL
   Abdomen: Fundal height 34 cm; fundus is mildly tender and feels firm.
   Genitalia: Scant blood at the vaginal introitus.
   Extremities: WNL
   Neuro/psych: WNL

3. What are your initial orders?
   Pulse oximetry, IV fluids (e.g., lactated Ringer), CBC, chem 8, PT/PTT, blood type and screen, urine toxicology, fetal ultrasound, fetal monitoring, obstetric-gynecology consult.
   Advance clock: Blood type O positive, Hb 11.3 g/dL, ultrasound reveals placental abruption, fetal monitoring reveals late decelerations. Other studies WNL except urine toxicology, which is positive for cocaine.

4. What are your follow-up actions?
   Group B Strep prophylaxis, cesarean section delivery with obstetrics-gynecology, child protection services, social work consult, counseling (including drug and tobacco counseling).
   Advance clock: Case ends.
   Critical actions: Early IV access and fluid resuscitation, fetal ultrasound, fetal monitoring, CBC, blood type and screen, toxicology screen, emergent obstetrics consult, social work consult, counseling.
   Discussion: A pregnant woman in the third trimester who experiences vaginal bleeding may have any of the following: early onset of labor, bloody show, placental abruption, placenta previa, uterine rupture, or vasa previa. Placenta previa is abnormal implantation of the placenta in the lower uterine segment. The classical presentation is painless vaginal bleeding with or without contractions. Placental abruption is abnormal separation of the placenta before delivery. The classical presentation is painful vaginal bleeding with contractions. Uterine rupture often occurs in patients with prior cesarean sections who attempt vaginal delivery or have sustained abdominal/uterine

trauma. Vasa previa is a rare obstetric emergency where fetal blood vessels (usually from abnormal umbilical cord insertion) block the cervical os. Like placenta previa it typically presents with painless vaginal bleeding and fetal bradycardia/distress.

Patients should undergo a thorough physical examination. If placenta previa is suspected, speculum and digital examinations are contraindicated because they can cause hemorrhage. Laboratory tests should assess hemoglobin/hematocrit, PT/PTT, and alloimmunization (Rh) status. RhoGAM should be given if fetal-maternal hemorrhage has occurred and the mother is Rh negative. Fetal ultrasound is very reliable in diagnosing placenta previa, although it is not sensitive enough to rule out placental abruption.

Continuous fetal monitoring can assess fetal distress or stability. In placental abruption, a fetus at less than 34 weeks of gestation can be delivered vaginally if stable or via cesarean section if unstable. In this patient, late decelerations indicate fetal distress so emergent cesarean section is indicated. Placental abruption can cause DIC, so coagulation parameters should be monitored.

Diagnosis: Placental abruption.

CASE 76

HPI: A 70-year-old woman presents to the ED with a headache. The headache was gradual in onset and is located in the right temporal region. It has continued to worsen over the last 12 hours and seems to worsen when the patient tries to eat. She has never had a previous headache like this. She denies fevers or neck stiffness, but she reports muscle aches at her shoulders and hips. She has had no visual changes or recent trauma.

Vital signs: Temperature 98.0°F (36.7°C), pulse 71 beats/min, BP 118/75 mm Hg, RR 16 breaths/min.

Additional history: No medical history. No tobacco, drugs, or alcohol use. No recent psychosocial stressors.

1. What is the differential diagnosis?
   Giant cell arteritis (temporal arteritis), intracerebral hemorrhage, neoplasm, tension headache, migraine.

2. What components of the physical examination do you perform?
   General appearance, skin, lymph nodes, HEENT, cardiovascular, lungs, abdomen, genitalia, extremities, neuro/psych.
   Physical examination:
   General: No acute distress.
   Skin/lymph nodes/HEENT: Tenderness over the right temporal artery.
   Cardiovascular: WNL
   Lungs: WNL
   Abdomen: WNL
   Genitalia: WNL
   Extremities: Tenderness over shoulders and hips.
   Neuro/psych: WNL. 20/20 visual fields bilaterally. No blurriness.

3. What are your initial orders?
   Pulse oximetry, CBC, chem 8, ESR, CRP, noncontrast head CT scan.
   Advance clock: ESR 110 mm/hr, CRP 10 mg/dL, other studies WNL.

4. What are your follow-up actions?
   High-dose prednisone, admit to ward, temporal artery biopsy (reveals temporal arteritis), rheumatology consult, repeat ESR, counseling.
   Advance clock:
   Symptoms greatly improved.
   Case ends.
   Critical actions: HEENT/neurologic exam, ESR and/or CRP, immediate prednisone, temporal artery biopsy.
   Discussion: New onset of headaches in the elderly should prompt a thorough evaluation for underlying pathology. This patient's historical features of new onset temporal headache with jaw claudication are suggestive of temporal arteritis (giant cell arteritis). The presence of temporal artery tenderness further suggests the diagnosis, especially in the setting of elevated ESR/CRP. For individuals younger than 50 years, temporal arteritis almost never occurs; the mean age at diagnosis is 70 years. The patient's history of proximal muscle pain also indicates she may have polymyalgia rheumatica, which frequently coexists with temporal arteritis (approximately 50% of patients with temporal arteritis also have or develop polymyalgia rheumatica). Temporal artery biopsy is indicated for formal diagnosis, but treatment with corticosteroids should not be delayed because biopsy results are not significantly altered if biopsy is performed within 1 to 2 weeks of starting therapy. If treatment is delayed, spread to the ophthalmic artery can cause irreversible vision loss. Serial ESR measurement can track the response to treatment. Any visual symptoms warrant consultation with an ophthalmologist. High-dose prednisone (1 mg/kg) is maintained for at least 2 weeks but less than 4 weeks, and a glucocorticoid taper is subsequently initiated.
   Diagnosis: Temporal arteritis (giant cell arteritis).

CASE 77

HPI: A 29-year-old woman presents to the ED because of epigastric abdominal pain that radiates to her back. The pain was gradual in onset but has been constant and severe for 8 hours. The patient has had nausea and vomiting but denies fever or diarrhea.

Vital signs: Temperature 99.0°F (37.2°C), pulse 105 beats/min, BP 135/85 mm Hg, RR 16 breaths/min.

Additional history: No medical history. No recent trauma. No use of tobacco, alcohol, or drugs.

1. What is the differential diagnosis?
   Peptic ulcer disease, cholelithiasis, cholecystitis, pancreatitis, esophageal spasm, AAA.

2. What components of the physical examination do you perform?
   General appearance, HEENT, cardiovascular, lungs, abdomen.
   Physical examination:
   General: Moderate distress due to pain, dry mucous membranes.
   HEENT: WNL
   Cardiovascular: Mild tachycardia.
   Lungs: WNL
   Abdomen: Tenderness to epigastric palpation without rebound or guarding.

3. What are your initial orders?
   Pulse oximetry, cardiac/BP monitor, CBC, chem 14, lipase, UA, urinary pregnancy test, morphine, ondansetron, IV LR, NPO.
   Advance clock:
   Lipase 1129 U/L, all other laboratory tests WNL.
   Pain moderately improved.

4. What are your follow-up actions?
   Right upper quadrant ultrasound, IV fluids, IV pain medication, fasting lipid panel (reveals extremely elevated triglycerides [1900 mg/dL]), LDH, lactate. Admit to ICU. IV insulin drip with glucose checks and glucose supplementation as necessary; consider D5 or D10 IV drip. Q1hr glucose, q4hr chem 14. Gemfibrozil PO once triglycerides less than 500. Advance diet as tolerated. Counseling on lifestyle modifications. Referral to preventative cardiology for hyperlipidemia management; consider genetic counselor referral.
   Advance clock: Case ends.
   Critical actions: Abdominal examination, lipase, fasting lipid panel, abdominal ultrasound, IV fluids.
   Discussion: This patient has epigastric abdominal pain radiating to the back. A focused physical examination and laboratory assessment for intraabdominal pathology reveal a lipase level that is diagnostic of pancreatitis (three times the upper normal limit). All patients with pancreatitis should receive IV fluids, pain control, and antiemetics. They should initially be NPO (although there is increasing evidence that early feeding as tolerated leads to shorter hospitalizations). Glucose and electrolytes (especially calcium) should be closely monitored. A diagnosis of pancreatitis should trigger evaluation of the cause. In the United States, gallstones, alcohol, medications, and triglycerides are the most common identifiable causes. Alcohol and medications can be ruled out by history. Gallstones should be evaluated using ultrasound, and triglycerides can be identified with lipid panel measurement.
   As triglyceride levels increase above 500 mg/dL, there is a progressive risk of pancreatitis. Severe hypertriglyceridemia is treated with apheresis or insulin infusion (same infusion regimen as DKA). This is because insulin is normally secreted in the "fed" state and promotes fat storage (since fat mobilization is not needed if you are fed!). This decreases serum triglyceride levels and helps resolve the pancreatitis. Once triglycerides are less than 500 mg/dL, patients can be transitioned to gemfibrozil PO to continue triglyceride control. In this case, an LDH test was ordered to calculate a Ranson score for prognosis. A CT abdomen/pelvis with IV contrast can be considered in cases of diagnostic uncertainty, suspected complications (such as necrotizing pancreatitis, pseudocyst, abscess, sepsis, hemoperitoneum), or lack of clinical improvement. Patients may be safely discharged home when pain is controlled, vital signs and electrolytes are normalized, and they are tolerating food. Patients with gallstone pancreatitis should have cholecystectomy with common bile duct exploration, intraoperative cholangiogram, and/or ERCP during the same hospitalization if they are surgical candidates. Patients with necrotizing pancreatitis are often treated with prophylactic antibiotics to prevent superinfection.
   Diagnosis: Pancreatitis.

CASE 78

HPI: A 71-year-old man presents to the ED with 10/10 intensity periumbilical abdominal pain. One hour before his arrival he was walking to the kitchen when he had sudden onset of abdominal pain radiating to his back. The patient felt dizzy at that time and had to lie down. The pain has been constant since then.

Vital signs: Temperature 98.8°F (37.1°C), pulse 110 beats/min, BP 100/75 mm Hg, RR 20 breaths/min.

Additional history: 25–pack-year smoker, hypertension on hydrochlorothiazide, hyperlipidemia on simvastatin.

1. What is the differential diagnosis?
   AAA rupture, ACS, pancreatitis, mesenteric ischemia, acute abdominal embolism, retroperitoneal hematoma, small bowel obstruction (SBO).

2. **What components of the physical examination do you perform?**
General appearance, HEENT, cardiovascular, lungs, abdomen, extremities, rectal.
Physical examination:
General: Diaphoretic. Visible discomfort from pain.
HEENT: WNL
Cardiovascular: Tachycardia.
Lungs: WNL
Abdomen: Palpable pulsatile abdominal mass. Severe tenderness to palpation.
Extremities: WNL
Rectal: WNL

3. **What are your initial orders?**
Pulse oximetry, BP/cardiac monitoring, CBC, chem 8, LFTs, lipase, coagulation panel, UA, troponin, ECG, blood type and crossmatch, CXR, abdominal ultrasound.
Advance clock:
Ultrasound: 7-cm AAA with periaortic fluid and free intraperitoneal fluid.
All other studies WNL

4. **What are your follow-up actions?**
Surgical consult, surgical repair of AAA.
Admit to ICU; check vital signs every 2 hours, CBC every 4 hours, chem 8 in the morning.
Counseling: activity, diet, smoking cessation.
Advance clock: Case ends.
Critical actions: Abdominal examination, surgical consult, surgical repair of AAA.
Discussion: This patient has a ruptured AAA, as evidenced by the 7-cm aortic aneurysm with periaortic fluid and free intraperitoneal fluid. The chief complaint and physical examination should prompt you to stabilize the patient and order a rapid imaging modality such as ultrasound or a CT scan to assess for an aneurysm. IV fluids and blood products can be used to treat hypotension, although there is evidence that the BP should be kept relatively low as long as the patient is stable to prevent further bleeding. An immediate surgical consult and repair are required. The patient should be admitted to the ICU after the surgery. A number of other routine tests can (and should) be ordered, but you should not wait for the results before proceeding with emergent surgical management.

An AAA is an abdominal aortic diameter of greater than 3 cm. Prophylactic surgical or endovascular repair is generally indicated for any symptomatic aneurysm, an aneurysm larger than 5 cm, or a rapidly enlarging aneurysm ($\geq$ 0.5 cm in 6 months or $\geq$1 cm in 1 year). Smaller AAAs can be monitored with serial ultrasound or CT scans. One-time screening is recommended for men of 65 to 75 years of age who have ever smoked. Most AAAs are caused by atherosclerosis, but some are caused by connective tissue disorders such as Marfan syndrome and Ehlers-Danlos syndrome. The most common modifiable risk factors are cigarette smoking and hypertension. The mortality rate for ruptured AAAs is very high, and the condition should always be considered in any older patient with abdominal pain, flank pain, back pain, hypotension, or syncope. A ruptured AAA can be mistaken for renal colic in older patients and is a common exam mislead. Remember that new onset kidney stone in an older patient without a history of nephrolithiasis is uncommon; hematuria can even be the presenting symptom for ruptured AAAs.
Diagnosis: AAA.

CASE 79

HPI: A 76-year-old man presents to the ED with palpitations. He says he has been having palpitations on and off for a week. Recently he has felt his heart racing extremely fast and has been feeling increasingly weak and short of breath. The patient denies chest pain, fever, and loss of consciousness. He has never had similar symptoms before.
Vital signs: Temperature 98.2°F (36.8°C), pulse 155 beats/min, BP 115/80 mm Hg, RR 17 breaths/min.
Additional history: History of hypertension on hydrochlorothiazide. No drug, tobacco, or alcohol use.

1. **What is the differential diagnosis?**
Stable tachycardia: AF, atrial flutter, supraventricular tachycardia (SVT), sinus tachycardia, stable primary or secondary ventricular tachycardia.

2. **What components of the physical examination do you perform?**
General appearance, HEENT, cardiovascular, lungs, abdomen, extremities.
Physical examination:
General: Mild distress due to palpitations.
HEENT: WNL
Cardiovascular: Tachycardic, irregularly irregular rhythm.
Lungs: WNL
Abdomen: WNL
Extremities: WNL

3. What are your initial orders?

Pulse oximetry, cardiac/BP monitor, ECG, CBC, chem 8, troponin, TSH, CXR.

Advance clock:

ECG reveals irregularly irregular narrow complex tachycardia without P waves.

Other studies WNL.

4. What are your follow-up actions?

Atrioventricular (AV) nodal blocking agent (e.g., metoprolol, diltiazem), anticoagulation (e.g., rivaroxaban), admit patient to ward, morning ECG, CBC, chem 8, PT/PTT, TTE, counseling.

Advance clock:

TTE reveals dilated right atrium without valvular pathology. ECG reveals continued atrial fibrillation.

Heart rate 98 beats/min, patient's symptoms greatly improved.

Case ends.

Critical actions: Cardiac examination, ECG, rate-controlling agent, anticoagulation therapy.

Discussion: The patient has AF with rapid ventricular response (RVR). Any patient with hemodynamic instability and AF with RVR should undergo immediate synchronized cardioversion. Select patients who have been in AF for less than 48 hours can also undergo cardioversion with low risk of thromboembolism and subsequent stroke.

Because this patient is stable and has been in AF for longer than 48 hours, he is not a good candidate for cardioversion. His symptoms of weakness and shortness of breath are probably due to his RVR, and because he does not have underlying causes of tachycardia (e.g., GI bleed, sepsis, CHF), he will benefit from rate control with an AV nodal blocking agent (usually metoprolol or diltiazem).

The major long-term risk associated with AF is thromboembolic disease. This can manifest as stroke, mesenteric ischemia, or limb ischemia. The $CHADS_2$-VASc score can be used to calculate the long-term risk of stroke. Points are assigned for the presence of CHF ($+1$), hypertension ($+1$), age 65 to 74 ($+1$) or 75 or older ($+2$), diabetes ($+1$), stroke/TIA/thromboembolism ($+2$), vascular disease history (MI, PAD, aortic plaque; $+1$). Patients with a score of 0 or 1 may take aspirin for stroke prevention, whereas patients with two or more risk factors qualify for anticoagulation therapy (usually with a DOAC or warfarin). This patient has two risk factors (age and hypertension), so he qualifies for anticoagulation therapy. Another management option in this case would involve TEE followed by synchronized or pharmacologic cardioversion if no cardiac thrombus is present. Even if patients undergo rhythm control with cardioversion, they should be assessed for anticoagulation using a $CHADS_2$-VASc score. Not all patients with new onset AF need hospital admission, but you should generally favor a conservative approach on Step 3.

Secondary causes of AF such as electrolyte abnormalities, hyperthyroidism, and structural cardiac problems such as valvular disease or atrial enlargement should be investigated for all new diagnoses of AF. Long-term rate control (to keep the heart rate at <110 beats/min) is beneficial and should be targeted.

Diagnosis: AF with RVR.

CASE 80

HPI: A 23-year-old woman presents to clinic because it has been 9 weeks since her last menstrual period. She usually has periods regularly every 28 days that last for 4 days with a moderate flow. She had menarche at 13 years of age and has never been pregnant. The patient is sexually active with one male partner and intermittently uses condoms. She has no history of sexually transmitted infection. She has never had a Pap smear.

Vital signs: Temperature 98.2°F (36.8°C), pulse 77 beats/min, BP 108/70 mm Hg, RR 14 breaths/min.

Additional history: No medical history. Drinks three beers daily. No tobacco or drug use.

1. What is the differential diagnosis?

Amenorrhea due to pregnancy, PCOS, hypothyroidism, hypothalamic amenorrhea/anovulation, pituitary adenoma, premature ovarian failure.

2. What components of the physical examination do you perform?

General appearance, skin, lymph nodes, HEENT, cardiovascular, lungs, abdomen, genitalia, extremities, neuro/psych.

Physical examination:

General: No acute distress.

Skin/lymph nodes/HEENT: WNL

Cardiovascular: WNL

Lungs: WNL

Abdomen: WNL

Genitalia: WNL

Extremities: WNL

Neuro/psych: WNL

3. What are your initial orders?

Urinary pregnancy test.

Advance clock: Urinary pregnancy test positive. The patient states that this is a desired pregnancy.

4. What are your follow-up actions?

CBC, chem 8, blood type and screen, Pap smear, RPR, *Chlamydia/Gonococcus* screening, hepatitis B surface anti-gen, HIV antibody test, rubella serology, varicella antibody, TSH, purified protein derivative, HbA$_{1c}$, UA, urine culture, fetal ultrasound, folic acid PO, obstetrics-gynecology consult, counseling (including alcohol cessation), follow-up in 4 weeks.

Advance clock:

Ultrasound reveals intrauterine pregnancy, dating consistent with last menstrual period.

Case ends.

Critical actions: Pregnancy test, fetal ultrasound, counseling.

Discussion: Although the differential for amenorrhea is broad, you should always consider pregnancy first. A thor-ough physical examination is indicated for amenorrhea, although it rarely can establish the cause on its own. Urine and serum tests for beta-hCG are extremely sensitive and specific for pregnancy.

Once you have determined the patient has a desired pregnancy, early prenatal care is important. Establishing dates is most accurate by counting from the first day of the last menstrual period (if known). If this date is not known, an ultrasound can estimate the gestational age. Although various guidelines and practitioners have slightly different recommendations, a conservative approach to laboratory testing includes CBC, blood type and screen, UA, urine culture, rubella status, hepatitis B, HIV, syphilis, gonorrhea, *Chlamydia,* Pap smear, TSH, and HbA$_{1c}$. Folic acid supplementation is indicated, although ideally it should have been started before the pregnancy occurred. Thorough counseling is indicated for all patients. Routine follow-up is usually scheduled every 4 weeks for the first 28 weeks, every 2 weeks from 28 to 36 weeks, and weekly after 36 weeks.

Diagnosis: Uncomplicated pregnancy.

CASE 81

HPI: A 27-year-old man presents to the ED with acute onset of chest pain and shortness of breath. Twenty minutes ago, he was watching television when he noticed sudden onset of shortness of breath. His chest pain is severe and worsens every time he inhales deeply.

Vital signs: Temperature 97.7°F (36.5°C), pulse 125 beats/min, BP 82/60 mm Hg, RR 32 breaths/min.

Additional history: No medical history. An 8–pack-year smoking history.

1. What is the differential diagnosis?

Pulmonary embolism, pericarditis, tension pneumothorax, aortic dissection, ACS.

2. What components of the physical examination do you perform?

General appearance, cardiovascular, lungs.

Physical examination:

General: Severe respiratory distress, pale.

Cardiovascular: Tachycardic, weak peripheral pulses.

Lungs: Trachea is deviated. No breath sounds on the right side, right side hyperresonance on percussion.

3. What are your initial orders?

Needle thoracostomy, pulse oximetry, oxygen, normal saline, BP/cardiac monitor.

Advance clock:

A rush of air is heard after needle placement, the patient's symptoms greatly improve, and his breathing normalizes.

O$_2$ saturation was 70% prior to needle thoracostomy and now 100%, repeat vital signs WNL.

4. What are your follow-up actions?

Chest tube, CXR, morphine, ECG, CBC, chem 8, admit to inpatient unit, surgery consult, repeat CXR in morning, counseling.

Advance clock:

Repeat CXR with resolved pneumothorax. Chest tube to water seal shows no air leak. Laboratory tests WNL.

Case ends.

Critical actions: Lung examination, immediate needle thoracostomy, chest tube, CXR after chest tube placement.

Discussion: The patient's history of acute onset of pleuritic chest pain and shortness of breath should alert you to a likely pneumothorax. A simple pneumothorax is a nonexpanding collection of air between the visceral and pari-etal pleura without respiratory or hemodynamic instability. A tension pneumothorax is an expanding pneumothorax with respiratory or hemodynamic compromise. Tension pneumothorax usually leads to some of the following signs: unilateral absence of breath sounds, deviated trachea, hyperresonance on percussion, distended neck veins, hypoxia, and hypotension. This patient has a primary spontaneous tension pneumothorax, often seen in thin young men who develop subpleural blebs or who smoke. Timing is extremely important in this case. As soon as the absent breath sounds are noted, the patient should be treated immediately with needle thoracostomy. There should be no delay for laboratory analysis, imaging, or a complete physical examination. Once the patient has been stabilized, a chest tube should be placed and a CXR should be ordered to confirm placement. A surgical consult is also appropriate. If the case continues, admit the patient for monitoring and maintain the chest tube until the pneumothorax has resolved and the chest tube to water seal has no air leak. The classical teaching for a needle decompression was 2nd intercostal space in the midclavicular line but subsequent data showed that the needle decompression in that space was often unsuccessful. Newer recommendations are to perform needle decompression in the same location as the chest tube would be placed (4th/5th intercostal space, anterior/midaxillary line), as it is a shorter distance between the chest wall and the pleural cavity.

   Diagnosis: Tension pneumothorax.

CASE 82

HPI: A 59-year-old male presents to clinic complaining of gradual-onset right knee pain over the past 7 months. The pain is an ache that is usually present but worsens on exercise. The patient has had mild stiffness of the joint over the previous months. He denies fever, weight loss, or trauma.

Vital signs: Temperature 98.6°F (37.0°C), pulse 75 beats/min, BP 125/73 mm Hg, RR 14 breaths/min.

Additional history: No medical history. No use of tobacco, alcohol, or drugs.

1. What is the differential diagnosis?

   OA, ligamentous injury, meniscal tear, RA, gouty arthritis, pseudogout, bursitis.

2. What components of the physical examination do you perform?

   General appearance, skin, HEENT, cardiovascular, lungs, abdomen, genitalia, extremities, neuro/psych.

   Physical examination:
   General: No acute distress.
   Skin/HEENT: WNL
   Cardiovascular: WNL
   Lungs: WNL
   Abdomen: WNL
   Genitalia: WNL
   Extremities: Antalgic gait. Decreased range of motion with crepitus in the right knee. No joint line tenderness. Negative anterior drawer, posterior drawer, and Lachman tests.
   Neuro/psych: WNL

3. What are your initial orders?

   Knee x-ray.

   Advance clock: X-ray reveals joint space narrowing with osteophytes, subchondral sclerosis, and subchondral cysts. Other studies WNL.

4. What are your follow-up actions?

   Acetaminophen, physical therapy, NSAIDs, counseling.

   Advance clock:
   The patient's symptoms are greatly improved.
   Case ends.

   Critical actions: Extremity examination, acetaminophen and/or NSAID.

   Discussion: This patient has monoarticular arthritis consistent with OA according to his history and physical examination. Plain x-ray films also reveal the four classic radiographic findings for OA: (1) joint space narrowing, (2) osteophytes, (3) subchondral sclerosis, and (4) subchondral cysts. Although every monoarticular arthritis should be considered a septic joint until proven otherwise, the patient's chronic course makes this extremely unlikely. A trial with acetaminophen with or without NSAIDs in conjunction with physical therapy are the first steps in strengthening the relevant muscles and improving flexibility. If the patient's symptoms were not controlled with these basic modalities, an MRI scan may be indicated to evaluate for ligamentous or meniscal injury of the knee. Other treatment modalities include weight loss and intraarticular glucocorticoids. The role of intraarticular glucocorticoids for osteoarthritis has come into question since a randomized placebo-controlled trial showed no benefit. For persistent pain resistant to the aforementioned therapies, referral to an orthopedist and evaluation for total knee arthroplasty are indicated.

   Diagnosis: OA.

CASE 83

HPI: A 52-year-old man arrives at the ED complaining of severe abdominal pain in the left lower quadrant for 10 hours. He has had two episodes like this in the past, but they were not as painful, and he chose not to seek medical attention. He denies nausea, vomiting, diarrhea, or blood in his stool.

Vital signs: Temperature 100.4°F (38.0°C), pulse 95 beats/min, BP 125/80 mm Hg, RR 14 breaths/min.

Additional history: No medical history. No use of tobacco, alcohol, or drugs.

1. What is the differential diagnosis?

   Diverticulitis, acute appendicitis, GI malignancy, IBD, UTI, prostatitis, constipation, SBO, abdominal hernia, abdominal abscess.

2. What components of the physical examination do you perform?

   General appearance, HEENT, cardiovascular, lungs, abdomen.

   Physical examination:
   General: No acute distress.
   HEENT: WNL
   Cardiovascular: WNL

Lungs: WNL
Abdomen: Severe tenderness over left lower quadrant. No rebound or guarding.

3. What are your initial orders?
Pulse oximetry, cardiac/BP monitor, CBC, chem 8, LFTs, lipase, blood cultures, lactate, UA, morphine, acetaminophen.
Advance clock:
O_2 saturation 100%.
WBC $\times$ $10^3/\mu L$ count 12.2, all other tests WNL.
Pain and fever improved, but the patient continues to have moderate pain in the left lower quadrant.

4. What are your follow-up actions?
CT scan of the abdomen/pelvis with IV contrast (reveals diverticulitis without phlegmon, stricture, or obstruction). Start amoxicillin-clavulanate PO or a combination of ciprofloxacin and metronidazole for 10 days. Counseling before discharge (particularly dietary counseling to increase fiber uptake or fiber supplements such as psyllium), follow-up in 1 week. Colonoscopy at 6 weeks.
Advance clock: Case ends.
Critical actions: Abdominal examination, amoxicillin-clavulanate (or other appropriate antibiotics), follow-up colonoscopy.
Discussion: This patient has left lower quadrant pain suggestive of acute abdominal pathology, including diverticulitis. It is reasonable to order a set of laboratory tests and treat his pain and fever first, but because he has severe tenderness without a known diagnosis of diverticulosis, a CT scan of the abdomen/pelvis is important to evaluate for other pathology. The CT scan reveals diverticulitis without complications (perforation, phlegmon, stricture, obstruction), the patient's pain is well controlled, and he does not have a high fever. Because these conditions are met, oral antibiotics and discharge home are appropriate. If he had a high fever, complications revealed by the CT scan, severe pain, or other concerning features, inpatient admission with IV antibiotics (e.g., ceftriaxone/metronidazole) would be more appropriate. An abscess requires interventional radiology or surgical drainage. A stricture or obstruction requires a surgical consult.

After an episode of diverticulitis is treated, all patients need colon cancer screening with colonoscopy because carcinoma of the colon with perforation can mimic diverticulitis clinically and on CT scans. Colonoscopy should be avoided during active diverticulitis because of the increased risk of perforation. A nonurgent surgical consultation is appropriate for recurrent cases of diverticulitis.
Diagnosis: Diverticulitis.

CASE 84

HPI: A 43-year-old-man with a medical history of schizophrenia is brought to the ED by ambulance. He is accompanied by his caregiver, who explains that this morning the patient was found in bed unresponsive and sweating. When she tried to rouse him, she noticed he felt "stiff as a board." His symptoms of schizophrenia had been under moderate control after his physician recently doubled his dose of haloperidol. Before presentation, the patient was interactive and ambulatory. His prior auditory hallucinations had resolved.
Vital signs: Temperature 104.2°F (40.1°C), pulse 115 beats/min, BP 164/94 mm Hg, RR 24 breaths/min.
Additional history: No other medical history or medications. No use of drugs, tobacco, or alcohol.

1. What is the differential diagnosis?
Neuroleptic malignant syndrome, meningitis, encephalitis, sepsis, catatonic schizophrenia, malignant hyperthermia, serotonin syndrome, dystonic reaction.

2. What components of the physical examination do you perform?
General appearance, HEENT, cardiovascular, lungs, abdomen, extremities, neuro/psych.
Physical examination:
General: Ill-appearing man, diaphoretic, tremulous. Protecting his airway without increased WOB.
HEENT: WNL
Cardiovascular: Tachycardic, otherwise WNL.
Lungs: Tachypneic.
Abdomen: WNL
Extremities: Lead pipe rigidity of all extremities.
Neuro/psych: Eyes open, nonresponsive to questioning, moves extremities in response to pain.

3. What are your initial orders?
Pulse oximetry, CBC, chem 14, serum CK, UA, CXR, CSF studies (protein, glucose, cell count, Gram stain and culture), discontinue haloperidol, acetaminophen, lactated Ringer IV, lorazepam, bromocriptine, dantrolene. Cooling measures.
Advance clock: Laboratory tests reveal CK 3670 U/L. UA positive for myoglobin. All other studies WNL.

4. What are your follow-up actions?
Serial laboratory tests: CK, chem 14, CBC. Aggressive IV hydration, passive vs active cooling, lower BP if very elevated, electrolyte repletion, cardiac monitoring, heparin to prevent DVTs

Admit to ICU.

Advance clock: Case ends.

Critical actions: Neurologic examination, discontinuation of haloperidol, supportive measures (cooling and IV fluids), ICU admission, consideration of bromocriptine/dantrolene.

Discussion: Neuroleptic malignant syndrome is a rare emergent condition caused by the use of dopamine antagonists (usually antipsychotic agents). In NMS dopamine antagonism at the hypothalamus causes autonomic dysfunction remembered by the mnemonic FEVER: *f*ever, *e*ncephalopathy, *v*itals unstable, *e*levated enzymes, and *r*igidity (lead pipe). Any patient on antipsychotic medication may be affected. Higher risk is associated with high-potency drugs, high dosage, or rapid escalation of dosing of antidopaminergic medications.

    The differential diagnosis is broad for any patient with hyperthermia and altered mental status. Meningitis should be considered and generally should be evaluated using a lumbar puncture. Other infectious causes should be evaluated via UA and CXR. Other toxic causes should be investigated where indicated (e.g., serotonin syndrome, malignant hyperthermia [inhaled anesthetics/succinylcholine], alcohol withdrawal). Treatment for neuroleptic malignant syndrome is primarily supportive, with airway protection, IV fluids, cooling measures, and assessment for rhabdomyolysis. In cases of severe muscle rigidity, treatment is started with benzodiazepines (e.g., lorazepam) and consideration of bromocriptine (dopamine agonist) and dantrolene (skeletal muscle relaxant).

    Diagnosis: Neuroleptic malignant syndrome.

CASE 85

HPI: A 52-year-old white female presents to her primary care doctor for a BP check. She has had no recent medical issues, but her BP has been elevated the last two times she was in the office. It has remained elevated despite dietary changes and increased exercise.

Vital signs: Temperature 97.1°F (36.5°C), pulse 78 beats/min, BP 158/98 mm Hg, RR 16 breaths/min.

Additional history: No medical history. Smokes one pack of cigarettes daily.

1. What is the differential diagnosis?

   Essential hypertension, hyperthyroidism, renal artery stenosis, pheochromocytoma.

2. What components of the physical examination do you perform?

   General appearance, skin, lymph nodes, HEENT, lungs, cardiovascular, abdomen, extremities, neuro/psych.

   Physical examination:

   General: No acute distress.

   Skin/lymph nodes/HEENT: WNL

   Cardiovascular: WNL

   Lungs: WNL

   Abdomen: WNL

   Extremities: WNL

   Neuro/psych: WNL

3. What are your initial orders?

   CBC, chem 8, ECG, lipid panel, UA, first-line antihypertensive agent (e.g., hydrochlorothiazide), follow-up in 1 month, counseling (diet, exercise, smoking cessation).

   Advance clock: Repeat BP 152/92 mm Hg. All studies WNL.

4. What are your follow-up actions?

   Add a second antihypertensive agent (e.g., lisinopril, atenolol, amlodipine), follow-up in 1 month.

   Advance clock:

   Repeat BP 120/80 mm Hg, no new symptoms.

   Case ends.

   Critical actions: First-line antihypertensive agent, add a second agent if BP not controlled; provide counseling, schedule follow-up.

   Discussion: Stage 1 hypertension is defined as BP 140 to 159/90 to 99 mm Hg measured on more than one occasion. Stage 2 hypertension is defined as BP 160/100 mm Hg or greater. To diagnose hypertension, BP should be measured twice on each of two separate office visits. Stage 1 hypertension can be managed initially with a trial of diet modification and exercise. In patients with stage 2 hypertension or comorbidities (e.g., diabetes or renal disease), early pharmacologic management is preferred.

       Because this patient has no comorbidities there are many reasonable first-line options, including thiazide diuretic (e.g., hydrochlorothiazide or chlorthalidone), dihydropyridine calcium channel blocker (e.g., amlodipine or nifedipine), or ACE inhibitor (e.g., lisinopril or enalapril). The patient's BP is still not controlled at the follow-up visit, so a second agent should be added. Note that beta-blockers (e.g., atenolol) are rarely appropriate for monotherapy but are reasonable as a second agent. If the patient had presented with stage 2 hypertension (BP >160/100 mm Hg), two agents could be started simultaneously. See Chapter 4 for more detail.

       Diagnosis: Essential hypertension.

CASE 86

HPI: A 56-year-old man presents to the ED because of five episodes of coffee ground emesis over the past 8 hours. He has had two episodes like this in the past 12 months, but never so severe. The patient has also noted a black, tarry quality to his stool. He began to feel weak and dizzy so he called 911.

Vital signs: Temperature 98.6°F (37.0°C), pulse 119 beats/min, BP 115/75 mm Hg, RR 16 breaths/min.

Additional history: Never sought medical care previously. Drinks 1 pint of vodka daily. No NSAID use.

1. **What is the differential diagnosis?**
   Bleeding varices, bleeding peptic ulcer, gastric cancer, erosive gastritis, Mallory-Weiss tear.

2. **What components of the physical examination do you perform?**
   General appearance, HEENT, cardiovascular, lungs, abdomen, rectal.
   Physical examination:
   General: Pale, temporal wasting, scleral icterus.
   HEENT: WNL
   Cardiovascular: Tachycardic.
   Lungs: WNL
   Abdomen: Soft, nontender, moderate distention with shifting dullness and positive fluid wave.
   Rectal: Melena.

3. **What are your initial orders?**
   Pulse oximetry, cardiac/BP monitor, CBC, chem 8, LFTs, PT/PTT, blood type and crossmatch, lipase/amylase, IV lactated Ringer, IV pantoprazole, IV ceftriaxone, IV octreotide, ondansetron, NPO.
   Advance clock:
   Hb 6.0 g/dL, INR 1.3, total bilirubin 2.3 mg/dL
   Reassess: The patient's vital signs have normalized and symptoms improved.

4. **What are your follow-up actions?**
   RBC transfusion, gastroenterology consult, upper GI tract endoscopy, admit to ICU, CBC every 4 hours, abdominal ultrasound. Decrease CBC frequency when stabilized and discontinue ceftriaxone and octreotide. Transition to oral PPI. Abdominal ultrasound (to confirm cirrhosis). Counseling before discharge, including alcohol cessation. Follow-up in 1 week.
   Advance clock: Case ends.
   Critical actions: Abdominal examination, IV fluids, upper GI tract endoscopy, pantoprazole, octreotide, ceftriaxone, counseling.
   Discussion: This patient has an upper GI tract bleed. After a focused physical examination, IV fluids and blood products should be given as needed until his vital signs improve. An IV PPI (e.g., pantoprazole) should also be started. Given the patient's stigmata for liver disease (temporal wasting, scleral icterus, shifting dullness and fluid wave), variceal bleeding should be assumed until proven otherwise. Octreotide is indicated for variceal bleeds for splanchnic vasoconstriction. Prophylactic antibiotics (e.g., ceftriaxone) should be given to all patients with cirrhosis and an upper GI tract bleed since they decrease infections and provide a mortality benefit. Upper GI tract endoscopy with variceal ligation is the definitive management and should not be delayed. If the case continues, you can admit the patient to the medicine floor (if his hemodynamics are stable) vs the ICU (if he remains hemodynamically unstable), monitor for improvement, deescalate care, image for cirrhosis with ultrasound, and schedule close follow-up. When the patient is stable, he should be given counseling, including alcohol cessation, and follow up with hepatology in the outpatient setting.
   Diagnosis: Upper GI tract bleed.

CASE 87

HPI: A 31-year-old woman presents to clinic complaining of watery diarrhea for the past 14 days. She complains of approximately four loose, foul-smelling stools daily. The patient has mild cramping abdominal pain but denies blood or mucus in her stool. She has had no fever or vomiting. She returned from a business trip to South America 2 weeks ago.

Vital signs: Temperature 97.7°F (36.5°C), pulse 90 beats/min, BP 122/82 mm Hg, RR 17 breaths/min.

Additional history: No medical history. No tobacco, alcohol, or drug use.

1. **What is the differential diagnosis?**
   Giardiasis, amoebiasis, traveler's diarrhea (enterotoxigenic *E. coli* [ETEC]), foodborne illness, intestinal parasitism, malabsorption/bacterial overgrowth, *C. difficile*.

2. **What components of the physical examination do you perform?**
   General appearance, skin, lymph nodes, HEENT, cardiovascular, lungs, abdomen, extremities, neuro/psych.
   Physical examination:
   General: No acute distress.
   Skin/lymph nodes/HEENT: WNL

Cardiovascular: WNL
Lungs: WNL
Abdomen: Hyperactive bowel sounds; no tenderness, rebound, or guarding.
Extremities: WNL
Neuro/psych: WNL

3. **What are your initial orders?**
Pulse oximetry, stool ova and parasites, stool culture, stool *Giardia* antigen, *C. difficile* toxin, counseling (including oral hydration).
Advance clock: *Giardia*-antigen positive, stool ova and parasites positive for *Giardia*, other laboratory tests WNL.

4. **What are your follow-up actions?**
Metronidazole PO, counseling, oral hydration, follow-up in 2 weeks.
Advance clock: Case ends.
Critical actions: Abdominal examination, stool ova and parasites, metronidazole, counseling.
Discussion: This patient has diarrhea after travelling abroad. Infectious sources should be at the top of your differential diagnosis. Most cases of diarrhea are due to viral illness. Viral gastroenteritis is usually self-limited and does not necessitate any laboratory evaluation. In this case, the prolonged time course, associated cramping, indicate a possible parasitic cause and should trigger a laboratory evaluation with stool studies. This patient's studies are positive for *Giardia*, which can be treated with metronidazole. A similar case presentation may appear for many patients with infectious diarrhea. The physical examination and laboratory evaluation are all the same. If this patient happened to be positive for *Entamoeba histolytica,* the treatment would be the same (metronidazole). If the case were consistent with ETEC (2–4 days of profuse watery diarrhea while traveling), the patient could be treated with azithromycin or ciprofloxacin. If it were most consistent with a viral cause (e.g., norovirus, rotavirus), the patient could be treated with oral hydration alone.
   Diagnosis: Acute diarrhea due to giardiasis.

CASE 88

HPI: A 25-year-old woman presents to the ED with severe abdominal pain in the left lower quadrant and scant vaginal bleeding that has progressively worsened over the past 5 hours. She has never had similar symptoms before. She denies fevers, vomiting, and diarrhea.
Vital signs: Temperature 98.2°F (36.8°C), pulse 110 beats/min, BP 100/70 mm Hg, RR 18 breaths/min.
Additional history: No medical history, sexually active with one male partner.

1. **What is the differential diagnosis?**
PID, ectopic pregnancy, threatened abortion, fibroids, endometriosis, appendicitis, diverticulitis, ovarian torsion, ruptured ovarian cyst.

2. **What components of the physical examination do you perform?**
General appearance, skin, HEENT, cardiovascular, lungs, abdomen, genitalia.
Physical examination:
General: Moderate distress secondary to pain.
Skin/HEENT: WNL
Cardiovascular: Tachycardic.
Lungs: WNL
Abdomen: Tenderness over left lower quadrant.
Genitalia: Scant blood from closed os, tenderness over left adnexa.

3. **What are your initial orders?**
Pulse oximetry, BP/cardiac monitor, urinary pregnancy test, IV fluids, CBC, chem 8, PT/PTT, blood type and screen.
Advance clock:
Pulse 120 beats/min, BP 90/60 mm Hg.
Positive urinary pregnancy test, hemoglobin 10.1 g/dL, blood type O negative.

4. **What are your follow-up actions?**
Serum beta-hCG (4200 mIU/mL), pelvic ultrasound (free pelvic and peritoneal fluid, empty uterus). RhoGAM, obstetrics-gynecology consult for laparoscopy (left salpingectomy performed), admit to inpatient unit, continuous monitoring, CBC every 4 hours, counseling.
Advance clock: Case ends.
Critical actions: Abdominal/genitalia examination, beta-hCG, pelvic ultrasound, blood type and screen, RhoGAM, laparoscopy.
Discussion: This Rh-negative woman has a ruptured ectopic pregnancy. The differential diagnosis is initially broad; however, early assessment for pregnancy greatly narrows the possibilities. After initial stabilization, you should quickly confirm the pregnancy is ectopic with a pelvic ultrasound that shows an empty uterus. Occasionally the ectopic pregnancy itself can be visualized in the fallopian tubes on ultrasound, but this is unnecessary for

diagnosis. An empty uterus with a beta-hCG level above the discriminatory zone (the exact number is a moving target but perhaps as high as 3,500 mIU/mL for transvaginal studies) corresponds to a high degree of suspicion for an ectopic pregnancy, and an urgent obstetrics-gynecology consult is required. Because this patient has unstable vital signs and free peritoneal fluid according to ultrasound, the ectopic pregnancy has probably already ruptured and will require urgent laparoscopy with obstetrics-gynecology. Stable patients with small, unruptured ectopic pregnancies qualify for methotrexate therapy, and beta-hCG levels are carefully monitored during this time. Attempted pregnancy is also not advised for 6 months after an ectopic pregnancy due to interference with beta-hCG monitoring. Because this patient is Rh negative, she should be treated with RhoGAM to prevent alloimmunization. Of note, RhoGAM is given to Rh-negative women at 28 weeks and during episodes of fetal-maternal hemorrhage.

Diagnosis: Ruptured ectopic pregnancy.

CASE 89

HPI: A 76-year-old man presents to clinic with a chief complaint of fatigue. He has been increasingly tired over the past 5 months and recently felt as if he could barely walk outside to collect his mail. He denies fever, shortness of breath, and chest pain. He has noticed a slight maroon color to his stool recently.

Vital signs: Temperature 97.7°F (36.5°C), pulse 90 beats/min, BP 120/85 mm Hg, RR 19 breaths/min.

Additional history: No medical history. No tobacco, drugs, or alcohol use.

1. What is the differential diagnosis?

Lower GI tract bleeding due to colorectal cancer, angiodysplasia, diverticulosis, AV malformation, hemorrhoids. Upper GI tract bleeding due to peptic ulcer disease, gastritis, varices, malignancy.

2. What components of the physical examination do you perform?

General appearance, skin, lymph nodes, HEENT, cardiovascular, lungs, abdomen, rectal, extremities, neuro/psych.

Physical examination:
General: No acute distress.
Skin/lymph nodes/HEENT: WNL
Cardiovascular: WNL
Lungs: WNL
Abdomen: WNL
Rectal: Maroon stool, no palpable masses.
Extremities: WNL
Neuro/psych: WNL

3. What are your initial orders?

Pulse oximetry, CBC, chem 8, PT/PTT, LFTs, fecal occult blood test, type and cross.
Advance clock: Hb 9.0 g/dL, MCV 65 fL, heme-positive stool, laboratory tests otherwise WNL.

4. What are your follow-up actions?

Ferritin, total iron-binding capacity (TIBC), serum iron, start iron supplementation (e.g., ferrous sulfate), gastroenterology consult for colonoscopy.
Advance clock: Ferritin is low, TIBC is high, serum iron is low. Colonoscopy reveals adenocarcinoma in the ascending colon.

5. What are your follow-up actions?

Surgical consult, CT abdomen/pelvis with contrast (large mass in the ascending colon without local invasion), CT chest without contrast (no distant metastases), carcinoembryonic antigen (CEA; elevated)

Advance clock: Case ends.

Critical actions: Abdominal/rectal examination, hemoglobin, colonoscopy, surgical consult.

Discussion: This patient has an ambiguous chief complaint of fatigue, but the historical component of maroon stools indicates that anemia arising from a GI bleed is the likely cause. His microcytic anemia and heme-positive stool provide further evidence. His iron studies indicate that his microcytic anemia is secondary to iron deficiency. Unexplained iron-deficiency anemia in nonmenstruating adults should trigger an evaluation for blood loss, especially colon cancer. Colonoscopy is the test of choice to diagnose colon cancer and may identify other sources of bleeding such as diverticular hemorrhage, hemorrhoids, and AV malformations. On colonoscopy, a biopsy should be obtained for any suspicious lesions.

In this case, adenocarcinoma of the ascending colon was diagnosed on colonoscopy. Adenocarcinomas account for 98% of colorectal cancer cases. They arise from adenomatous polyps that can be detected on screening colonoscopy. Recall that right-sided colon cancers tend to bleed, and left-sided colon cancers tend to obstruct (leading to the classical "pencil-thin" stools). When malignancy is detected, a surgical consult should be considered if the disease is localized, and the patient is able to tolerate surgery because resection is the only possibility of a cure. If the case continues, a CT imaging may be helpful in assessing local invasion and metastases. Colon cancer tends to metastasize to the liver and lungs. CEA testing may be ordered to establish a preoperative baseline.

Diagnosis: Microcytic anemia secondary to colon cancer.

CASE 90

HPI: A 32-year-old man presents to clinic because of 4 months of diarrhea and abdominal pain. He reports waxing and waning of mild lower abdominal cramps that are relieved by defecation. He passes up to five loose stools per day that are occasionally streaked with mucus. The symptoms are worse during the day and seem to disappear at night. There is no blood in his stool, and he denies weight loss, fever, nausea, or vomiting. He has not had any recent travel or dietary changes.

Vital signs: Temperature 97.9°F (36.3°C), pulse 82 beats/min, BP 135/85 mm Hg, RR 17 breaths/min.

Additional history: No medical history. No use of tobacco, alcohol, or drugs.

1. What is the differential diagnosis?

Lactose intolerance, infectious diarrhea, Crohn disease, ulcerative colitis, irritable bowel syndrome (IBS), microscopic colitis, celiac disease.

2. What components of the physical examination do you perform?

General appearance, skin, lymph nodes, HEENT, cardiovascular, lungs, abdomen, genitalia, rectal, extremities, neuro/psych.

Physical examination:
General: No acute distress.
Skin/lymph nodes/HEENT: WNL
Cardiovascular: WNL
Lungs: WNL
Abdomen: WNL
Genitalia/rectal: WNL
Extremities: WNL
Neuro/psych: WNL

3. What are your initial orders?

Pulse oximetry, CBC, chem 8, LFTs, lipase, TSH, stool culture, stool ova and parasites, *Giardia* antibody, transglutaminase antibody.

Advance clock: All studies WNL.

4. What are your follow-up actions?

Counseling (high-fiber diet, lactose-free diet, avoid caffeine), colonoscopy, follow-up in 4 weeks.

Advance clock:
Colonoscopy WNL. The patient's symptoms are improved.
Case ends.

Critical actions: Abdominal examination, counseling.

Discussion: This patient has abdominal pain and diarrhea that are consistent with IBS. He meets the Rome IV criteria of at least two of the following associated with recurrent abdominal pain over 1 day per week in the last 3 months: (1) pain related to defecation (either improving or increasing), (2) associated with a change in stool frequency, and (3) associated with a change in stool form (appearance). The history and physical examination lack red flags such as weight loss, hematochezia, nocturnal symptoms, and worsening symptomatology. Laboratory studies also lack red flags such as anemia and electrolyte disturbances. A physical examination, reassurance, and counseling are the most important aspects of this case. Limited diagnostic studies can evaluate for anemia, hyperthyroidism, *Giardia*, infectious diarrhea, and celiac disease. A colonoscopy is warranted for any concerning signs/symptoms and to evaluate for the possibility of IBD. However, other invasive studies should be avoided. If the diarrhea is not improved by counseling alone, a trial of loperamide may be indicated. IBS is primarily treated with lifestyle modifications: (1) dietary avoidance of FODMAPs (fermentable olig-, di-, and monosaccharide and polyols) and occasionally lactose and gluten avoidance, (2) avoidance of flatulence-producing foods (beans, onions, celery, carrots, raisins, bananas, apricots, prunes, Brussel sprouts, wheat germ, pretzels, bagels, etc.), (3) physical activity (20–60 min of vigorous activity three to five times per week).

Persistent symptoms may warrant trial of a TCA (amitriptyline) or antispasmodic agent (dicyclomine). Persistent symptoms despite conservative therapies may warrant referral to a gastroenterologist for further evaluation.

Diagnosis: IBS.

CASE 91

HPI: A 25-year-old man presents to the ED because of palpitations of 1 hour in duration. They occurred suddenly when he was watching television. He says his heart feels as if it is racing extremely fast. The patient has never had similar symptoms before. He denies chest pain or shortness of breath. He has had no loss of consciousness.

Vital signs: Temperature 98.6°F (37.0°C), pulse 205 beats/min, BP 110/80 mm Hg, RR 17 breaths/min.

Additional history: No medical history. No use of drugs, tobacco, or alcohol.

1. What is the differential diagnosis?

Stable tachycardia: AV nodal reentrant tachycardia, AV reciprocating tachycardia, atrial flutter, AF, multifocal atrial tachycardia, ventricular tachycardia, sinus tachycardia.

2. What components of the physical examination do you perform?

General appearance, HEENT, cardiovascular, lungs, extremities.

Physical examination:

General: Mild distress due to palpitations.

HEENT: WNL

Cardiovascular: Tachycardia, regular rhythm.

Lungs: WNL

Extremities: WNL

3. What are your initial orders?

Pulse oximetry, cardiac/BP monitor, ECG, vagal maneuvers

Advance clock:

ECG reveals regular narrow-complex tachycardia without P waves with a ventricular rate of 205 beats/min. Vagal maneuvers have no effect.

4. What are your follow-up actions?

Adenosine IV (the patient's heart rate normalizes). CBC, chem 8, serum magnesium, repeat ECG. Cardiology consult. Counseling. Follow-up in 2 days.

Advance clock:

Repeat ECG shows normal sinus rhythm without evidence of preexcitation.

Case ends.

Critical actions: Cardiac examination, ECG, vagal maneuvers, adenosine, synchronized cardioversion if the patient becomes unstable, counseling.

Discussion: Reentry SVT refers to a collection of regular narrow complex tachycardias without P waves. These conditions include AV nodal reentrant tachycardia (AVNRT), atrioventricular reentrant tachycardia (AVRT), and others. The specific rhythms are difficult to distinguish but treated similarly, therefore the umbrella term *reentry SVT* is usually sufficient. Reentry SVT usually occurs spontaneously, although it may be triggered by stimulants, exercise, or alcohol. The most common presenting symptom is palpitations. Other symptoms such as angina or loss of consciousness represent unstable tachycardia and warrant a more aggressive approach. Because the patient is stable, vagal maneuvers such as the Valsalva maneuver can be attempted. The REVERT trial showed a much more effective vagal maneuver where you have the patient sitting up, have them attempt to blow the plunger out of a syringe, and then lie them flat and raise their legs. If these fail, adenosine should be used to attempt to convert the heart to a sinus rhythm. Adenosine administration can be repeated three times. Adenosine is successful in inducing cardioversion in most cases. If it fails, however, an AV nodal blocking agent can be used, such as a nondihydropyridine calcium channel blocker (diltiazem) or a beta-blocker (metoprolol).

If at any point the patient becomes unstable (angina, hypotension, loss of consciousness), adenosine administration may be tried, but you should proceed quickly to synchronized cardioversion. A repeat ECG after the episode has resolved can screen for underlying dysrhythmias such as the preexcitation seen in Wolff-Parkinson-White syndrome. Patients with a single episode of well-tolerated AVNRT may not require any further treatment. Diltiazem and metoprolol are usually first-line agents for chronic suppressive therapy. In patients with poorly tolerated SVT, definitive management with catheter ablation should be considered. These decisions should be made in conjunction with a cardiologist. Patients with uncomplicated reentry SVT without significant comorbidities may be discharged home with close cardiology follow-up. Poorly tolerated reentry SVT or the presence of significant comorbidities may warrant admission for monitoring.

Diagnosis: SVT.

CASE 92

HPI: A 46-year-old man presents to clinic complaining of 1 week of back pain. He had been lifting boxes when he felt acute onset of right lower backache. The pain has been persistent ever since. He denies numbness, weakness, fever, urinary retention, and fecal incontinence.

Vital signs: Temperature 97.2°F (36.2°C), pulse 75 beats/min, BP 108/70 mm Hg, RR 16 breaths/min.

Additional history: No medical history. No drug or alcohol use. Smokes one pack of cigarettes daily.

1. What is the differential diagnosis?

Muscle strain, sciatica, lumbar radiculopathy, vertebral compression fracture, herniated disc, neoplasm, paraspinal abscess.

2. What components of the physical examination do you perform?

General appearance, skin, lymph nodes, HEENT, cardiovascular, lungs, abdomen, rectal, neuro/psych, musculoskeletal.

Physical examination:

General: No acute distress.

Skin/lymph nodes/HEENT: WNL

Cardiovascular: WNL
Lungs: WNL
Abdomen: WNL
Rectal: WNL
Musculoskeletal: Tenderness to palpation over the right paraspinal muscles. Decreased range of motion at hips secondary to pain.
Neuro/psych: WNL

3. What are your initial orders?
Counseling (including smoking cessation), ibuprofen, acetaminophen, follow-up in 1 month.
Advance clock:
The patient's symptoms have greatly improved.
Case ends.
Critical actions: Extremities/neurologic examination, analgesia (NSAIDs or acetaminophen)
Discussion: This patient has acute onset of lower back pain consistent with muscle strain. His history and physical examination lack red flags such as IV drug use, trauma, malignancy, neurologic signs and symptoms, weight loss, night sweats, or symptoms lasting for longer than 4 weeks. These red flags are reasons to order imaging such as an x-ray, CT, or MRI. In this low-risk setting, pursuit of advanced imaging may lead to deduction of points from your score. Analgesia is important in this case. Because the patient has not tried any medications, it is appropriate to start with an NSAID or acetaminophen. A short course of a muscle relaxant (baclofen) could be added as a second agent for incomplete relief of symptoms. If this case revealed cord compression, cauda equina syndrome, or a significant neurologic deficit, then MRI and an emergent neurosurgical consult would be indicated.
    Diagnosis: Muscle strain.

CASE 93

HPI: A 25-year-old woman presents to clinic 4 months after she was assaulted and robbed at knifepoint. Although she suffered no significant physical trauma, she reports she has had difficulty concentrating since the event. When she tries to go to sleep, the experience seems to play over repeatedly in her head. She has even stopped leaving her house at night for fear the event might occur again. She denies suicidal or homicidal ideation. She has experienced no audio or visual hallucinations.
Vital signs: Temperature 97.7°F (36.5°C), pulse 75 beats/min, BP 125/70 mm Hg, RR 17 breaths/min.
Additional history: No medical history. No tobacco, alcohol, or drug use.

1. What is the differential diagnosis?
Posttraumatic stress disorder (PTSD), acute stress disorder, major depressive disorder, adjustment disorder, generalized anxiety disorder.

2. What components of the physical examination do you perform?
General appearance, skin, lymph nodes, HEENT, cardiovascular, lungs, abdomen, extremities, neuro/psych.
Physical examination:
General: No acute distress.
Skin/lymph nodes/HEENT: WNL
Cardiovascular: WNL
Lungs: WNL
Abdomen: WNL
Extremities: WNL
Neuro/psych: No focal neurologic deficits. Normal mood and affect.

3. What are your initial orders?
Psychiatry consult, follow-up in 2 weeks, therapy, counseling, SSRI.
Advance clock:
The patient's symptoms are improved.
Case ends.
Critical actions: Neurologic/psychologic examination, therapy, counseling, SSRI.
Discussion: This patient presents to clinic after a traumatic event with difficulty in concentrating, intrusive thoughts, and avoidance behaviors that interfere with her functioning. Because these symptoms have lasted for longer than 1 month, the patient meets criteria for PTSD. Other symptoms of PTSD include hyperarousal and emotional numbing. Similar symptoms lasting for less than 4 weeks do not meet the criteria for PTSD and instead fall under the diagnosis of acute stress disorder. Inciting events include any major trauma that was experienced personally or witnessed. Events include acts of war, terrorism, physical assault, sexual assault, and serious accidents. The lifetime prevalence of PTSD is higher in women (10%) than men (5%). Risk factors include preexisting psychiatric disorders, including anxiety, depression, and substance abuse. The evaluation for PTSD can be limited to a history and physical examination, with laboratory testing only needed if suspicion is raised for underlying pathology.

Treatment includes counseling and therapy by a mental health specialist. SSRIs are first-line pharmacotherapy and should be started at a low dose and slowly uptitrated as needed. The patient should be followed up regularly as an outpatient to assess for improvement. Patients often suffer from relapses of these episodes intermittently throughout their lives and should be monitored by their primary care physician or psychiatrist. If they develop suicidal or homicidal ideation, they require hospitalization.

    Diagnosis: PTSD.

CASE 94

HPI: A 57-year-old man is brought by ambulance to the ED because of chest pain and shortness of breath. Thirty minutes before his arrival he was mowing the lawn when he noticed retrosternal chest pressure that radiated to his left arm. His pain was 8/10 and improved minimally with rest. When the pain did not resolve he called 911.

Vital signs: Temperature 98.2°F (36.8°C), pulse 76 beats/min, BP 155/78 mm Hg, RR 16 breaths/min.

Additional history: 15–pack-year smoker, hyperlipidemia on atorvastatin.

1. **What is the differential diagnosis?**
   ACS, aortic dissection, pulmonary embolism, pneumothorax, cardiac tamponade, pericarditis.

2. **What components of the physical examination do you perform?**
   General appearance, HEENT, cardiovascular, lungs, abdomen.
   Physical examination:
   General: Diaphoretic. Visible discomfort because of chest pain.
   HEENT: WNL
   Cardiovascular: WNL
   Lungs: WNL
   Abdomen: WNL

3. **What are your initial orders?**
   Pulse oximetry, BP/cardiac monitor, aspirin, sublingual nitroglycerin, morphine, CBC, chem 8, ECG/troponin every 6 hours, CXR.
   Advance clock: ECG reveals ST elevation in leads V_2 through V_6 and ST depression in leads II, III, and aV_f. Troponin elevated. Other studies WNL.

4. **What are your follow-up actions?**
   Immediate cardiology consult, cardiac catheterization, admit to ICU.
   Anticoagulation therapy (e.g., heparin), antiplatelet agent (e.g., ticagrelor), beta-blocker (e.g., metoprolol), ACE inhibitor (e.g., lisinopril), statin (e.g., simvastatin), TTE, troponin/ECG every 6 hours, lipid panel, TSH, CBC, chem 8 in the morning, counseling (including smoking cessation and diet).
   Advance clock: Case ends.
   Critical actions: Aspirin, nitroglycerin, and ECG early. Immediate cardiology consult, and cardiac catheterization after ECG result. Anticoagulation therapy, beta-blocker, and antiplatelet agent.
   Discussion: This patient is having an acute ST-elevation MI (STEMI). The history alone should trigger an immediate workup for ACS. An immediate ECG should be ordered, and prompt treatment with aspirin should not be delayed. Standard laboratory tests can also be ordered as long as they do not interfere with the evaluation and treatment of the patient. Nitroglycerin is given for relief of chest pain unless (1) right ventricular infarction is suspected, (2) hypotension or bradycardia is present, or (3) a phosphodiesterase inhibitor (e.g., sildenafil) was used in the previous 24 to 48 hours. As soon as the ECG reveals a STEMI, you should consult cardiology and order cardiac catheterization. Note that even though you have not yet received the results of many laboratory tests, you should proceed to cardiac catheterization (i.e., do not advance the clock before you order cardiac catheterization). The other laboratory results will become available later. If the case does not end after catheterization, continue inpatient ICU management of the STEMI, including anticoagulation therapy (heparin or enoxaparin), an antiplatelet agent (ticagrelor), a beta-blocker (metoprolol), an ACE inhibitor (lisinopril), a statin, echocardiography, laboratory monitoring, risk factor modification, and counseling.
       Diagnosis: STEMI.

CASE 95

HPI: A 23-year-old woman at 11 weeks of gestation (gravida 1 para 0) presents to clinic complaining of vaginal bleeding. The bleeding started approximately 6 hours previously and has included passage of clots and mild abdominal cramping. The pregnancy has been uncomplicated up to this point. The patient takes no medications other than a prenatal vitamin supplement.

Vital signs: Temperature 98.6°F (37.0°C), pulse 81 beats/min, BP 115/80 mm Hg, RR 15 breaths/min.

Additional history: No past medical history. No use of tobacco, drugs, or alcohol. No fertility treatment was used to achieve this pregnancy.

1. **What is the differential diagnosis?**
   Threatened abortion, inevitable abortion, incomplete abortion, complete abortion, missed abortion, septic abortion, vaginal trauma (e.g., intimate partner violence).

2. **What components of the physical examination do you perform?**
   General appearance, skin, lymph nodes, HEENT, cardiovascular, lungs, abdomen, genitalia, extremities, neuro/psych.
   Physical examination:
   General appearance: No acute distress.
   Skin/lymph nodes/HEENT: WNL
   Cardiovascular: WNL
   Lungs: WNL
   Abdomen: WNL
   Genitalia: Scant blood pooling from open os.
   Extremities: WNL
   Neuro/psych: WNL

3. **What are your initial orders?**
   Pulse oximetry, CBC, blood type and screen, fetal ultrasound.
   Advance clock: Blood type O negative; ultrasound reveals an intrauterine pregnancy with no fetal cardiac activity. Other studies WNL.

4. **What are your follow-up actions?**
   Counseling, RhoGAM, misoprostol, follow-up after 1 week.
   Advance clock: Case ends.
   Critical actions: Pelvic examination, fetal ultrasound, blood type and screen, RhoGAM.
   Discussion: The most immediate concern for first-trimester vaginal bleeding is to evaluate for ectopic pregnancy. An intrauterine pregnancy visualized on ultrasound is usually sufficient to rule out ectopic pregnancy (the exception being in the setting of fertility treatment, for which heterotopic pregnancies are more common). Septic abortion typically presents with fever, tachycardia, cool extremities, heavy vaginal bleeding, abdominal/pelvic pain, nausea/vomiting, and cervical motion tenderness. First-trimester vaginal bleeding is categorized as threatened abortion (os closed, viable intrauterine fetus); inevitable abortion (os open); incomplete abortion (partial passage of products of conception); complete abortion (complete passage of products of conception); missed abortion (fetal demise without passage of products of conception), or septic abortion (intrauterine infection). Threatened abortion is managed expectantly, and there is no definitive evidence that any medication or behavioral change prevents miscarriage. Inevitable abortion, incomplete abortion, and missed abortion can be managed expectantly, medically (misoprostol), or surgically (dilation and curettage/evacuation). The particular approach is largely based on patient preference. Septic abortion should be managed by stabilizing the patient, obtaining cultures, broad-spectrum antibiotic therapy (e.g., clindamycin IV and gentamycin IV), and immediate procedural evacuation of the products of conception. Blood type should be determined for all gravid women, and RhoGAM should be administered to Rh-negative women at about 28 weeks of pregnancy or for any antenatal events that are likely to cause fetal-maternal hemorrhage (e.g., amniocentesis, spontaneous or therapeutic abortions, abdominal trauma).
   Diagnosis: Inevitable abortion.

CASE 96

HPI: A 7-year-old boy presents to the ED with shortness of breath and wheezing that has gradually worsened over the previous 5 hours. He has never had similar symptoms before. He has had no fever, cough, or sick contacts. His vaccinations are up to date.
Vital signs: Temperature 98.1°F (36.7°C), pulse 85 beats/min, BP 110/80 mm Hg, RR 24 breaths/min.
Additional history: Medical history of eczema and allergic rhinitis.

1. **What is the differential diagnosis?**
   Foreign body aspiration, pneumonia, asthma, bronchitis.

2. **What components of the physical examination do you perform?**
   General appearance, HEENT, cardiovascular, lungs, abdomen.
   Physical examination:
   General: Mild increased WOB.
   HEENT: WNL
   Cardiovascular: WNL
   Lungs: Tachypnea, diffuse wheezing in bilateral lung fields, subcostal retractions, increased expiratory phase. No stridor.
   Abdomen: WNL

3. What are your initial orders?

Pulse oximetry, BP/cardiac monitor, albuterol inhaled, ipratropium inhaled, prednisone PO, CXR, peak flow.

Advance clock:

The patient's symptoms are greatly improved.

CXR: No infiltrate; mildly hyperinflated lungs.

4. What are your follow-up actions?

Repeat the pulmonary examination (decreased wheezing, improved air movement, no increased WOB). Monitor vital signs. Discharge home with albuterol inhaler, steroids, counseling, follow-up after 1 week.

Advance clock: Case ends.

Critical actions: Lung examination/reexamination, pulse oximetry and/or oxygen measurement, albuterol, steroids, counseling.

Discussion: The patient's atopic history (eczema and allergic rhinitis), physical examination, CXR findings, and response to treatment are all consistent with an acute episode of asthma. Asthma is characterized by recurrent and reversible obstruction of the airways caused by inflammation and bronchospasm. The presenting symptoms are wheezing, chest tightness, and shortness of breath. Severe exacerbations are characterized by respiratory distress with tachypnea, increased WOB, and use of accessory muscles. It is important to identify and address common triggers when possible. These include respiratory infections, exercise, environmental allergies, and gastric reflux. Initial management of acute asthma exacerbations includes oxygen as needed, along with inhaled albuterol (beta$_2$-agonist) and ipratropium (anticholinergic). These inhaled medications are fast acting and address reversible bronchospasm. Steroids are indicated for incomplete response to inhaled medications and are almost always indicated in exacerbations requiring a trip to the ED. Steroids address the inflammatory component of asthma. CXRs are generally unnecessary for recurrent asthma exacerbations, but CXR is indicated in "first-time wheezers" to evaluate for other etiologies. Antibiotics are only given if bacterial infection is suspected or present, unlike COPD treatment in adults. If the patient does not significantly improve, continuous nebulizers should be given, and IV magnesium can be tried to further address bronchospasm. Admission is indicated for refractory symptoms, hypoxia, and respiratory distress. Patients with hypoxic or hypercapnic respiratory failure despite aggressive management will require endotracheal intubation in addition to continued treatments. Mechanical ventilation can be dangerous in these situations, however, given the tendency for air trapping. This can lead to complications from barotrauma and volutrauma. Patients with mild to moderate exacerbations with sustained and significant improvement can be discharged home with follow-up. If the case continues to the outpatient setting, the patient may eventually need to start inhaled corticosteroids for frequent exacerbations.

Diagnosis: Asthma.

INDEX

A

ABCDEs
  of moles, 124
  of trauma, 16
ABCs (airway, breathing, circulation), 58
  in shock, 58
Abdomen, acute condition of, 83
Abdominal aortic aneurysm (AAA), 72, 295
Abdominal trauma
  blunt, management of, 97
  penetrating, management of, 97
Abetalipoproteinemia, 197, 199f
Abnormal uterine bleeding (AUB), 259–260
  differential diagnosis of, 259
  follow-up actions for, 260
  initial orders for, 259
  physical examination for, 259
Abortion, 181
Abruptio placentae, 174
Abscess, 130
Acetaminophen
  overdose of, 19, 90
  toxicity of, 19, 232
Achalasia, 80
Achlorhydria, 82
Acid-base disorders, 153–157
Acid burns, 38, 134–135
Acidosis
  causes of, 153
  serum, on potassium and calcium levels, 153
Acne, 123
  treatment options for, 123
Acromegaly, 146
Acute bowel infarction, 66–67
Acute kidney injury (AKI)
  categories of, 149
  causes of, 149
  intravenous contrast and, 150
  intrinsic, 150
  postrenal, 149–150
  signs and symptoms of, 149
Acute laryngotracheitis, 51–52, 51f
Acute myelogenous leukemia (AML), 245
  differential diagnosis of, 244
  follow-up actions for, 245
  initial orders for, 245
  physical examination for, 244–245
  treatment of, 245
Acute rejection, of transplanted kidney, 151
Acute respiratory distress syndrome (ARDS), 45
Acute urinary retention, symptoms and management of, 211
Acyclovir, for HSV-1 primary infection, 238
ADAMTS13 deficiency, 246
Addison disease, 230
  in shock, 58
Adenomyosis, 161
Adenosine deaminase deficiency, 214

Adhesions, in small bowel obstruction, 86
Adjustment disorder, 101–102
Admission rate bias, 16
Adnexal mass, 162
Adolescence
  causes of death in, 6
  disorders originating in, 104–105
  normal development in, 5–6
Adrenal disorders, 141–144
Adrenal insufficiency, 230
  causes of, 143–144
  diagnosis of, 144
  signs and symptoms of, 143
  type of, 143
Adrenal tumors, 141
Adrenocorticotropic hormone (ACTH), 142–143, 231
Adulthood
  normal development in, 6–8, 6t
  vaccines in, 6, 6t
Adults
  cerebellar findings in, 33
  neck mass in, 79
Afterload, 56
Age
  dementia and, 9
  milestones of, 1–2t
  pattern of development and, 2
  rapidly growing segment of population, 8
Aging
  female sexual function changes and, 8
  hearing and vision changes and, 8
  male sexual function changes and, 8
Airway, breathing versus, in trauma protocol, 16–17
Airway obstruction, 53
Akathisia, definition of, 100
Albuterol/ipratropium, for COPD exacerbation, 283
Alcohol, 63
  abuse, epidemiology of, 106
  as cause of cirrhosis and esophageal varices, 89
  chronic intake of, disease and conditions caused by, 106
  effects on pregnancy, 191
  hypoglycemia, 147
Alcoholism
  treatment of, 106
  vitamin, mineral, and electrolyte deficiencies in, 93
Alcohol withdrawal, 278
  differential diagnosis of, 278
  follow-up actions for, 278–279
  initial orders for, 278
  physical examination for, 278
  stages of, 106
  treatment of, 106
Alkali burns, 134–135
Alkaline burns, 38
Alkaline phosphatase
  elevated levels of, 88
  in Paget disease, 114

Page numbers followed by f refer to figures and by t to tables.